MEDICINE RECALL

MEDICINE RECALL

EDITOR

JAMES D. BERGIN, M.D.
Assistant Professor of Medicine
University of Virginia
Charlottesville, Virginia

ASSISTANT EDITORS

WILLIAM MAYNARD, M.D.
Chief Medical Resident
University of Virginia
Charlottesville, Virginia

CHRISTINA PRILLAMAN, M.D.
Chief Medical Resident
University of Virginia
Charlottesville, Virginia

MOHAN NADKARNI, M.D.
Clinical Assistant Professor of Medicine
University of Virginia
Charlottesville, Virginia

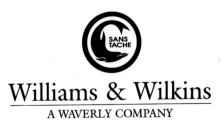

Williams & Wilkins
A WAVERLY COMPANY

BALTIMORE • PHILADELPHIA • LONDON • PARIS • BANGKOK
BUENOS AIRES • HONG KONG • MUNICH • SYDNEY • TOKYO • WROCLAW

Editor: Elizabeth Nieginski
Managing Editor: Amy G. Dinkel
Marketing Manager: Rebecca Himmelheber
Development Editor: Melanie Cann
Production Coordinator: Danielle Hagan
Text/Cover Designer: Karen S. Klinedinst
Typesetter: Port City Press, Inc.
Printer/Binder: Port City Press, Inc.

Accurate indications, adverse reactions and dosage schedules for drugs are provided in this book, but it is possible that they may change. The reader is urged to review the package information data of the manufacturers of the medications mentioned.

Printed in the United States of America

First Edition

Library of Congress Cataloging-in-Publication Data

Medicine recall / editor, James D. Bergin; assistant editors, William Maynard, Christina Prillaman, Mohan Nadkarni. — 1st ed.
    p.   cm. — (Recall series)
  Includes index.
  ISBN 0–683–18098–3
  1. Internal medicine—Examinations, questions, etc. 2. Internal medicine—Outlines, syllabi, etc. I. Bergin, James D. II. Series.
  [DNLM: 1. Medicine—examination questions. WB 18.2 M4895 1997]
RC58.M48 1997
616′.0076—dc21
DNLM/DLC
for Library of Congress   97–11939
                                              CIP

The publishers have made every effort to trace the copyright holders for borrowed material. If they have inadvertently overlooked any, they will be pleased to make the necessary arrangements at the first opportunity.

To purchase additional copies of this book, call our customer service department at **(800) 638-0672** or fax orders to **(800) 447-8438.** For other book services, including chapter reprints and large quantity sales, ask for the Special Sales department.

Canadian customers should call **(800) 665-1148,** or fax **(800) 665-0103.** For all other calls originating outside of the United States, please call **(410) 528-4223** or fax us at **(410) 528-8550.**

Visit Williams & Wilkins on the Internet: http://www.wwilkins.com or contact our customer service department at **custserv@wwilkins.com.** Williams & Wilkins customer service representatives are available from 8:30 am to 6:00 pm, EST, Monday through Friday, for telephone access.

                                            97 98 99 00 01
                                  1 2 3 4 5 6 7 8 9 10

Dedication

This book is dedicated to my parents; to my wife, Leslie; and to my children, Christopher and Laura.

Contents

Contributors

CARDIOLOGY
Mical Kupke, Medical Student, class of 1996
Mark A. Mitchell, M.D., Fellow
James D. Bergin, M.D., Assistant Professor of Medicine

PULMONOLOGY
Annie Chang, Medical Student, class of 1996
Steven Koenig, M.D., Assistant Professor of Medicine
Mark Robbins, M.D., Assistant Professor of Medicine

NEPHROLOGY
Caroline Shen, Medical Student, class of 1996
Sarah Warren, M.D., Resident
Suzanne Schmidt, M.D., Resident
Crystal A. Gadegbeku, M.D., Fellow
Karl G. Koenig, M.D., Assistant Professor of Medicine

GASTROENTEROLOGY
Catherine Matthews, Medical Student, class of 1997
George F. Goldin, M.D., Fellow
Cynthia M. Yoshida, M.D., Assistant Professor of Medicine

HEMATOLOGY
Lara B. H. Evans, Medical Student, class of 1996
Donald V. Woytowitz, M.D., Fellow
John E. Humphries, M.D., Assistant Professor of Medicine

ONCOLOGY
Donald V. Woytowitz, M.D., Fellow
Susan Miesfeldt, M.D., Assistant Professor of Medicine

INFECTIOUS DISEASE
Vanessa Shami, Medical Student, class of 1996
Nathan M. Thielman, M.D., Fellow
Carol A. Sable, M.D., Assistant Professor of Medicine

ENDOCRINOLOGY
Stephen Wehibe, Medical Student, class of 1996
Lisa Asnis, M.D., Fellow
Stacey Gildersleeve, M.D., Fellow

Carmen Pastor, M.D., Fellow
Nikhita Shah, M.D., Fellow
Christopher G. Zitnay, M.D., Fellow
Alan Dalkin, M.D., Assistant Professor of Medicine

ALLERGY AND IMMUNOLOGY
Meg R. Reitmeyer, M.D., Resident
Sulaiman AlGazlan, M.D., Fellow
Lisa M. Wheatley, M.D., Assistant Professor of Medicine

RHEUMATOLOGY
James Worledge, Medical Student, class of 1996
Barbara True, M.D., Fellow
Carolyn Brunner, M.D., Professor of Medicine

NEUROLOGY
Barnett R. Nathan, M.D., Resident
William T. Garret, M.D., Fellow
Russell H. Swerdlow, M.D., Fellow
Nathan B. Fountain, M.D., Fellow

PSYCHIATRY
Timothy J. Kane, M.D., Resident

DERMATOLOGY
Rebecca Rudd, Medical Student, class of 1996
R. Carter Grine, M.D., Resident
Barbara Braunstein Wilson, M.D., Associate Professor of Dermatology

PHARMACOLOGY
Katherine A. Michael, Pharm D.
Rebecca H. Hockman, Pharm D.

THE CONSULTANT
Adam Hill, Medical Student, class of 1996
Mohan Nadkarni, M.D., Clinical Assistant Professor of Medicine

DISEASES RESULTING FROM ENVIRONMENTAL AND
CHEMICAL CAUSES
Meg R. Reitmeyer, M.D., Resident
Rebecca H. Hockman, Pharm D.
Katherine A. Michael, Pharm D.
James D. Bergin, M.D., Assistant Professor of Medicine

Preface

I remember when Lorne Blackbourne came to my office to discuss this book. He commented on the success of his book, *Surgical Recall*, and suggested to me that *Medical Recall* (later renamed *Medicine Recall*) would be a tremendous project. He advised me that the project would be simple if I would surround myself with some of the superb people at the University of Virginia. I followed his advice (although it was far from simple) and I believe that we have produced an excellent teaching tool in the model of *Surgical Recall*. The framework for each subspecialty team was a medical student, a fellow, and an attending. The chapters progress from the basics to more advanced medicine and from the usual to the urgent and emergent. The authors were asked to frame questions as they had heard them (medical students) or as they had taught them on rounds (fellows and attendings). Our intention was to put together a book that could be conveniently carried and used as a study guide and source of information by medical students and residents. I hope that you will agree that we have achieved this goal.

Acknowledgments

I would like to acknowledge the work of Lorne Blackbourne, who inspired the Recall series. I would also like to acknowledge the efforts of the contributors who have made this book possible.

Section I

Overview

1   Introduction

Medical Recall is written in the same vein as *Surgical Recall* and other books in the *Recall* series. The contributing authors have written questions from the attending, fellow, resident, and student level about material covered while on rounds. The book is organized in a self-study/quiz format with questions on the left and answers on the right. The right-hand column should be covered while reading through the book. The chapters in this pocket-sized guide are organized by systems, with section abbreviations and definitions preceding each discussion. When applicable, a list of appropriate landmark clinical trials follows the discussion.

CLINICAL PEARLS

1. Always sit down when talking to the patient. Physicians who stand at the doorway while talking appear to be in a hurry. A physician who sits with the patient is perceived as having spent more time with the patient than the physician who spends an equal amount of time or longer while standing. This also allows the physician to be at the same physical level as the patients, that is, not talking down to them.
2. Ask before sitting on the patient's bed. This is the patient's private space (the patient is allowed to keep few personal belongings, particularly clothes, after being admitted).
3. Ask before using the patient's first name. If you use the patient's first name, you should use your own as well; otherwise you may be perceived as arrogant.
4. Respect the patient's **modesty.** Always use curtains, gowns, and other appropriate coverings.
5. The patient's **confidentiality** should be maintained beyond the patient's room (e.g., the patient's case should not be offhandedly discussed in elevators, while eating, or while traveling to and from work); the patient's family or friends or others may overhear.
6. Always speak in terms with which the patient is familiar. A patient with cancer may be better able to understand lay terms rather than terms such as "malignancy" and "tumor." Because many physicians may care for the same patient and may use different terms, it may be preferable to have one physician be the primary deliverer of information.
7. Identify important family members (e.g., who holds power of attorney) early in the patient's care. Having all important family members present during the history and when following up on tests saves repetition and prevents misconceptions that occur when the information is relayed among family members.

8. After making comments to a patient, it is often helpful to ask the patient to repeat back the substance of your message. This allows you to correct any misconceptions and to check the patient's understanding.

9. When delivering bad news, it is often best to diminish the patient's anxiety by sitting and delivering the information without delay. Because much of the remainder of the conversation will be forgotten, it is often best to return to the patient later to review important data.

10. Always find out the patient's occupation. This may impact the patient's present illness, and the patient's recovery may necessitate that job modifications be made.

11. Find out whether tobacco and alcohol are used liberally in the workplace or at home by other family members. If so, are there steps that can be taken where avoidance of specific locations would help the patient discontinue these habits?

12. Depression is common. Approximately 60% of medical patients have depression as an important aspect of their illness.

13. Heart disease, smoking-related illness, and cancer are common illnesses. One or more of these should always be considered in the differential diagnosis.

14. A common illness presenting in an uncommon fashion is more common than an uncommon illness presenting in a common fashion. (In other words, when you hear hoof beats, always think of horses, not zebras.) Furthermore, the diagnosis should be in the differential in 80% of the cases after a careful history, in 10% of cases after the physical examination, and in 10% of cases after laboratory results are known.

15. Never talk disparagingly about your colleagues. Talking in a disparaging fashion about referring colleagues only undermines the patient's confidence in the referring physician or in you. If the patient has had a long-term relationship with the referring physician, the patient may trust the other physician's word over yours, regardless of who is right. On the attending level, talking poorly about another physician may eventually sever a referral source.

16. Before ending an interview or discussion with a patient, always ask whether the patient has questions (and not as you are going to the door).

PRESENTING ON ROUNDS

While presenting on rounds, it is extremely important that you be thoroughly familiar with your patients. As a student, you will not have a large number of patients and, therefore, should be able to keep all their data (e.g., medications, tests) in order. It is imperative that you see your patients before formal rounds in the morning. If you have not seen your patient, however, you must be truthful. It is better to give no information than wrong information.

It is extremely important to be thought of as a team player. Getting ahead and showing one's knowledge by stepping on the heads of colleagues is never appreciated. Although you may receive higher marks for knowledge, you will always receive lower marks for professional behavior. It is easy to recognize people with substantial knowledge, so you should not worry about "shining through."

Essential elements to follow-up presentations in the morning include the following:

A summary of the patient's course over the past 24 hours and, commonly, a 1- to 2-sentence summary of the patient's admission course

Current vital signs, including intake and output when appropriate

Physical examination, focusing on the pertinent positive and negative findings and any appropriate follow-up laboratory testing

Your plan for the patient's day, even if it is incorrect (it is always important to make a formulation and present it to the team)

Diagnostic possibilities, starting with what you think is the most likely and ending with the least likely.

Section II

The Specialties

2
Cardiology

ABBREVIATIONS

AAA	Abdominal aortic aneurysm
ACE	Angiotensin-converting enzyme
AF	Atrial fibrillation
AI	Aortic insufficiency
AIVR	Accelerated idioventricular rhythm
AMI	Acute myocardial infarction
APB	Atrial premature beat
AS	Aortic stenosis
ASA	Acetylsalicylic acid
ASD	Atrial septal defect
AV	Atrioventricular
BBB	Bundle branch block
BP	Blood pressure
BSA	Body surface area
CABG	Coronary artery bypass grafting
CAD	Coronary artery disease
CHB	Complete heart block
CHD	Congenital heart disease

CHF	Congestive heart failure
CI	Cardiac index
CMV	Cytomegalovirus
CO	Cardiac output
COPD	Chronic obstructive pulmonary disease
CVA	Cerebrovascular accident
CVP	Central venous pressure (also RA pressure)
DCA	Directional coronary atherectomy
DM	Diabetes mellitus
DORV	Double outlet right ventricle
DP	Dipyridamole
ECG	Electrocardiogram
ESR	Erythrocyte sedimentation rate
GXT	Graded exercise test
HDL	High-density lipoprotein
HOCM	Hypertrophic obstructive cardiomyopathy (also IHSS)
HR	Heart rate
HTN	Hypertension
IABP	Intraaortic balloon pump
ICD	Implantable cardioverter-defibrillator
IE	Infective endocarditis
IHD	Ischemic heart disease

IHSS	Idiopathic hypertrophic subaortic stenosis (also HOCM)
IMA	Internal mammary artery
IMI	Inferior myocardial infarction
JVD	Jugular venous distention (also JVP)
JVP	Jugular venous pressure (also JVD)
LA	Left atrium
LAD	Left anterior descending artery or left axis deviation
LAFB	Left anterior fascicular block
LBBB	Left bundle branch block
LCx	Left circumflex artery
LDL	Low-density lipoprotein
LPFB	Left posterior fascicular block
LV	Left ventricle
LVED	Left ventricular end-diastolic
LVEDP	Left ventricular end-diastolic pressure
LVEF	Left ventricular ejection fraction
LVES	Left ventricular end-systolic
LVESP	Left ventricular end-systolic pressure
LVH	Left ventricular hypertrophy
MAP	Mean arterial pressure
MET	Metabolic equivalent
MI	Myocardial infarction
MR	Mitral regurgitation

MS	Mitral stenosis
MUGA	Multigated acquisition
MVP	Mitral valve prolapse
PA	Posteroanterior or pulmonary artery
PAOP	Pulmonary artery occlusion pressure
PCWP	Pulmonary capillary wedge pressure (also PC, PAOP)
PDA	Posterior descending artery
PMI	Posterior myocardial infarction or point of maximal impulse
PND	Paroxysmal nocturnal dyspnea
PS	Pulmonic stenosis
PTCA	Percutaneous transluminal coronary angioplasty
PVR	Pulmonary vascular resistance
PVRI	Pulmonary vascular resistance index
RA	Right atrium
RAD	Right axis deviation
RBBB	Right bundle branch block
RCA	Right coronary artery
RV	Right ventricle
RVEF	Right ventricular ejection fraction
RVH	Right ventricular hypertrophy
saECG	Signal-averaged ECG
SVR	Systemic vascular resistance

SVRI	Systemic vascular resistance index
SVT	Supraventricular tachycardia
TEE	Transesophageal echocardiogram
TGA	Transposition of the great arteries
tPA	Tissue plasminogen activator
TS	Tricuspid stenosis
TTE	Transthoracic echocardiogram
VF	Ventricular fibrillation
VLDL	Very low-density lipoprotein
VPB	Ventricular premature beat (also PVC, VPC)
VSD	Ventricular septal defect
VT	Ventricular tachycardia

DEFINITIONS

Orthopnea	Difficulty breathing in the recumbent position
Paroxysmal nocturnal dyspnea (PND)	Patients awaken after 1–2 hours of sleep because of acute shortness of breath
Trepopnea	Positional dyspnea that is generally noted in either the left or right lateral decubitus position; may be seen with a ball-valve effect of a left or right atrial mass (e.g., thrombus, myxoma)
Platypnea	Dyspnea that occurs only in the upright position
Hemoptysis	Coughing up of blood
Cheyne-Stokes respiration	Respiration characterized by a rapid deep-breathing phase followed by periods of apnea

Myocardial stunning	Prolonged depressed function of viable myocardium caused by a brief episode of severe ischemia (myocardium can recover with time if recurrent ischemic events are prevented)
Hibernating myocardium	Chronically depressed function of viable myocardium due to severe chronic ischemia (which can be reversed by revascularization)
Angina	A squeezing sensation in the chest caused by a number of illnesses
Stable angina	A predictable pattern of angina onset and offset that is stable over time
Unstable angina	A change in the patient's normal pattern of angina onset or offset, probably due to plaque rupture
Accelerated angina	Angina that occurs at lower levels of exertion or that takes longer to resolve with rest or nitroglycerin; although technically, accelerated angina fits the definition of unstable angina, accelerated angina usually occurs over a longer period of time and is probably due to progression of atheromatous coronary disease without plaque rupture, whereas unstable angina occurs in a more abrupt fashion
Q-wave infarct	Infarct in which Q waves evolve on ECG (implies larger MI; also called transmural infarct)
Non–Q-wave infarct	Infarct in which Q waves do not evolve on ECG (implies smaller infarction; also called nontransmural or subendocardial infarct)

HISTORY AND PHYSICAL EXAMINATION

HISTORY

Why is a history of chest pain important?	Chest pain is common and there are several causes of chest pain that are lethal and require early recognition. A

careful history is the most important aspect in the workup of chest pain.

What structures are in the chest?

Heart, pericardium, and other vasculature
Lungs and pleura
Esophagus
Mediastinal structures

What structures are around the chest?

Chest wall
Neck
Other musculoskeletal structures
Stomach, liver, spleen, gallbladder, pancreas, and transverse colon

What is Levine's sign?

Clenched fist over the midsternum

What seven historical features of chest pain must be identified to differentiate cardiac pain from noncardiac pain?

Think **PQRST:**
   Precipitating factors—pain that follows exertion, exposure to cold, or meals suggests angina; pain that **follows** retching or a twisting movement suggests alternative causes
   Quality—sustained squeezing or pressure may be described as "a heavy feeling," "tightness," "an elephant sitting on my chest," "band-like," or "not sharp"
   Radiation and location—pain may be central, left-, or right-sided (a specific location suggests alternative causes); radiation may extend to the neck, left arm, or right arm
   Relief—nitroglycerin relieves most angina in 2–5 minutes (a longer duration suggests MI or other causes); relief with leaning forward (positional effects) suggests pericarditis, relief with antacids suggests gastrointestinal causes
   Risk factors—family history, gender, tobacco use, diabetes, hyperlipidemia, HTN, and obesity are risk factors
   Symptoms—associated symptoms, such as dyspnea, nausea, vomiting, belching, diaphoresis, and

palpations all suggest angina;
patients often express a sensation of
impending doom or total denial
Time and duration—very brief
(seconds) episodes are not angina;
prolonged (hours) episodes may
indicate infarction or other causes
(e.g., pericarditis, dissection)

What are the major cardiovascular causes of chest pain that you cannot miss or forget?

Myocardial ischemia, MI, aortic dissection, aortic aneurysm, and pulmonary emboli

What are some other cardiovascular causes of chest pain?

MVP, pericarditis, pulmonary HTN

List some noncardiovascular causes of chest pain.

Gastrointestinal (e.g., esophageal spasm, reflux, and rupture; stomach, duodenum, or gallbladder disease)
Pleura and lung conditions (e.g., pneumothorax, pleural adhesions)
Shoulder-hand syndrome, shoulder girdle
Diseases of the chest wall (e.g., thrombophlebitis, herpes zoster infection, costochondritis)
Diseases of the spine and mediastinum

What are some important causes of hemoptysis?

MS, pulmonary infarction, Eisenmenger's complex, aortic aneurysm, pneumonia, pulmonary carcinoma, vasculitis, and tuberculosis

What are some of the causes of dyspnea?

CHF, anginal equivalent, arrhythmias, cardiac tamponade, COPD, pneumonia, pneumothorax, restrictive lung disease, pulmonary embolism, pulmonary HTN, airway obstruction, interstitial lung disease, and adult respiratory distress syndrome
Anemia and thyroid disease
Deconditioning and chest wall weakness (muscle or nerve disease)
Psychogenic cause (anxiety) and malingering

PHYSICAL EXAMINATION

How is the width of a BP cuff determined?	The width should be approximately 40% of the circumference of the limb in which the BP is being measured. Using an inappropriately sized cuff results in inaccurate measurement. An undersized BP cuff results in an overestimated BP measurement; an oversized BP cuff results in an underestimated BP measurement.
How accurate is a BP cuff?	±5 mm Hg
How close should the right and left arm pressures be?	Within 10 mm Hg
What is arcus senilis?	Circumferential light ring around the iris, which is frequently associated with hypercholesterolemia if present in patients younger than 50 years
What is ectopia lentis and what is it associated with?	Dislocated lenses; homocystinuria or Marfan's syndrome
What are the causes of blue sclera?	Ehlers-Danlos syndrome, osteogenesis imperfecta, and Marfan's syndrome, which are all associated with aortic root dilation or aneurysm and/or MVP
What are plaques of Hollenhorst?	Orange-yellow plaques secondary to cholesterol emboli seen in arterioles on fundoscopic examination
What are the causes of clubbing?	Cyanotic CHD Pulmonary disease (e.g., hypoxia, lung cancer, bronchiectasis, cystic fibrosis) IE Biliary cirrhosis Regional enteritis Familial clubbing
What is abdominal-jugular (also called hepatojugular) reflux?	An increase in JVP of greater than 3 cm H_2O with 10–30 seconds of periumbilic pressure, which is associated with right or left ventricular failure, tricuspid regurgitation, or any cause of elevated CVP or PCWP

Where is the normal PMI found?	At the fifth to sixth intercostal space at the midclavicular line
What causes an S1?	Closure of the mitral–tricuspid valve
What causes an S2?	Closure of the aortic–pulmonic valve
What causes an S3?	Unknown, but it occurs in patients with volume overloaded hearts (RV or LV) or hyperdynamic circulation; it may also be a normal variant in patients younger than 40 years of age
What causes an S4?	An S4 is caused by organized atrial contraction into a stiff ventricle (i.e., it does not occur in AF). When an S4 is present, the following should be considered: LVH (HTN, AS, HOCM), RVH, IHD, hyperdynamic circulation, acute valvular regurgitation, and restrictive cardiomyopathy.
With respect to gallops, what do Tennessee and Kentucky represent?	The sequence in the cardiac cycle for an S4 is TEN-nes-see (i.e., S4 precedes S1); the sequence in the cardiac cycle for an S3 is ken-tuck-Y (i.e., S3 follows S2).
How are S3 and S4 gallops best heard?	By using the bell of the stethoscope over the apex (S3) or the left sternal border (S4)
When does cyanosis occur?	When the concentration of deoxyhemoglobin in the blood is greater than 5 mg/dl
What are the two main categories of cyanosis?	Central and peripheral. In central cyanosis, decreased arterial oxygen saturation is due to right to left shunting, impaired ability of hemoglobin to bind oxygen (e.g., in methemoglobinemia or abnormal hemoglobin variants), or impaired pulmonary function. Peripheral cyanosis is secondary to cutaneous vasoconstricion caused by low CO or exposure to cold.

What are the causes of peripheral edema?	Chronic venous insufficiency Obstruction Thrombosis Heart failure (high and low output) Constrictive pericarditis Nephrotic syndrome Hepatic cirrhosis Angioneurotic edema Myxedema Lymphatic obstruction
What is the normal JVP?	Less than 6–8 cm H_2O
What is the formula for converting cm H_2O to mm Hg?	cm H_2O × 0.75 = mm Hg
List the waveforms seen on the jugular venous tracing.	a, c, and v waves and x and y descents
Identify the various waveforms and their timing or event in the cardiac cycle.	a—atrial contraction c—tricuspid closure v—ventricular systole x—descent of the ventricle y—passive ventricular filling
List the five major causes of pronounced a waves.	1. Pulmonary HTN 2. Mitral valve disease 3. Pulmonary embolus 4. Cor pulmonale 5. TS or atresia
What is the major cause of pronounced v waves?	Tricuspid regurgitation
How high is the JVP if the earlobes have a bobbing motion while the patient is sitting?	Greater than 15 cm H_2O
How is a mean BP calculated?	[systolic pressure + (2 × diastolic pressure)]/3
What causes cannon A waves?	Atrial contraction against a closed tricuspid valve

What heart rhythms do cannon A waves suggest?	CHB and VT
What is Kussmaul's sign?	Increased JVP with inspiration
What is the differential diagnosis of Kussmaul's sign?	Constrictive pericarditis versus RV infarction or failure
What is pulsus paradoxus?	An exaggeration of a normal response; present when the systolic pressure declines more than 10–12 mm Hg during inspiration and during normal breathing
What is the differential diagnosis of pulsus paradoxus?	Pericardial tamponade, constrictive pericarditis, restrictive cardiomyopathy, COPD (exacerbation), asthma (exacerbation), superior vena cava obstruction, pulmonary embolus, hypovolemic shock, pregnancy, and obesity
What is pulsus alternans?	Alternating weak and strong pulse beats
What is the differential diagnosis of pulsus alternans?	Severe CHF, anything causing rapid respiratory rates, pericardial tamponade
What is a bisferiens pulse?	A pulse waveform with two upstrokes
List five causes of a bisferiens pulse.	AI, IHSS, exercise, fever, PDA
With what are the following findings associated?	
Pulsus tardus	Obstruction to LV outflow (valvular AS or nonvalvular AS)
Pulsus parvus	Reduced LV stroke volume
Pulsus parvus et tardus	Severe AS
Bisferiens pulse (both peaks in systole)	Conditions in which a large stroke volume is ejected rapidly from the LV (aortic regurgitation, combined AS and AI), hypertrophic cardiomyopathy, hyperkinetic circulation, normal variant

Dicrotic pulse (first peak in systole, second peak in diastole—based on the relation to S2)

Hypotension, fever with decreased SVR, tamponade, severe heart failure, hypovolemic shock

Pulsus alternans

Severe LV dysfunction and a regular rhythm

Pulsus bigeminus

Bigeminy (LV function can be normal)

What is the pulse pressure?

The systolic BP minus the diastolic BP; index = (systolic BP − diastolic BP)/ (systolic BP)

What are causes of a wide pulse pressure?

Aortic regurgitation, PDA, truncus arteriosus, CHB, sinus bradycardia, fever, anemia, strenuous exercise, thyrotoxicosis, AV fistulas, and hot weather

What are causes of a narrow pulse pressure?

CHF, AS, and dehydration

Why measure the BP in both arms and a leg?

For the diagnosis of subclavian stenosis, aortic dissection, and aortic coarctation

How do you distinguish systolic murmurs from diastolic murmurs?

Listen to the murmur with your fingers on either the carotid or brachial pulse. Murmurs heard during pulsation are systolic; those without pulsation are diastolic.

What tones are heard with the bell of the stethoscope?

Low tones (i.e., the murmur of MS and S3 and S4 gallops)

What tones are heard with the diaphragm of the stethoscope?

Mid- and high-pitched tones (e.g., murmurs of MR, AS, and AI)

In what order do you hear the aortic and pulmonic closure sounds and why?

Aortic first, then pulmonic. The pressure head in the aorta is higher in the pulmonary artery, and the LV is activated earlier than the RV.

List the murmur rating scale.	I—only heard under optimal listening conditions II—mild to moderately loud murmur III—moderate to loud murmur IV—murmur with an associated thrill V—murmur heard with the edge of the stethoscope touching the chest VI—murmur heard with the stethoscope 1 cm off the chest Diastolic murmurs are often scaled 1–4.

With what are the following findings associated?

Widely split S1	TS, Ebstein's anomaly, RBBB, LV pacing
Soft S1	MR
Fixed split S2	RBBB, PS, ASD, pulmonary atresia, MR, pulmonary HTN
Paradoxic split S2	PDA (left to right shunt), tricuspid regurgitation, LBBB, AS, IHD

With what are the following findings associated?

Retinal changes (AV nicking, copper wiring)	HTN
Reduced pulses, bruits	Atherosclerotic vascular disease
Laterally displaced PMI	Cardiomegaly
Unilaterally reduced breath sounds	Pneumothorax, pneumonia, pleural effusion
Distended neck veins	CHF, restrictive or constrictive cardiomyopathy, tamponade
Distended or pulsatile liver	Right-sided heart failure, tricuspid regurgitation
Absent leg hair	Peripheral vascular disease
Diagonal earlobe creases	CAD

Xanthelasma	Hyperlipidemia
High palate, hyperextendable joints	Marfan's syndrome

CORONARY ARTERY DISEASE

What is CAD?	Narrowing of the coronary arteries
What is the incidence of CAD?	On an annual basis in the United States, 5.4 million people are diagnosed with CAD, and CAD is responsible for 550,000 deaths per year.
What are the three ways that CAD presents?	1. Angina (one third) 2. Infarction (one third) 3. Sudden death (one third)
What are the standard CAD risk factors?	Male gender, age, tobacco use, DM, HTN, family history of premature CAD, hypercholesterolemia, low HDL, peripheral vascular disease, carotid artery disease, obesity, and sedentary lifestyle
What are the major modifiable CAD risk factors?	Tobacco use, HTN, hypercholesterolemia (LDL, HDL), and DM
Modification of which of these factors results in decreased risk of cardiovascular events?	Probably all four
In patients with angina, why is a workup always necessary?	To discriminate between low- and high-risk groups
What exercise variables are associated with low- and high-risk groups?	Low-risk group—has good functional status (very active, can exercise greater than 10 minutes on Bruce protocol, has ECG changes relatively late during exercise test) High-risk group—has poor functional status (limited activity due to angina, exercise limited to less than 10 minutes on a stress test, has ECG changes relatively early during exercise test)

What is perfusion pressure?

The coronary perfusion pressure equals the MAP minus the LVEDP.

What factors can lower perfusion pressure?

Coronary perfusion pressure—
   hypotension, coronary stenosis
High LVEDP—hypertrophy (HTN
   < AS), CHF, MR, and AR

How is coronary flow determined?

(perfusion pressure)/(vascular resistance)

What happens when coronary flow is critically reduced?

Myocardial ischemia (angina or infarction) results. This can be due to factors that decrease perfusion pressure or increase vascular resistance [e.g., CAD, significant ventricular hypertrophy (HTN, AS)].

What is preload?

The LV blood volume present immediately prior to ventricular systole

What is afterload?

The amount of pressure against which the ventricle pumps

What is the difference in the coronary histopathology of chronic stable angina and acute coronary syndrome?

In stable angina, there is significant luminal narrowing by a plaque that consists of smooth muscle and lipid-laden macrophages, and there is an intact endothelium. In acute coronary syndrome (unstable angina or MI), there is significant luminal narrowing by a complicated plaque consisting of smooth muscle and lipid-laden macrophages, and there is a disrupted endothelium with luminal thrombus (a ruptured plaque).

List several factors that contribute to ischemia in unstable angina or MI.

Relatively decreased O_2 supply (caused by anemia, hypoxia, coronary narrowing from plaque with or without thrombus)
Increased O_2 demand (caused by tachycardia, HTN, high myocardial wall tension)

What is the 1%, 3% rule in cholesterol management?

A 1% lowering in cholesterol level results in a 3% lowering in mortality rate.

How are the different types of hyperlipoproteinemia classified?

Type I—increased chylomicrons, normal cholesterol, increased triglycerides

Type IIA—increased LDL and cholesterol; normal triglycerides and VLDL

Type IIB—increased LDL, VLDL, and triglycerides

Type III—floating β-lipoprotein; increased cholesterol and triglycerides

Type IV—increased VLDL and triglycerides; normal to increased cholesterol

Type V—increased chylomicrons, VLDL, and cholesterol; greatly increased triglycerides; reduced LDL

Which is the most common hyperlipidemia?

Type IIB

What is LP(a)?

A derivative of LDL that is substantially more atherogenic than LDL alone

How much fat is in the average American diet?

35%–40% of all calories ingested

What is the first step in treating hyperlipidemia?

Controlling exercise and diet. By reducing the fat content of foods ingested to 20%–25% of the total calories taken in, a reduction of 15% in LDL cholesterol can be achieved.

What are the other treatment options for hyperlipidemia?

HMG-CoA reductase inhibitors (e.g., fluvastatin, lovastatin, pravastatin, simvastatin)

Bile-acid sequestrants (e.g., cholestyramine, colestipol)

Nicotinic acid

Fibric acid derivatives (e.g., gemfibrozil, clofibrate, fenofibrate)

What are the side effects of:
   HMG-CoA reductase inhibitors?

Constipation, myositis (< 1%; more frequent with drug combinations such as gemfibrozil and cyclosporine), hepatitis (< 3%)

Bile-acid resins?	Gastrointestinal complaints (e.g., constipation, bloating)
Niacin?	Flushing, pruritus, hepatitis, hyperglycemia
Fibric acid derivatives?	Gastrointestinal complaints, hepatitis

What are the treatment goals for patients with elevated plasma LDL?

Patients with fewer than two risk factors	< 160 mg/dl of LDL in plasma
Patients with two or more risk factors	< 130 mg/dl of LDL in plasma
Patients with DM plus microvascular disease or known atherosclerotic disease	< 100 mg/dl of LDL in plasma

ACUTE MYOCARDIAL INFARCTION (AMI)

What is an AMI?	Interruption of blood flow to a portion of the heart that results in myonecrosis
What is the incidence of AMI?	1.5 million people per year; accountable for 25% of all deaths in the United States
What is the correct triage decision when a patient has typical chest pain consistent with unstable angina or infarction, several cardiac risk factors, and a normal ECG?	Admission of the patient to the hospital. The ECG confirms the diagnosis of an acute syndrome but it is not the deciding factor (i.e., history is more important).
How is the diagnosis of an AMI made?	By identifying symptoms, ECG changes (ST segment depression or elevation, Q waves), and increased serum levels of cardiac isoenzymes
List the spectrum of ECG findings in angina.	Normal, T-wave inversions, ST segment depression, ST segment elevation

Name five cardiac isoenzymes.	Creatine kinase (CK), lactate dehydrogenase (LDH), aspartate aminotransferase (AST), troponin I, troponin T
Name seven causes of CK elevation.	1. AMI 2. Myocarditis 3. Rhabdomyolysis (trauma, status epilepticus, surgery, severe prolonged exercise) 4. Polymyositis or muscular dystrophy 5. Devastating brain injury 6. Familial elevation 7. Renal injury
Name four causes of CK-MB elevation.	AMI, cardiac surgery, muscular dystrophy, and myocarditis
Name four causes of CK-BB elevation.	Brain injury or Reye's syndrome, uremia, malignant hyperthermia, and small intestine necrosis
Name six causes of LDH elevation.	1. AMI 2. Hemolytic anemia, pernicious anemia, or sickle cell crisis 3. Large pulmonary embolus 4. Renal infarction 5. Prosthetic heart valves 6. Hepatic injury
Which isoenzyme elevates first after an AMI?	Troponin I and T and CK-MB elevate within hours; LDH elevates within 24 hours; and AST elevates within 2–3 days.

TREATMENT (CORONARY SYNDROMES)

How do you treat: **Stable angina?**	Low-risk patients: antianginal medications (e.g., ASA, nitroglycerin), β blockers, calcium channel blockers, and risk factor modification High-risk patients: in addition to the medications listed for patients with a low-risk profile, consider cardiac catheterization or myocardial nuclear perfusion imaging to determine whether the patient would benefit from revascularization (e.g., patients with significant three-vessel disease or

left main coronary disease may
require revascularization)

Unstable angina?

Oxygen, correction of metabolic factors
(e.g., anemia), ASA with or without
heparin, β blockers, nitroglycerin
(generally intravenously), risk
stratification (when the patient's
condition is stable with myocardial
nuclear perfusion imaging or cardiac
catheterization), and risk factor
modification

Non–Q wave MI?

Oxygen, ASA with or without heparin,
nitroglycerin intravenously, β blockers,
diltiazem; early during recovery—risk
stratification (early, with cardiac
catheterization, or later, with myocardial
nuclear perfusion imaging) to determine
the need for revascularization; risk factor
modification

Q wave MI?

Consider thrombolytic therapy or
primary angioplasty in addition to ASA,
heparin, nitroglycerin, and β blockers;
early during recovery—risk stratification
with cardiac catheterization or
myocardial nuclear perfusion imaging to
determine the need for revascularization;
risk factor modification. Note: the heart
prefers blood over drugs.

**With regard to Q wave
versus non–Q wave MI,
which is associated with a
higher in-hospital
mortality rate?**

Q wave MI

**Of the two, which has a
higher reinfarction rate
within the first 12 months?**

Non–Q wave MI (reinfarction occurs in
20% of medically treated cases; this
equalizes the mortality rate difference at
12 months)

**Which drugs save lives in
patients with AMI?**

tPA and streptokinase, ASA, β blockers,
ACE inhibitors

What is the treatment of choice for a patient with AMI and shock?	Primary angioplasty
What are the common thrombolytic agents?	tPA, streptokinase, anosylated plasminogen streptokinase activator complex (APSAC), and urokinase
What are the indications for thrombolysis?	ST segment elevation in two contiguous ECG leads in patients with pain onset within 6 hours who have been refractory to sublingual nitroglycerin (with or without heparin) and who have no contraindications; therapy may also be beneficial in patients presenting at 6–12 hours and perhaps at 12–24 hours
What are four contraindications to thrombolysis?	1. Recent trauma or surgery 2. Recent stroke or transient ischemic attack (TIA) 3. Significant HTN: systolic pressure > 200 mm Hg, diastolic pressure > 120 mm Hg 4. Prolonged cardiopulmonary resuscitation (CPR)
What are other important medications used in the treatment of an MI?	Aspirin, β blockers, nitrates, and narcotics
What are contraindications to the use of β blockers?	Brittle diabetes, severe peripheral vascular disease (unopposed alpha activity), significant asthma, COPD, known allergic reaction, and severe heart failure
What are contraindications to calcium channel blockers?	Heart failure (for diltiazem, nifedipine, verapamil), significant AV block or bradycardia (for diltiazem, verapamil), known allergic reaction (for all), and AMI (for nifedipine)

MECHANICAL COMPLICATIONS OF MYOCARDIAL INFARCTION

List two causes of new murmurs following an AMI.	MR and VSD

List six mechanical complications that may follow an AMI.

1. Left ventricular aneurysm
2. Left ventricular rupture. If the free wall is contained, there is a pseudoaneurysm; if it is not contained, the patient dies. Septal rupture is a VSD.
3. Papillary muscle rupture (acute MR)
4. Thromboembolus
5. Reinfarction or extension
6. Pericardial effusion or tamponade

What is the incidence of ruptured papillary muscle in patients who die following AMI?

1%–5% in patients who die of AMI

When does a ruptured papillary muscle typically occur?

2–10 days after the MI. Primarily, the posterior papillary muscle is involved.

What is the mortality rate associated with papillary muscle rupture?

70% within 24 hours, 90% within 2 weeks (if unrepaired)

What is the treatment for papillary muscle rupture?

Afterload reduction with nitroprusside or IABP and surgery after stabilization

What is the incidence of VSD following AMI?

< 1%; accountable for 2% of deaths following AMI

When does a VSD typically occur?

9–10 days after MI

What is the mortality rate for VSD?

25% in 24 hours; 90% in 2 months

What is the treatment for VSD?

Same as for papillary muscle rupture (afterload reduction with nitroprusside or IABP and surgery after stabilization)

What is the incidence of left ventricular rupture following AMI?

More common than VSD or papillary muscle rupture; accountable for up to 25% of fatal AMIs

When does left ventricular rupture typically occur?

50% of cases within 5 days of AMI; 90% within 2 weeks

What is the mortality rate for left ventricular rupture?

> 95%

What is the treatment for left ventricular rupture?

Immediate surgery with volume replacement, repeated pericardiocentesis, or open chest resuscitation if needed

How can acute MR due to papillary muscle rupture be differentiated from an acute VSD?

Patient history—Patients with VSDs have little or no orthopnea early after the event, whereas patients with acute MR often have severe orthopnea.

Auscultation—A VSD is best over the sternum. The MR murmur can be heard at the apex but frequently radiates superiorly in posterior leaflet papillary muscle ruptures and posteriorly in anterior leaflet papillary muscle ruptures.

Echocardiogram and Doppler testing—These are probably the best ways to differentiate acute MR due to papillary rupture from an acute VSD.

Right heart catheterization with measurement of the oxygen saturation in the various chambers—An increase in oxygen saturation by more than 5% between chambers is consistent with a shunt (i.e., VSD). For example, the following percentages are consistent with a shunt (VSD) at the RV: RA O_2 saturation 61%, RV O_2 saturation 75%, PA O_2 saturation 78%, arterial saturation 95%.

Can the amount of left to right shunting be estimated in a VSD (or ASD)?

Yes. Variables include arterial O_2 saturation (ART sat), RA O_2 saturation (RA sat), and PA O_2 saturation (sat):
Shunt (Qp/Qs) = (ART sat − RA sat)/
                (ART sat − PA sat)
Using the percentages listed in the example: Qp/Qs = (95 − 61)/(95 − 78) = 2/1 shunt. In other words, there is two times more pulmonary blood flow than systemic blood flow with the shunt at the RV (normal 1:1).

What factors predispose to pulmonary embolism after MI?

LV failure, arrhythmias, old age, obesity, and immobility

What are preventive measures against pulmonary embolism after MI?

Early ambulation after AMI and therapy with low-dose heparin (5000 units subcutaneously twice daily)

What is the incidence of arterial embolism?

Old studies (from 1973) cite 2%–5% incidence to the brain, kidneys, and limbs from a mural thrombus overlying the infarcted area. Highest risk is seen with thrombi that project into the LV cavity.

List five causes of chest pain following an AMI.

Reinfarction, infarct extension, recurrent ischemia, pericarditis, and noncardiac causes (e.g., gastrointestinal)

How is an RV infarct recognized?

Hypotension associated with an IMI (especially when preload-reducing agents such as diuretics, nitrates, and narcotics have been administered), elevated JVP, distended liver, and clear lungs

What is the first therapy for hypotension or shock associated with:
An IMI?

Volume and remove nitrates

An AMI?

Administer vasopressors or inotropes, consider IABP and PTCA, and use hemodynamic monitoring

What is the prognostic significance of VF early after an AMI (within 24 hours)?

None

What is the prognostic significance of VF late after an AMI (longer than 24 hours)?

The mortality rate significantly increases due to recurrent VF, which requires evaluation and long-term treatment.

After the patient's discharge from the hospital, what nonpharmacologic therapy should be considered?	Cardiac rehabilitation
List the goals of cardiac rehabilitation.	To promote a healthier lifestyle (by giving assistance with tobacco cessation, low-fat cooking, and BP monitoring) To help patients start or maintain an exercise program in a controlled environment To help patients achieve an improved functional status through an exercise program To help patients cope with the psychological stresses associated with MI To help patients understand the limits (if any) that their coronary disease imposes

ICU FORMULAS

What are the normal filling pressures?	
RA pressure or CVP	0–8 mm Hg (mean)
RV pressure	15–30/0–8 mm Hg (systolic/diastolic)
PA pressure (PA)	15–30/3–12 mm Hg (systolic/diastolic)
PCWP	3–12 mm Hg (mean)
What other terms are used to describe the PCWP?	PAOP, PC pressure, wedge pressure
What is the PCWP?	Approximation of the left atrial and left ventricular pressure during ventricular filling
What is the PCWP useful for?	For determining the volume status of the patient (i.e., PCWP > 12 = volume overloaded; PCWP < 3 = volume depleted)

What are three sources of error encountered when measuring pressures with a fluid-filled catheter (e.g., arterial line, Swan-Ganz catheter)?

1. Deterioration in frequency response—Check for air in the catheter or transducer.
2. Catheter whip—As the catheter is hit by the pulse wave, motion is generated, increasing systolic pressures and lowering diastolic pressures (i.e., the mean pressure is unaltered). This can also be tested for in arterial lines by inflating a BP cuff proximal to the line; as the cuff is deflated, the pressure that corresponds to the first pressure wave recorded on the arterial line is the true systolic pressure.
3. Catheter impact—Catheter impact is caused by a valve or other structure hitting the catheter.

How is CO calculated?

CO = [HR (beats/min)] × [stroke volume (ml/beat)]/(1000 ml/L)

What is the normal CO?

5 ± 1 L/min

How is CI calculated?

CI = CO/BSA

What is the normal CI?

3 ± 0.5 L/min/m^2

How is SVR calculated?

SVR = [systemic BP (mean) – RA (mean)]/CO × 80 dyne-cm-sec^{-5}

What is the normal SVR?

1200 ± 300 dyne-cm-sec^{-5}

What does the SVR measure?

Left ventricular afterload

How is the SVRI calculated?

SVRI = SVR × BSA (i.e., SVR/CI)

What is the normal SVRI?

2100 ± 500 dyne-cm-sec^{-5} × m^2

How is the PVR calculated?

PVR = [PA (mean) – PCWP (mean)]/CO × 80 dyne-cm-sec^{-5}

What is the normal PVR?

100 ± 50 dyne-cm-sec^{-5}

How is the PVRI calculated?	PVR × BSA
What is the normal PVRI?	170 ± 70 dyne-cm-sec^{-5} × m^2 (i.e., PVR/CI)
What are Wood units used for?	For heart transplant evaluations: PVR/80 (ideal < 4). The PVR = [PA (mean) – PCWP (mean)]/CO.

DETERMINATION OF CARDIAC OUTPUT

What is the thermodilution method?	Injection of a known quantity and temperature of fluid into the RA and measurement of the bolus transit time
Name nine pitfalls of the thermodilution method.	1. Low outputs (outputs < 2.5 L/min average a 35% overestimation) 2. Tricuspid regurgitation 3. Improper technique (i.e., slow injection, incorrect volume) 4. Intracardiac shunts (VSD) 5. Extracardiac shunts (AV fistula) 6. Cold patients 7. Distal tip of the catheter in the main PA 8. Changes in blood viscosity (anemia or polycythemia) 9. Invasive insertion
What is the Fick method?	Measurement of the oxygen extraction
What variables are needed for this calculation?	Patient's hemoglobin (Hgb) Oxygen saturation of the PA (PA O$_2$) and aorta (Ao O$_2$) Oxygen consumption (generally estimated at 100–150 ml/m^2)
What is the Fick equation?	CI = [oxygen consumption × 10]/[(Ao O$_2$ sat – PA O$_2$ sat) × (Hgb × 1.36)]
Name five pitfalls of the Fick equation.	1. Intracardiac shunts 2. Difficult measurement of oxygen consumption (generally estimated) 3. Incorrect data (e.g., estimated PA O$_2$ saturation versus measured, which is a problem with some blood gas

machines that estimate the saturation based on a nomogram for arterial blood)
4. Invasive insertion
5. PA sample drawn too quickly, which pulls pulmonary capillary (oxygenated) blood into the sample

In general, a PA O_2 saturation of > 65% is consistent with a normal CO and a PA O_2 saturation > 80% is consistent with some type of left-to-right shunting.

How can errors in CO determination affect SVR?

The SVR, PVR, and so on are calculated numbers, and errors in pressure or CO measurements affect these numbers. For example, a patient with a normal CO of 6.0 L/min and significant tricuspid regurgitation may have a measured CO of 3.0 L/min. This would double the calculated SVRI and may result in inappropriate treatment.

CENTRAL AND PERIPHERAL VASCULAR DISEASE

What is the incidence of CAD in patients with peripheral vascular disease, carotid disease, or AAA?

Normal coronaries— < 10%
Mild CAD—Approximately 30%
Moderate CAD—Approximately 30%
Severe CAD—Approximately 30%
 (5%–10% are inoperable)

What is the diameter of a normal *ascending* aorta?

3 cm

What is the diameter of a normal *descending* aorta (at the level of the renal arteries)?

< 2 cm

What percentage of aortic aneurysms are confined to the abdominal aorta?

75%

What percentage of the general population has an abdominal aortic aneurysm?

1%–4%

What is the mortality rate for a recognized rupture of an abdominal aortic aneurysm?

50%–80%

What are the symptoms and signs of thoracic aneurysms?

They are generally asymptomatic and are seen on chest radiograph. There may be associated symptoms and signs of compression of contiguous structures (e.g., cough, dyspnea, dysphagia, hoarseness). Less commonly, there is deep throbbing chest pain or back pain (often secondary to erosion of the aorta into contiguous structures).

What is the survival rate for medically treated symptomatic thoracic aneurysms?

25% at 5 years

What are causes of aortic arch aneurysms?

Connective tissue diseases (e.g., Marfan's syndrome, Ehlers-Danlos syndrome), HTN, infectious causes (e.g., syphilis), endocarditis

What are the common classifications for dissecting aortic aneurysms?

DeBakey
    Type I—involves the ascending aorta and beyond
    Type II—involves the ascending aorta only
    Type III—involves the aorta distal to the left subclavian artery
Daily (Stanford)
    Type A—involves the ascending aorta (including retrograde extension from the descending aorta)
    Type B—involves the descending aorta only
This classification is useful in that type A dissections need immediate surgery whereas type B dissections are treated medically unless there is evidence of continued dissection (pain) or organ or limb ischemia. Less than 40% of these aneurysms require surgery.

What are the causes of aortic dissections?

Marfan's syndrome and other connective tissue abnormalities (Ehlers-Danlos)

Cystic medial necrosis (without overt Marfan syndrome)

Bicuspid aortic valves and aortic coarctation (predisposing factors to dissection)

Pregnancy (with 50% of dissections occurring in women younger than 40 years old during the last trimester of pregnancy; often associated with coronary dissection)

Trauma, possibly causing a tear in the aorta at the isthmus

What type of pain is usually described during aortic dissection?

Tearing, stabbing, ripping

Anterior chest pain (almost universal for proximal dissections)

Back pain (present in > 90% of patients with involvement of the descending aorta, whether type A or B dissection)

What are the common physical examination features of a dissecting aorta?

Shock, although, initially, 50% of patients are hypertensive

Pulse deficits (right to left difference; occurs in 50% of proximal dissections and may occur in distal dissection secondary to compression of the subclavian artery)

Aortic regurgitation (50% of patients with proximal events; may cause severe, rapid onset CHF)

Neurologic deficits

What process involving the ascending aorta is associated with aortic coarctation?

Aortic dissection or rupture

What are the causes of hypotension during an aortic dissection?

Cardiac tamponade

Intrapleural or intraperitoneal rupture

Pseudohypotension (impingement on the brachiocephalic vessels by the dissecting hematoma interfering with BP measurement)

What are the typical features of patients with Marfan's syndrome?

Arachnodactyly, high-arched palate, thoracic cage deformities, lax ligaments, decreased muscle mass, subluxation or dislocation of lenses, aortic aneurysms, myxomatous changes of the aortic or mitral valves

What is a mycotic aneurysm?

An aneurysm resulting from damage to the aortic wall secondary to an infection (generally bacterial)

What are the symptoms and signs of abdominal aortic aneurysms?

They are generally asymptomatic and are noted during physical examination or some imaging test; otherwise, symptoms may include abdominal fullness or abdominal or back pain. Aortic rupture is recognized by severe back and abdominal pain and by hypotension or frank hemorrhagic shock appearance. Most patients have a palpable pulsatile abdominal aorta.

What percentage of abdominal aneurysms larger than 6 cm will rupture by 1 year?

50% (the larger the aneurysm the greater the percentage); 80% if symptomatic

At what rate do abdominal aneurysms expand?

0.25–0.50 cm/year; after the aneurysm reaches 4–5 cm, the rate of expansion and rupture increases

What is Takayasu's disease?

Also called pulseless disease, Takayasu's disease is inflammation and then scarring of the aorta, major branches, and pulmonary arteries, leading to occlusion (hence pulselessness) or pulmonary HTN if the pulmonary arteries are involved.

What is the cause of Takayasu's disease?

Takayasu's disease is thought to be secondary to an autoimmune process. It affects women 9:1 over men.

What are the associated constitutional symptoms?

Fever, night sweats, malaise, weight loss, Raynaud's phenomenon, angina, MI, CHF, pericarditis

In a patient older than 50 years of age with unilateral headache and scalp tenderness, what connective tissue disease must be considered and why?

Temporal arteritis because, if undiagnosed, it may lead to blindness

How is the diagnosis of arteritis made?

Elevated ESR and positive temporal artery biopsy

What is the treatment for arteritis?

Corticosteroids

If a bruit is heard over one carotid but not over the other, is it safe to assume that the nonbruit side is free of disease?

No, the nonbruit side may be tightly stenosed or occluded.

What are the "Ps" of acute arterial occlusion?

Pain, paresthesias, paralysis, pallor, pulselessness, poikilothermy

What are indications for immediate intervention in patients with peripheral vascular disease?

Resting pain, cyanosis, neurologic deficits

What noninvasive index is used to determine the degree of peripheral vascular impairment?

The ankle–brachial index (ABI). An ABI consistent with claudication is < 0.7; a limb-threatening ABI is < 0.4.

Where are neuropathic ulcers usually seen?

The toes

Where are venous ulcers usually seen and what is their usual course?

The medial malleolar area; these ulcers usually resolve and recur.

What therapies for peripheral vascular disease are available?

Heparin, thrombolytic therapy, angioplasty, surgical bypass

What should you think of in a patient who complains of claudication symptoms but has good distal pulses or good ABIs?

Spinal stenosis

What symptoms suggest spinal stenosis?

Spinal stenosis tends to improve with walking and worsen with sitting, and is generally accompanied by some back trauma history.

What is Raynaud's phenomenon?

Cold or emotionally induced digital ischemia

With what is Raynaud's phenomenon associated?

Primary thromboangiitis obliterans, cryoglobulinemia, occupational trauma, collagen vascular diseases (e.g., systemic lupus erythematosus, polyarteritis), frostbite, sympathetic hyperactivity, and thoracic outlet syndrome

How is livido reticularis recognized?

Regional blushing intermixed with vasospasm

What are the causes of livido reticularis?

Systemic lupus erythematosus, polyarteritis nodosa, and cholesterol embolization

How is livido reticularis treated?

Alpha or calcium channel blockers and ACE inhibitors

What peripheral vascular disease is associated with tobacco use in younger males (< 30 years of age)?

Buerger's disease (thromboangiitis obliterans). Other associated symptoms are superficial phlebitis, Raynaud's phenomenon, and calf claudication. Unlike atherosclerotic disease, the upper extremities are usually involved. **These patients must quit smoking.**

Where are the common arterial entrapment sites?

Superficial femoral artery, popliteal artery, and thoracic outlet

How is the diagnosis of thoracic outlet syndrome made?

When the arm is abducted to 90 degrees and externally rotated, paresthesias and numbness occur, a bruit is heard over the supraclavicular fossa, and symptoms resolve when the arm is returned to baseline position.

What is repetitive trauma and what are the areas involved with injury?

Injuries occur with repetitive tasks and frequently involve the hands and wrists; this is becoming a significant problem.

What is Buerger's sign?

Rubor when the extremity is in the dependent position, pallor when it is elevated

What does Buerger's sign indicate?	Venous disease
What dermatologic clues suggest venous rather than arterial disease?	Patients with venous disease usually have thick scaly skin; those with arterial disease usually have thin shiny skin.
What are the risk factors for venous thrombosis?	Stasis, trauma, and altered coagulation (e.g., that caused by oral contraceptives, malignancies, and factor deficiencies)
How is venous thrombosis treated?	With heat, elevation, heparin, and warfarin (Coumadin)
What is plethysmography?	A method of looking at venous emptying
What may also be confused with deep venous thrombosis?	Lymphedema secondary to lymphatic outflow obstruction (lymphangitis, neoplasm, adenopathy, or surgical removal)

CARDIOVASCULAR PROCEDURES

CHEST RADIOGRAPHY

What six structures need to be identified on an ICU chest radiograph?	1. Lines—correct location and heart chamber 2. Tubes—correct location 3. Bones—lytic lesions and fractures 4. Lungs—infiltrates, effusions, and air 5. Heart—size and shape (e.g., water-bottle shape indicates pericardial effusion) 6. Diaphragms—symmetrical or obscured
What is the cardiothoracic ratio?	The ratio of the maximum heart width to the maximum inner dimension of the thorax measured on the PA film. Normal is < 50%.

On the PA chest film, what are the silhouette structures on the patient's right side of the mediastinum?	From superior to inferior:
	    Superior vena cava
	    Ascending aorta
	    RA
	    Inferior vena cava

On the PA chest film, what are the silhouette structures on the patient's left side of the mediastinum?	From superior to inferior:
	    Left subclavian artery and vein
	    Aortic arch
	    PA
	    LA
	    LV

What are the causes of a widened mediastinum?	Aortic aneurysm or dissection AS (post-stenotic dilatation) Uncoiled aorta of the elderly

ELECTROCARDIOGRAM

What are the common uses of the ECG?	Diagnosis of rhythm disorders, ischemia, pericarditis, electrolyte abnormalities, and drug toxicity
In what order should you read an ECG?	Rate Rhythm Intervals Axis Hypertrophy Ischemia Infarction
What leads are considered the limb leads?	I, II, III, aVR, aVL, and aVF
What leads are considered the precordial leads?	V_1–V_6
What are the inferior leads?	II, III, and aVF
What are the anterior leads?	V_1–V_4
What are the lateral leads?	V_5–V_6, I, and aVL
What are the right-sided precordial leads?	V3R and V4R
What are the right precordial leads useful for?	To confirm an RV infarct

What does the P wave represent?

Atrial depolarization (the first half is from the RA; the second half is from the LA)

What leads are best used to see the P wave?

II, III, aVF, V_1, and V_2

At a standard paper speed of 25 mm/sec, what does one small box on the ECG represent?

Horizontal = 40 msec (0.04 sec); vertical = 1 mm (0.1 mV)

What is the normal size of the P wave?

< 120 msec (3 boxes)—if longer, consider LA enlargement
< 0.25 mV (2.5 boxes)—if taller, consider RA enlargement

What is P mitrale?

It is consistent with enlargement of the LA and is recognized by a notched P wave in leads II, III, aVF, V_1, or V_2. Other signs of left atrial enlargement include a wide P wave (> 120 msec) and a biphasic P wave in V_1.

What is P pulmonale?

It is consistent with enlargement of the RA and is recognized by a P wave > 0.25 mV in lead II.

What does the QRS complex represent?

Ventricular depolarization

What does the T wave represent?

Ventricular repolarization; the area under the T wave equals the area under the QRS complex (i.e., people with high QRS voltage, or hypertrophy, have larger T waves).

Where is the atrial repolarization (i.e., the atrial T wave)?

Hidden in the QRS complex

What is the 300, 150, 100 rule?

The 300, 150, 100 rule is used to quickly calculate the rate on the ECG. The HR = 1500/number of small boxes between R waves or 300/number of large boxes:

Table 2–1.   Calculating the Heart Rate on the ECG

Number of Large Boxes	Time	Rate (bpm)
1	200 msec	300
2	400 msec	150
3	600 msec	100
4	800 msec	75
5	1 msec	60
6	1.2 sec	50

What is the PR interval?

The distance from the beginning of the P wave to the beginning of the QRS complex

What is the normal range for the PR interval?

120–200 msec (3 to 5 boxes)

List three causes of a short PR interval.

1. Accelerated AV conduction
2. Tachycardia
3. Accessory AV pathway (e.g., Wolff-Parkinson-White syndrome)

List four causes of a long PR interval.

1. High vagal tone
2. AV conduction system degenerative disease
3. IHD
4. Drugs that impair AV conduction (e.g., β blockers and digoxin)

What is the QRS interval?

The distance from the beginning of the QRS complex to the end of the QRS complex

What is the normal range for the QRS interval?

60–120 msec (1.5–3 boxes). A conduction delay is present if the QRS is ≥ 110 msec, and a BBB is present if the QRS is ≥ 120 msec.

What is the QT interval?

The distance from the beginning of the QRS complex to the end of the T wave

What is the normal range for the QT interval?

The range varies by HR; however, the QT should be less than half of the QRS to QRS interval (RR interval).

What is the QTc?

The corrected QT interval (corrects for the HR)

$$QTc = \frac{QT}{\sqrt{RR}}$$

Why is it important to measure intervals?

The measurement allows determination of blocks (e.g., first-degree or RBBB).

What prolongs the PR interval?

AV blocks

What prolongs the QRS interval?

BBBs
Premature ventricular beats
LVH
Preexcitation syndromes (e.g., Wolff-Parkinson-White syndrome)
Electrolyte abnormalities (e.g., hyperkalemia)
Paced beats
Medications (e.g., amiodarone, procainamide, tricyclic antidepressants)

What prolongs the QT interval?

Medications [tricyclic antidepressants, antiarrhythmics (e.g., quinidine, procainamide, amiodarone), terfenadine plus macrolide antibiotics (e.g., erythromycin)]
Electrolyte deficiencies (e.g., potassium, magnesium, calcium)
Congenital long QT
IHD
Hypothermia
MVP
Intracranial events (e.g., subarachnoid hemorrhage)

What is a normal ECG QRS axis?

-10 degrees to 100 degrees (or, simply, 0 degrees to 90 degrees)

How do you calculate the ECG axis?

Locate the most isoelectric lead (QRS deflection above and below the line is the same). Then, locate the positive lead 90 degrees from the isoelectric lead. That is the axis. For example, if the isoelectric lead is located at lead aVL (-30 degrees) and the positive 90-degree lead is lead II, then the axis is 60 degrees.

What is the I, aVF rule?

From the previous example, if leads I and aVF are both more positive than negative, then the axis is normal.

What is a significant Q wave?

40 msec or one third the height of the QRS. The Q wave represents previous MI. Some areas tend to lose Q waves over time—inferior infarctions lose Q waves approximately 50% of the time; anterior infarctions lose Q waves less than 10% of the time.

Describe the QRS complex in the following:
RBBB

QRS > 120 msec
rSR' pattern in V_1
Deep slurred S wave in V_6, I

LBBB

QRS > 120 msec
All negative in V_1
All positive in V_6, I

LAFB

QRS < 120 msec (unless associated with an RBBB)
LAD (more than -45 degrees)
Small Q waves in I, aVL
R waves in II, III, aVF (i.e., no IMI)

LPFB

QRS < 120 msec (unless associated with an RBBB)
RAD (more than 120 degrees)
Small Q waves in II, III, aVF
R waves in I, aVL (i.e., no lateral myocardial infarction)

What is the most common combination for hemiblock plus BBB?

RBBB plus LAFB
QRS > 120 msec
rSR' in V_1
Left axis (> -45 degrees)
R waves in II, III, aVF

What BBB pattern is seen for paced beats (transvenous pacemaker)?

LBBB. If an RBBB pattern is observed, consider septal perforation by the wire.

List six criteria for LVH.

1. (S in V_1 or V_2) + (R in V_5 or V_6) > 35 mm
2. Any QRS in V_5–V_6 > 25 mm
3. R in aVL > 12 mm
4. R in aVF > 20 mm
5. S in aVR > 14 mm
6. (R in I) + (S in III) > 25 mm

List three criteria for RVH.

1. R in V_1 > 5 mm
2. RAD
3. Deep S in V_5 or V_6

Name nine causes of ST elevation.

1. AMI
2. Ventricular aneurysm
3. Pericarditis
4. Myocardial contusion
5. Prinzmetal's angina
6. Early repolarization
7. Hypothermia (Osbourne J wave)
8. Hyperkalemia
9. Artifact
ST elevation is also occasionally seen with LBBB, LVH, myocardial neoplasms, and hypertrophic myopathies.

Name five causes of ST depression.

1. Acute posterior MI
2. Ischemia
3. Digitalis
4. LVH
5. BBB

Name nine important causes of T-wave inversion.

1. Ischemia
2. Electrolyte abnormalities
3. Medications (digitalis)
4. BBB
5. Myocarditis
6. Pericarditis
7. "Juvenile" T waves
8. Subarachnoid hemorrhages
9. After a VPB and some tachycardias

List three causes of hyperacute T waves.

1. Hyperkalemia
2. Other acute metabolic derangements
3. Acute ischemia

What does the S1S2S3 pattern (i.e., S waves in leads I, II, and III) or the S1Q3T3 pattern (i.e., S wave in lead I and Q wave and inverted T wave in lead III) suggest?	Acute pulmonary embolus causing acute RV strain (seen in approximately 10% of cases)
What is electrical alternans?	Alternating ECG voltage beat by beat
What are the four causes of electrical alternans?	1. Digitalis toxicity 2. Rapid respiratory rates 3. Large pericardial effusion 4. Reentrant tachycardias
In patients with AF who are on digoxin, and who present with a regular rhythm, what rhythms should be considered?	Sinus Junctional, especially if other medications such as verapamil, quinidine, or amiodarone have been added (all of which increase the digoxin level)

SIGNAL-AVERAGED ELECTROCARDIOGRAPHY

What is signal-averaged ECG (saECG)?	An ECG technique used to improve signal-to-noise ratio so that late ventricular afterpotentials (the substrate responsible for some VTs) can be detected
When is saECG helpful?	saECG is helpful when you suspect that a patient's symptoms are caused by VT and you want to risk stratify a patient for risk of VT and sudden death. A patient with a normal LVEF and a normal saECG has a low risk of VT and sudden death. A patient with a low LVEF and an abnormal saECG has a high risk of VT and sudden death (approximately 30% at 1 year of follow-up).

HOLTER MONITORING, EVENT RECORDER

What is a Holter monitor?	A device that a patient wears for 24–48 hours; it records a continuous ECG rhythm strip and ST segment shift from two ECG leads

When is a Holter monitor helpful?	When you suspect that a patient's symptoms are due to an arrhythmia. Some monitors can detect ischemia by recording ST segment shifts.
What is an event recorder?	A device that a patient wears for an extended period of time (weeks) that records a patient's rhythm for a given time interval before and after the patient activates the device. (The patient must be able to activate the device.)

TILT TABLE

What is the tilt table test used for?	To test for vasovagal syncope
How is a tilt table test performed?	The patient is strapped to a table and the table is tilted to 70 degrees from horizontal for 45 minutes with continuous ECG and arterial BP monitoring. A positive test is a decreased HR and BP with reproduction of syncope.

ECHOCARDIOGRAPHY

What are some indications for echocardiography?	To assess chamber size (left and right atrium, left and right ventricle) To assess RV and LV function To assess the cause of a new murmur (especially after MI) To assess the heart valves for stenosis, regurgitation, and vegetation To look for intracardiac thrombus and pericardial effusion and tamponade To assess proximal great vessel disease (ascending aortic dissection) To assess congenital cardiac anomalies (e.g., ASD, VSD)
What are the major advantages of transthoracic echocardiography (TTE)?	It is noninvasive and carries no risk. It can be done at the bedside. It can be used to estimate PA pressure, which can be followed up over time.

What are some disadvantages of TTE?

Acoustic windows are not obtained in all patients (e.g., patients with COPD). Only an indirect assessment of intracardiac pressures can be obtained.

What are some indications for transesophageal echocardiography (TEE)?

Inadequate transthoracic windows
Intraoperative assessment of valvular repair
Assessment of aortic arch

What are some disadvantages of TEE?

It is invasive and there is risk of esophageal injury.
It is not available at all centers.
Operators require more advanced training.

Can stenotic valves be assessed by Doppler sonography?

Yes. The peak gradient across the valve corresponds to the pressure drop. Gradients greater than 50 mm Hg across the aortic valve suggest significant AS and gradients greater than 10–15 mm Hg across the mitral valve suggest significant MS. The mitral valve area can be estimated using the pressure half-time formula; the aortic valve area can be estimated using the continuity equation.

Can regurgitant valves be assessed using Doppler techniques?

Yes. All the valves can be imaged and regurgitation quantitated.

What is the Doppler technique used to estimate the PA pressure?

The Bernoulli equation: $4v^2$ + RA pressure. If the Doppler velocity is 3 m^2 and you estimate the RA pressure at 10 mm Hg, then the PA pressure (assuming no PS) is $4 \times (3)^2 + 10 = 46$ mm Hg. This can be a convenient, noninvasive way of following up patients with pulmonary HTN.

How are shunts detected?

Color flow and pulsed Doppler sonography can identify abnormal flows (e.g., ASD and VSD). Agitated saline or Albunex, a contrast agent, can be rapidly injected into a peripheral vein while the heart is imaged. If there is an ASD, then contrast can be seen flowing from the RA to the LA. Often, shunts are bidirectional and flow into the RA of noncontrasted blood, which creates a contrast-negative jet.

STRESS TESTING

Why would you obtain a stress test?

To determine whether a patient has coronary disease

To determine the extent of coronary disease in a patient with known disease (risk stratification)

To assess functional status

To assess response to antianginal or antihypertensive therapy

To enable determination of an exercise prescription (e.g., after infarction)

What is the Bruce protocol?

Also called a maximum stress test, the Bruce protocol applies 3-minute stages of progressing speed and elevation of the treadmill.

What other protocols are there?

There are several—Naughton, Ellestad, modified Bruce, and so on—all of which use variations of smaller increments in workload, shorter duration, and less elevation of the treadmill.

What are some contraindications to exercise stress testing [i.e., a graded exercise test (GXT)]?

Uncontrolled HTN

Decompensated CHF

AMI or unstable angina

Critical AS

Severe idiopathic subaortic stenosis

Uncontrolled arrhythmia or heart block

Inability to walk on treadmill due to neurologic or musculoskeletal abnormalities or to vascular disease

Acute myocarditis or pericarditis

Acute systemic illness

What are the alternatives to a GXT?

Dobutamine or DP testing with radionuclide perfusion scan. Some centers are evaluating adenosine infusions. Pacing can also be used.

What are indications for pharmacologic testing?

The indications are the same as for the GXT, except pharmacologic testing is for patients who cannot exercise due to musculoskeletal disease, neurologic disease, or vascular disease. Pharmacologic testing does not give information on functional status or the efficacy of antianginal therapy.

What are contraindications to DP testing?

Significant asthma, COPD, and recent CVA. Caffeine and theophylline compounds must be withheld before testing.

What are contraindications to dobutamine testing?

Significant HTN and known catechol-induced arrhythmias

What variables indicate a high-risk GXT?

Inability to exercise or poor exercise performance (< 5 METs) due to a cardiac reason

Significant ECG changes within the first 3–6 minutes

Extensive ischemic changes (> 2-mm ST segment depression, many leads involved)

Decrease in BP or flat BP response to exercise

Significant arrhythmias

Where is the coronary stenosis if a patient undergoes a GXT and has the following:

3-mm inferolateral ST depression

Nonspecific finding

3-mm anterior ST elevation

LAD (ST elevation outside the anterior leads is not predictive of stenosis location)

How is the maximum HR determined?

220 – age

What is a MET?

A metabolic equivalent: 3.5 ml O_2/min/m^2. It takes 1 MET for a person to sit quietly.

How much should the HR increase during a GXT?	10 bpm/stage (a delay may be noted in athletes and patients taking β blockers)
How much should the BP increase during a GXT?	10 mm Hg/stage (a delay may be noted in athletes)
What is the sensitivity and specificity for GXT?	65% and 65%
List the causes of false-positive GXT results.	Female gender, hyperventilation, MVP, LVH, digitalis

RADIONUCLIDE IMAGING

In general terms, what are scintigraphic scans (Tl201, MIBI) used for?	To provide functional assessment of coronary flow and to identify exercise-induced pulmonary edema
How are scintigraphic scans performed?	Approximately 1 minute before termination of stress, the isotope is injected. Images of immediate post-stress scans are then compared with resting scans.
Why does thallium provide useful information?	It behaves like potassium; that is, it is taken up by viable cells.
Describe the thallium image of ischemia.	In the stress views, there is little tracer uptake in a region; in the delayed images, the defect resolves or improves.
Describe the thallium image of an infarct.	In the stress and delayed views, there is a persistent regional decrease in tracer uptake.
What are the sensitivity and specificty for GXT plus radionuclide perfusion scan?	85%–90% and 85%–90%
What variables indicate a high-risk radionuclide myocardial perfusion scan?	Increased lung uptake (thallium scans) Cardiac enlargement with exercise Reversible perfusion defects in multiple vascular territories

What are indications for radionuclide ventriculography (MUGA)?

A rest study is used to assess LVEF with or without RVEF; an excercise study is used to assess evidence of exercise-induced ischemia.

How does MUGA work?

Red blood cells are removed from the body and labeled with pyrophosphate. The labeled cells are then returned to the patient and technetium is injected into the patient. The technetium binds to the pyrophosphate-labeled cells. The gamma rays are then tracked. LVEF = (LVED counts + LVES counts)/LVED counts

What are the limitations of MUGA?

Large regional wall motion abnormalities can be missed if the LVEF is calculated only from the left anterior oblique projection.

ELECTROPHYSIOLOGIC TESTING

List the indications for electrophysiologic testing.

To study unexplained syncope
To assess a patient at high risk for VT
To determine the mechanism of SVT
To assess response to antiarrhythmic medications
To assess the feasibility of catheter ablation

PACEMAKERS

List the indications for use of a temporary pacemaker.

Symptomatic bradycardia, second-degree AVB type II, CHB, a new bifascicular block in the setting of AMI, and the prevention of bradycardia-dependent VT

What are the indications for implantation of permanent pacemakers?

Symptomatic bradycardia, prolonged sinus pauses (> 3 seconds, symptomatic; > 5 seconds, asymptomatic), second-degree AVB type II, CHB, the prevention of arrhythmias in patients with a long QT interval, and, possibly, HOCM

How can arrhythmias be treated nonsurgically?

Percutaneous ablation (destruction) of a critical portion of the cardiac conduction system so that an arrhythmia cannot be initiated or propagated

Patients with an ICD usually suffer from what arrhythmia?

VT or VF

What do the letters in a three-letter pacemaker code represent?

The first letter is the chamber or chambers paced. The second letter is the chamber or chambers sensed. The third letter is the mode of response to a sensed event.

What are the pacemaker response modes?

Inhibition. The pacemaker is inhibited from pacing if a QRS complex is sensed.
Triggering. The pacemaker triggers a paced beat if a complex is sensed.
Dual. Both inhibition and triggering occur.

What does the letter R after a three-letter pacemaker code represent?

It indicates that the pacemaker is rate responsive; that is, the pacemaker increases the pacing rate in response to some physiologic event (e.g., changes in respiratory rate, CO_2 level, or motion).

What does a VVI-R pacemaker do?

V = ventricular lead for pacing
V = senses intrinsic ventricular activity
I = inhibits pacing when an intrinsic sensed event occurs
R = responds to activity (i.e., rate responsive)

What does a DDD pacemaker do?

D = paces both the RA and the RV
D = senses both the RA and the RV
D = inhibits and triggers. That is, if an atrial event is sensed, the pacemaker inhibits an atrial paced beat and triggers a ventricular paced beat if a ventricular beat is not sensed; if a ventricular event is sensed, it inhibits both atrial and ventricular paced beats.

CARDIAC CATHETERIZATION

What are the three major coronary arteries?	1. LAD (left anterior descending) 2. LCx (left circumflex) 3. RCA (right coronary artery)
Which artery supplies the anterior wall, septum, and the anterolateral wall?	Left anterior descending coronary artery
Which artery supplies the inferior wall, inferior septum, and RV?	RCA
Which artery supplies the posterior wall and posterolateral wall (and the inferior wall if dominant)?	Circumflex coronary artery
What branches come off the LAD?	Diagonals and septal perforators (septals)
What branches come off the circumflex?	Obtuse marginals (generally three)
What branches come off the RCA?	Acute marginals, PDA, posterolateral
What does "right dominant" mean?	The PDA comes off the RCA. This occurs in 90% of cases. The other 10% of the time, the PDA comes from the LCx (left dominant).
What are the indications for cardiac catheterization?	To assess coronary anatomy To assess the degree of valvular stenosis and regurgitation To assess pericardial disease (e.g., constriction and tamponade) To assess for restrictive cardiomyopathy To assess for CHD To determine the cause of postinfarct angina To assess anatomy after non–Q-wave MI or Q-wave MI

What are the important complications of cardiac catheterization?

Allergic contrast reaction, bleeding, infection, renal failure, 1/1000 incidence of stroke, MI, arrhythmias, cardiac perforation, and death

What are the benefits of cardiac catheterization?

It provides a map of all vessel stenoses, distal vessels, collaterals, and left ventricular function. It also provides information as to the severity of valvular regurgitation, allows calculation of stenotic valve areas, and directly measures intracardiac pressures.

Has PTCA been shown to reduce the rate of MI?

No

What is PTCA effective for?

Alleviating symptoms in patients with stable or unstable angina
Decreasing the mortality rate in patients with acute transmural MI

What is the downside of PTCA?

There is a 6-month restenosis rate after PTCA of approximately 33%; however, if there is no evidence of restenosis at 6 months, then restenosis does not occur.

How can restenosis be treated?

Redilatation is successful approximately 90% of the time. After the first episode, the re-restenosis rate increases; at some point, CABG should be considered (depending on the lesion and symptoms). Note: Most restenosis presents as recurrent angina, not infarction.

What is the complication rate of PTCA?

Less than 2%–4%

What other interventional coronary procedures are there?

DCA—cuts atheroma out of the vessel
Laser—burns atheroma
Rotoblator—device spins at > 20,000 RPM to emulsify plaque
Stents

What is valvuloplasty?

Repair of a heart valve. It can be done in an open fashion by a surgeon or percutaneously using a balloon in the cardiac catheterization laboratory.

What is an IABP?

An intraaortic balloon pump is a device, generally inserted through the femoral artery into the descending aorta. The device inflates during diastole, augmenting coronary blood flow, and deflates during systole, causing a reduction in afterload.

What is an IABP used for?

To provide temporary hemodynamic support (by increasing the mean BP)
To treat reversible causes of CHF
As a bridge to transplant
For support following CABG or valve surgery
For pain control with unstable angina
To treat refractory arrhythmias

What are three contraindications to an IABP?

1. Significant aortic regurgitation
2. Aortic dissection
3. Severe peripheral vascular disease

Where should you compress an artery after removing an IABP (or any other arterial catheter)?

1–2 cm proximal to the skin puncture site. Note: The needle enters the skin at an angle so the arterial puncture site is proximal to the skin site.

CORONARY ARTERY BYPASS GRAFTING

What are the common indications for CABG?

Three-vessel CAD with reduced LV function
Two-vessel CAD with a proximal LAD stenosis
Left main coronary disease
Palliation of symptoms (angina)

What are the common vascular conduits for CABG surgery?

IMA (right to the LCx or RCA, left to the LAD); can be removed from the subclavian for a free graft
Saphenous veins
Gastroepiploic artery
Superficial epigastric vessel
Radial artery

What percent of IMA grafts are patent after 10 years?

> 90%–95%

What percent of saphenous vein grafts are patent after 10 years?	60%
What is the CABG operative *mortality* rate?	1%–2%, although the rate varies according to comorbid conditions
What are the mechanisms of chest pain reduction after CABG?	Restoration of blood flow to the myocardium, MI, placebo effect, and denervation

VALVULAR SURGERY

What are the common indications for valve replacement or repair?	Critical AS or MS and palliation of symptomatic valvular regurgitation
In patients undergoing mitral valve surgery, why is it important to maintain the subvalvular apparatus?	It helps maintain normal ventricular geometry.

VALVULAR HEART DISEASE

What are the cardiac manifestations of acute rheumatic fever?	Carditis (highest frequency in patients younger than 3 years old; rare in patients older than 25 years old), myocarditis (with or without pericarditis), and valvulitis Acute MR secondary to left ventricular dysfunction or valvulitis
What are the Jones criteria?	Screening criteria for the diagnosis of acute rheumatic fever. Patients with two major and one minor criteria or one major and two minor criteria have a high probability of acute rheumatic fever.
What are the major Jones criteria?	Carditis, erythema marginatum, chorea (St. Vitus' dance), polyarthritis, subcutaneous nodules
What are the minor Jones criteria?	Fever, arthralgia, elevated ESR or positive C-reactive protein, previous rheumatic fever or rheumatic heart disease, and prolonged PR interval. There is also supporting evidence for a preceding streptococcal infection, that is,

history of recent scarlet fever, positive throat culture for group A streptococcus, or increased ASO titers or titers for other streptococcal antibodies.

After someone contracts rheumatic fever, how long does it take before important valvular changes occur (e.g., significant MS)?

15–20 years

What are the *common* systolic murmurs?

AS, MR, and VSD

What are the *common* diastolic murmurs?

Aortic regurgitation and MS

What are the *common* continuous murmurs?

PDA and the combination of AS and AI

What are the volume overload valve lesions?

MR and AI

What is the response of the ventricle to volume overload?

The ventricle primarily dilates.

What are the pressure overload valve lesions?

AS and MS

What is the response of the ventricle to the pressure overload of AS?

The ventricle primarily hypertrophies.

What are the common bioprosthetic valves?

Hancock, Carpentier, and homograft (human valve tissue)

Why is immunosuppression not required for tissue valves?

The valves are fixed in glutaraldehyde; there is no active surface protein.

What are the common metal valves?

Bjork-Shiley, Lillehi-Caster, Medtronic Hall, St. Judes, and Starr-Edwards

How long do tissue valves last?

There is a 30% failure rate at 15 years.

How long do metal valves last?

The known life of the Starr-Edwards is greater than 25 years. Presumably, metal valves can last indefinitely.

What medication is required after placement of a metal valve?

Warfarin (Coumadin)

In whom should anticoagulation be avoided?

Young children, older persons (especially those prone to falling), young women who desire to bear children, and patients with a history of peptic ulcer disease or bleeding diathesis (in whom a tissue valve would be required)

What is the main concern in taking care of a patient with a valvular lesion?

Determining when (if ever) surgery is necessary. If the patient is referred to surgery too soon, the patient may be exposed to an unnecessary surgical risk and to the risks associated with anticoagulation (where applicable) and the prosthetic valve.

What is the risk of late patient referral?

Irreversible ventricular failure

What is the appropiate antibiotic prophylaxis for nonsterile procedures in patients with heart defects?

If the patient is not allergic to penicillin, amoxicillin (3 g before and 1.5 g afterward) are given for the procedure. For patients who are allergic to penicillin, erythromycin or clindamycin are substitutes. For patients with metal prosthetic valves, vancomycin plus gentamicin is given.

AORTIC STENOSIS

What are the common causes of AS?

1. Rheumatic (< 25% of cases have aortic valve involvement without significant mitral valve involvement)
2. Congenital (bicuspid and unicuspid)
3. Calcific

Is age helpful in determining the cause of AS?

Yes. If the patient is younger than 30 years, the cause is congenital. If the patient is between 30 and 70 years, the cause is rheumatic or bicuspid. If the patient is older than 70 years, the cause is calcific.

What is the normal aortic valve area?

2–3 cm^2

What valve area is considered to be critically narrowed?

< 0.7 cm^2 (< .5 cm^2/m^2)

What are the symptoms and signs of AS?

Think **ASC** (AS complications):
    Angina (approximately 5-year survival after developing)
    Syncope (approximately 3-year survival)
    CHF (approximately 1-year survival)

What is the expected survival rate in patients with symptoms and a critical aortic valve area?

90% mortality at 1 year

What are the physical examination findings of severe AS?

Low pulse pressure, sustained apical impulse, delayed pulse peak, and low amplitude (pulsus parvus et tardus; best appreciated at the brachial artery)
S4; S3 if in CHF
Ejection click
Diamond-shaped systolic murmur (the later the peak, the tighter the valve)
Reduced (or absent) A2
Delayed A2 closure (or paradoxic splitting of A2P2)
Mild AI (severe AS and severe AI cannot occur together)

What are the usual echocardiographic findings?

LVH
Decreased aortic valve leaflet movement (bicuspid aortic valve)
Doppler gradient > 50 mm Hg

What hemodynamic findings are observed at heart catheterization?

Elevated PC pressure and a gradient between the LV and aortic (or femoral artery) systolic pressure

What is an easy formula to calculate the aortic valve area?

$$\text{Aortic valve area} = \frac{CO}{\sqrt{\text{Peak LV systolic pressure} - \text{peak Ao systolic pressure}}}$$

AORTIC REGURGITATION

What are the common causes of AI?	Rheumatic causes, connective tissue disorders (e.g., Marfan's syndrome, Ehlers-Danlos syndrome), arthritis (Reiter's, rheumatoid arthritis, systemic lupus erythematosus), Takayasu's aortitis, congenital (bicuspid) causes, association with dissections, endocarditis, syphilitic causes, trauma, and acute rheumatic fever
Why is acute AI difficult to diagnose?	The murmur is soft due to the rapid equalization of the aortic diastolic pressure and the LVEDP.
What are the common physical findings of chronic severe AI?	Wide pulse pressure (if pulse pressure is less than 50 mm Hg or aortic diastolic pressure is greater than 70 mm Hg, then the AI is probably not severe) Decrescendo diastolic murmur
Name the common signs associated with AI.	Corrigan's pulse (rapid increase and decrease) DeMusset's sign (head bob with pulsations) Pistol shot pulses Duroziez's murmur (femoral artery systolic and diastolic murmur) Mueller's sign (uvula bobs) Quincke's sign (nail-bed pulsation) Hill's sign (augmented femoral artery systolic and diastolic pressure)
What is the Austin-Flint murmur?	It occurs in severe AI. The regurgitant jet strikes the anterior leaflet of the mitral valve, causing it to move into the mitral inflow and causing relative MS.

What is the treatment for AI?	Medical—antibiotic prophylaxis prior to dental and genitourinary procedures, digoxin, diuretics, and afterload reduction Surgical—valve replacement
When is surgery needed for patients with AI?	This is a difficult decision. Some studies have shown improved survival when the LV is greater than 75 mm at end diastole or greater than 55 mm at end systole.

MITRAL STENOSIS

What are the common causes of MS?	Rheumatic, congenital, vegetative, calcific
What is the normal mitral valve area?	4–6 cm^2
What are some nonvalvular causes of LV inflow obstuction?	Atrial myxoma and LA thrombus
What are the common symptoms and historical features of MS?	Dyspnea, fatigue, palpitations, hemoptysis, hoarseness, chest pain, seizures, and CVA. It often manifests during pregnancy.
What are the common physical findings of MS?	A diastolic rumble that increases with exercise and is heard best in the left lateral decubitus position Increased S1 Opening snap—The closer the A2 opening snap interval, the tighter the valve Presystolic augmentation of the rumble Malar flush Peripheral cyanosis Elevated JVD (when right heart failure occurs) v wave on jugular inspection All signs increase with exercise and pregnancy.

What is the treatment for severe MS?	Medical—Rate control if in AF, anticoagulation, diuretics, and percutaneous balloon mitral valve commissurotomy Surgical—Mitral valve repair or replacement. Generally, if the valve is not heavily calcified or the submitral apparatus is not severely affected, the valve is repaired.

MITRAL REGURGITATION

What are the common causes of MR?	Rheumatic causes, MVP, left ventricular dilatation (multiple causes), calcific (annular) causes, endocarditis, papillary muscle dysfunction or rupture, connective tissue disorders (e.g., Marfan's syndrome, Ehlers-Danlos syndrome, osteogenesis imperfecta, systemic lupus erythemotosus), and other congenital causes (e.g., corrected transposition, endocardial fibroelastosis, partial AV canal, and cleft leaflet)
How common is MVP?	It depends on the definition. Probably 10%–15% of women and 5% of men have some degree of bowing of the anterior leaflet of the mitral valve. People at risk for endocarditis are those with a murmur and, most likely, only those with myxomatous valve leaflets.
What is the classic description of an MVP murmur?	Mid to late systolic click and murmur. Any maneuver that shrinks the LV cavity, that is, decreases the preload or afterload (e.g., by sitting or standing up) causes the click and murmur to occur earlier; any maneuver that increases the cavity size, that is, increases preload or afterload, causes the click and murmur to occur later (e.g., by raising the legs up or gripping the hands).
What is the typical body habitus for patients with MVP?	Pectus excavatum, asthenic features, and straight back

Do all patients with MVP need antibiotic prophylaxis?	No, probably only those with a murmur
How does left ventricular cavity dilatation cause MR?	Cavity enlargement of any cause (e.g., dilated cardiomyopathies and multiple MIs) results in a stretch of the mitral annulus and consequent leaflet noncoaptation. Enlargement of the ventricle also causes malposition of the papillary muscle structure and leaflet malcoaptation.
How does CAD cause MR?	1. Recurrent MIs lead to left ventricular dilatation. 2. Papillary muscle infarction causes papillary muscle dysfunction or disruption, leading to leaflet malcoaptation.
What population is most commonly affected by mitral annular calcification?	Older women
What historical feature is common to patients with acute MR?	Acute pulmonary edema
What historical features are common to patients with chronic MR?	Dyspnea, fatigue, and, eventually, symptoms and signs of left ventricular dysfunction (e.g., orthopnea, PND, and edema)
What is the most common cause of palpitations in patients with significant MR?	Atrial fibrillation
What are the common physical examination findings of acute MR?	Respiratory distress, rales, JVD, possible absence of holosystolic murmur (similar to acute AI), and normal-sized heart and pulmonary congestion shown on chest radiograph

Where does the murmur of acute MR radiate?	The location depends on the mitral leaflet involved and the mechanism. If the murmur is secondary to AMI with papillary muscle dysfunction and involves the anterior leaflet, the regurgitant jet is reflected to the back. With the same mechanism and involvement of the posterior leaflet, the regurgitant jet is reflected superiorly (e.g., to the clavicular region).
What are the common physical examination findings of chronic MR?	Holosystolic murmur radiating to the apex and pulses with an abrupt upstroke and shorter duration
What are the common physical examination and radiographic findings of severe MR?	S3 gallop, rales, JVD, liver distention, and edema; chest radiograph shows an enlarged heart with or without pulmonary congestion
What factors determine survival in patients with MR?	Factors depend on the cause—CAD or cardiomyopathy increases the mortality rate; acute MR with cardiogenic shock is associated with a 60%–80% mortality rate

INFECTIVE ENDOCARDITIS

What is IE?	Infection of the endocardial surface of the heart, most commonly the valves; microorganisms are present
How does acute endocarditis differ from subacute endocarditis?	Acute endocarditis is a fulminant infection with fever, leukocytosis, toxicity, and death occurring in days to less than 6 weeks. It is caused by more virulent organisms such as *Staphylococcus aureus, Streptococcus pneumoniae,* and *Streptococcus pyogenes.* Subacute endocarditis is more common in patients with prior valvular disease and has a more indolent course characterized by fever, weight loss, constitutional symptoms, and death occurring in 6 weeks to 3 months.
What is the incidence of IE?	< 1/1000 hospital admissions

What are the risk factors for IE?

Most structural cardiac defects including the following:

CHD (e.g., PDA, VSD, coarctation of the aorta, bicuspid aortic valve, tetralogy of Fallot, and pulmonary stenosis)

Rheumatic heart disease

Degenerative cardiac lesions

Intracardiac pacemakers or intracardiac prostheses

Intravascular access procedures in ill hospitalized patients

Intravenous drug use

MVP with regurgitation

What are the symptoms and signs of IE?

Almost any organ can be involved, but symptoms are due to four basic processes: (1) infectious process on the valve, (2) bland or septic embolization, (3) sustained bacteremia, and (4) circulating immune complexes. Symptoms and signs include fever, constitutional symptoms, murmur in greater than 85% of cases (new or changing murmur is uncommon, occurring in less than 10% of cases), peripheral manifestations in less than 50% of cases, musculoskeletal symptoms, CHF, emboli, and neurologic symptoms.

What are the peripheral manifestations of IE?

Splinter hemorrhages, Roth's spots, petechiae, Osler's nodes, and Janeway lesions

Identify each of the following lesions:
Osler's nodes

Arteriolar intimal proliferation with extension into the capillaries. They may have associated thrombosis and necrosis. They appear as small, painful nodules on the pads of the fingers and toes.

Janeway lesions

Septic emboli that appear as painless, macular lesions on the palms and soles

Roth's spots

Lymphocytes surrounded by edema and hemorrhage on the retina. They appear as white lesions surrounded by erythema and are usually near the optic disk. They are uncommon, occurring in less than 5% of cases, and can be seen in other diseases.

Splinter hemorrhages

Linear red to brown streaks found in the nail beds. They may also occur with trauma and are more suggestive of IE if they are close to the nail matrix.

Petechiae

Local vasculitis or emboli. They appear as red, nonblanching lesions on the buccal mucosa, soft palate, conjunctivae, or extremities.

What laboratory results suggest endocarditis?

Commonly noted but not diagnostic are the following findings: anemia (70%–90% of cases), thrombocytopenia, leukocytosis or leukopenia, elevated ESR (90%–100% of cases), and abnormal urinalysis with proteinuria, hematuria, and red blood cell casts.

What is the role of blood cultures in diagnosing IE?

It is the single most important diagnostic test because IE is a continuous, low-grade bacteremia. In two thirds of patients, all blood cultures are positive. The first two blood cultures yield a pathogen more than 90% of the time. Three sets of specimens should be drawn within 24 hours, but no more than two vials should be drawn from one site at one time. Cultures should be held for 21 days (for fastidious organisms).

What other diagnostic tests can be used?

TTE may define the valve involved by the presence of a vegetation and demonstrate valvular dysfunction or the presence of a complication. Sensitivity varies so a negative study does not rule out IE.

TEE is more sensitive (95% versus 65% for TTE). Consider TEE when TTE is negative and there is suspicion of IE.

What are the pathogens involved in IE?

Streptococci (viridans streptococci, enterococci, among others)

Staphylococci (*S. aureus*; coagulase-negative)

Gram-negative bacilli (uncommon, high mortality rate)

Fungi

Miscellaneous bacteria

Culture-negative cause

Streptococci and staphylococci cause approximately 90% of all cases of IE.

How likely is endocarditis if a blood culture is positive for the following:

Streptococcus mutans?

15 cases of IE for every 1 case of bacteremia without valvular involvement

Streptococcus sanguis?

3 cases of IE for every 1 case of bacteremia without valvular involvement

Enterococci?

Equal likelihood of IE or bacteremia without valvular involvement

Group A Streptococcus?

Only 1 case of IE for every 7 cases of bacteremia without valvular involvement

What is culture-negative endocarditis?

Culture-negative endocarditis occurs when the results of routine blood cultures are negative. Possible explanations for negative findings on blood cultures include subacute right-sided endocarditis, mural endocarditis, timing [cultures drawn at the end of a chronic course (> 3 months)], prior antibiotic use, slow-growing fastidious organisms (HACEK, nutritionally variant streptococci), fungal infection, obligate intracellular pathogens, noninfectious endocarditis, or the wrong diagnosis.

What are the general principles of treatment?

1. Parenteral antibiotics with sustained bactericidal activity should be selected.
2. The course of therapy should be extended.
3. Static antibiotics are ineffective.

4. Combination therapy has a rapid cidal effect.
5. The patient should be closely monitored (e.g., by ECG) and may require ICU admission.
6. Antibiotic therapy should be based on susceptibility tests.
7. Blood cultures should be repeated to document clearing.
8. Anticoagulation is associated with bleeding complications and should be avoided.
9. There should be rapid access to a cardiothoracic surgeon.

What is the specific treatment for the following:

Pencillin-susceptible streptococci

Penicillin with or without an aminoglycoside (use an aminoglycoside initially; consider stopping if the pathogen is susceptible)

Penicillin-resistant streptococci

Penicillin with an aminoglycoside

Enterococci

Penicillin or ampicillin plus gentamicin

S. aureus

Nafcillin with or without gentamicin (consider using for the first 5 days to clear blood faster, then stop the gentamicin if the pathogen is sensitive to penicillin)

Methicillin-resistant S. aureus (MRSA) and coagulase-negative staphylococci

Vancomycin (consider rifampin and gentamicin)

Prosthetic valve endocarditis caused by staphylococci

Vancomycin plus rifampin and gentamicin or, if susceptible, nafcillin plus rifampin and gentamicin

Culture-negative endocarditis

Ampicillin plus gentamicin with or without vancomycin
Vancomycin plus cefotaxime and gentamicin

What are the indications for surgery?	Refractory CHF Uncontrolled infection Significant valvular dysfunction Repeated systemic embolization Ineffective antimicrobial therapy (against, e.g., fungi) Resection of a mycotic aneurysm Most cases of prosthetic valve endocarditis Local suppurative complications with conduction abnormalities
Who should receive endocarditis prophylaxis?	Patients with prosthetic valves, rheumatic valvular disease, MVP with regurgitation, bicuspid aortic valve or another congenital heart defect, history of bacterial endocarditis, calcified aortic or mitral valve, or hypertrophic cardiomyopathy
For which procedures should prophylaxis be given?	Procedures that are likely to produce bacteremia, such as dental procedures with gingival bleeding, upper respiratory and oropharyngeal procedures, genitourinary manipulations, gastrointestinal procedures, obstetric–gynecologic interventions, and manipulation of septic foci. Sterile procedures do not require specific prophylaxis. Each procedure should be evaluated individually.
What prophylaxis should be given?	For dental, oral, or upper respiratory tract procedures in adults, 3 g of amoxicillin should be given 1 hour before and 1.5 g should be given 6 hours after the procedure. For genitourinary, gynecologic, and gastrointestinal procedures, 2 g of ampicillin should be given intravenously plus 1.5 mg/kg of gentamicin should be given 30 minutes before and 8 hours after the procedure. Other regimens exist for high-risk patients (e.g., those with prosthetic valves) and pencillin-allergic patients

PROSTHETIC VALVE ENDOCARDITIS

What is the incidence of prosthetic valve endocarditis?	< 3% of valve replacements; 2% in the first year, 1% per year thereafter
Which pathogens cause prosthetic valve endocarditis?	Early (< 60 days)—*Staphylococcus epidermidis*, gram-negative bacilli, *S. aureus*, and diphtheroids Late (> 60 days)—Viridans group streptococci (more like native valve endocarditis)
What is the treatment for prosthetic valve endocarditis?	Antibiotics as described for IE, but, commonly, valve replacement is required for cure

ARRHYTHMIAS

COMMON ARRHYTHMIAS

What is a first-degree block?	PR interval > 200 msec
What is a second-degree block?	Variable PR interval (progressive lengthening) = Wenkebach or Mobitz I Dropped beats (fixed PR interval with dropped beats) = Mobitz II
What is a third-degree block?	Dissociation of atrial and ventricular activity due to complete block at the AV node
What are the basic mechanisms of cardiac arrhythmias?	Reentry, automaticity, and triggered activity
List the three common mechanisms for SVT.	1. AV node reentry 2. Atrial flutter with rapid ventricular response 3. AV reciprocating tachycardia (accessory pathway)
What is the diagnosis in a patient with a narrow QRS complex and regular tachycardia?	SVT

What is the differential diagnosis in a patient with a narrow QRS complex and an irregular tachycardia?

AF, multifocal atrial tachycardia, and sinus tachycardia with frequent APBs

What is the diagnosis in a patient with a wide QRS complex and regular tachycardia?

VT; however, VT often has a warm-up and a cool-down period that may not be perfectly regular

What is the best question to ask to determine whether a patient has an SVT with aberrancy or VT?

"Have you had a heart attack?" If the answer is "yes," then the rhythm is a VT; if the answer is "no," consider SVT.

What causes a wide bizarre complex tachycardia?

Hyperkalemia and drug toxicity (especially type IC drugs)

Name seven causes of ectopy (atrial and ventricular)

1. Ischemia
2. Reperfusion following thrombolytic therapy (the classic example is AIVR, also known as slow VT)
3. Electrolyte abnormalities (potassium, calcium, magnesium)
4. Hypoxia
5. Monitoring lines (e.g., Swan-Ganz catheters, CVP lines)
6. Medications (e.g., β agonists, antiarrhythmics)
7. Endogenous catechols (e.g., pain, anxiety)

Surgical therapy may be indicated for what arrhythmias?

VT associated with a resectable aneurysm (aneurysmectomy with or without endocardial resection)
AF refractory to medical therapy (Maze procedure)

ANTIARRHYTHMIC MEDICATIONS

Name three class Ia antiarrhythmics.

Quinidine, procainamide, disopyramide

Name three class Ib antiarrhythmics.

Lidocaine, mexiletine, tocainide

Name a class Ic antiarrhythmic.	Flecainide
What are the class II antiarrhythmics?	β blockers
Name four class III antiarrhythmics?	Amiodarone, bretylium, sotalol (also a β blocker), and ibutilide
What are the class IV antiarrhythmics?	Calcium channel blockers
List two agents with mixed antiarrhythmic activity.	Sotalol (class II and III) and propafenone (class II, III, and Ic)
What causes quinidine syncope?	Torsades de pointes
What is torsades de pointes?	A polymorphic VT
What is a cause of arthritis in patients taking procainamide?	Drug-induced lupus reaction
What large group of patients should avoid disopyramide?	Men (urinary retention is caused by the anticholinergic effect)

What antiarrhythmics cause the following:

Prolonged QT (torsades de pointes)	Ia, III
Central nervous system toxicity including seizures	Ib, III
Pulmonary fibrosis, hepatitis, thyroid dysfunction, and corneal deposits	III (amiodarone)
Exacerbation of asthma	II, III (sotalol, propafenone)

What two groups of patients should not receive flecainide?	Patients with structural heart disease (e.g., CAD and previous MI) Patients with reduced left ventricular function

ATRIAL FIBRILLATION

In patients taking digoxin, the addition of which common (cardiovascular) medications requires a digoxin dose adjustment?	Quinidine, verapamil, and amiodarone [also affects warfarin (Coumadin) levels]. All increase the serum digoxin level.
In the diagnosis of new-onset AF, what does *PIRATES* stand for?	**P**ulmonary disease including pulmonary embolism **I**diopathic disease (including idiopathic HTN) or **I**nflammatory disease (including pericarditis and pericardial trauma or surgery) **R**heumatic valvular heart disease **A**therosclerotic CAD **T**hyrotoxicosis **E**thanol consumption (holiday heart syndrome) **S**ick sinus syndrome
What issues must be addressed in every patient with AF?	1. Stability 2. Rate control 3. Anticoagulation 4. Antiarrhythmic drugs 5. Cardioversion
How do you treat AF in a patient with hypotension and dyspnea?	Direct electrical cardioversion (synchronized if possible)
What medications are used to control the ventricular rate of AF?	Digoxin, β blockers, and calcium channel blockers (diltiazem and verapamil)
What is the stroke rate in patients with AF?	10%–20%; consider cardioversion or use warfarin (Coumadin) or ASA

EMERGENT TREATMENT—PROTOCOLS

What is the presumptive diagnosis in a patient with a wide complex, regular tachycardia and no pulse?	VT

What is your first intervention?	In rapid succession, defibrillation with 200 J, 200–300 J, and 360 J
What is the diagnosis in a patient with a wide complex, regular tachycardia who is comfortable, awake, and has a pulse?	VT or SVT with a BBB
What is your first intervention?	Intravenous lidocaine or procainamide
If the monitor shows sinus rhythm but the patient is unresponsive and has no pulse, what is the diagnosis?	Pulseless electrical activity [formerly known as electromechanical dissociation (EMD)]
What are the reversible causes of this syndrome?	Hypoxemia, hypovolemia, pneumothorax, pulmonary embolism, acidosis, and cardiac tamponade
How is bradycardia with hypotension treated?	Atropine or a temporary pacemaker if atropine is ineffective

SYNCOPE

What percentage of syncope cases are:	
Cardiovascular?	10%–25% (mortality rate at 12 months = 30%)
Noncardiovascular?	40%–60% (mortality rate at 12 months = 12%)
Unknown?	50%–70% (mortality rate at 12 months = 6%)
List nine noncardiac causes of syncope.	Vasovagal, orthostatic, TIA, CVA, seizure, psychogenic, hypoglycemic, hyperventilation, pulmonary embolus
List five cardiac causes of syncope.	AS, CAD catastrophic event (e.g., ventricular free wall rupture or acute VSD), dissecting aortic aneurysm, congenital lesions, dysrhythmias

CARDIOMYOPATHIES

MYOCARDITIS

What are the causes of myocarditis?

Coxsackie A and B, influenza B and A, and echovirus, among others. In South and Central America, Chagas disease [trypanosomal infection following the bite of a reduviid bug (bedbug)] is the most common cause of myocarditis.

Why is the muscle injured in myocarditis?

It is uncertain, but there may be a close human leukocyte antigen match between the virus protein and the myocardium, causing an autoimmune type injury.

How common is myocarditis?

It is uncommon, although the numerator and denominator are unknown. (Not everyone with a viral infection undergoes echocardiography.)

What is the natural history of the process in myocarditis?

50% recovery at 6 weeks to 6 months

What elements predict recovery?

Short time interval between disease onset and presentation as well as fairly low filling pressures (e.g., PC pressure < 20 mm Hg)

Do steroids help in the treatment of myocarditis?

There are no good studies to answer this question.

GENERAL CARDIOMYOPATHIES

What is a cardiomyopathy?

A disease of the heart **muscle,** causing impaired function

What is CHF?

A syndrome characterized by dyspnea that is secondary to an elevation of left or right atrial pressure, or both

What are the common symptoms associated with CHF?

Dyspnea, orthopnea, PND, palpitations

What is the New York Heart Classification?

An assessment of a patient's functional classification as follows:
    Class I—no symptoms, tolerates strenuous exercise
    Class II—dyspnea on strenuous exertion
    Class III—dyspnea on routine, light activity
    Class IV—dyspnea at rest

What are the common findings in patients with CHF?

Sinus tachycardia, elevated JVP, lateral PMI, S3 or S4 gallop, distended liver (sometimes pulsatile), and edema

What are the three types of cardiomyopathy?

Dilated, hypertrophic, and restrictive

Why are ischemic myopathies not a true diagnosis?

Technically, ischemic myopathies are due to coronary disease and are not a primary muscle problem; however, as infarcts occur, the ventricle remodels, so muscle changes do occur. Therefore, this term is acceptable.

What is the common feature explaining dyspnea in all types (dilated, hypertrophic, restrictive) of cardiomyopathies?

Elevated left atrial pressure

What is low output heart failure?

Because heart failure is a syndrome, low output heart failure represents inadequate blood flow to maintain the normal metabolic needs of the body. Common causes include any of the cardiomyopathies (except MR and AI).

What are the causes of high output heart failure?

Causes include MR, AI, beriberi, thyrotoxicosis, sepsis, any AV shunt (Paget's, renal shunts, Osler-Weber-Rendu), and severe anemia.

List ten potentially reversible causes of a dilated cardiomyopathy.

1. Alcoholic cardiomyopathy
2. Hypocalcemia, hypokalemia, hypophosphatemia
3. Hemochromatosis (although usually restrictive)
4. Pheochromocytoma
5. Myocarditis

6. Sarcoid heart disease
7. Lead poisoning
8. Selenium deficiency
9. Uremic cardiomyopathy
10. Ischemic cardiomyopathy

What are the classic physical signs of left ventricular dysfunction?

Distended neck veins, lateral PMI, S3 gallop, murmurs of MR or tricuspid regurgitation, rales, distended and possibly pulsatile liver, and edema. Note: Edema is found in the most dependent site, which is frequently the sacrum in hospitalized patients. These signs are helpful only when they are positive; that is, patients may have significant heart failure without a gallop or rales, for example.

What is the mechanism of MR in dilated cardiomyopathies?

As the ventricle enlarges, the mitral valve annulus stretches and the papillary muscles become malaligned, preventing the leaflets from coapting.

List the common chest radiograph features of dilated cardiomyopathies.

Cardiomegaly, Kerley B lines, venous congestion or cephalization, and pulmonary edema

What is the significance of a narrow pulse pressure in a patient with cardiomyopathy?

A pulse pressure index of less than 25% is associated with a CI of less than 2 L/min/m^2.

What are common inotropic agents?

β agonists (dobutamine, epinephrine, dopamine in moderate doses, isoproterenol)
Phosphodiesterase inhibitors (milrinone, amrinone)
Digoxin

Can different inotropic agents be used together?

Yes. β agonists, phosphodiesterase inhibitors, and digoxin all work through different pathways.

What are potential cardiovascular side effects of inotropic medications?

Arrhythmias (e.g., sinus tachycardia, VT, VF), hypotension (all vasodilate), and tolerance secondary to β-receptor downregulation

What are ACE inhibitors used for?

First-line therapy for any patient with a reduced ejection fraction

What are some potential side effects of ACE inhibitors?

Hypotension, renal failure (in patients with bilateral renal artery stenosis), hyperkalemia, allergic reactions (the most serious of which is angioedema), and cough. ACE receptor blockers may have a role in CHF and have been associated with fewer side effects but have not been approved for use, as yet, in CHF.

If ACE inhibitors are not tolerated, what drug combination is generally used?

Hydralazine and isosorbide

List the "reversible" causes of dilated cardiomyopathies.

Spontaneous improvement in left ventricular function occurs in 50% of patients with myocarditis and alcoholic and peripartum cardiomyopathies. Reasonably low filling pressures at catheterization and a short illness duration are predictive of recovery.

TRANSPLANT

What is three-drug immunosuppressive therapy?

Cyclosporine, azathioprine, and prednisone

What medications lower cyclosporine levels?

Dilantin, phenobarbital, rifampin, and isoniazid

What medications increase cyclosporine levels?

Macrolides (e.g., erythromycin), ketoconazole, itraconazole, diltiazem, and amiodarone

What medications may potentiate renal dysfunction when used with cyclosporine?

Aminoglycosides, amphotericin, nonsteroidal antiinflammatory agents

What side effects does azathioprine cause?

Bone marrow toxicity (leukopenia) and hepatic toxicity (potentiated by allopurinol)

Name six side effects of steroids.	Glucose intolerance, adrenal insufficiency if acutely withdrawn, cataracts, osteoporosis, cushingoid appearance, and skin fragility
What medication should not be used to treat bradycardia after heart transplantation?	Atropine
What medications should be used to treat bradycardia after heart transplantation?	Epinephrine and isoproterenol
What medication should not be used to treat SVT after heart transplantation?	Digoxin. The long-term use of β blockers is generally discouraged because these agents reduce exercise tolerance.
Why are tachy- and bradydysrhythmias treated differently in heart transplant recipients?	The heart is denervated; that is, vagolytic (atropine) and vagotonic (digoxin) agents are not effective.
Can a heart transplant patient have a heart attack?	Yes, CAD is a manifestation of chronic rejection. Approximately 50% of heart transplant patients have some evidence of CAD at 5 years. This is usually significant in only 5% of cases.
Does reinnervation ever occur?	Yes, 75% of heart recipients show some sympathetic reinnervation after 1 year.
Does reinnervation have any practical implication?	Yes, patients who undergo reinnervation have improved exercise performance (faster HR response), and some recipients in whom CAD develops complain of chest pain.
How long can a donor heart remain ischemic?	Approximately 4 hours (thus limiting the distance one can travel to obtain donor organs)
When are infections most common after any transplant?	In the first 3–6 months

What type of infections (other than a "cold") are most common after transplantation?	Bacterial (common) and atypical bacterial, followed by viral, fungal, and protozoal
What organ systems are most frequently involved with CMV?	Gastrointestinal (e.g., stomach and colon) Lung (e.g., resulting in pneumonitis) Other (e.g., heart and eyes) CMV infections can also stimulate the immune system and therefore are frequently associated with rejection.
When is rejection most common for any organ after transplantation?	In the first 1–2 months
What factors are important for successful heart, lung, and heart–lung transplantation?	ABO compatibility and approximate size match
What noninfectious process can masquerade with fever and an infiltrate following organ transplantation?	Transplant-associated B cell lymphoma, which occurs in 1%–5% of patients over time (frequency depends on the organ transplanted)
What is the most important factor limiting successful organ transplantation?	Lack of donors

ASSIST DEVICES

What is the most common assist device used in treatment of cardiomyopathy?	IABP
What are the disadvantages of balloon pumps?	They may cause ischemia of the leg where they are inserted. Insertion in the femoral artery severely limits mobility and may be associated with infection. The level of support is only moderate.

What two types of flow patterns are associated with left ventricular assist devices?	Continuous and pulsatile
What are the disadvantages of continuous flow?	All devices tend to cause hemolysis and may cause end-organ failure over time (1–2 weeks).
What are the disadvantages of pulsatile flow?	The devices tend to be more complex to insert and must be larger than the continuous flow devices due to the size of the pumping chamber.

PERICARDIAL DISEASE

EFFUSIONS AND TAMPONADE

What is the differential diagnosis of a pericardial friction rub?	Idiopathic cause, infectious cause, AMI, recent MI, postpericardiotomy syndrome (Dressler's syndrome), uremia, cancer, radiation, autoimmune disease, drug use, trauma, dissecting aortic aneurysm, and chylopericardium
What are the most common causes of pericardial disease?	Postoperative (i.e., following median sternotomy) AMI Idiopathic Uremia Infectious (e.g., viral, acute bacterial, fungal, or other infections, such as toxoplasmosis and Lyme disease) Radiation Autoimmune Other inflammatory disease (e.g., sarcoidosis, amyloidosis) Neoplasia Drug use (e.g., hydralazine and procainamide) Trauma Dissecting aortic aneurysm Myxedema
What is Dressler's syndrome?	Fever, pericarditis, and pleuritis occuring weeks to months after AMI. It may have an immunologic basis (different from pericarditis immediately after MI).

What is postpericardiotomy syndrome?

Inflammation of the pericardium and sometimes the pleura occurring in as many as 30% of patients 2–4 weeks after open heart surgery

What are the symptoms and signs of acute pericarditis?

Those of the underlying etiology. Retrosternal or precordial chest pain is usually pleuritic in nature and worsens with deep inspiration, lying down, or movement, causing dyspnea.

What relieves this pain?

Leaning forward, sitting up, and breathing shallowly

What is the most important physical finding of pericarditis?

Pericardial friction rub, which is heard best at the apex with the patient leaning forward

What does the ECG show?

In the acute phase, there is diffuse ST segment elevation that is most prominent in leads V_5–V_6 and I–II. ST elevation in V_6 is usually more than 25% the T-wave amplitude. Isoelectric or depressed ST in V_1 is common. PR segment depression in II, aVF, and V_4–V_6 may be seen.

What are infectious causes of pericardial disease?

Most common: spread of abscess and infection with coxsackie B, echovirus, influenza, herpes simplex virus, *S. aureus, S. pneumoniae,* and *Histoplasma capsulatum*
Acute rheumatic fever
Pleuropulmonary foci from trauma or surgery

What is one of the most consistent clinical findings with pericardial tamponade?

Pulsus paradoxus, which is not specific to tamponade. It may be found in constrictive pericarditis, restrictive cardiomyopathy, shock, pulmonary embolism, asthma, and tension pneumothorax.

When is pulsus paradoxus absent in tamponade?

During hypovolemia, low-pressure tamponade, and with LVH

What else is found on physical examination of pericardial tamponade?	Decreased systolic BP, narrow pulse pressure, distended neck veins with rapid "x" descent and attenuated "y" descent on examination of jugular venous pulsations, tachycardia, and "distant" heart sounds
What may be seen on ECG examination of pericardial tamponade?	Electrical alternans, low-voltage QRS complexes, ST elevation, and PR depression as seen with pericarditis
When should tamponade be suspected in the hemodynamically compromised patient?	After blunt or penetrating chest trauma, open heart surgery, or cardiac catheterization When there is suspected or known pericarditis, intrathoracic neoplasm, or dissecting aortic aneurysm When there is unexplained hypotension
What is the treatment for tamponade?	Volume expansion with normal saline increases CO and BP, but is, at best, a temporary measure. Pericardiocentesis can be lifesaving.

CONSTRICTIVE PERICARDITIS

What process causes constrictive pericarditis?	A chronic process of repair after pericardial injury. This may cause a fibrous thickening of pericardium that constricts the normal filling of the chambers.
What are predisposing factors?	Acute pericardial injury, cardiac trauma, pericardiotomy, and infectious pericarditis
What are symptoms and signs of constrictive pericarditis?	Similar to CHF (e.g., fatigue and dyspnea) Clear lungs (usually) Normal or small heart Kussmaul's sign (elevation of JVP with inspiration) Rapid "y" descent on jugular venous pulsations
What are the ECG findings for constrictive pericarditis?	No specific features

CHRONIC PERICARDITIS

How is chronic pericarditis recognized?	Chronic pain following a bout of acute pericarditis
What are the symptoms and signs of chronic pericarditis?	Dyspnea and fatigue associated with edema Hepatic distention
What is the treatment for chronic pericarditis?	Treatment is generally difficult due to the chronic nature of the disease. Search for an underlying cause (e.g., infection). Chronic diuretic use and nonsteroidal antiinflammatory drugs are the mainstays of treatment. Steroid use should be avoided, if possible. Other agents such as colchicine, azathioprine, and other immunosuppressants may be helpful.

CONGENITAL HEART DISEASE

What are the causes of cyanotic CHD with each of the following: **Increased PA flow**	Complete TGA Taussig-Bing anomaly Truncus arteriosus Total anomalous pulmonary venous return Univentricle Common atria Tetralogy of Fallot with pulmonary atresia and collaterals Tricuspid atresia with a VSD
Normal or decreased PA flow	Tricuspid atresia PA atresia with intact ventricular septum Ebstein's anomaly Single LV with PS IVC to LA shunt Tetralogy of Fallot PS with an ASD, TGA, or DORV
PA HTN	Eisenmenger's syndrome DORV TGA

Total anomalous pulmonary venous return
Hypoplastic left heart syndrome

What is tetralogy of Fallot?   VSD, overriding aorta, RVH, and infundibular stenosis

What is the pentalogy of Fallot?   Same as tetralogy of Fallot but with an ASD

What is Eisenmenger's syndrome?   Any CHD with consequent pulmonary HTN (e.g., ASD, VSD, PDA, and AP window)

If a parent has a CHD, what is the likelihood of that parent's offspring having a congenital heart defect?   Approximately 5%

List four sequelae of cyanotic CHD.   Hyperuricemia, increased blood viscosity, paradoxical embolism, and cerebral abscess (secondary to infected embolus)

What is the procedure used to diagnose the majority of patients with CHD?   Echocardiography

What findings suggest significant CHD in the adult?   Two or more of the following:
1. Continuous murmur
2. Cyanosis with or without clubbing and polycythemia
3. Chamber enlargement
4. Chest radiograph findings of increased pulmonary vasculature or abnormal heart silhouette
5. ECG abnormalities

What are the acyanotic forms of CHD seen in adults?   Bicuspid aortic valve, supraaortic or subaortic valvular stenosis, aortic coarctation, valvular PS, ASD, PDA, and corrected TGA

What are the cyanotic forms of CHD seen in adults?   Tetralogy of Fallot, Eisenmenger's syndrome, and Ebstein's anomaly

NEOPLASMS

What percentage of neoplasms involving the heart are benign?	75% (25% are malignant)
Is the heart more likely to be involved as the primary or secondary site for a neoplasm?	Secondary neoplasms occur 20–40 times more commonly than primary tumors.
What are the most common benign heart tumors?	Myxoma (40%) Lipoma (15%) Papillary fibroelastoma (10%) Rhabdomyoma (5%)
What are the most common malignant heart tumors?	Angiosarcoma (30%) Rhabdomyosarcoma (20%) Mesothelioma (20%)
What is the location of most myxomas?	LA (75%). Myxomas in children are found in increased frequency in the ventricle.
What is the classic examination feature of a myxoma?	A tumor plop (occurs when the patient shifts position)
What percentage of metastatic tumors affect the myocardium?	5%
What percentage of metastatic tumors affect the pericardium?	10%
What metastatic tumors most frequently involve the heart (endocardium, myocardium, and pericardium)?	Bronchogenic carcinoma, breast cancer, leukemias, and lymphomas
What are common features of tumors involving the pericardium?	Pericarditis (pain) Pericardial effusions and tamponade Atrial arrhythmias Pericardial constriction

What are common features of tumors involving the myocardium?	Atrial and ventricular arrhythmias (tachycardias and heart block), CHF, angina and infarction, cavity obliteration, valve obstruction and damage, and ECG changes (STT changes)

MAJOR TRIALS

Table 2–2   Major Trials

Trial name	Question	Result
GISSI	Streptokinase vs placebo in acute MI	Streptokinase associated with better survival, especially when given early (< 3 hours)
ISIS-2	Streptokinase vs ASA vs Streptokinase + ASA vs placebo	Streptokinase and ASA each associated with better survival (effects were comparable and additive)
GUSTO	tPA + intravenous heparin vs streptokinase + intravenous heparin vs streptokinase + subcutaneous heparin vs tPA + streptokinase in acute MI	tPA + intravenous heparin = best survival
VHeFT	Hydralazine + isosorbide vs prazosin vs placebo in mild–moderate CHF	Hydralazine + isosorbide associated with better survival
VHeFT-2	Hydralazine vs enalapril in moderate CHF	Enalapril associated with better survival
SOLVD	Enalapril vs placebo in mild–moderate or asymptomatic CHF	Enalapril reduced mortality rate and progressive CHF
PAMI	PTCA vs tPA in acute MI	PTCA reduced mortality > tPA
SAVE	Captopril vs placebo following acute MI	Improved survival in patients receiving captopril
CONSENSUS	Enalapril vs placebo in severe CHF	Patients receiving enalapril had improved survival
TIMI-I	tPA vs streptokinase in 90-minute vessel patency in acute MI	tPA patency 62%; streptokinase patency 31%
TIMI-II	Comparison of invasive vs conservative strategy following acute MI	No difference between infarction or mortality rate at 42 days
TIMI-III	Comparison of invasive vs conservative (tPA) strategy vs heparin in unstable angina	No difference among groups

3

Pulmonology

ABBREVIATIONS

ABG	Arterial blood gas
ABPA	Allergic bronchopulmonary aspergillosis
AFB	Acid-fast bacillus
AIDS	Acquired immune deficiency syndrome
ANCA	Antinuclear cytoplasmic antibodies
ARDS	Adult respiratory distress syndrome
ASD	Atrial septal defect
BAL	Bronchoalveolar lavage
BiPAP	Bilevel positive airway pressure
BO	Bronchiolitis obliterans (also obliterative brochiolitis)
BOOP	Bronchiolitis obliterans with organizing pneumonia
CF	Cystic fibrosis
CHF	Congestive heart failure
CMV	Cytomegalovirus
CNS	Central nervous system
COPD	Chronic obstructive pulmonary disease
CPAP	Continuous positive airway pressure
CSA	Central sleep apnea

C-T	Connective tissue
CT	Computed tomography
DLCO	Diffusion capacity of carbon monoxide
DVT	Deep venous thrombosis
EDS	Excessive daytime sleepiness
FEV$_1$	Forced expiratory volume in 1 second
FVC	Forced vital capacity
HIV	Human immunodeficiency virus
HSP	Hypersensitivity pneumonitis
HTN	Hypertension
ILD	Interstitial lung disease
INR	International normalized ratio
IPF	Idiopathic pulmonary fibrosis
IPG	Impedance plethysmography
IVDA	Intravenous drug abuse
LDH	Lactate dehydrogenase
LFT	Liver function test
OSA	Obstructive sleep apnea
PA	Pulmonary artery
PC	Pressure control
PCP	*Pneumocystis carinii* pneumonia
PE	Pulmonary thromboembolism
PEEP	Positive end-expiratory pressure
PFT	Pulmonary function test

PMN	Polymorphonuclear neutrophils
ppd	Purified protein derivative
PPH	Primary pulmonary hypertension
P-R	Pulmonary–renal
PS	Pressure support
PSG	Polysomnogram
PTT	Partial thromboplastin time
RDI	Respiratory disturbance index
RV	Right ventricle
SLE	Systemic lupus erythematosus
TB	Tuberculosis
TLC	Total lung capacity
VSD	Ventricular septal defect
WBC	White blood cell count

HISTORY AND PHYSICAL EXAMINATION

What questions should be asked of any patient with lung disease?	Think **OLD EQQS** (onset, location, duration, exacerbation, quality, quantity, associated symptoms)
What is hemoptysis?	Coughing up of blood
What are the four main causes of hemoptysis?	Bronchogenic carcinoma, bronchiectasis, rheumatic mitral valve disease, and TB
What should be determined on past medical history?	Past medical events, previous hospitalizations, and previous immunizations
What parts of the social history are vital?	History of smoking, drug use, sexual activity, travel, and work exposure

How can you tell that a patient's FEV₁ is decreased to 30% or less?

The patient uses accessory muscles for inspiration.

What does an increased anteroposterior diameter signify?

Pulmonary hyperinflation

How do patients with emphysema breathe?

They take only small breaths and exhale through pursed lips.

What does asymmetric chest expansion indicate?

There is volume restriction on the side with reduced expansion such as is seen with pleural effusions, bronchial obstruction, and pneumothorax.

What does symmetrically impaired chest expansion indicate?

Restrictive lung disease or an early sign of ankylosing spondylitis

What is the significance of paradoxical breathing?

It is a sign of diaphragmatic weakness or overwork in severe chronic COPD. The patient may need mechanical ventilation.

What causes the trachea to deviate?

Lobar atelectasis causes the trachea to deviate toward the side of atelectasis. The trachea deviates away from the side of a tension pneumothorax or pleural effusion.

How do you interpret an increase in tactile fremitus?

There is a direct solid communication from the bronchus, through the lung, out to the chest wall (i.e., consolidation). A decrease means that there is bronchial obstruction or that the lung is displaced from the chest wall by air, fluid, or scar in the pleural space.

How do you interpret changes in the volume of breath sounds?

Similarly to changes in tactile fremitus

What causes bronchial breath sounds to be heard in the periphery?

Any solid matter that has replaced the usual acoustic phenomena caused by air-filled alveoli

What causes percussion to be dull?	Consolidation of underlying lung parenchyma, fluid in the pleural space, and pleural thickening
What physical signs can be observed with a pleural effusion?	Dullness over the fluid area, decreased expansion, decreased tactile fremitus, decreased breath sounds, bronchial breathing, and egophony above fluid level. With massive effusions, the trachea shifts away from the affected side.

OBSTRUCTIVE LUNG DISEASE

CHRONIC OBSTRUCTIVE PULMONARY DISEASE

What is COPD?	Chronic irreversible destruction of the lungs resulting in decreased expiratory air flow
What is emphysema?	Abnormal permanent enlargement in air spaces and destruction of alveolar walls caused by imbalance of proteases and antiproteases
What is chronic bronchitis?	Chronic sputum production every day for at least 3 months per year for 2 consecutive years
What is a pink puffer?	A patient with severe emphysema and hypoxemic, hypercarbic respiratory failure
What is a blue bloater?	A patient with cyanosis and normal PCO_2. Most patients' condition falls between a pink puffer and blue bloater.
List three risk factors for COPD.	Smoking, genetic predisposition, and air pollution
What are the symptoms of COPD?	Shortness of breath, wheezing, coughing, and sputum production
What are the signs of COPD?	Hyperresonance, prolonged expiration, pursed lip breathing, decreased breath sounds, expiratory wheezing, and absence of clubbing

What is cor pulmonale?

COPD with right heart failure (e.g., edema, jugular venous distention, and hepatic distention)

What laboratory test results are significant for COPD?

PFTs—reduced FEV_1/FVC ratio ($< 70\%$)

Increased TLC and residual volume

Reduced DLCO—contrasts with asthma, which is characterized by a normal or high DLCO

Hyperinflation and low, flat diaphragms shown on chest radiograph

What is the first laboratory test to check when looking for a genetic cause of COPD?

α_1-Antitrypsin levels. The threshold level is 80 mg/dL (11 μmol/L), which is 35% predicted. Below this level, patients have increased risk of emphysema.

What is the pathologic change that occurs with α_1-antitrypsin disease?

Panacinar lower lobe emphysema

What other organ systems are affected in α_1-antitrypsin disease?

The liver, rarely (cirrhosis)

What are the indications for replacement therapy with Prolastin (α_1-antitrypsin)?

Obstructive lung disease ($FEV_1 < 80\%$ predicted), serum α_1 levels less than 80 mg/dl, age older than 18 years, and smoking abstinence

What pathologic changes occur with cigarette smoking?

Upper lobe centrilobular emphysema

What is a bulla?

Airspace greater than 1 cm

What is a bleb?

Intrapleural collection of air

What is the chronic treatment of COPD?

Patients should stop smoking. Initial drug therapy includes inhaled ipratropium and a β agonist. Theophylline and steroids may be beneficial. Inhaled steroids are of questionable value.

What is the acute treatment of COPD?

Give oxygen if the O_2 saturation is less than 90%. Check ABG for hypercarbia. Give nebulized albuterol. Intravenous steroids (0.5 mg/kg) every 6 hours for 3 days is recommended. Consider giving antibiotics.

What is the mechanism of action and effect of theophylline?

Phosphodiesterase inhibition, leading to increased levels of intracellular cyclic adenosine monophosphate, causing bronchodilation, enhanced mucociliary clearance, stimulation of the respiratory drive, improved cardiac function, and augmented diaphragmatic strength

List the side effects of theophylline.

Nausea, vomiting, tremors, seizures, arrhythmias, diuresis, and sleep disturbance

Which medications increase theophylline levels?

Macrolide antibiotics, cimetidine, and quinolones

What medical conditions increase theophylline levels?

Cirrhosis and heart failure

Why is overly aggressive nutritional therapy dangerous?

Intake of increased calories may lead to increased oxygen consumption and increased CO_2 production, leading to increased ventilatory requirements.

What antibiotics can be used for outpatient exacerbation of COPD?

Trimethoprim–sulfamethoxazole (cost-effective), amoxicillin–clavulanate, tetracycline, and erythromycin (beware of a theophylline interaction)

What is the most common precipitant of acute respiratory failure?

Infection

When is oxygen therapy indicated?

When the room air PO_2 is less than 56 mm Hg or the PO_2 is less than 60 mm Hg in a patient with polycythemia or cor pulmonale. Oxygen may cause worsening hypercarbia by worsening V/Q mismatch, not by decreasing respiratory drive.

Which is more rapidly lethal, hypoxemia or hypercarbia?	Hypoxemia kills.
What vaccinations should be given to patients with COPD?	Pneumovax (every 5–6 years) and influenza vaccine (yearly in the fall)
What is the long-term prognosis for COPD patients hospitalized on mechanical ventilation who are discharged to home?	50% 1-year mortality rate
What are the indications for lung transplantation?	$FEV_1 < 30\%$ Room air $PO_2 < 55$ mm Hg on RA Weight loss
What is the survival rate after transplantation?	75% at 1 year; 60% at 2 years
What is lung shaving?	Lung volume reduction surgery that removes emphysematous lung tissue to improve pulmonary mechanics

ASTHMA*

What is asthma?	Clinically reversible airflow obstruction and wheezing
What is the pathophysiology of asthma?	Inflammation of the airways
What is the prevalence of asthma?	5% of the general population
What are the risk factors for asthma?	History of atopy and allergy
What are asthma symptoms?	Wheezing, shortness of breath, and cough
What are the signs of asthma?	Wheezing, diaphragm retraction, decreased breath sounds, and cough

---

* In collaboration with M. Reitmeyer, S. AlGazlan, and L. Wheatley

What else can cause wheezing?

Important other causes of wheezing are upper airway obstruction, laryngospasm, tracheal stenosis and webbing, foreign body aspiration, heart failure (pulmonary edema), and COPD.

What are the most common causes of chronic cough?

Asthma, postnasal drip, gastroesophageal reflux, postviral sequelae, and sequelae of pertussis (after up to 4–6 weeks)

How is asthma diagnosed?

The diagnosis requires demonstration of reversible obstructive airway disease.

How is obstruction determined?

An FEV_1/FVC ratio of < 75%

How is reversibility demonstrated?

1. ≥ 15% increase in FEV_1 on spirometry after administration of a β agonist
2. ≥ 15% increase in FEV_1 over time with antiinflammatory–bronchodilator therapy
3. ≥ 20% variability in peak flow measurements
4. Hyperreactivity on methacholine testing

Is allergy testing useful in treating asthma?

Asthma is an allergic disease in the majority of young adults with asthma, and, when feasible, allergen avoidance is the treatment with the fewest adverse effects. Allergy testing should be considered in any patient whose asthma is difficult to control, although it is less likely to be helpful in patients older than 50 years of age.

Which allergens should be tested for?

The allergens that are most important in asthma are indoor allergens, including dust mite, animal dander, and cockroach antigens. Other important allergens include alternaria, which is associated with an increased risk of fatal and near fatal asthma attacks in the Midwest, and aspergillus because of the syndrome of ABPA. Pollen allergies are usually more obvious to the patient and therefore are less of a problem.

What is the treatment for mild asthma?

β Agonist bronchodilator on an as-needed basis, implying its use less than three times a week

What is the treatment for moderate asthma?

Inhaled antiinflammatory (e.g., steroids, cromolyn, or nedocromil), β agonist as needed, zafirlukast (Accolate), and theophylline (third line, serum peak levels 5–15 μg/ml)

What is the treatment for severe asthma?

Treatment is the same as for moderate asthma plus oral steroids are given at the lowest dose tolerated; corticosteroid-sparing agents are given if the side effects are less than those of steroids.

What agents have been used as corticosteroid sparing?

Methotrexate, gold, cyclosporine, and hydroxychloroquine. Studies have failed to show a benefit of corticosteroid-sparing agents over steroids, but, in selected patients, these agents may be useful.

Is allergen immunotherapy useful?

Only in patients with mild to moderate asthma. The risk of death is too high in patients with more severe disease. Contraindications also include initiation during pregnancy and β-blocker therapy.

What is the role of aspirin as an allergen in asthma?

Aspirin is generally tested by escalating challenges. Testing of aspirin for an asthmatic reaction is dangerous and should be done in a monitored unit. Similarly, aspirin desensitization is performed using graduating doses and is similarly dangerous. It is, however, effective in controlling asthma in some patients. There is little evidence to suggest that aspirin desensitization is effective for urticaria.

Is cromolyn useful in acute asthma?

No. Cromolyn is not a bronchodilator; rather it works by inhibiting histamine release. It works as a noncorticosteroid antiinflammatory agent, and it takes up to a week for there to be improvement.

Are mucolytics useful?

There is no evidence that acetylcysteine helps; rather it may be an irritant and worsen cough. Intravenous hydration is not helpful either.

What are the physical findings in severe asthma?

Pulse > 120 bpm, pulsus paradoxus > 20 mm Hg (decrease in systolic blood pressure with inspiration), respiratory rate > 30 breaths per minute, use of accessory muscles, silent chest, altered mental status, and fragmented speech

What is the treatment in the emergency room for severe asthma?

Nebulized bronchodilators every 20 minutes, intravenous steroids (40–125 mg methylprednisolone every 6 hours), and oxygen

What are the indications for hospital admission?

Failure to respond to emergency room therapy after 4 hours, hypoxemia, altered mental status, and peak flow less than 25% predicted (see findings in severe asthma)

What are the indications for intubation?

Intubation is based on clinical indications. These patients are very difficult to mechanically ventilate because of hyperinflation and airway resistance. Intubate if hypoxemia and hypercarbia develop with severe fatigue.

Which patients are at high risk for asthma-related death?

Patients who have undergone previous intubation, who have had two or more hospitalizations in 1 year, three or more emergency room visits in 1 year, or recent steroid withdrawal, who have a history of asthma syncope, or who have serious psychiatric disorders

What should a peak flow meter be used for?

To follow up a patient's condition at home (patients may have a decrement in airflow and be unaware of the change) and to provide information about a patient's response to therapy in the emergency room

What is the management of exercise-induced asthma?

Inhaled β agonists used 5–60 minutes before exercise. Cromolyn is also useful.

Has the rate of deaths due to asthma declined in the past 10 years?

No. The mortality rate in the United States has increased.

What subgroup of the population is at high risk for asthma death?

Inner city minorities and men

Do β agonists increase the risk of death?

Some studies suggest that high doses of β agonists may be associated with increased mortality.

What is the most important drug regimen to be given to patients who are discharged from the emergency room after an asthmatic episode?

Steroid taper with close follow-up

Is Primatene mist useful?

No. It is essentially inhaled epinephrine.

What are some areas of work associated with occupational asthma?

Laboratory work; work in pharmaceutical and food industries; sawmill, plastic, and metal work; farming; cosmetology (e.g., beauticians), longshoring, and clothing manufacture

How is occupational asthma diagnosed?

Having the subject follow peak flows at home and at work may be helpful in some situations, but objectivity is hard to verify. Determination of a specific IgE to an agent in the workplace is useful, as is a challenge test when possible.

What is HSP?

Immunologically mediated ILD of known cause, occurring in susceptible individuals secondary to repeated exposure to an organic dust or other agent

Is HSP the same as occupational asthma?

No. Although HSP is found in some of the same professions as occupational asthma, it is immunologically and clinically distinct. Both diseases are characterized by cough, but HSP also causes fevers and lymphadenopathy, as well as restrictive lung disease, decreased DLCO, and pulmonary fibrosis. HSP is not IgE-mediated, whereas occupational asthma generally is.

How is HSP diagnosed?

The major finding is precipitating antibodies to an antigen appropriate to the patient's history. BAL may also be helpful because there is an increase in CD8+ T cells as opposed to the increase in CD4+ T cells seen in sarcoidosis.

What is the treatment for HSP?

Avoidance of allergens and corticosteroid therapy

BRONCHIECTASIS*

What is bronchietasis?

Chronic irreversible destruction and dilation of bronchioles caused by inflammatory destruction of muscular and elastic components of the bronchial walls

What are the causes of bronchiectasis?

Infections (e.g., influenza and TB)
Genetic factors (e.g., CF, α_1-antitrypsin deficiency, immotile cilia, Young's syndrome, B-cell dysfunction)
ABPA and yellow-nail syndrome

What are the signs of bronchiectasis?

Recurrent cough, hemoptysis, and purulent sputum

What diagnostic tests are useful in establishing bronchiectasis?

Sputum test
Bronchography (the former gold standard has been replaced by thin-cut CT)
Chest radiograph showing "tram tracks"
Bronchoscopy
Fine-cut chest CT

What is the treatment for bronchiectasis?

Medical treatment— treat as for CF patients; use chest clearance techniques, antibiotics, and DNAse
Surgical treatment— if the disease is isolated, surgical treatment may be useful

---

* In collaboration with M. Reitmeyer, S. AlGazlan, and L. Wheatley

What is ABPA?

Allergic bronchopulmonary aspergillosis is a syndrome of severe, refractory asthma with central bronchiectasis and recurrent pulmonary infiltrates because of hypersensitivity to aspergillus found in the lung. Without adequate treatment, ABPA may progress to irreversible obstructive disease or fibrotic, restrictive disease.

What are the diagnostic criteria for ABPA?

1. Demonstration of specific IgE to aspergillus (by skin testing or radioallergosorbent test)
2. Elevated total IgE to greater than or equal to 1000 n/ml
3. Eosinophilia greater than or equal to 8%
4. Positive precipitin to aspergillus
5. Elevated specific IgG to aspergillus
All criteria but the first may be absent in remission.

What is the treatment for ABPA?

At first, give 0.5 mg/kg of oral prednisone per day for 2 weeks; then give the same amount on an alternate day basis for 2–3 months. Thereafter, the regimen is tapered as symptoms allow. Following up the total IgE level is useful because a doubling of the level over the baseline generally indicates a relapse, often with pulmonary infiltrates.

INTERSTITIAL LUNG DISEASE

What is interstitial lung disease?

ILD is a heterogeneous, diverse group of disorders that involve alveolar and perialveolar tissue. The body's initial response to the disease process is typically inflammation (alveolitis); if the process becomes chronic, fibrosis and scarring may occur. There are approximately 200 causes of ILD.

What are the six main groups of ILD in the immunocompetent host?

1. IPF
2. C-T diseases and P-R syndrome
3. Environmental diseases
4. Granulomatous diseases

5. Inherited diseases
6. Miscellaneous diseases

Which C-T diseases and P-R syndromes cause ILD?

C-T disease— SLE, rheumatoid arthritis, ankylosing spondylitis, progressive systemic sclerosis, Sjögren's syndrome, and polymyositis–dermatomyositis

P-R syndromes—Goodpasture's syndrome, Wegener's granulomatosis, allergic angiitis, and Churg-Strauss granulomatosis

Which environmental substances cause ILD?

Inorganic dusts—asbestos, silica, coal, and beryllium

Organic dusts—cotton (byssinosis)

Toxic gases and fumes—nitrogen dioxide

Which ILDs are associated with granulomas?

Known causes—HSP, beryllium, silica, and medications (e.g., methotrexate)

Unknown causes—sarcoidosis, Langerhans' cell granulomatosis (eosinophilic granuloma), granulomatous vasculitides (Wegener's, Churg-Strauss), and bronchocentric granulomatosis

Which inherited diseases cause ILD?

Tuberous sclerosis, Hermansky-Pudulak syndrome, neurofibromatosis, metabolic storage disorders (e.g., Gaucher's, Nieman-Pick), and hypocalciuric hypercalcemia

Which miscellaneous diseases cause ILD?

BO with or without organizing pneumonia (BOOP), eosinophilic pneumonia, drugs, radiation, lymphangioleiomyomatosis, respiratory bronchiolitis, alveolar proteinosis, veno-occlusive disease, lymphangitic carcinomatosis, idiopathic pulmonary hemosiderosis, gastrointestinal or liver diseases (inflammatory bowel disease, primary biliary cirrhosis, chronic active hepatitis), graft versus host disease (bone marrow transplant), lymphocytic infiltrative diseases, and alveolar microlithiasis

What are the symptoms of ILD?	Dyspnea (typically chronic and progressive), exercise intolerance, and cough (typically nonproductive)
What are the signs of ILD?	Tachypnea, crackles (sometimes "Velcro-like"), clubbing, and cor pulmonale
What do the following history and physical examination findings suggest in association with ILD?	
Farmer	Farming is associated with HSP.
Coal miner	Coal mining is associated with pneumoconiosis.
Pigeon breeding	HSP
Bleomycin	Drug-induced ILD
Extrapulmonary symptoms and signs	Sarcoidosis, C-T disease, P-R syndrome
Clubbing	Associated almost exclusively with IPF and asbestosis
What is a pneumoconiosis?	Lung disease that occurs secondary to exposure to inorganic dusts. The most common pneumoconioses are asbestosis, silicosis, and coal workers' pneumoconiosis.
What pulmonary diseases are associated with asbestos exposure?	Disease with pleural involvement (e.g., effusion, calcification, localized plaque, diffuse thickening, and mesothelioma), ILD and fibrosis, round atelectasis, and bronchogenic carcinoma (in smokers)
What is asbestosis?	The ILD and fibrosis associated with exposure to asbestos
What is Caplan's syndrome?	The association of rheumatoid arthritis and pulmonary nodules in patients with pneumoconiosis, particularly coal workers' pneumoconiosis

What infection is an individual with silicosis at an increased risk for?

TB

What is farmer's lung?

A form of HSP that results from repeated exposure to thermophilic actinomycetes found in moldy hay, silage, or grain

What is progressive massive fibrosis?

Also known as complicated pneumoconiosis, progressive massive fibrosis is said to exist when the small, rounded opacities associated with simple silicosis or coal workers' pneumoconiosis coalesce to form irregular masses greater than or equal to 1 cm in diameter. Typically, symptoms and PFT abnormalities are minimal until progressive massive fibrosis supervenes; the only treatment is transplantation.

What is sarcoidosis?

A multisystemic disorder of unknown cause, characterized by the presence of noncaseating granuloma in involved organs

What are the four most common organs involved with sarcoidosis?

1. Lung (90%–95%)
2. Lymph nodes (80%–95%)
3. Skin (20%–50%)
4. Eye (20%–50%)

What ILD is most commonly associated with hilar or mediastinal adenopathy?

Sarcoidosis

What is alveolar proteinosis?

A rare disorder in which proteinaceous material resembling surfactant is deposited in alveoli and bronchioles

What is Hamman-Rich disease?

Also known as acute interstitial pneumonia, Hamman-Rich disease is an interstitial pneumonitis with a rapidly progressive course, with recovery (often complete) or death occurring within several weeks to a few months. Diffuse alveolar damage occurs as in ARDS.

Bronchiolitos obliterans   *Bronchiolitis obliterans with organizing pneumonia*

What are BO and BOOP?

Both are relatively nonspecific manifestations of bronchiolar injury due to a variety of causes, including infections, drugs, toxins, and C-T diseases. BO is also associated with transplantations (bone marrow, heart–lung, and lung).

What pulmonary function abnormalities occur with BO and BOOP?

BO is obstructive and BOOP is restrictive.

What are the natural history features of BO and BOOP?

BO is progressive and steroid unresponsive. BOOP is steroid responsive.

What are the radiographic features of BO and BOOP?

BO features are normal or show hyperinflation. BOOP radiographs show patchy airspace opacities, often bilateral and often with a "ground glass" appearance.

What are the pathologic features of BO and BOOP?

BO is associated with mural fibrosis, obliteration of the bronchial lumen, and airway obstruction. BOOP is associated with intraluminal fibrosis in the distal airways, alveolar ducts, and peribronchiolar alveoli.

What diagnostic tests are used for ILD?

1. Chest radiograph, which is normal in 10% of cases
2. High-resolution CT scan, which is more sensitive than a chest radiograph, and allows selection of the best biopsy site. It is possibly helpful for diagnosis and for assessing disease activity.
3. PFTs, which are typically "restrictive," showing decreased lung volumes and DLCO
4. Screens for antibody to nuclear antigens, rheumatoid factor, ANCA, anti-glomerular basement membrane (GBM) antibodies, angiotensin-converting enzymes (ACEs), and HSP
5. Biopsy of extrathoracic disease (e.g., lymph nodes and skin)

6. Bronchoscopy with BAL and transbronchial biopsy
7. Open lung biopsy, which is more invasive yet more reliable than bronchoscopy

How is the diagnosis of ILD made?

1. Thorough history and physical examination
2. Chest radiograph and PFTs
3. Laboratory evaluation and extrapulmonary biopsy based on the preceding information
4. If no additional information is needed and the ILD is not progressing, then periodic follow-up is indicated.
5. If additional information is needed or there is progression of disease, then bronchoscopy or open lung biopsy may be necessary. If bronchoscopy is chosen, but results are nondiagnostic or inconsistent with clinical data, then open lung biopsy may be performed.

What ILD is most readily diagnosed by bronchoscopy with transbronchial biopsy?

Sarcoidosis

What is therapy for ILD?

The following therapy options depend on the diagnosis and clinical circumstances:
1. No action
2. Removal or avoidance of the cause
3. Prednisone (1–1.5 mg/kg)
4. Cyclophosphamide (2 mg/kg)
5. Azathioprine (2 mg/kg)
6. Alternatives (e.g., colchicine and penicillamine), although there are limited data on these alternative therapies
7. Transplantation (criteria include DLCO < 30%; room air PaO_2 < 60 mm Hg; limited activity)

When giving prednisone, cyclophosphamide, or azathioprine, determine whether the patient is "responsive" after 3–6 months based on symptoms, chest radiograph, and static PFTs with or without exercise; if the patient is responsive, consider tapering medication after 1 year. Note: The survival rate associated with ILD is worse than that associated with other lung diseases; therefore, patients with this diagnosis listed for transplant are given 90 days additional time.

What should you think of if your patient's illness worsens during treatment with Cytoxan and prednisone?

Infection or pneumonitis

If hematuria recurs when following up a patient with a P-R syndrome, what should you consider?

Relapse, bladder cancer, and cystitis (associated with Cytoxan)

CYSTIC FIBROSIS

What is CF?

A genetic disorder resulting in inspissated secretions in the lungs, pancreas, and reproductive tract

What is the incidence of CF?

1/2500 births in the white population; 1/17,000 in the black population

What are the genetic characteristics of CF?

Autosomal recessive
Clinically silent carrier state

What is CFTR?

Cystic fibrosis transmembrane conductance regulator, an apical protein that acts as a chloride channel. Defective CFTR leads to clinical CF. The gene was discovered in 1989 by Collins and Tsui.

What is the carrier rate for the gene?

1/40 whites

What makes the diagnosis of CF?

Clinical syndrome and positive sweat chloride test or two genetic mutations associated with CF

What is the survival rate associated with CF?

As of 1996, median survival was 30 years.

How many patients with CF are older than 18 years of age?

34%

What are the symptoms of CF?

Purulent cough, hemoptysis, recurrent sinusitis, failure to thrive, diarrhea, and steatorrhea

What are the signs of CF?

Clubbing, low weight gain, and nasal polyps

What laboratory tests are performed for CF?

Chest radiograph—shows hyperinflation, bronchiectasis, and reticular nodular fibrosis; rarely shows atelectasis or pneumothorax

PFTs—early, shows obstructive lung disease; late, shows restrictive lung disease

Sweat chloride test—shows > 60 mEq/L of chloride in sweat

What is a sweat chloride test?

Pilocarpine iontophoresis. Sweat is collected and chloride measured.

What are the causes of false-positive sweat tests?

Eczema, edema, adrenal insufficiency, and hypothyroidism

What are the other affected organ systems in patients with CF?

Pancreas, reproductive tract, sinuses, and sweat glands

What does the pancreatic insufficiency lead to?

Malabsorption and steatorrhea

What vitamins are often deficient in CF?

Fat-soluble vitamins A, D, E, and K

What is the therapy for pancreatic disease in CF?

Enzyme replacement (e.g., lipase, amylase, protease). Titrate to decrease steatorrhea. Avoid overdosing enzymes. Consider H_2-blocker to improve enzyme efficacy.

How common is infertility in CF?

In men, 99% are infertile from obstructive azoospermia. Women are relatively infertile secondary to cervical mucus changes and undernutrition.

Should patients take salt tablets to avoid heat prostration?

No.

What are common organisms found in the sputum of patients with CF?

Staphylococcus aureus, Haemophilus influenzae, and *Pseudomonas aeruginosa*

What is the usual chronic therapy for CF patients?

Antibiotics, chest physiotherapy, DNAse, and oxygen

What is DNAse (Pulmozyme)?

DNAse (Pulmozyme) is a genetically engineered product identical to native DNAse, which enzymatically cleaves DNA in the airways. DNA from degrading PMNs increases secretion viscosity.

What antibiotics should be used for patient exacerbations?

An intravenous anti-*Pseudomonas* β lactam (e.g., ceftazidime or piperacillin) and aminoglycoside (e.g., gentamicin or tobramycin). The goal is for aminoglycoside peaks (30 minutes after infusion) to be 8–10 μg/ml and trough levels to be less than 2 μg/ml.
For chronic maintenance, inhaled antibiotics (e.g., gentamicin or tobramycin, 40–80 mg inhaled twice daily) reduce frequency of hospitalizations.
Chronic suppressive antibiotics include trimethoprim–sulfamethoxazole, tetracycline, amoxicillin clavulanate, and quinolones. Note: Quinolones rapidly induce resistance.

What is the risk of pneumothorax in CF?

20% lifetime risk

What is the management of hemoptysis?	Treat infection, correct any clotting abnormality, and consider vitamin K. Encourage cough. Consult radiology for bronchial artery embolization. Intubate as a last resort.
What is the management of respiratory failure in CF?	Oxygen and possibly BiPAP nasal ventilation. Intubate only if a reversible problem caused the respiratory failure or if the patient is close to transplant. Patients are very difficult to mechanically ventilate because of their thick secretions, airway resistance, and hyperinflation.
What are the indications for lung transplantation in patients with CF?	$FEV_1 < 30\%$ predicted, $PO_2 < 60$ mm Hg on room air, and weight loss
Why do these patients require "double" (bilateral sequential) lung transplants?	A single lung transplant would be the equivalent of immunosuppressing a septic patient because the nontransplanted lung is chronically infected.
What are transplant outcomes?	More than 500 patients with CF have undergone "double" lung transplant. The 1-year survival rate is 75%–80%. Most patients have more productive, healthier lives. Other CF problems (e.g., pancreatic disease and sinusitis) continue to be problems.

PULMONARY THROMBOEMBOLISM AND DEEP VENOUS THROMBOSIS

What are DVT and PE?	DVT is a clot present in a "deep" vein of the lower extremities (popliteal vein and above). PE is occlusion of a pulmonary artery by a detached fragment of thrombus from another source. Greater than 95% of PEs arise from the deep veins of the lower extremities; less common sources include pelvic veins, upper extremity veins, and mural thrombi in the right side of the heart.

What is the incidence of DVT and PE?

DVT—5 million per year in the United States

PE—third most common cardiovascular disease in the United States, trailing only coronary artery disease and stroke. Based on epidemiologic and autopsy data, the incidence likely exceeds 500,000 per year and the diagnosis is probably missed more than 70% of the time. There should be a low threshold of suspicion for pursuing the diagnosis of PE in anyone with a compatible clinical history.

What are the risk factors for DVT and PE?

Virchow's triad—stasis, abnormalities of or injury to the vessel wall, and alterations of the blood coagulation and fibrinolytic system

Major predisposing factors—immobilization, surgery lasting more than 30–60 minutes (particularly hip, knee, and pelvic surgery), malignancy, trauma to the lower extremities, estrogen therapy, stroke, CHF, obesity, postpartum status (less than or equal to 3 months), and history of thromboembolism

What are the primary hypercoagulable states?

Antithrombin III, protein C, and protein S deficiencies

Activated protein C resistance

Anticardiolipin antibody syndromes including lupus anticoagulation

Abnormal fibrinogen function and fibrinolytic activity

What are the clinical indicators of a primary hypercoagulable state?

Family history of thrombosis, recurrent thrombosis without an obvious predisposing factor, thrombosis at an unusual anatomic site (e.g., artery), thrombosis at a young age, and resistance to conventional antithrombotic therapy

What are the symptoms of DVT and PE?

DVT—pain, swelling or fullness, and redness of the lower extremity, pain in the lower extremity worsened by standing or walking, and fever

PE—dyspnea (the most common and reliable symptom, but it may be absent), pleuritic chest pain, hemoptysis, cough, palpitations, wheezing, syncope, and "angina-like" chest pain (uncommon)

What are the signs of DVT and PE?

DVT—edema, increased girth, tenderness, erythema, cyanosis (occasionally), palpable cord, venous engorgement of the feet, Homan's sign (i.e., pain in the back of the leg with flexion of the ankle), fever, and tachycardia

PE—tachypnea (the most common and reliable sign, but it may be absent), tachycardia, diaphoresis, fever (uncommon without infection or infarction), localized crackles, wheeze, pleural friction rub, cyanosis, and signs of pulmonary HTN and cor pulmonale (see discussion of signs of pulmonary HTN); also think of PE when there is a history of repetitive, otherwise unexplained supraventricular tachycardia or unexplained worsening of CHF or COPD

What is a pulmonary infarct?

An area of dead lung tissue that occurs in less than 10% of emboli because the lung is supplied with oxygen by three sources— airway, pulmonary arterial circulation, and bronchial arterial circulation. It is more likely to occur with CHF, COPD, and mitral stenosis. The classic presentation includes hemoptysis, pleuritic chest pain, and pleural-based wedge-shaped infiltrate on chest radiograph.

What diagnostic tests are used for DVT and PE?

For both DVT and PE, the presence of D-dimers (established by enzyme-linked immunosorbent assay) indicates activation of coagulation or fibrinolysis.

The finding is nonspecific but very sensitive.

For DVT

The gold standard is ascending contrast venography. Less invasive tests include IPG and Doppler ultrasound ("duplex"), which are very sensitive and specific for DVT but not for calf vein thrombosis.

For PE

ABG results classically show hypoxemia and hypocapnia, but even the finding of a normal A-a gradient does not rule out the diagnosis.

Chest radiograph usually shows some abnormality, such as atelectasis, parenchymal infiltrate, elevated diaphragm, pleural effusion, pleural-based opacity, Westermark's sign (prominent central pulmonary artery with decreased pulmonary vascularity), cardiomegaly, or pulmonary edema (uncommon).

Electrocardiogram findings are abnormal in most cases, usually with nonspecific ST segments or T-wave abnormalities. Uncommon findings include atrial flutter or fibrillation, premature atrial contractions, premature ventricular contractions, and evidence of acute pulmonary HTN (e.g., P-pulmonale, rightward axis, right bundle branch block, and right heart "strain").

Ventilation-perfusion scanning (V/Q scanning) is useful.

Pulmonary angiogram, which is invasive, is the gold standard.

What are the four basic V/Q scan patterns and how are they used clinically?

1. Normal—rules out significant PE
2. Low probability—nondiagnostic and depends on the pretest probability, often requiring further evaluation
3. Intermediate (indeterminant) probability—nondiagnostic and depends on the pretest probability, often requiring further evaluation
4. High probability—"diagnostic" of PE in most circumstances

What is the likelihood of PE if the VQ scan is one of the following:

    Low probability   < 10%–20%

    Intermediate probability   40%–50%

    High probability   > 90%

How useful are noninvasive methods of diagnosis (e.g., V/Q scan) for DVT and PE?
The symptoms, signs, and "screening" laboratory data associated with both DVT and PE are neither specific nor sensitive. For PE, their greatest usefulness is in ruling out other diagnoses (e.g., pneumothorax and myocardial infarction). Have a low threshold for pursuing the diagnosis of PE in a patient with a compatible clinical history.

How is the diagnosis made for DVT?
IPG or Doppler ultrasound; venography if results are questionable

How is the diagnosis made for PE?
1. Determination of the pretest probability of disease
2. V/Q scan if the pretest probability indicates further workup is needed
3. IPG or Doppler ultrasound of lower extremities if the V/Q scan is not normal and there is high pretest probability and if the V/Q scan plus the pretest probability indicate further workup is needed
4. Pulmonary angiogram if the V/Q scan results plus the pretest probability indicate further workup is needed, despite negative IPG or Doppler ultrasound of the lower extremities

When the suspicion for PE is so high that nothing short of a pulmonary angiogram will be helpful, it should be the only test done.

Why is either IPG or Doppler ultrasound of the lower extremities, which are diagnostic tests for DVT, part of the diagnostic workup for PE?
Because therapy for DVT and PE is the same, a positive study allows treatment to be initiated after a much less invasive procedure.

What is the purpose of determining pretest probability?

Because this estimate influences the likelihood of PE, it helps determine the extent of the workup to be done.

What is the treatment for PE and DVT?

1. Supplemental oxygen (for PE)
2. Intravenous heparin for 5–10 days (goal = PTT 1.5–2.5 times normal), followed by oral Coumadin (goal = INR 2–3) for 3–6 months
3. Inferior vena cava filter (e.g., Greenfield filter) for patients who have failed anticoagulation (rare) or in whom anticoagulation is contraindicated (i.e., patients with active gastrointestinal bleeding)
4. Thrombolysis (indications are not based on prospective studies)
5. Surgical embolectomy for hemodynamically unstable patients (PE) who are unresponsive to thrombolysis or with a contraindication to thrombolysis (as for thrombolysis, there are no prospective studies)

When should thrombolysis be considered?

DVT— when iliac veins are involved
PE— when hemodynamically unstable patients are unresponsive to maximal medical management

What is the INR?

International normalized ratio. INR is preferable to "fraction of PT control" because of the considerable variability in commercial thromboplastin

What is the recommended starting heparin regimen?

80 U/kg bolus plus 18 U/kg/hr intravenous infusion (5000 U or 10,000 U bolus followed by an intravenous infusion rate of 1000 U/hr often leads to inadequate initial anticoagulation)

PULMONARY HYPERTENSION

What is pulmonary HTN?

Increased PA pressures and pulmonary vascular resistance, measured as a mean PA pressure > 20 mm Hg

How is pulmonary HTN classified?

As precapillary and postcapillary and as primary and secondary

What are the precapillary causes of pulmonary HTN?
  Primary (pulmonary vascular destruction or obstruction)

PPH, vasculitis, PE, sickle cell disease, chronic portal HTN, and toxins (intravenous drugs, cocaine, anorexic agents, L-tryptophan)

  Secondary (pulmonary parenchymal involvement)

Sarcoidosis, IPF, C-T disease, airway involvement (e.g., emphysema), hypoxic vasoconstriction (high altitude, sleep apnea syndrome, neuromuscular diseases, and thoracic-cage abnormalities), and mechanical obstruction

What are the postcapillary causes?

Cardiac—left ventricular failure, mitral valve disease, and left atrial obstruction (e.g., myxoma and cor triatriatum)
Pulmonary—pulmonary veno-occlusive disease and anomalous pulmonary venous return
Mediastinum—fibrosis, aneurysms, and neoplasm

What is primary pulmonary HTN?

The diagnosis made after all other causes of pulmonary HTN have been excluded. Pathologically, primary pulmonary arteriopathy has features of plexogenic and thrombotic arteriopathies but it is not pathognomonic.

Who is affected by pulmonary HTN?

Females twice as often as males. Patients most commonly present in the third and fourth decades of life, although the age range of affected persons is from infancy to older than 60 years.

What is the mortality rate?

The natural history is unknown because the disease is initially asymptomatic. However, functional class is a good predictor of survival: class II and III, 3.5 years; class IV, 6 months.

What are the symptoms of pulmonary HTN?

Dyspnea, exercise intolerance, fatigue, chest discomfort, and syncope, particularly with exertion

What are the signs of pulmonary HTN?

Elevated jugular venous pressure with prominent A wave (decreased right ventricular compliance) or V-wave tricuspid regurgitation)

RV heave

Right-sided S3 and S4, increased P2, and pulmonary ejection click

Murmurs of tricuspid regurgitation or pulmonary insufficiency

Hepatomegaly, ascites, and edema

What findings may be demonstrated on the following diagnostic tests?

Chest radiograph

Enlarged RV and PAs, parenchymal lung disease, and Kerley B lines (CHF or pulmonary veno-occlusive disease)

Electrocardiogram

Characteristics of right ventricular hypertrophy (axis > 90 degrees), RSR' in V_1 and V_2, prominent R in V_1 and S in V_6 (incomplete right bundle branch block pattern), and P-pulmonale

Echocardiogram

Right ventricular, left ventricular, and valvular dysfunction; atrial myxoma; ASD; estimate of PA pressures

PFTs

Parenchymal, airway, and pulmonary vascular disease; hypoxemia; hypercapnia

V/Q scanning

Thromboemboli

CT scan of the chest

ILD (high-resolution CT); large central PEs and vascular abnormalities (spiral CT)

Cardiac catheterization

Congenital heart disease, valvular heart disease, and elevated PA pressures

What other laboratory tests may be useful in detecting pulmonary HTN?

C-T disease serologic tests and LFTs

What other testing should be considered?	Sleep study—for sleep-disordered breathing Open lung biopsy (controversial)—only when disease is of unclear etiology and data suggest a cause other than PPH
What is the first step in the diagnostic algorithm for unexplained pulmonary HTN?	Obtain a chest radiograph 1. Parenchymal opacities indicate restrictive lung disease (confirm with PFTs; FVC < 50%), pulmonary veno-occlusive disease, or CHF (investigate with echocardiography with or without catheterization). 2. Look for thoracic cage abnormalities. If lung fields are clear, then perform PFTs.
How do PFTs help in patients with clear lung fields?	They may show an obstructive pattern (e.g., COPD—FEV_1 < 1 L/30% predicted), a restrictive pattern (e.g., neuromuscular diseases and possible PPH), or a normal pattern with or without decreased DLCO.
How are ABG tests helpful in patients with normal PFTs?	They may show hypercapnia (e.g., central alveolar hypoventilation, sleep-disordered breathing, and neuromuscular diseases), normocapnia, or hypocapnia
If the patient has clear lung fields, normal PFTs, and normocapnia or hypocapnia, what is the next test?	V/Q scan 1. High probability strongly suggests pulmonary embolus. 2. Less than high probability but segmental or larger defects indicate a need for a pulmonary arteriogram. 3. Normal or patchy nonsegmental defects on V/Q scan or normal pulmonary angiogram indicate the need for an echocardiogram with or without cardiac catheterization to look for primary cardiac disease (e.g., ASD).
What is the treatment for pulmonary HTN?	1. Supplemental oxygen for hypoxemia 2. Diuretics for edema 3. Digoxin for RV failure

4. Chronic anticoagulation for chronic thromboemboli and PPH
5. Vasodilators (e.g., prostacyclin) for PPH, which should be initiated only in the setting of hemodynamic monitoring because they can cause profound hypotension and death
6. Transplantation (lung or heart–lung)

What are the criteria for transplant for pulmonary HTN?

Predicted 2-year survival < 50%
PA systolic pressure > 60 mm Hg
Symptoms of right-sided heart failure

PULMONARY NEOPLASMS (SEE ONCOLOGY)

SLEEP-RELATED BREATHING DISORDERS

What are sleep-related breathing disorders?

A group of disorders characterized by decreases in airflow that occur only during sleep or that are significantly worsened by sleep. Examples include OSA, CSA, and hypoventilation syndromes such as the obesity–hypoventilation syndrome. Note: Sleep can adversely affect patients with a variety of other diseases, including COPD, neuromuscular diseases (e.g., muscular dystrophy), and disorders of the thoracic cage (e.g., kyphoscoliosis).

What is pickwickian syndrome?

Often used interchangeably with obesity–hypoventilation syndrome, the label is given to obese patients who have an elevated $PaCO_2$ (hypoventilate) during the day; however, the term is probably best reserved for massively obese patients with EDS, hypercapnia, hypoxia, polycythemia, pulmonary HTN, and cor pulmonale.

What is hypopnea?

A decrease in airflow by at least 50% that lasts for at least 10 seconds. An apnea is complete or near complete cessation of airflow that lasts at least 10 seconds.

What is the difference between obstructive and central apnea?

In obstructive apnea, there is no airflow with persistent respiratory effort.
In central apnea, there is no airflow with no associated respiratory effort (presumably secondary to the absence of the central drive to breathe).
Mixed apnea is a combination of the two.

What is Cheyne-Stokes respiration?

A pattern of central apnea, characterized by periodic, regular waxing and waning of ventilation. During the waning phase, there is frank apnea. Major causes include CHF, CNS lesions, renal failure, and high altitude.

What is the RDI?

Average number of respiratory events per hour of sleep.
The RDI is the average number of apneic plus hypopneic episodes per hour of sleep. The apnea index, hypopnea index, and RDI are all measures of the severity of sleep-disordered breathing.

How is sleep apnea defined?

RDI > 4

What is sleep apnea syndrome?

Sleep apnea (RDI > 4) plus some physiologic consequence (e.g., EDS)

What is the incidence of OSA?

Much more common than previously thought. Twenty-four percent of men and 9% of women have sleep apnea; 4% of men and 2% of women have sleep apnea syndrome.

What are the risk factors for sleep apnea?

Obesity, anatomic abnormality of the upper airway (e.g., retrognathia or micrognathia), neuromuscular disease (e.g., polymyositis), hypothyroidism, acromegaly, alcohol use, sedative use, nasal congestion, and sleep deprivation. Note: A patient does not have to be obese to have sleep apnea, but one or more of the stated predisposing factors must be present.

What are the symptoms and signs of sleep apnea?	They are secondary to either arousals from sleep or hypoxemia and hypercapnia. Note: The patient does not have to desaturate to have very significant, symptomatic sleep apnea.
What are some of the consequences of repeated arousal from sleep?	Falling asleep unintentionally (e.g., while driving), personality changes (from irritability to depression and frank psychosis), intellectual deterioration (i.e., decreased memory), visual–motor incoordination, impotence, insomnia, restless sleep, and awakening choking or gagging
What are some of the consequences of hypoxia and hypercapnia?	Polycythemia, pulmonary HTN, cor pulmonale, chronic hypercapnia, morning and nocturnal headache, CHF, nocturnal arrhythmias, nocturnal angina, systemic HTN
What clinical factors are particularly good discriminators for OSA?	Although not definitive, the absence of snoring makes the diagnosis of OSA very unlikely; likewise, OSA is improbable if the patient is not obese (body mass index > 25 kg/m^2) and does not have pulmonary HTN, witnessed apneas, and EDS. The fewer of these characteristics the patient has, the less likely the diagnosis is.
What makes the diagnosis of OSA?	Nocturnal PSG, or sleep study
What kind of information is obtained from a PSG?	Sleep staging, airflow measurement, respiratory effort, electrocardiographic data, oximetry, and periodic limb movements
What is the therapy for sleep apnea?	General—weight reduction, aggressive treatment of nasal congestion, sufficient sleep, alcohol and sedative avoidance, and treatment of thyroid disease, neuromuscular disease, or acromegaly OSA—nasal CPAP or BiPAP

CSA or hypoventilation syndromes—
nasal BiPAP or nasal volume
ventilator
Hypoxemia—supplemental oxygen
(alone or combined with nasal CPAP,
BiPAP, or volume ventilator)
Tracheotomy is only rarely required and
should be considered a last resort.
Rapid eye movement–sleep
suppressant drugs (i.e., tricyclic
antidepressants) should be used only
in select cases. Respiratory stimulants
(e.g., progesterone and acetazolamide)
should also only be used in select
cases.

**What is the difference
between CPAP and BiPAP?**

With CPAP, the inspiratory and
expiratory pressures are and must be the
same; with BiPAP, the inspiratory
positive airway pressure and the
expiratory positive airway pressure can
vary; consequently, you can ventilate a
patient with BiPAP.

**When would you consider
using BiPAP instead of
CPAP?**

When a patient has difficulty tolerating
CPAP or when the patient has CSA or is
hypoventilating

BRONCHITIS AND PNEUMONIAS*

BRONCHITIS

What is bronchitis?

Inflammation of the tracheobronchial
tree

**What are the pathogens of
bronchitis?**

Most commonly, respiratory viruses.
Bacterial pathogens include *Bordatella
pertussis*, *Mycoplasma pneumoniae*, and
Chlamydia pneumoniae.

**What are the symptoms
and signs of bronchitis?**

Cough is the prominent symptom that
typically persists after the other
symptoms of the underlying viral
infection subside. Dyspnea is usually
present only if patients have underlying
COPD. On lung examination, rhonchi or
coarse rales may be heard.

---

* In collaboration with N. Thielman, V. Shami, and C. Sable

How is the diagnosis of bronchitis made?	Cough is a symptom associated with a variety of pulmonary diseases; other causes must be ruled out before the diagnosis of acute bronchitis is made.
What is the treatment for bronchitis?	Symptomatic, directed at controlling cough. If a specific pathogen (*M. pneumoniae, B. pertussis,* or *C. pneumoniae*) is identified, antibiotic treatment (with erythromycin or tetracycline for these organisms) can be used.

PNEUMONIA*

What is pneumonia?	Infection of the lung parenchyma
What is the incidence of pneumonia?	Approximately 4 million episodes per year; approximately 1 million hospitalizations per year; approximately 50,000 deaths per year
What is typical versus atypical pneumonia?	Typical pneumonia is infection produced by pyogenic bacteria that live in the nasopharynx. Atypical pneumonia is caused by organisms inhaled from the environment that are not apparent on Gram stain and are not susceptible to cell wall active antibiotics.
What are the symptoms and signs typical of pneumonia?	Classic history—acute onset of pulmonary symptoms, that is, dyspnea, pleuritic chest pain, purulent cough, fever, shaking chills, and rusty sputum Segmental pulmonary consolidation seen on chest radiograph
What are symptoms and signs of atypical pneumonia?	Onset is less abrupt, cough is usually nonproductive, and pleuritic chest pain is uncommon. Extrapulmonary symptoms may predominate (e.g., headaches, myalgias, nausea, and diarrhea). Diffuse bilateral infiltrates are seen on chest radiograph.

---

* In collaboration with N. Thielman, V. Shami, and C. Sable

What is the presentation of pneumonia in elderly patients?

Pneumonia in elderly patients frequently presents atypically. Many patients are afebrile or hypothermic. Cough and sputum may be absent. Sometimes, the only change is in mental status.

What diseases can mimic community-acquired pneumonia?

HSP, chronic eosinophilic pneumonia, BOOP, drug-induced pneumonitis, systemic vasculitis, and lung cancer

What clinical signs suggest chlamydial pneumonia?

Hoarseness and fever starting first, with respiratory tract symptoms not appearing for a few days

What symptoms and signs can suggest mycoplasmal pneumonia?

Ear pain, bullous myringitis, and persistent nonproductive cough

What symptoms and signs can suggest legionnaires' disease?

Elevated temperature, CNS and gastrointestinal abnormalities, bradycardia, elevated serum transaminases, and hypophosphatemia

What should be sought in the physical examination for pneumonia?

Fever, poor dentition (suggesting mixed infection), splinting on the side of bacterial pneumonia, rales, and consolidation (suggesting bacterial infection)

What are the risk factors for pneumonia?

Smoking, alcohol use, endotracheal intubation, nasogastric intubation, respiratory therapy, hypoxemia, acidosis, toxic inhalation, pulmonary edema, uremia, malnutrition, immunosuppression, mechanical obstruction, diabetes mellitus, splenectomy, advanced age, and decreased level of consciousness or other factors that increase the risk of aspiration

What is the pathogenesis of pneumonia?

Aspiration of upper airway organisms Inhalation of airborne organisms from other people (*Mycoplasma*, influenza), soil, or water (*Legionella*, *Histoplasma*) or animals (Q fever, psittacosis)

Note: In up to 50% of cases, a specific cause is not determined despite extensive evaluation.

What are the most common causes of typical pneumonia?

S. pneumoniae, H. influenzae, Moraxella catarrhalis, polymicrobial agents (including anaerobes), aerobic gram-negative bacilli, *S. aureus*, TB, and endemic fungi (*Cryptococcus, Aspergillus, Histoplasmosis, Candida, Coccidioides*)

What are the most common causes of atypical pneumonia?

M. pneumoniae, C. pneumoniae, influenza, parainfluenza, adenovirus, *Legionella, Coxiella burnetii* (Q fever), and *Chlamydia psittaci*

What are the most common causes of nosocomial pneunomia?

Gram-negative bacilli (e.g., *P. aeruginosa, Klebsiella pneumoniae, Escherichia coli*, and *Enterobacter*) and *S. aureus*

What are predisposing factors to nosocomial pneumonia?

Severity of underlying illness, previous hospitalization, intubation, indwelling urethral catheterization, recent thoracic or abdominal surgery, and use of broad-spectrum antibiotics

What is the most common cause of community-acquired pneumonia in the following patients:
    An alcoholic

Pneumococcus. Alcoholics also have a higher incidence of pneumonia caused by gram-negative organisms, *S. aureus*, and aspiration (anaerobic).

    A patient with HIV

Pneumococcus. Patients with HIV also have a higher incidence of pneumonia caused by *Pneumocystis carinii*.

Who is likely to be infected with *Mycoplasma*?

Young adults, especially if living in close quarters

Who is likely to be infected with *Moraxella*?

Cigarette smokers, COPD patients, diabetics, patients with malignancies, alcoholics, and patients taking corticosteroids. Such infection is rare in normal adults.

Who is likely to be infected with *Legionella*?

Elderly patients, cigarette smokers, patients with COPD, transplant recipients, persons taking corticosteroids, and patients with hairy cell leukemia

Why are elderly patients more susceptible to development of pneumonia?

Older persons aspirate more frequently, and there is an increased amount of gram-negative flora in 20% of elderly persons.

What is the most common cause of secondary pneumonia following influenza?

S. pneumoniae; also consider *S. aureus*

What pathogens are likely to infect asplenic patients?

S. pneumoniae and *H. influenzae*

What are the complications and pathogens associated with severe pneumonia?

Approximately 10% of patients require admission to the intensive care unit for respiratory (and often, multisystemic) failure with or without hemodynamic shock. The most common pathogens are *S. pneumoniae* and *Legionella pneumophila*, but it may also be caused by gram-negative bacilli or *M. pneumoniae*.

What are complications of anaerobic pneumonia?

If untreated, necrosis and cavitation

What is the mortality rate of community-acquired pneumonia?

5%–25%

What laboratory and diagnostic tests are useful for establishing the diagnosis of pneumonia?

Routine laboratory tests, not for determining the cause of pneumonia but for prognosis and determination of the need for hospitalization

ABG in hospitalized patients or in patients being considered for hospitalization

Sputum Gram stain and culture (sensitivity and specificity vary)

Viral cultures, not for the initial evaluation unless the epidemiologic study suggests viral infection (e.g., influenza)

Blood cultures in hospitalized patients

Thoracentesis in patients with a pleural effusion

Serology tests, not for initial or routine workup but for retrospective diagnosis and epidemiologic study

Chest radiograph. Lobar consolidation, cavitation, and effusion suggest bacterial pneumonia. Diffuse bilateral involvement suggests *Pneumocystis carinii* pneumonia, *Legionella* infection, or virus. If the superior segment of the lower lobe or posterior segment of the upper lobe is involved, consider aspiration.

Invasive procedures (e.g., bronchoscopy), reserved for the initial evaluation of severely ill patients or those who are immunocompromised (there is a much wider differential diagnosis)

What findings on Gram stain are associated with the following:

Pneumococcal pneumonia	Gram-positive oval-shaped diplococci
S. aureus	Gram-positive cocci in clusters, chains, and pairs
***H. influenzae* pneumonia**	Gram-negative coccobacilli and many PMNs
M. catarrhalis	Gram-negative cocci, singly or in pairs
Neisseria meningitidis	Gram-negative cocci that are indistinguishable from *M. catarrhalis*
Gram-negative bacillary pneumonia	Gram-negative rods
Anaerobic pneumonia	Numerous white cells with an abundant variety of organisms
Mycoplasma pneumoniae	Numerous white cells, mouth flora

Legionella	Numerous white cells and mouth flora; organisms not visible
In general, how is pneumonia treated?	Based on age and severity of disease or underlying illness Age younger than 60 years or outpatient— macrolide (e.g., erythromycin) Age 60 years or older or patient with underlying disease— second-generation cephalosporin, β lactam or β lactamase inhibitor, or trimethoprim–sulfamethoxazole with or without erythromycin Hospitalized patients—third-generation cephalosporin or β lactam or β lactamase inhibitor with or without erythromycin Severe disease—erythromycin plus third-generation cephalosporin
How do you treat the following infections: **Pneumococcal pneumonia**	Penicillin sensitive— 1.2–2.4 million U intravenously/day Intermediate—12 million U intravenously/day Resistant—vancomycin, ceftriaxone, or cefotaxime, if sensitive Alternatives—erythromycin or first-generation cephalosporins, clindamycin
***H. influenzae* pneumonia**	Ampicillin, if penicillin-sensitive; tetracycline, doxycycline, trimethoprim–sulfamethoxazole, second- and third-generation cephalosporins, chloramphenicol, amoxicillin–clavulanate, or azithromycin
M. catarrhalis	Tetracycline or doxycycline, trimethoprim–sulfamethoxazole, cephalosporins, amoxicillin–clavulanate, sulbactam, macrolides, or fluoroquinolones
Meningococcal pneumonia	Penicillin if identity is certain; otherwise, use chloramphenicol, cephalosporins,

tetracycline, erythromycin, trimethoprim–sulfamethoxazole to cover for *Moraxella* as well

S. *aureus* pneumonia

Methicillin sensitive— nafcillin, oxacillin, vancomycin, first-generation cephalosporin

Methicillin-resistant infection

Vancomycin

Legionella

Erythromycin

Gram-negative bacillary pneumonia

Aminoglycoside plus cephalosporin or anti-pseudomonal penicillin until the organism is identified

Anaerobic pneumonia

Penicillin, 6–10 million U intravenously/day; clindamycin, 300 mg by mouth four times per day; metronidazole, 500 mg by mouth three times a day, plus penicillin, amoxicillin–clavulanate, or sulbactam

***Mycoplasma* pneumonia**

Erythromycin, 500 mg four times per day, or doxycycline, 100 mg twice daily

Who should be hospitalized?

The decision to admit patients to the hospital depends on the risk factors associated with increased complications and mortality rate. These include age older than 65 years, underlying medical diseases, or presence of physical or laboratory findings consistent with more severe disease.

How long should treatment last?

For bacterial pneumonia, generally 7–10 days. *M. pneumoniae* and *C. pneumoniae* infection as well as *Legionella* infection often require longer therapy (10–14 days and 21 days, respectively).

How is response assessed?

Some improvement should be seen in 72 hours in normalizing temperature and WBC. Physical examination findings may persist for longer than 7 days and the chest radiograph shows a return to normal in only approximately 50% of patients by 4 weeks.

What if the patient is not improving?	Treatment may be for the wrong pathogen or with the wrong drug or wrong dose. Also, the patient may be immuncompromised (e.g., HIV-positive).
What is aspiration pneumonia?	There are three different processes: chemical pneumonitis, bronchial obstruction secondary to particulate matter, and bacterial aspiration pneumonia. Bacterial aspiration usually develops slowly over days and may evolve into necrotizing pneumonia, abscess, or empyema.
What are the pathogens involved in aspiration pneumonia?	Anaerobes alone are responsible for 50% of cases; aerobic bacteria are involved in another 40%.
Who is susceptible to recurrent pneumonia?	Children with defects in white blood cell function and Ig, congenital defects in cilia, and CF Adults with structural abnormalities including bronchiectasis, sequestration, malignancy, AIDS, or underlying respiratory disease or who have received a transplant

NOSOCOMIAL PNEUMONIA*

What is the incidence of nosocomial pneumonia?	It is the second leading cause of nosocomial infection (> 250,000 episodes per year) and the number 1 cause of death from nosocomial infection in the United States.
What are the risk factors for nosocomial pneumonia?	Hospital stay in the intensive care unit, intubation or other respiratory tract instrumentation, decreased mental status, thoracic or abdominal surgery, obesity, poor nutrition, smoking history, alcohol use, intravenous drug use, underlying pulmonary disease, and CHF
What pathogens are associated with nosocomial pneumonia?	Multiple organisms are usually the cause, and bacteria are most common. These are sometimes divided into "early" and "late" pathogens.

---

* In collaboration with N. Thielman, V. Shami, and C. Sable

Early (first 3 days in the hospital)—*S. pneumoniae, Moraxella, H. influenzae*
Late—Gram-negative bacilli or *S. aureus*

What laboratory and diagnostic tests are useful in establishing nosocomial pneumonia?

Complete blood count, Gram stain and culture of sputum or endotracheal aspirate, bronchoscopy with BAL and biopsy, chest radiograph

How is the diagnosis of nosocomial pneumonia made?

History, physical examination, and laboratory tests. Diagnosing pneumonia in intubated patients is more difficult because of bacterial colonization. In such patients, consider the presence of fever, leukocytosis, change in quantity and character of sputum, change in oxygenation, and new infiltrate on chest radiograph.

What is the treatment for nosocomial pneumonia?

Administration of antibiotics and aggressive pulmonary toilet. Address risk factors, if possible. Several antibiotic combinations are adequate. The prevalence of bacteria in the individual hospital should be taken into consideration. Possible combinations of antibiotics include the following, among others:
1. Ceftazidime and gentamicin
2. Ticarcillin clavulanate and gentamicin
3. Clindamycin and ceftazidime

MYCOBACTERIUM TUBERCULOSIS*

What is the incidence of TB?

> 1.7 billion people in the world are infected with TB. There are 8 million new cases of TB per year, and TB causes 3 million deaths per year.

What groups are at risk for TB?

Immigrants from regions with high endemic rates of TB, homeless persons, persons with low socioeconomic status and lack of access to health care, and persons in close contact with active TB Persons with the following medical conditions: HIV infection, substance abuse problems (e.g., IVDA and

---

* In collaboration with N. Thielman, V. Shami, and C. Sable

alcohol), diabetes mellitus, end-stage
renal disease, hematologic malignancies,
silicosis, and weight greater than 10%
below ideal body weight

How is TB transmmitted?   Airborne droplet

What are the clinical   Pulmonary disease is most common with
manifestations of TB?   prolonged and productive cough,
                        chest pain, night sweats, fatigue,
                        anorexia, and weight loss
                    Extrapulmonary TB occurs in
                        approximately 1 in 6 cases and may
                        involve the CNS, bone, genitourinary
                        system, lymph nodes, or
                        gastrointestinal tract

What screen is used for   Mantoux skin test (5TU ppd).
infection?   **Induration** is read at 48 to 72 hours.

Who should be tested?   People in the risk groups listed

What groups are
considered to have a
positive ppd test if the
induration is one of the
following:
    > 5 mm but < 10 mm   Persons with known or suspected HIV
                        infection, close contacts of persons with
                        active TB, persons with a chest
                        radiograph suggestive of old TB,
                        intravenous drug users, persons with
                        silicosis

    > 10 mm but < 15 mm   Persons with medical conditions as listed
                        for risk factors, intravenous drug users,
                        persons with known HIV infection;
                        foreign-born persons from high endemic
                        areas, medically underserved and low-
                        income persons, residents of long-term
                        care facilities, children younger than 4
                        years old, and local high-prevalence
                        groups (e.g., migrant workers)

    > 15 mm   Everyone

What is preventive   Isoniazid (INH) plus or minus vitamin
therapy? B_6 for 6 months (1 year if HIV positive)

Who should receive preventive therapy?

Persons with a positive skin test regardless of age if they are known or suspected to be HIV positive or are close contacts of persons with active TB, if their chest radiograph is suggestive of TB and inadequate treatment, or if they are intravenous drug users, have certain medical conditions, or have undergone recent skin test conversion

Persons with a positive skin test who are younger than 35 years old if they are foreign born where TB is prevalent, medically underserved, have a low income, are residents of long-term care facilities, are younger than 4 years old, or are members of local high-prevalence groups

How is the diagnosis of active TB made?

History and physical examination, Mantoux skin test, chest radiograph, AFB smear, and culture of sputum or other involved site

What diagnostic tests are used for TB?

Polymerase chain reaction of cerebrospinal fluid and DNA probes of positive cultures

What is the treatment for TB?

Four drugs empirically—INH, rifampin, pyrazinamide (PZA), and ethambutol (or streptomycin) unless INH resistance is known to be < 4%

How long should therapy last?

Drug susceptibility must be tested on all initial isolates. If there is susceptibility to all agents, ethambutol can be stopped and INH, rifampin, and PZA can be continued. At 2 months, PZA can be stopped and 6 total months with INH and rifampin should be completed. Other regimens are required if drug resistance is present.

What is MDR-TB?

Multidrug-resistant TB, defined as resistant to both INH and rifampin

Why is MDR-TB important?	Different drug regimens are needed for a longer time. Cure rates are much lower than for susceptible TB.
What is the association between HIV and TB?	Active TB is more likely to develop in HIV-positive patients once infected (50% first year versus 5%–15% in general; 8%–10% per year versus 0.3% per year). TB can develop at any time in patients with HIV. Lower CD4 counts are associated with atypical disease and such patients are less likely to have a positive ppd and more likely to have extrapulmonary TB. INH preventive therapy should be given for 1 year to all HIV-positive patients with a positive ppd. Treatment of disease is the same four-drug regimen given for 9 months.
Which HIV-positive patients should be tested?	All HIV-positive patients for TB and all TB-positive patients for HIV

PLEURAL EFFUSIONS

What are pleural effusions?	Collections of fluid in the pleural space
What is normally in the pleural space?	Only a thin film of fluid. The pleural space is a potential rather than a real space.
What are the symptoms and signs of a pleural effusion?	Small effusions can be asymptomatic and be an incidental finding on chest radiograph. Larger effusions may cause dyspnea, nonspecific discomfort, and cough.
What are the physical signs of pleural effusion?	< 500 ml— minimal findings > 500 ml— dullness to percussion, decreased fremitus, and decreased breath sounds over fluid area > 1500 ml— egophony, bronchial breath sounds at fluid level, decreased expansion, and mediastinal shift away from the side of effusion

What can cause fluid to accumulate?	Abnormal hydrostatic and osmotic pressures Increased capillary permeability Decreased lymphatic drainage
What are examples of abnormal hydrostatic and osmotic pressures?	High pulmonary venous pressure (CHF) and hypoalbuminemia
What would cause an increase in capillary permeability?	Inflammation, which can be infectious or noninfectious
What can cause lymphatic dysfunction?	High venous pressures (e.g., CHF and superior vena caval syndrome) and obstruction (e.g., malignancies)
How is the etiology of pleural effusion determined?	Thoracentesis and pleural fluid analysis
What tests should be ordered on pleural fluid?	Pleural fluid LDH, protein, glucose, pH, cell count, WBC and differential, amylase, culture, Gram stain, special stains as indicated, and cytologic study (if suspecting neoplasm)
What are the two categories of pleural effusions?	Transudative and exudative
Give some examples of transudative effusions.	CHF, nephrotic syndrome, cirrhosis, ascites, starvation, hydronephrosis, peritoneal dialysis, superior vena cava obstruction, and Meigs' syndrome (pleural effusion with ovarian tumors)
Give some examples of exudative effusions.	Infectious pleurisy (usually viral), parapneumonia, malignancy, and PE. Other common examples are TB, trauma, collagen vascular disease, abdominal disease. Unusual causes include esophageal rupture, drug induced, asbestos, Dressler's syndrome, chylothorax, uremia, radiation therapy, sarcoid, yellow nail syndrome, myxedema, and CHF (usually transudate).

What defines a transudate?

Protein < 3 g/dl
Pleural/serum protein < 0.5
Pleural/serum LDH < 0.6

What defines an exudate?

Any one of the following:
Protein > 3 g/dl
Pleural/serum protein > 0.5
Pleural/serum LDH > 0.6
Absolute LDH > 2/3 upper limit of
    serum value

What is seen on chest radiograph?

Blunting of the costophrenic angle with
small amounts of fluid; larger amounts
can have dense lung field opacification
with a concave meniscus.

What is the earliest radiographic sign of pleural effusion?

Loss of posterior sulcus on lateral chest
film

What is the minimal amount of fluid to show on chest film?

If upright, 300–500 ml
If lying with affected side up, < 100 ml
As little as 10–15 ml with careful
    positioning

What is a subpulmonic effusion?

Pleural effusion localized to the
diaphragmatic region that presents only
as subtle abnormalities in the contour of
the hemidiaphragm

How do you confirm the presence of a subpulmonic effusion?

Obtain a lateral decubitus film or do an
ultrasound.

What is the best way to localize a loculated pleural effusion?

Ultrasound

When is a pleural biopsy needed?

To diagnose unexplained exudative
effusions or suspected cases of TB and
malignancy

When is bronchoscopy indicated?

If the patient has a parenchymal
abnormality on chest film or CT scan or
to rule out an obstruction if atelectasis is
associated with effusions

**What should be suspected
with the following:**

    **A pleural glucose < 20
    mg/dl**

Rheumatoid arthritis, occasionally
cancer, and infection

    **An increased amylase
    level**

Pancreatitis and esophageal rupture

    pH < 7.2

Empyema secondary to infection

    **Predominance of
    lymphocytes?**

TB, fungal infection, myxedema, and
malignancy

    PMNs

Bacterial pneumonia, pulmonary
infarction, empyema, rheumatic fever,
rheumatoid arthritis, pulmonary abscess,
SLE, scleroderma, and coxsackie A virus

    Eosinophils

Contusions, pulmonary infarctions,
induced pneumothorax, Hodgkin's
disease, echinococcus, rheumatoid
arthritis, and Löffler's disease (a high
eosinophil count is usually due to air or
blood in the pleural space)

    Brown exudative fluid

Amebic liver abscesses and old
cholesterol effusions

    Recurrent effusions

Asbestosis

    Blood-tinged fluid

Pulmonary infarction, pleural
carcinomatosis, and TB

**What is the treatment for
pleural effusion?**

Treatment of the underlying disease. Up
to 1500 ml of fluid may be removed for
symptomatic relief, but removal of more
may cause cardiovascular collapse.

What is an empyema?

Frank pus in the pleural space with the
following parameters:
WBC > 5000 cells/mm^3
Protein > 3 g/dl
Glucose < 40 mg/dl
LDH > 600 mg/dl
pH < 7.0

What is a hemothorax?	Blood in the pleural space, usually from trauma
What is a chylothorax?	Milky effusion that has a high lipid content, usually caused by traumatic or neoplastic process involving the thoracic duct
What is a cholesterol effusion?	Presence of cholesterol crystals in pleural fluid, also known as chyliform or pseudochylous effusion
What causes a cholesterol effusion?	Long-standing chronic pleural effusion
What is significant about a cholesterol effusion?	It indicates an underlying process that should be sought.
Which drugs can cause effusions?	Frequently, hydralazine, procainamide, isoniazid, phenytoin, chlorpromazine Infrequently, nitrofurantoin, bromocriptine, dantrolene, procarbazine
When is a chest tube needed?	In cases of empyema
What is pleurodesis?	Instillation of an irritative agent (e.g., tetracycline or bleomycin) in the pleural space to obliterate it and to prevent the reaccumulation of effusions. It is usually done for large recurrent symptomatic malignant effusions.
What complications are associated with pleural effusions?	Acute—pneumothorax Chronic—pleural fibrosis, resulting from organization of the pleural effusion. Extensive fibrosis can pull the trachea to the affected side (late finding).

IMMUNOSUPPRESSED PATIENTS

LUNG TRANSPLANTATION

What are the indications for lung transplantation?	End-stage lung disease with a life expectancy of less than 24 months (e.g., COPD, IPF, and CF). Due to long waiting times, late patient referral can be a significant problem.

When should bilateral sequential lung transplantation be considered?

Bilateral sequential lung transplants are reserved for patients with pulmonary sepsis (e.g., CF and bronchiectasis) and pulmonary HTN of any cause; all other patients receive single lung transplants.

What are the characterisitics of a donor?

Brain dead
Family consent given
Minimal lung disease
< 20 pack-year smoking history
PO_2 > 350–400 mm Hg on 100% FIO_2 and minimal PEEP
Minimal secretions on bronchoscopy

How are donors and recipients matched?

Matched for blood group (ABO), size, and, often, CMV status

What ischemic times are allowable for the donor lungs?

6–8 hours

What complications need to be watched for in the immediate post–lung transplant period?

Bleeding, air leak, and bronchial anastomotic dehiscence

What drug therapy is used for immunosupression following lung transplantation?

Cyclosporine, azathioprine, and prednisone

What are side effects of cyclosporine?

Renal disease, elevated LFTs, hyperkalemia, hypomagnesemia, tremors, hirsutism, HTN, cholestasis, and elevated cholesterol

Which drugs increase cyclosporine levels?

Diltiazem, ketoconazole, and erythromycin

What are the side effects of prednisone?

Hyperglycemia, osteoporosis, adrenal suppression, cataracts, and poor wound healing

What are the side effects of azathioprine?

Leukopenia, thrombocytopenia, alopecia, hepatitis, and pancreatitis

What are the side effects of OKT3?

Hypotension, pulmonary edema, and long-term, lymphoproliferative disorders

How is acute rejection recognized?

Diffuse pulmonary infiltrates in the transplanted lungs, decreased PO_2, rales, cough, dyspnea, low-grade fever. The gold standard diagnosis is perivascular infiltrate of lymphocytes on transbronchial biopsy.

What patients are at highest risk for acquiring CMV?

Seronegative patients receiving seropositive organs

When are patients at highest risk for acquiring CMV?

3–6 months after transplantation

What infection commonly occurs during the first 3 months after transplantation?

Bacterial bronchitis

What is BO?

A destructive airway process leading to obstructive lung disease. It is generally seen 1 year after transplantation and is the most frequent cause of death following the first year after transplantation.

How is BO diagnosed?

BO is diagnosed by a 20% decline in FEV_1.

What is posttransplant lymphoproliferative disorder?

It is related to the total dose of immunosuppresion and possibly Ebstein-Barr virus infection in a naive host.

What diseases recur in the transplanted lung?

Sarcoid, giant cell interstitial pneumonitis, and lymphangioleiomyomatosis

What is the most common pulmonary problem in bone marrow transplantation?

Interstitial pneumonitis

ACQUIRED IMMUNODEFICIENCY SYNDROME

What type of immunodeficiency is involved in HIV?

T-cell deficiency

What are the common pathogens in neutropenic patients?

Staphylococcus, *Enterobacteriaceae, Pseudomonas, Bacteroides fragilis, Candida, Aspergillus*

What are the most common respiratory infections in AIDS?

Pneumococcus and *Pneumocystis carinii* (PCP)

When does PCP occur?

When the CD4 count decreases to below 200

What is the clinical picture of PCP?

Fever, cough, dyspnea, and diffuse interstitial or alveolar infiltrates

What is the radiographic appearance of the chest in an AIDS patient with PCP on inhaled pentamidine?

Often, the disease is isolated to upper lobes.

How is the diagnosis of PCP made?

Induced sputum is 50%–80% sensitive and BAL is 90% sensitive. In patients receiving prophylaxis, the yield is lower. Transbronchial biopsy may help in diagnosing atypical or recurrent cases.

What is the therapy for PCP?

Either trimethoprim–sulfamethoxazole or pentamidine. There are many adverse reactions to trimethoprim–sulfamethoxazole, including rash, fever, and elevated aminotransferase levels, thus limiting its use. Alternatives include trimethoprim–dapsone, clindamycin–primaquine, and atovaquone. Corticosteroids are recommeded if PO_2 < 70 mm Hg or alveolar–arterial gradient > 35 mm Hg.

What is the prophylaxis for PCP?

Prophylaxis is recommended after an episode of PCP or when CD4+ counts are less than 200/m³. Regimens include:
1. Oral trimethoprim–sulfamethoxazole three times weekly, or

2. Trimethoprim–dapsone 3 times
   weekly, or
3. Inhaled monthly pentamidine

What types of bacterial pneumonia affect AIDS patients?

Encapsulated bacteria such as *S. pneumoniae* and *H. influenzae*

What AIDS patients are at risk for *Myocobacterium avium-intracellulare* infection?

Patients with CD4 counts < 100

What is Kaposi's sarcoma?

Often a purple skin lesion that can occur in lung also. It may present as infiltrates, interstitial disease, effusions, lymphadenopathy, or endobronchial involvement. Hemorrhage may occur. Gallium scans are negative, unlike those for infections and lymphoma.

What is the principal CNS diagnosis in AIDS patients?

Cryptococcal meningitis, toxoplasmic encephalitis, progressive multifocal encephalopathy, herpes encephalitis, and brain abscess

CRITICAL CARE

What is shock?

Defect in tissue perfusion or failure to remove metabolites

What are the phases of shock?

1. Compensated hypotension (blood flow to brain, heart, liver, and kidney is maintained)
2. Decompensated hypotension (end-organ malperfusion)
3. Irreversible shock (microcirculatory failure and cell death)

What are general indications for intubation?

Severe respiratory distress (e.g., respiratory rate > 40 breaths per minute)
PO_2 < 60 on 100% face mask
Elevated PCO_2 with pH < 7.2
Severe CHF
Obtundation

How much should an FIO_2 increase with nasal cannula?

FIO_2 increases 3%–4% per liter

What size tube is used for intubation?

For adult men, 8 mm
For adult women, 7.5 mm

Why is tube size important for weaning?

Resistance, which affects the patient's work, is directly related to tube length and tube radius to the fourth power.

What should the initial ventilator settings be?

FIO_2 = 100%
Tidal volumes = 7–8 ml/kg
Respiratory rate = 8–16 breaths/min

What is assist control?

Volume-limited ventilation. With every breath the patient initiates, the ventilator delivers a predetermined (by physician) volume. If there is no spontaneous breathing, the ventilator delivers a minimum predetermined number of breaths. It is important to set peak inspiratory flow above patient demand to avoid patient intolerance.

What is IMV?

Volume-limited ventilation. The patient can take spontaneous breaths but receives a set number of coordinated breaths. The patient receives a predetermined (by physician) number of breaths if there is no spontaneous breathing.

What is pressure support (PS)?

Pressure-limited ventilation. With every spontaneous breath, the ventilator delivers an additional boost of a set pressure. CAUTION: There is no backup rate. PS should be used only when patients have an adequate drive to breathe.

What determines the tidal volume in PS ventilation?

Lung compliance. If lung compliance decreases (lung is more stiff), the tidal volume may become smaller, thus reducing minute ventilation. PS ventilation does not guarantee a fixed minute ventilation.

What is pressure control (PC)?	Pressure-limited ventilation. Unlike for PS, a rate can be given. This is a very uncomfortable mode and often (but not always) requires sedation and chemical muscle relaxation. Minute ventilation may change if lung compliance changes.
What is a reverse I:E ratio?	Normal ventilation has a shorter inspiratory time (I) than expiratory time (E). A reverse I:E gives a longer inspiratory (I) time. This mode may allow better oxygenation in patients with stiff lungs (e.g., ARDS).
What is permissive hypercapnia?	Purposely allowing PCO_2 to increase in order to limit peak airway pressure. The technique is used in patients at risk for barotrauma.
What is PEEP?	Positive-end expiratory pressure, which perhaps splints the airways open
Can PEEP be used to tamponade mediastinal bleeding after coronary artery bypass graft?	No. That is a common myth.
Is there such a thing as physiologic PEEP?	No. In spontaneously breathing humans, there is no positive pressure at end expiration.
How should hypoxemia be corrected?	Increase FIO_2, tidal volume, and PEEP
How can hypercarbia be corrected?	Increase minute ventilation (increase rate, tidal volume, or both).
How do you calculate an A-a gradient?	Simplified method: $PAO_2 - PaO_2$ $PAO_2 = 7 \times FIO_2$ $PaO_2 = PO_2 - (PCO_2 \times 1.25)$ Normal is < 20.
What are causes of shunting?	ARDS, pulmonary emboli, pneumonia, other alveolar filling (e.g., blood, fluid), ASD, and VSD

Where should the distal tip of the endotracheal tube be seen on chest radiograph?	4–5 cm above the carina
What are the common complications of mechanical ventilation?	Barotrauma, pneumothorax, pneumomediastinum, tracheomalacia, sinusitis, and decreased cardiac output
What are chest radiograph signs of a pneumothorax?	Most are anterior. Look for a deep sulcus sign, sharp heart border, absent lung markings, pleural reflection, or a mediastinal shift.
What is dynamic compliance?	Tidal volume/(peak pressure – PEEP); indicates airway resistance
What is static compliance?	Tidal volume/(plateau pressure – PEEP); reflects parenchymal disease
What could cause dynamic compliance to increase out of proportion to static compliance?	Bronchospasm, plugging, selective intubation of the right main-stem bronchus
What is auto-PEEP?	Positive airway pressure present at end of expiration.
What danger is associated with auto-PEEP?	Hyperinflation, autocycling, and pneumothorax
What is the best mode for weaning patients?	There is no best mode. Multiple studies have not shown a clear advantage of any one technique. Possible methods include T-piece, intermittent mandatory ventilation, PS, and assist control.
What parameters indicate successful weaning?	Vital capacity > 10 ml/kg Negative inspiratory force > 25 cm H_2O Minute ventilation (to maintain PCO_2 = 40) less than 10 L/min.
What are causes of weaning failure?	Increased ventilatory requirements, increased dead space, increased CO_2 production, overfeeding, muscle weakness, hypophosphatemia, excessive work of breathing, too small an ET tube, respiratory alkalosis, and hypoxemia

What is often the first sign of weaning failure?

Increased respiratory rate or paradoxical abdominal motion

When should a ventilator patient have a tracheostomy?

Generally at 2–3 weeks, but there is no hard and fast rule. Early tracheostomy may be considered in patients requiring prolonged ventilator support (e.g., quadriplegic patients). Tracheostomy can also facilitate a difficult-to-wean patient.

What are risk factors for prolonged paralysis after the use of neuromuscular blockers?

Renal failure, steroid use, female gender, and hypomagnesemia

What noninvasive modes of ventilation are available?

Negative pressure methods such as the iron lung from the polio days or a negative pressure vest. Positive pressure includes nasal BiPAP ventilation.

What are appropriate situations for use of BiPAP?

OSA, muscle weakness, COPD, and CF. Requires an alert, cooperative patient. BiPAP can be used with a respiration rate.

If you press the "silent alarm" button on a beeping ventilator, what is your obligation?

You should stay with the patient until the alarm resets. If the patient becomes disconnected from the ventilator, there will be no alarm and the patient could be in a life-threatening situation.

4

Nephrology

ABBREVIATIONS

ABG	Arterial blood gas
ACE	Angiotensin-converting enzyme
AIDS	Acquired immune deficiency syndrome
AIN	Acute interstitial nephritis
ANA	Antineutrophil antibody
ANCA	Antineutrophil cytoplasmic antibody
ARF	Acute renal failure
ASO	Antistreptolysin O
ATN	Acute tubular necrosis
BP	Blood pressure
BUN	Blood urea nitrogen
CBC	Complete blood count
CHF	Congestive heart failure
CNS	Central nervous system
CrCl	Creatinine clearance
CRF	Chronic renal failure
CT	Computed tomography
CVA	Cerebrovascular accident
DKA	Diabetic ketoacidosis

DM	Diabetes mellitus
DN	Diabetic nephropathy
ECG	Electrocardiogram
EDTA	Ethylenediaminetetraacetic acid
ESRD	End-stage renal disease
ESWL	Extracorporeal shock wave lithotripsy
FE$_{Na}$	Fractional excretion of sodium
FE$_{urea}$	Fractional excretion of urea
GBM	Glomerular basement membrane
GFR	Glomerular filtration rate
HIV	Human immunodeficiency virus
HPF	High-powered field
IVP	Intravenous pyelography
JVD	Jugular venous distention
MPGN	Membranoproliferative glomerulonephritis
MRI	Magnetic resonance imaging
NSAIDs	Nonsteroidal antiinflammatory drugs
PAN	Polyarteritis nodosa
P$_{Na}$	Plasma sodium concentration
P$_{Cr}$	Plasma creatinine concentration
PSGN	Post-streptococcal glomerulonephritis
PT	Prothrombin time
PTH	Parathyroid hormone

PTT	Partial thromboplastin time
PVD	Peripheral vascular disease
RBC	Red blood cell
RF	Rheumatoid factor
RPGN	Rapidly progressive glomerulonephritis
RTA	Renal tubular acidosis
SIADH	Syndrome of inappropriate secretion of antidiuretic hormone
SLE	Systemic lupus erythematosus
SPEP	Serum protein electrophoresis
TB	Tuberculosis
TPN	Total parenteral nutrition
U_{Cr}	Urine creatinine concentration
U_{Na}	Urine sodium concentration
UOP	Urine output
U_{osm}	Urine osmolality
UPEP	Urine protein electrophoresis
UTI	Urinary tract infection
WBC	White blood cell

HISTORY AND PHYSICAL EXAMINATION

What are the risk factors for the development of renal disease?	DM (including its duration, how well it has been controlled, and whether or not retinopathy is involved) Hypertension (including its duration and how well it has been controlled) Coronary artery disease PVD Hypotension Contrast administration

What past medical history is important?

History of recurrent UTIs, SLE, hypertension, DM, baseline BUN/creatinine levels, GFR

What medication use is important?

ACE inhibitors, other BP medications, NSAIDs, antimicrobials, and diuretics

What family history is important?

Diabetes, hypertension, polycystic kidney disease, Alport's, and nephrolithiasis

What social history is important?

Tobacco use (correlation with Goodpasture's syndrome), drug ingestion, intravenous drug abuse, and HIV risk factors

What parameters are important to follow on a frequent basis in patients with renal impairment?

Weight, temperature, intake and output, BP, and filling pressures if the patient is in intensive care

What physical examination findings are important in patients with renal dysfunction in each of the following systems:

Head, ears, eyes, nose, and throat

Hemorrhage, exudates, hypertensive changes, and diabetic retinopathy

Neck

Jugular venous pressure

Chest

Rales

Cardiovascular structures

Pericardial rub, murmurs, and gallops

Abdomen

Flank tenderness, bruits, suprapubic tenderness or distention, and masses

Genitourinary structures

Prostate size or irregularity

Extremities

Edema and pulses

Skin

Rash, purpura, petechiae, and livedo reticularis

Neurologic structures

Mental status, sensation, and equal reflexes

Specifically with regard to hematuria, where is the problem if hematuria starts at the following:

Beginning of stream   Urethral lesion

End of stream   Bladder lesion

Throughout   Renal, ureteric, and diffuse lesions

Where is the source of hematuria in the following circumstances:

When there is "Coca-Cola" or cloudy urine   Suggestive of a glomerular source

When there are clots   Suggestive of a postrenal source

What other history is important in evaluating hematuria?   Use of prosthetic devices (e.g., valve or shunt) or presence of a bleeding diasthesis

What symptoms and signs are associated with hematuria?   Dysuria, urgency, frequency, photosensitivity, arthritis and arthralgias, rash, and pain (if unilateral flank pain occurs in men older than 50 years of age, consider renal cell carcinoma)

What medications are associated with hematuria?   Warfarin, heparin, and aspirin (exacerbation of bleeding)
Cyclophosphamide (hemorrhagic cystitis)

What findings on urinalysis are associated with hematuria?   Normal findings are < 2 RBC/HPF; microscopic hematuria findings are > 3 RBC/HPF.
In nephritic hematuria, dysmorphic red cells or red cell casts and mild proteinuria (glomerular bleeding) are found.
When there is distal pathology, normal red cells and clots are seen.

What laboratory tests are ordered for hematuria?   Blood chemistry tests, BUN, creatinine, CBC, PT and PTT, and hemoglobin electrophoresis (in blacks). Serologic results depend on presentation (e.g., ANA, complement, ASO, anti-GBM, and ANCA), especially if there are signs of systemic disease.

What history is important in evaluating proteinuria?

DM (with or without retinopathy), hepatitis, syphilis, pregnancy, HIV and associated risk factors, malignancy, fever, hypertension, and recent infections

What are the usual symptoms of proteinuria?

Rash, arthralgias, swelling, and dyspnea

What physical examination findings are associated with proteinuria?

Hypertension, edema, ascites, and hepatosplenomegaly

In proteinuria, what findings are made on urinalysis?

Nephritis, when there is associated hematuria or RBC casts

Nephrosis, when there are oval fat bodies, fatty casts, or free fat droplets, which suggest glomerular origin and strongly indicate a distinct pathologic process

Tubulointerstitial disease, associated with mild proteinuria (< 2 g), leukocytes, granular casts without hematuria, or fat droplets

What laboratory tests are ordered for proteinuria?

Blood chemistry tests, BUN, and creatinine. Serologic results depend on presentation (e.g., ANA, RF, complement, hepatitis, lipids, HIV).

24-hour protein analysis—normal, < 100–150 mg; nephritic, 150–3500 mg; nephrotic, greater than or equal to 3.5 g

CrCl

UPEP and SPEP (for multiple myeloma)

Serologies depend on presentation (ANA, RF, complement, hepatitis, lipids, HIV)

EVALUATION OF KIDNEY FUNCTION

What serum tests estimate renal function?

BUN and creatinine

What is the normal range of BUN?

7–18 mg/dl

What agents and conditions not associated with renal function result in an increase in the BUN level?

High-protein diet, gastrointestinal bleeding, steroids, dehydration, and some antibiotics (e.g., tetracyclines)

What conditions not associated with renal function result in a decrease in the BUN level?

Low-protein diet, liver disease, sickle cell anemia, and pregnancy

Which is a more accurate measure of renal function, BUN level or creatinine level?

Creatinine level. Up to 50% of BUN can be reabsorbed, whereas only a very small amount of creatinine is secreted.

What conditions not associated with renal function result in an increase in the creatinine level?

DKA and ingestion of meats and drugs

Which drugs inhibit tubular secretion of creatinine?

Cimetidine, aspirin, and trimethoprim

How can GFR be estimated?

Cockroft-Gault formula:

$$\frac{(140 - age) \times (lean\ body\ weight\ in\ kg)}{(Serum\ creatinine\ mg/dl) \times 72}\ [\ \times 0.85\ (for\ women)]$$

What is CrCl?

A more sensitive measure of GFR involving a urine collection as follows:

$$\frac{(urine\ Cr\ in\ mg/dl) \times (volume\ of\ urine\ in\ ml)}{(serum\ Cr\ in\ mg/dl) \times (minutes)}$$

GFR of less than 20 ml/min may be overestimated by CrCl secondary to the amount of creatinine that is secreted by the tubules.

What is a normal CrCl?

For men, 97–137 ml/min; for women, 88–128 ml/min

How much creatinine determines adequate urine collection?

For men, 18–24 mg/kg/day of urine creatinine; for women, 13–18 mg/kg/day of urine creatinine

What procedure estimates GFR?	Renal scan with technetium diethylenetriamine pentaacetic acid (^{99}mTc-DTPA). This substance is freely filtered by the glomerulus.

IMAGING TECHNIQUES

What differential diagnoses are suggested by renal calcification on an abdominal film?	Kidney stones, calcified neoplasms, nephrocalcinosis, papillary necrosis, TB, trauma, and cortical necrosis
How is a renal ultrasound helpful?	Detects renal size, masses, cysts, hydronephrosis, abscess or hematoma, renal vein thrombosis, and renal artery stenosis Localizes kidney for invasive procedures
What do CT and MRI detect?	Renal masses, trauma, hemorrhage, and calcification
When are CT and MRI evaluations helpful?	When ultrasound evaluation is limited by obesity and bowel gas and when used to localize the kidney. MRI is more useful for evaluating adrenal masses (e.g., pheochromocytoma and renal vein thrombosis).
What is arteriography useful for?	For detecting atherosclerosis, fibromuscular dysplasia and stenosis, vasculitis, and arteriovenous fistula For selective renal vein sampling for renin For treating renovascular hypertension with angioplasty
What is venography useful for?	For detecting renal vein thrombosis
What is IVP?	Radiopaque dye is administered intravenously and concentrates in the kidney and collecting system. Serial radiographs are obtained after instillation of the dye.
What is IVP useful in detecting?	Kidney size and shape, calyces, obstruction, medullary sponge kidney, papillary necrosis, and pyelonephritis

What are the relative contraindications to IVP?

Contrast allergy, renal insufficiency, dehydration, DN, arrhythmias, CHF, and pregnancy

What is retrograde pyelography?

Radiopaque dye is administered through a cystoscopically placed catheter.

How does retrograde pyelography differ from IVP?

Gives more detail for filling defects and possibly less risk of ARF

Gives additional information on obstructing lesions and for selective cytologic cultures

Excludes obstruction if all noninvasive studies are negative

What is a cystourethrogram?

Cystography is performed after radiopaque dye is administered through a catheter to fill the bladder.

What is a cystourethrogram used for?

Detecting vesicoureteral reflux (usually used in children)

Evaluating bladder function prior to kidney transplantation

Evaluating pelvic trauma, fistula, level of urinary incontinence, posterior urethra, and stricture

What is ^{99}Tc-DTPA used for?

Use of ^{99}Tc-DTPA with serial imaging measures radioactive counts to evaluate flow to the kidney and ability of the kidney to excrete the radioactive substance.

What does ^{99}Tc-DTPA detect?

Renovascular hypertension (asymmetric perfusion), infarction, embolism, perfusion, and excretion in the transplanted kidney

What is a furosemide renogram?

Use of ^{99}Tc-DTPA and Lasix (furosemide) to cause a diuresis that leads to immediate dilution of the isotope, or washout, in the nonobstructed kidney. There is no washout in the obstructed kidney.

ACUTE RENAL FAILURE

What is ARF?

Abrupt decline in the ability of one or both kidneys to excrete waste products resulting in the accumulation of nitrogenous wastes

What is the incidence of ARF?

Occurs in approximately 5% of all hospitalized patients, more common in the intensive care unit

What are the presenting symptoms and signs of ARF?

Decreased UOP, mental status changes, gastrointestinal symptoms, evidence for volume overload, pericarditis, increased BUN and serum creatinine, hyperkalemia, acidosis, hypocalcemia, hyperphosphatemia, and abnormal urinalysis

At what GFR does creatinine increase?

When GFR decreases to < 20%–40% of normal

How much does the creatinine increase daily in patients with ARF?

An increase by 0.5–1.0 mg/dl indicates total renal failure. If the creatinine level increases more rapidly than 1.0 mg/dl/day, search for causes of muscle destruction or a hypercatabolic state.

How much is the daily increase in BUN level in ARF?

10–20 mg/dl indicates total renal failure, but this measurement is less specific than measurement of creatinine.

How can the causes of renal failure be grouped?

Prerenal, renal, and postrenal

What is FE_{Na}?

Fractional excretion of sodium; demonstrates the ratio between urine and serum sodium with relation to urine flow and GFR

How is FE_{Na} calculated?

$FE_{Na} = (U_{Na} \times P_{Cr})/(P_{Na} \times U_{Cr}) \times 100$

What is the significance of the FE_{Na} value?

$FE_{Na} < 1\%$ indicates avid salt retention consistent with a prerenal state.
$FE_{Na} > 2\%$ indicates a renal cause of ARF.

How do diuretics affect FE_{Na}?	They elevate the FE_{Na}, so that when they are given, fractional excretion of urea must be used.
How is a FE_{urea} calculated?	$FE_{urea} = (U_{urea} \times P_{Cr})/(P_{urea} \times U_{Cr}) \times 100$
What is the significance of the FE_{urea} value?	$FE_{urea} < 35\%$ indicates a prerenal cause of ARF $FE_{urea} > 35\%$ indicates a renal cause of ARF

PRERENAL AZOTEMIA

What are the risk factors for prerenal azotemia?	Dehydrating conditions (e.g., vomiting and diarrhea) and cardiac dysfunction with poor renal perfusion
What are the causes of prerenal azotemia?	Hypovolemia, cardiac failure, peripheral vasodilation (e.g., sepsis), renal vasoconstriction, and fluid losses through skin from extensive burns
What is the incidence of prerenal azotemia?	At least 50% of all cases of ARF
What are the symptoms and signs of prerenal azotemia?	Thirst, weight loss, decreased UOP, dizziness, dyspnea and peripheral edema in CHF; orthostasis, oliguria, tachycardia, JVD and rales in CHF
What laboratory parameters are used to establish prerenal azotemia?	BUN:Cr > 20:1 High urine specific gravity (≥ 1.020) Normal sediment or occasional hyaline and granular casts $U_{osm} > 500$ $U_{Na} < 20$ Urine$_{Cr}$:plasma$_{Cr} > 40:1$ $FE_{Na} < 1\%$
What does renal ultrasound show in patients with prerenal azotemia?	Kidneys of normal size and echogenicity
What diagnostic tests are used for prerenal azotemia?	Volume challenge Right heart catheter measurement of the pulmonary capillary wedge and cardiac output

What is the treatment for prerenal azotemia?	Volume replacement, generally with normal saline, to maintain UOP at 1–2 ml/min (pressors and inotropic drugs may be required)

RENAL FAILURE

What are the major causes of renal failure?	Toxins or ischemia leading to ATN, acute glomerulonephritis, AIN, and vascular diseases
What is ATN?	Acute tubule cell necrosis resulting from an insult that produces a sudden decrease in GFR
What causes ATN?	Ischemia, drugs or toxins, pigment (including hemoglobin and myoglobin), cholesterol emboli, and crystal disease
What is the incidence of ATN?	10%–50% of ARF cases depending on the patient population selected
What drugs and other agents can cause ATN?	Aminoglycosides, amphotericin B, contrast media, chemotherapeutic agents, organic solvents, cyclosporine, and heavy metals
What are the risk factors for ATN?	Advanced age, volume depletion at the time of renal injury, DM, and coadministration of multiple nephrotoxins
What are the symptoms of ATN?	Asymptomatic, or symptoms of uremia (i.e., lethargy, nausea, vomiting, abdominal pain, and anorexia) or CHF and low cardiac function
What are the signs of ATN?	Oliguria (anuria is rare), volume overload, azotemia, signs of uremia, metabolic disarray, acidosis, livedo reticularis, and rash
What are the findings on urinalysis for ATN?	Brownish pigmented granular casts, cellular debris, renal tubular epithelial cells, hematuria, occasionally crystals, and other cellular casts

What laboratory tests should be ordered for the workup of ATN?	Tests for electrolytes, urine electrolytes, and urine myoglobin
Are RBC casts usually present in renal failure?	RBC casts are typically absent in ATN, and they are present in acute glomerulonephritis.
What are the urinary indices for ATN?	$U_{osm} < 350$ mosm/kg H_2O $U_{Na} > 40$ mEq/L $U_{Cr}:P_{Cr} < 20:1$ $FE_{Na} > 1\%$ (usually $> 2\%$)
What are the urinary indices in uric acid nephropathy?	$U_{uric\ acid}:U_{Cr} > 1$ is consistent with uric acid nephropathy.
What does renal ultrasound show in ATN?	Normal or hypoechogenic kidneys (if ischemic)
What diagnostic tests are used for ATN?	Renal biopsy if the presentation is atypical or there is a mixed picture
What is the treatment for ATN?	Convert oliguric to nonoliguric failure with a loop diuretic, carefully maintain input equal to output, follow up and judiciously correct electrolyte abnormalities, and dialyze if necessary.
How is treatment directed when ARF is due to:	
Exogenous toxin?	Discontinuation of the toxin
Rhabdomyolysis?	Vigorous hydration, alkalinization of urine, and administration of mannitol if needed to increase UOP
Uric acid nephropathy?	Administration of allopurinol, hydration, and urine alkalinization
Ischemia?	Improvement of blood flow and discontinuation of ACE inhibitors and NSAIDs
Acute glomerulonephritis?	Imunosuppression in many cases (see Glomerular Disease section)

POSTRENAL AZOTEMIA

What are the causes of postrenal azotemia?
Renal obstruction, ureteral obstruction, bladder obstruction or disruption, and urethral obstruction

What is the most common renal cause?
Crystal deposition

What are the most common ureteral causes?
Calculi, blood clots, and intraperitoneal or retroperitoneal neoplasm

What are the most common bladder causes?
Traumatic rupture and stones

What is the most common urethral cause?
Prostatic hypertrophy (benign or malignant)

What is the incidence of postrenal azotemia?
Less than 10% of ARF cases

What are the risk factors for postrenal azotemia?
Advanced age and male gender, previous UTIs, pelvic or retroperitoneal surgery, and known intraabdominal mass lesion

What are the symptoms of postrenal azotemia?
Nocturia, urinary frequency, hesitancy, and inability to void

What are the signs of postrenal azotemia?
Enlarged prostate, palpable mass in the abdomen, palpable or percussible bladder, progressive renal failure particularly with wide fluctuations in UOP, and UTI

What laboratory test is ordered for postrenal azotemia?
Urine culture

What are the urinalysis findings in cases of postrenal azotemia?
Normal

What are typical renal ultrasound findings?
Hydronephrosis and possibly an enlarged bladder

What diagnostic tests are ordered for postrenal azotemia?	Foley catheter insertion, possibly IVP to demonstrate ureteral patency, and ultrasound or abdominal CT scan
What is the treatment for postrenal ARF of renal origin?	Dissolution of stones
What is the treatment for postrenal ARF of ureteral origin?	Percutaneous stent placement and removal of obstructing mass
What is the treatment for postrenal ARF of urethral origin?	Indwelling catheter and transurethral prostatectomy

GENERAL MANAGEMENT OF ACUTE RENAL FAILURE

What are the guidelines for treatment of ARF?	Exclude all treatable causes of decreased renal function, discontinue potentially nephrotoxic agents, establish UOP with diuretics, limit intake of nitrogen, monitor water and renal excretion of electrolytes, provide adequate nutrition to avoid catabolism, dose all medications based on renal function, and perform dialysis as needed.
When should you treat acidosis?	When serum HCO_3^- < 15 mEq/dl
When should you treat hyperkalemia?	When the serum potassium level equals or exceeds 6.5 mEq/dl or when there are ECG changes
When is acute dialysis indicated?	Acute dialysis is indicated in the presence of volume overload with compromise (e.g., pulmonary edema) that does not respond to diuretics, refractory hyperkalemia, severe acidosis that does not respond to treatment with bicarbonate, symptomatic uremia, and for the removal of some toxins. Think **A, E, I, O, U:** **A**cidosis **E**lectrolytes—hyperkalemia and hyperphosphatemia

Intoxication (e.g., lithium, theophylline,
   and alcohol)
Overload (volume)
Uremia—pericarditis and weight loss

CHRONIC RENAL FAILURE

What is CRF?

Decreased renal function on the basis of progressive and irreversible nephron destruction

What is the incidence of CRF?

The incidence of CRF is uncertain but increasing. Nearly 200,000 patients are being treated for ESRD in the United States.

What are the risk factors for CRF?

Family history of renal disease, DM, hypertension, increased age, African-American descent

What are the major causes of CRF?

DM (30%), hypertension (30%), glomerulonephritis (15%), polycystic kidney disease, and obstructive uropathy

What is uremia?

A clinical syndrome occurring in patients with overt renal failure

What are symptoms of uremia?

Lethargy, malaise, pruritus, anorexia, nausea, vomiting, impotence, leg cramping, dyspnea, and poor concentration

What are signs of uremia?

Ecchymoses, pallor, edema, rales, pleural effusions, hypertension, pericardial friction rub, cardiomegaly, and mental status changes

At what GFR does uremia occur?

Less than 20% of normal

How long must GFR be decreased to consider renal failure to be chronic?

Diagnosis can be made after 3–6 months of known decreased GFR.

What laboratory tests are indicated for patients with CRF?

Complete blood count and serum biochemistry profile (will reveal normochromic normocytic anemia, hypocalcemia, hyperkalemia, hyperphosphatemia), urinalysis, 24-hour urine test for protein and CrCl, and serum PTH level

What are the urinalysis findings for CRF?

Broad casts (> 2 WBCs in diameter), dilation and hypertrophy of the remaining nephrons, and proteinuria with or without hematuria

What is typically seen on renal ultrasound?

Bilaterally small (< 9 cm) and scarred kidneys

If normal or large kidneys are seen on renal ultrasound, what diagnoses should be suspected?

Polycystic kidney disease, amyloid, and DM

What diagnostic tests are ordered for CRF?

Radiographs for evidence of renal osteodystrophy (late finding) and IVP, which may also demonstrate decreased kidney size

What is the treatment for CRF?

Correct any reversible factors (see discussion of ARF), maintain normal electrolytes with supplementation and dietary restrictions, and avoid nephrotoxins.

What amount of acid is generated daily?

1 mEq/kg/day

What elements should be restricted in patients with CRF?

Potassium (salt substitutes are often high in potassium and are not recommended), protein, sodium, phosphorus, and fluids

What elements should be supplemented in patients with CRF?

Calcium, erythropoietin, vitamin D, and bicarbonate

When is dialysis indicated?
When there is persistent metabolic disarray despite use of restrictions and supplements, worsening acidosis, volume overload with pulmonary edema, pericardial friction rub, neuropathy, decreased mental status, and debilitating fatigue

How is remaining kidney function preserved?
BP control, possibly glucose control in diabetics, decrease in dietary protein, and avoidance of nephrotoxic drugs. Patients with CRF presenting with a sudden acute decline in renal function always require evaluation for reversible causes of ARF superimposed on their chronic disease.

What is ESRD?
Irreversible decrease in renal function requiring replacement therapy in the form of either dialysis or renal transplantation

What are the most common causes of ESRD?
DM (25%), hypertension (25%), glomerulonephritis (15%), and polycystic kidney disease (5%)

What is hemodialysis?
Filtering of blood by diffusion across a semipermeable membrane to remove toxins while adding required substances

What are the advantages of hemodialysis?
Hemodialysis clears dialyzable substances most effectively and can usually be done in three weekly sessions.

What are the disadvantages of hemodialysis?
Hemodialysis requires indwelling arteriovenous access and generally requires patients to visit a dialysis center.

What complications are associated with hemodialysis?
Shunt infection, hypotension, and chronic blood loss

What is peritoneal dialysis?
Instillation of dialysate solution into the peritoneal cavity, allowing toxins to passively diffuse into solution for removal

What are the advantages of peritoneal dialysis?	Peritoneal dialysis may be done at home, the patient has more freedom to travel, and it is generally well tolerated.
What are the disadvantages of peritoneal dialysis?	Peritoneal dialysis has longer treatment times and must be done up to five times a day with continuous ambulatory peritoneal dialysis; clearance of toxins is occasionally inadequate.
What complications are associated with peritoneal dialysis?	Catheter tunnel infections and peritonitis
What are CAVH and CVVHD?	Continuous arteriovenous hemofiltration and continuous venovenous hemofiltration and dialysis (modes of continuous hemodialysis)
What are the advantages of continuous hemodialysis?	Continuous hemodialysis can remove very large amounts of extracellular fluid and there is less hypotension than in other types of hemodialysis.
What are the disadvantages of continuous hemodialysis?	Continuous hemodialysis runs 24 hours per day, requires significant monitoring, and is restricted to use in critically ill patients.
What is an option to dialysis for patients with ESRD?	Renal transplantation

SODIUM AND WATER BALANCE

WATER

What factors affect water balance?	Water intake, renal and extrarenal water losses, and antidiuretic hormone levels
What percentage of body mass is water?	60% of weight for men; 50% of weight for women
What proportion of total body water is intracellular versus extracellular?	Intracellular, two thirds; extracellular, one third

What is normal osmolality?	285–295 mOsm/kg H_2O
How is osmolality estimated?	Serum osmoles = $[2(Na^+) + (BUN/2.8) + (glucose/18)]$

HYPOVOLEMIA

What is hypovolemia?	Low total body water
What are the causes of hypovolemia?	Extrarenal losses—sweating and skin losses from fever, exercise, and increased work of breathing Gastrointestinal losses—diarrhea and vomiting Renal losses—diuretic use, glucosuria secondary to diabetes, diabetes insipidus, and adrenal insufficiency Blood loss—hemorrhage Extracellular fluid sequestration—burns, pancreatitis, peritonitis, and "third spacing"
What are signs of hypovolemia?	Poor skin turgor, dry mucous membranes, dry axilla, flat neck veins, tachycardia, and orthostatic hypotension
What laboratory tests are ordered for hypovolemia?	Serum electrolytes including BUN and creatinine, urine electrolytes and specific gravity, and total protein and hematocrit, which may be increased due to hemoconcentration
How do you determine the H_2O deficit?	H_2O deficit = $0.6 \times$ weight in kg $\times [(Na^+/140) - 1]$
What is the treatment for hypovolemia?	Correction of underlying cause (e.g., insulin drip in DKA) Crystalloid—lactated Ringer's solution and normal saline Colloid—albumin, fresh-frozen plasma, red cells, and hetastarch

HYPERVOLEMIA

What is hypervolemia?	Excess total body water

What are the causes of hypervolemia?	Nephrotic syndrome, CHF, cirrhosis, ARF, CRF, and hypoproteinemia
What are symptoms and signs of hypervolemia?	Shortness of breath at rest or with exertion, JVD, rales, S3, hepatojugular reflex, ascites, and pitting edema
What laboratory tests are ordered for hypervolemia?	Serum electrolytes, urine specific gravity, 24-hour urine for CrCl (renal failure), serum albumin, total protein, cholesterol (nephrotic syndrome), liver enzymes, and bilirubin (cirrhosis)
What other diagnostic procedures are helpful?	Echocardiogram and abdominal ultrasound (to evaluate for ascites and liver size)
What is the treatment for hypervolemia?	Diuresis, dialysis if the case is severe, and large-volume paracentesis if ascites is present (depends on the underlying disorder)

HYPONATREMIA

What is hyponatremia?	Serum Na^+ < 135 mEq/L
What are symptoms and signs of hyponatremia?	Confusion, lethargy, stupor, coma, nausea, vomiting, headache, irritability, muscle twitches, and seizures (usually when hyponatremia develops rapidly)
What is the first step in the treatment of hyponatremia?	Establish the volume status.
What laboratory test is crucial to the diagnosis?	Serum osmolality
What causes iso-osmotic hyponatremia?	Pseudohyponatremia (hyperlipidemia and hyperproteinemia), isotonic infusions (e.g., glycine, glucose, mannitol, sorbitol, and ethanol), and laboratory error
What is the treatment of iso-osmotic hyponatremia?	Correct lipids and protein

What causes hyperosmotic hyponatremia?

Hyperglycemia or hypertonic infusions (e.g., glucose and mannitol)

What is the treatment for hyperosmotic hyponatremia?

Correct hyperglycemia and discontinue hypertonic fluids:
[corrected Na^+ = 0.016 (measured glu – 100) + measured Na^+]
Or, to estimate, add 1.5 mEq/L for every 100 mg/dl that the glucose is over 200. For example, if the measured Na^+ = 125 mEq/L with a serum glucose of 800 mg/dl, then the corrected Na^+ is 125 + (6 × 1.5) = 134 mEq/L.

What causes hypo-osmotic hyponatremia?

Depends on volume status

What causes hypovolemic hypo-osmotic hyponatremia?

Urine Na^+ > 20; renal losses—RTA, adrenal insufficiency, diuretics, partial obstruction, and salt-losing nephropathy
Urine Na^+ < 10; extrarenal losses— vomiting, diarrhea, skin and lung loss, and pancreatitis

What is the treatment for hypovolemic hypo-osmotic hyponatremia?

Na^+ deficit = (0.6 × weight in kg) × (140 – Na^+) replaced as isotonic saline

What causes euvolemic hypo-osmotic hyponatremia?

Urine Na^+ < 10; H_2O intoxication—renal failure, SIADH, hypothyroidism, pain, emotion, drugs, and adrenal insufficiency

What is the treatment for euvolemic hypo-osmotic hyponatremia?

Water restriction. If SIADH is resistant to water restriction, demeclocyline can be used.

What causes hypervolemic hypo-osmotic hyponatremia?

Urine Na^+ < 10—nephrotic syndrome, cirrhosis, and CHF
Urine Na^+ > 20—ARF, CRF, and iatrogenic volume overload

What is the treatment for hypervolemic hypo-osmotic hyponatremia?

Water restriction

HYPERNATREMIA

What is hypernatremia?	Serum $Na^+ > 145$ mEq/L
What causes hypervolemic hypernatremia?	More sodium retained than water—administration of hypertonic Na^+-containing solutions (e.g., $NaHCO_3$), Na^+ tablets, hypertonic infusions, mineralocorticoid excess (e.g., Cushing's syndrome, Conn's syndrome, and congenital adrenal hyperplasia), high renin states, hypertonic hemodialysis, peritoneal dialysis, and replacement of hypotonic fluid losses with normal saline
What is the treatment for hypervolemic hypernatremia?	Diuretics to promote sodium and water excretion and water replacement
What causes isovolemic hypernatremia?	Insensible skin and respiratory loss and diabetes insipidus (central and nephrogenic)
What laboratory tests are ordered for hypernatremia?	BUN and creatinine, urine Na^+, and urine osmolality. In cases of isovolemic hypernatremia, perform a fluid deprivation test to distinguish central from nephrogenic diabetes insipidus.
How is the fluid deprivation test performed?	1. Withhold fluids the day or night before testing. 2. Measure serum osmols until 295 mosm/kg H_2O is reached. 3. Measure urine osmols until values do not increase further or 5% weight loss occurs. 4. Administer 5 U of subcutaneous or 10 μg of intranasal vasopressin. 5. One hour later, remeasure urine osmols. In central diabetes insipidus, there is no change in urine osmolality. In nephrogenic diabetes insipidus, there is an increase in urine osmolality with vasopressin.

What is the treatment for isovolemic hypernatremia?

Water replacement. The H_2O deficit is calculated as follows:
H_2O deficit = $(0.6 \times$ weight in kg$) \times [(Na^+/140) - 1]$

At what rate should the H_2O deficit be corrected?

Correct half of the deficit in 24 hours. The rate of correction should not exceed 1 mEq/L/hr in acute hypernatremia or 0.5 mEq/L/hr in chronic hypernatremia.

What causes hypovolemic hypernatremia?

Loss of more water than sodium as follows:
Renal losses—diuretics, osmotic diuresis (e.g., glucose, urea, and mannitol), non-oliguric ATN, ARF, and CRF
Gastrointestinal losses—vomiting, diarrhea, nasogastric suction
Excess sweating
Respiratory losses
Adrenal deficiencies

What are symptoms and signs of hypernatremia?

Lethargy, confusion, restlessness, seizures, coma, hyperreflexia, and spasticity. Neurologic symptoms are due to dehydration of brain cells.

What is the treatment for hypovolemic hypernatremia?

Initially, isotonic NaCl is given to restore extracellular volume; then hypotonic saline is given.

Is there a limit as to how fast the Na^+ can be corrected?

Yes. The rate of correction of plasma osmolality should not exceed 2 mosm/kg/hr.

What is the danger of correcting hypernatremia too quickly?

Central pontine myelinolysis

ELECTROLYTES

HYPOKALEMIA

What is hypokalemia?

Serum potassium < 3.5 mEq/L

What causes hypokalemia?

Decreased dietary intake

Gastrointestinal losses—vomiting, diarrhea, fistulas, villous adenoma, and ureterosigmoidostomy

Renal losses—metabolic alkalosis, diuretics, polyuric phase of ATN diuresis, hypomagnesemia, drugs (e.g., amphotericin, aminoglycosides, cisplatin, and penicillins), renal tubular diseases (e.g., RTA, leukemia, and Liddle's syndrome), and mineralocorticoid excess (e.g., primary aldosteronism, secondary aldosteronism, malignant hypertension, Bartter's syndrome, licorice ingestion, Cushing's syndrome, exogenous glucocorticoid, and ectopic adrenocorticotropic hormone)

Cellular shifts—hypokalemic periodic paralysis, alkalosis, insulin effect, beta-agonists, and theophylline toxicity

What are symptoms and signs of hypokalemia?

Neuromuscular—muscle weakness, paralysis, rhabdomyolysis, and hyporeflexia

Gastrointestinal—paralytic ileus

Renal—polyuria, polydipsia, and secondary decreased concentrating ability

Cardiac—ECG findings include T-wave flattening and inversion, U wave, and ST segment depression. Hypokalemia enhances cardiac toxicity of digitalis.

What laboratory tests are ordered for hypokalemia?

Serum electrolytes, urine electrolytes, and possibly an ABG. Additional tests include measurement of plasma renin, aldosterone, and urinary cortisol.

What is the treatment for hypokalemia?

Serum K^+ of 3.0 mEq/L indicates a K^+ deficit > 300 mEq; K^+ of < 2.0 mEq/L indicates a deficit $\geq$ 1000 mEq.

1. Correct existing metabolic acidosis due to possible RTA, DKA, and diarrhea.
2. Administer intravenous KCl at 10 mEq/hr peripherally or 20 mEq/hr

centrally only if the patient cannot take it orally, in life-threatening situations, or if there are ECG abnormalities.

3. Administer oral KCl (elixir or tablets). As a rule, 10 mEq of potassium orally or intravenously increases serum potassium by approximately 0.1 mEq/L if the patient has a normal GFR.

HYPERKALEMIA

What is hyperkalemia?

Serum potassium > 5.0 mEq/L

What causes hyperkalemia?

1. Pseudohyperkalemia—test tube hemolysis, ischemic blood draw
2. Redistribution—acidosis, insulin deficiency, tissue necrosis, periodic paralysis, drugs and toxins, hemolysis, rhabdomyolysis, burns
3. Excessive intake with decreased excretion—K^+ replacement, K^+-penicillin, salt substitutes, diet
4. Decreased renal excretion—K^+-sparing diuretics (e.g., spironolactone, triamterene, and amiloride), type IV RTA, renal insufficiency, NSAIDs, ACE inhibitors, aldosterone deficiency, acquired unresponsiveness to aldosterone

What drugs and toxins cause redistribution?

Arginine, digitalis, beta-blockers, and succinylcholine

What diseases cause aldosterone unresponsiveness?

Lupus, myeloma, AIDS, diabetes, interstitial nephritis, and sickle cell anemia

What drugs lead to aldosterone deficiency?

ACE inhibitors and NSAIDs

What are the symptoms and signs of hyperkalemia?

Weakness, paresthesias, flaccid paralysis, ventricular fibrillation, and cardiac arrest

What are the ECG findings in hyperkalemia?

Peaked T waves, flattened P waves, prolonged PR, and widened QRS complex

What laboratory tests are ordered for hyperkalemia?	BUN, creatinine, urine and serum electrolytes, WBC, platelet count, ABG for pH, hematocrit, and CrCl
What procedures are performed for hyperkalemia?	ECG and bladder catheterization or ultrasound to rule out obstruction
What electrocardiographic findings are seen in patients with severe hyperkalemia?	Absent P waves, widened QRS complexes, "sine wave" patterns, and arrhythmias
What is the treatment for severe cases of hyperkalemia?	Calcium gluconate, 10–30 ml in 10% solution intravenously (for membrane stabilization) Sodium bicarbonate, 50 mEq intravenously (shifts K^+ into cells) Glucose–insulin, 1 ampule D_{50} with 5 U regular insulin (shifts K^+ into cells) Sodium polystyrene sulfonate, 50–100 g enema with 50 ml 70% sorbitol and 100 ml tap water, or 20–40 g orally (removes excess K^+ through the gastrointestinal tract) Dialysis when the case is complicated by volume overload, acidosis, or severe uremia (removes K^+ from serum)
What is treatment for mild cases of hyperkalemia?	Oral sodium polystyrene
What is treatment for chronic cases of hyperkalemia?	K^+ restriction, loop diuretics, oral bicarbonate therapy, discontinuation of ACE inhibitors, NSAIDs, and mineralocorticoids

HYPOCALCEMIA

What is hypocalcemia?	Serum calcium < 8.5 mg/dl
What causes hypocalcemia?	Low PTH levels or impaired function of PTH—hypothyroidism, magnesium deficiency or excess, sepsis, and severe bone diseases

Vitamin D deficiency—pancreatic insufficiency, partial gastrectomy, intestinal bypass, and sprue
25(OH) D$_3$ deficiency—hypoparathyroidism, severe liver disease, and seizure medications
Magnesium deficiency
Pseudohypoparathyroidism
Calcium shifts, chelation, or precipitation—EDTA, citrate, calcitonin, albumin, ethylene glycol, toxic shock syndrome, hungry bones syndrome, tumor lysis syndrome, rhabdomyolysis, and iatrogenic

What are symptoms and signs of hypocalcemia?

Cardiovascular—hypotension, bradycardia, asystole, impaired contractility, QT prolongation, and T-wave inversion on ECG, and digitalis insensitivity
Respiratory—bronchospasm and laryngeal spasm
Neuromuscular—weakness, paresthesias, tetany, muscle spasm, Chvostek's and Trousseau's signs, hyperreflexia, and seizures
Psychiatric—anxiety, depression, irritability, confusion, dementia, and psychosis

What laboratory tests are ordered for hypocalcemia?

Calcium and albumin. Thirty percent to 60% of the total calcium is bound to albumin. For each gram of albumin below 4, add 0.8 to the calcium value to correct for hypoalbuminemia. Ionized calcium (not affected by albumin) is the physiologically active amount and the most accurate measurement. Normal range is 4.5–5.0 mg/dl). If ionized calcium is low, check magnesium, phosphorus, BUN, and creatinine to rule out ARF or CRF. Sometimes PTH is needed.

What is the treatment for symptomatic cases of hypocalcemia?

Calcium gluconate bolus intravenously (100–200 mg over 10 minutes) followed by 0.3–2 mg/kg/hr with frequent checks of ionized calcium. Hyperphosphatemia must be corrected first to prevent precipitation with the calcium. Low or high magnesium levels must be corrected as well.

What is the treatment for asymptomatic cases of hypocalcemia?

Oral calcium supplementation, 1 g/day of elemental calcium, and vitamin D replacement if deficient

HYPERCALCEMIA

What is hypercalcemia?

Serum calcium > 10.5 mg/dl

What causes 90% of cases of hypercalcemia?

Hyperparathyroidism and malignancies

What are the associated malignancies?

PTH-related protein producers—lung, esophagus, head and neck, renal cell, ovary, and bladder cancers
Vitamin D producers—lymphoma
Lytic metastases—multiple myeloma, breast, and prostate

What other endocrine disorders are associated with hypercalcemia?

Thyrotoxicosis, vasoactive intestinal polypeptide (VIP) tumors, pheochromocytoma, and adrenal insufficiency

What granulomatous diseases are associated with hypercalcemia?

Sarcoid, TB, histoplasmosis, coccidioidomycosis, berylliosis, and leprosy

What drugs are associated with hypercalcemia?

Vitamins A and D, thiazides, lithium, estrogens and antiestrogens, aminophylline, and aluminum intoxication (in CRF)

What are other causes of hypercalcemia?

Milk–alkali syndrome, immobilization, familial hypocalciuric hypercalcemia, TPN, and hemoconcentration. Think **CHIMPANZEES:**
Calcium supplementation intravenously (TPN)
Hyperparathyroidism (1°, 2°, 3°), hyperthyroidism
Idiopathic, iatrogenic immobility
Milk–alkali syndrome, metastases

Paget's disease, pheochromocytoma
Adrenal insufficiency, acromegaly
Neoplasms (colon, lung, breast, prostate,
multiple myeloma)
Zollinger-Ellison syndrome
Excessive vitamin D
Excessive vitamin A
Sarcoidosis, TB, histoplamosis

What are symptoms and signs of hypercalcemia?

Also known as "stones, bones, groans, and psychiatric overtones."
Cardiovascular—hypertension, bradycardia, first-degree AV block, increased repolarization, shortened QT interval
Gastrointestinal—constipation, anorexia, nausea and vomiting, peptic ulcer disease, pancreatitis
Renal—polyuria and polydipsia, nocturia, renal insufficiency, nephrolithiasis
Musculoskeletal—weakness, myopathy, osteoporosis, bone pain
Neurologic—decreased concentration, depression, confusion, psychosis, coma
Other—pruritus, metastatic calcification

What laboratory tests are ordered for hypercalcemia?

Calcium, albumin, alkaline phosphatase, magnesium, BUN, creatinine, 24-hour urine calcium, and PTH

What is the treatment for severe hypercalcemia?

1. Hydration with normal saline for repletion and to increase calcium excretion
2. Loop diuretic to enhance calciuria by inhibiting reabsorption in the thick ascending limb of the loop of Henle
3. Biphosphonates (e.g., etidronate, pamidronate, clodronate) to bind to hydroxyapatite and inhibit dissolution of crystals
4. Plicamycin to inhibit RNA synthesis in osteoclasts
5. Calcitonin to inhibit bone resorption, increase renal calcium excretion, and induce a rapid decrease in calcium
6. Gallium to reduce solubility of hydroxyapatite crystals

7. Glucocorticoids to counteract the action of vitamin D and to inhibit growth of neoplastic lymphoid tissue
8. Phosphate, which is restricted to use in extreme, life-threatening hypercalcemia and when all other measures fail because of its risk of precipitation with calcium

What is the treatment for mild hypercalcemia?

See steps 1 through 3 for treatment of severe hypercalcemia.

What is the treatment for chronic hypercalcemia?

Oral hydration and oral biphosphonate

HYPERPHOSPHATEMIA

What is hyperphosphatemia?

Serum phosphate > 5 mg/dl

What causes hyperphosphatemia?

1. Decreased renal excretion—dehydration, ARF, CRF
2. Enhanced tubular reabsorption—thyrotoxicosis, hypoparathyroidism, pseudohypoparathyroidism, abnormal circulating PTH, acromegaly, tumor calcinosis, rhabdomyolysis
3. Increased release of intracellular phosphate—bone metastases, tumor lysis syndrome, leukemia, lymphoma, hypercatabolism, respiratory acidosis, DKA, hemolysis
4. Administration of phosphate salts or vitamin D

What are symptoms and signs of hyperphosphatemia?

Pruritus; otherwise, symptoms are unremarkable

What laboratory tests are ordered for hyperphosphatemia?

Serum phosphate with other electrolytes, possibly thyroid function tests and PTH

What is the treatment for hyperphosphatemia?

Dietary phosphate restriction, phosphate binders (e.g., calcium acetate or carbonate), hydration to promote excretion, correction of acidosis, and D_{50} and insulin to shift phosphate into cells

HYPOPHOSPHATEMIA

What is hypophosphatemia?	Serum phosphate < 2.5 mg/dl
What level of serum phosphate induces symptoms?	< 1 mg/dl
What causes hypophosphatemia?	1. Increased excretion—hyperparathryroidism, RTA, diuretics, polyuric phase of ATN, following renal transplantation, extracellular volume expansion, Fanconi's syndrome, glycosuria 2. Defective vitamin D metabolism—vitamin D–dependent and vitamin D–deficient rickets, familial hypophosphatemia 3. Defective gastrointestinal absorption—malabsorption, vomiting and diarrhea, nasogastric suction, administration of phosphate binders, malnutrition 4. Cellular shifts—severe respiratory alkalosis, refeeding syndrome, alcohol withdrawal syndrome, toxic shock syndrome
What are symptoms and signs of hypophosphatemia?	Weakness, lethargy, irritability, depressed cardiac and respiratory function, hypotension, cardiac arrhythmias, red and white cell dysfunction, and skeletal demineralization
What laboratory tests are ordered for hypophosphatemia?	Other electrolytes, calcium, and ABG. A 24-hour urinary phosphate level < 100 mg/day suggests gastrointestinal losses or redistribution; levels > 100 mg/day suggest renal excretion (consider recovering PTH)
What is the treatment for hypophosphatemia?	Daily dietary intake of 1000 mg/day. If respiratory or cardiac depression or arrhythmia occurs, give 0.2 mmol/kg of KPO_4 or $NaPO_4$ intravenously over 6 hours with the goal of reaching a

phosphate level of 2.5 mg/dl. If
administered too rapidly, calcium
phosphate precipitation can result.

HYPOMAGNESEMIA

What is hypomagnesemia?

Serum magnesium < 1.8 mg/dl

**What causes
hypomagnesemia?**

1. Gastrointestinal—decreased intake or
   malabsorption
2. Increased renal losses—loop or
   thiazide diuretics, RTA, diuretic
   phase of ATN, DKA,
   hyperaldosteronism, hyperthyroidism,
   hyperparathyroidism
3. Drugs—ethanol, cyclosporine,
   amphotericin, digoxin, cisplatin,
   pentamidine, gentamicin, ticarcillin,
   carbenicillin

**What are symptoms and
signs of hypomagnesemia?**

Cardiovascular—arrhythmias (e.g., atrial
fibrillation and torsades de pointes),
prolonged PR and QT intervals,
T-wave flattening
Neuromuscular—weakness, seizures,
delirium, coma, hyperreflexia,
fasciculations, Chvostek's and
Trousseau's signs

**What other electrolytes,
when depleted, are
resistant to repletion when
Mg^{2+} is low?**

Potassium and calcium

**What laboratory tests are
used to evaluate
hypomagnesemia?**

Serum Mg^{2+} and 24-hour urine
collection for Mg^{2+} when gastrointestinal
causes are ruled out

**What Mg^{2+} level is
considered severely low?**

< 1 mg/dl or when the patient is
symptomatic

**What is the treatment for
severe hypomagnesemia?**

2 g $MgSO_4$ intravenously over 60
minutes with ECG and BP monitoring

**What is the treatment for
moderate
hypomagnesemia?**

6 g $MgSO_4$ intravenously infused over 6
hours, then titrated to the serum level

What is the treatment for mild hypomagnesemia?	420–840 mg magnesium oxide orally one to two times per day

HYPERMAGNESEMIA

What is hypermagnesemia?	Serum magnesium > 2.3 mg/dl
What causes hypermagnesemia?	1. Decreased renal function—CrCl < 30 ml/min 2. Increased intake—abuse of Mg^{2+}-containing antacids and laxatives by patients with renal insufficiency 3. Iatrogenic—overtreatment of hypomagnesemia
What are the symptoms and signs of hypermagnesemia?	Respiratory—respiratory depression, apnea Cardiovascular—hypotension, cardiac arrest, ECG findings (prolonged QRS complexes and QT intervals, heart block, peaked T waves) Gastrointestinal—nausea and vomiting Neuromuscular—paresthesias, somnolence, confusion, coma, hyporeflexia, paralysis, apnea
What laboratory tests are ordered for hypermagnesemia?	Serum magnesium, BUN, creatinine, and calcium
What does increased serum Mg^{2+} do to PTH?	Suppresses PTH secretion
What is the treatment for acute cases of hypermagnesemia?	Calcium infusion (increases excretion of magnesium), especially in the setting of cardiac conduction abnormalities Saline infusion with a loop diuretic (also increases excretion) Dialysis
What is the treatment for chronic hypermagnesemia?	Restriction of leafy green vegetables, grain, and dairy products and avoidance of magnesium-containing antacids and laxatives

ACID–BASE BALANCE

What tests are used to evaluate acid–base balance?	ABG and electrolytes

How do you rule out a laboratory error (i.e., is the ABG internally consistent)?	**[H⁺]**	**pH**
	25	7.60
	32	7.50
	40	7.40
	50	7.30
	63	7.20
	79	7.10
	100	7.00

What is a quick equation to verify a pH between 7.26 and 7.45?

$[H^+]$ = 80 – the last two digits of the pH

What is the normal pH?

7.38–7.42

What pH values determine acidemia and alkalemia?

Acidemia, pH < 7.38
Alkalemia, pH > 7.42

How do you determine whether a problem is metabolic or respiratory?

	Metabolic	**Respiratory**
Acidosis	HCO_3^- < 24	P_{CO_2} > 40
Alkalosis	HCO_3^- > 24	P_{CO_2} < 40

What is an anion gap?

The difference between the serum anions that are measured in a chemistry profile and the unmeasured anions

What is a normal anion gap?

< 10–12

How do you calculate the anion gap?

$Na^+ - [Cl^- + HCO_3^-]$

When anion-gap metabolic acidosis is present, how do you correct the HCO_3^- level to check for a secondary acid–base disturbance?

Corrected HCO_3^- = measured HCO_3^- + (anion gap - 12). If the corrected HCO_3^- > 24, then a metabolic alkalosis is also present; if the corrected HCO_3^- < 24, then both gap and nongap metabolic acidosis are present.

METABOLIC ACIDOSIS

Are the pH, P_{CO_2}, and HCO_3 high or low in metabolic acidosis?

pH, low; P_{CO_2}, low; HCO_3^-, low

What is appropriate compensation for metabolic acidosis?

Expected $P_{CO_2} = [1.5 \times HCO_3^-] + 8$ (± 2). If the expected P_{CO_2} is greater than the observed P_{CO_2}, then a respiratory alkalosis is also present; if the expected P_{CO_2} is less than the observed P_{CO_2}, then a respiratory acidosis is also present. (The expected P_{CO_2} should be equal to the last two digits of the pH.)

What is the differential diagnosis for anion-gap acidosis?

Think **MUDPILES**:
Methanol
Uremia
DKA, ketoacidosis
Paraldehyde
Iron, **I**soniazid (INH)
Lactic acidosis
Ethanol, ethylene glycol
Salicylates

What are the clues, symptoms, and signs of anion-gap acidosis?

Intoxication, history of ingestion or drug use, tinnitus, oliguria, fruity breath, renal failure, hypotension, shock, and tachypnea (Kussmaul's breathing)

What laboratory tests are ordered for anion-gap acidosis?

BUN, creatinine, glucose, serum and urine ketones, lactic acid, ethanol level, methanol level, salicylate level, osmolal gap, and urinalysis for oxalate crystals

What is the treatment for anion-gap acidosis?

Treatment is based on the underlying cause.

Which toxins can be removed with dialysis?

Methanol, ethanol, ethylene glycol, and salicylates

What is the differential diagnosis for nongap acidosis?

Think **HARDUPS**:
Hyperalimentation
Acetazolamide (any carbonic anhydrase inhibitor), amphotericin
RTA
Diarrhea
Ureteral diversions

Pancreatic fistulae
Saline resuscitation

What laboratory tests are ordered for nongap acidosis?	Urinary anion gap (U_{AG})
What is the equation to calculate the urinary anion gap?	$U_{AG} = (U_{Na} + U_K) - U_{Cl}$
How are negative and positive urinary anion gaps interpreted?	During normal kidney acidification, U_{AG} is negative because there is unmeasured cation excretion (i.e., NH_4^+); in impaired acidification, U_{AG} is positive.
What is treatment for nongap acidosis?	Discontinuation of culprit medications, treatment of underlying causes, and administration of low-dose oral HCO_3^- (e.g., Polycitra, sodium bicarbonate, and Shohl solution)
What is the differential diagnosis for a low anion gap?	Think **PLEAB:**

Paraproteinemias and multiple myeloma
    (nonsodium cations and
    underestimation of serum sodium)
Lithium intoxication (nonsodium cation)
Excessive calcium and magnesium
Albumin—hypoalbuminemia (reduced
    unmeasured cations)
Bromism (overestimation of chloride)

METABOLIC ALKALOSIS

In a primary metabolic alkalosis, are the pH, P_{CO_2}, and HCO_3^- expected to be high or low?	pH, high; P_{CO_2}, high; HCO_3^-, high
What are the categories of metabolic alkalosis?	Chloride-responsive and chloride-unresponsive
What is the differential diagnosis for the following: **Chloride-responsive metabolic alkalosis?**	Volume contraction, vomiting, nasogastric suction, and diuretics Post-hypercapnia state Hypokalemia, hypomagnesemia Carbenicillin, penicillin

Chloride-unresponsive metabolic alkalosis?	Adrenal disorders (e.g., glucocorticoid or mineralocorticoid excess) Exogenous steroids Alkali ingestion, Bartter's syndrome, or licorice ingestion
What are the symptoms and signs of metabolic alkalosis?	Muscle cramps, weakness, hypoxia, and cardiac arrhythmias
What laboratory tests are ordered for metabolic alkalosis?	Cl⁻, K⁺, Mg⁺, PO₄, urine electrolytes, and possibly a 24-hour urine collection for cortisol
What is the treatment for metabolic alkalosis?	Volume repletion with saline (in chloride responsive cases), correction of K⁺, Mg⁺, and PO₄ depletion, spironolactone for hyperaldosteronism, and treatment of the underlying process

RESPIRATORY ACIDOSIS

Are the expected pH, P_{CO_2}, and HCO_3^- values for respiratory acidosis high or low?	pH, low; P_{CO_2}, high; HCO_3^-, high
How much does the pH change with the increase in P_{CO_2}?	Δ pH = (P_{CO_2} - 40) × 0.03 if chronic Δ pH = (P_{CO_2} - 40) × 0.08 if acute > 0.03 but < 0.08 = acute superimposed on chronic respiratory acidosis
What is the differential diagnosis for respiratory acidosis?	CNS—sedatives, trauma, infection, neoplasm Pulmonary disease—pneumothorax, pleural effusion, chronic obstructive pulmonary disease, adult respiratory distress syndrome, pneumonia, pulmonary embolism, thoracic cage restriction (e.g., kyphosis, scleroderma, and injuries), improper ventilator settings Musculoskeletal disease—neuropathies and myopathies (e.g., Guillain-Barré syndrome, polio, myasthenia gravis, and muscular dystrophies)

What are the symptoms and signs of respiratory acidosis?

Headache, dyspnea, respiratory distress, increased intracranial pressure, tachypnea, and obtundation

What is the treatment for respiratory acidosis?

Restoration of adequate ventilation with intubation if necessary

RESPIRATORY ALKALOSIS

Are the expected pH, P_{CO_2}, and HCO_3 values high or low in a primary respiratory alkalosis?

pH, high; P_{CO_2}, low; HCO_3^-, low

How much does the pH change with the decrease in P_{CO_2}?

Δ pH = (40 - P_{CO_2}) × 0.03 if chronic
Δ pH = (40 - P_{CO_2}) × 0.08 if acute
> 0.03 but < 0.08 = acute superimposed on chronic respiratory alkalosis
Note: exact opposite of respiratory acidosis

What is the differential diagnosis for respiratory alkalosis?

CNS—increased respiratory drive, infection, CVA, trauma, increased chemoreceptor stimulation, anxiety
Pulmonary—pulmonary edema, pneumonia, pulmonary emboli, improper ventilator settings
Drugs—salicylates, catechols, progesterones
Sepsis, fever
Pregnancy, liver disease, anemia
Carbon monoxide toxicity

What are the symptoms and signs of respiratory alkalosis?

Hyperventilation, perioral and extremity paresthesias, muscle cramps, tachypnea, hyperreflexia, seizures, and cardiac arrhythmias

What is treatment for respiratory alkalosis?

Elimination of the underlying cause

NEPHROLITHIASIS

What is nephrolithiasis?

Solute precipitation from supersaturated urine leading to crystallization and stone formation along the urinary tract

What is the incidence of nephrolithiasis?

1%–5% in the United States, with recurrences commonly occurring every 2–3 years. The southeast region of the United States is called the "stone belt" in association with its climate and prevalent diet.

What dietary risk factors are associated with nephrolithiasis?

Decreased fluid intake, increased dairy intake, supplemental calcium and vitamins C and D, and malabsorptive syndromes

What other risk factors are associated with nephrolithiasis?

Multiple UTIs, gout, family history, hyperparathyroidism, steroids, history of RTA, and small bowel diseases or surgery

What are symptoms of nephrolithiasis?

Abrupt onset of severe flank pain, which can intensify over 15–30 minutes to cause nausea and vomiting and then remit (renal colic), with radiation of pain to the groin

What are the signs of nephrolithiasis?

Gross or microscopic hematuria, crystalluria, urine pH > 7.5 associated with struvite stones formed by bacteria producing urease (e.g., *Proteus* species)

What are the types of stones?

Calcium oxalate dihydrate stones (75%–85%)
Uric acid stones (5%–8%)
Struvite stones (10%–15%)
Cystine stones (1%)

What workup is necessary for nephrolithiasis?

Urine studies of calcium, sodium, oxalate, uric acid, citrate, and cystine, repeated urine cultures, and stone analysis
Serum calcium, ionized calcium, albumin, phosphate, alkaline phosphatase, bicarbonate, parathyroid hormone, and creatinine

What diagnostic tests are used for nephrolithiasis?

Radiographic study—detects radiopaque stones [85%–90% of stones made up of calcium phosphate, calcium oxalate, magnesium-ammonium phosphate (struvite), and cystine]. Radiolucent

stones are the 10%–15% of stones made up of uric acid.
IVP
Ultrasound

In general, what is the therapy for nephrolithiasis?

Avoid dehydration and use pain control when needed.

CALCIUM OXALATE STONES

What is absorptive hypercalciuria?

Intestinal hyperabsorption of calcium. Hypercalciuria results from increased filtered load and reduced renal reabsorption.

What is renal hypercalciuria?

Impairment in renal tubular reabsorption

What is the treatment for both absorptive hypercalciuria and renal hypercalciuria?

Thiazides and potassium citrate

What causes resorptive hypercalciuria?

Hyperparathyroidism (increased filtered load of calcium)

What is the treatment for resorptive hypercalciuria?

Parathyroidectomy

What causes hyperuricosuria?

Increased intake of purine-rich foods. Urate crystals form a nidus for calcium oxalate precipitation.

What is the treatment for hyperuricosuria?

Potassium citrate if uric acid excretion is low; allopurinol if uric acid excretion is high

What causes hyperoxaluria?

Intestinal hyperabsorption of oxalate, usually from small bowel inflammation, resection, or bypass

What is the treatment for hyperoxaluria?

Potassium citrate and magnesium gluconate

What are the causes of hypocitraturia?

Acidosis from strenuous exercise, RTA, high-protein diet, or idiopathic causes decrease citrate. Citrate in the urine inhibits crystallization of calcium salts.

What is the treatment for hypocitraturia?	Potassium citrate

OTHER STONES

What causes uric acid stones?	Increased intake of purine-rich foods, purine overproduction, and diarrheal illnesses
What is the treatment for uric acid stones?	Potassium citrate or D-penicillamine
What causes cystine stones?	Inborn error of metabolism and a low solubility constant
What is the treatment for cystine stones?	Low methionine diet, increased fluid intake, and potassium citrate
What causes struvite stones?	Magnesium-ammonium phosphate stones are caused by urea-splitting bacteria, most commonly *Proteus* (urine pH > 7.5). These may form staghorn calculus.
What is the treatment for struvite stones?	Eradication of infection
What is ESWL?	Ultrasound or laser shock waves directed at stone
What is percutaneous lithotripsy?	A percutaneous needle is passed through the collecting system and is used to guide a nephroscope, which either removes or pulverizes the stone.
What is a dormia basket extractor?	A basket used to extract stones
What treatment is used for stones in the following:	
Kidney	ESWL
Upper ureter	Push stone retrograde to renal pelvis for ESWL.
Midureter	Ureteroscope, J-stent

Lower ureter	Dormia basket extractor
Large stones	Percutaneous or open surgery

GLOMERULAR DISEASES

What is nephrotic range proteinuria?	Proteinuria > 3.5 g/day
What is nephrotic syndrome?	Proteinuria > 3.5 g/day, hypoalbuminemia, and edema
What are other manifestations of nephrotic syndrome?	Hyperlipidemia, hypertension, decreased renal function, hypercoagulability, and renal vein thrombosis
What is nephritic syndrome?	Hematuria, pyuria, cellular casts, and variable proteinuria
What is acute glomerulonephritis?	Rapid onset of hematuria, edema, hypertension, proteinuria, cellular casts, and decreased renal function
What is RPGN?	Hematuria, proteinuria, and cellular casts, with doubling of serum creatinine in less than 12 weeks

MINIMAL CHANGE DISEASE

What is minimal change disease?	The most common cause of nephrotic syndrome in children, occurring as an idiopathic or secondary disease. There are minimal histologic changes (normal glomeruli shown on light microscopy) and fusion of epithelial foot processes shown on electron microscopy.
What are the secondary causes of minimal change disease?	Lymphoma, leukemia, amyloidosis, and exposure to NSAIDs, lithium, gold, ampicillin, or rifampin
What is the clinical presentation of minimal change disease?	Normal to mildly reduced renal function, hematuria, and nephrotic syndrome

What is the treatment for minimal change disease?	Children—steroids (90% response rate) Adults—steroids (slightly less responsive than children, but some cases spontaneously resolve) Secondary causes—removal of the offending drug or agent, or treatment of the underlying disease

FOCAL SEGMENTAL GLOMERULOSCLEROSIS

What is focal segmental glomerulosclerosis?	A common cause of idiopathic nephrotic syndrome. Histologic study reveals segmental sclerosis of some of glomeruli.
What are secondary causes of focal segmental glomerulosclerosis?	AIDS (seen in blacks), heroin use, massive obesity, malignancy, and reflux nephropathy
What is the clinical presentation of focal segmental glomerulosclerosis?	Nephrotic syndrome or proteinuria, hematuria, hypertension, and renal insufficiency
What is the treatment for focal segmental glomerulosclerosis?	Less than one third of cases respond to steroids, and there may be recurrence in transplanted kidney.

DIABETIC NEPHROPATHY

In what proportion of type 1 and type 2 diabetic patients does nephropathy (DN) develop?	Type 1, 40%; type 2, 10% (more in certain ethnic groups)
What ethnic groups are predisposed to DN?	Blacks, Mexican-Americans, and Pima Indians
What is the histopathology of DN?	Nodular and diffuse glomerulosclerosis with increased mesangial matrix and GBM thickening
What is a Kimmelstiel-Wilson lesion?	Nodules in the mesangium extending into capillary wall. These lesions are pathognomonic for DN.

What is the clinical presentation of DN?	Asymptomatic Benign urine sediment Microalbuminuria (> 20 mg/day of albumin in urine; the earliest sign) Retinopathy already present when DN occurs in type 1 Retinopathy and DN not as tightly associated in type 2
What is the clinical course of DN?	An increase in GFR with overt proteinuria and hypertension. Eventually GFR decreases roughly 10 ml/min/yr.
What may prevent or reverse early DN?	Intensive glucose control
What may slow the rate of decline in GFR?	ACE inhibitors, strict BP control, protein restriction, and intensive glucose control

AMYLOIDOSIS AND LIGHT CHAIN DEPOSITION DISEASE

How common is the renal involvement in amyloidosis?	Occurs in 90% of primary and secondary cases
What is the histopathology of amyloidosis?	Diffuse glomerular deposition of hyaline and nodule formation Congo red staining reveals green birefringence on polarized light. Amyloid fibrils (AA) can be seen on electron microscopy.
How does light chain deposition disease differ from amyloidosis?	1. Light chain deposits cannot form amyloid fibrils. 2. There is a granular appearance on electron microscopy, commonly kappa light chain. 3. Immunofluorescence is strongly positive for light chains. (In amyloid, immunofluorescence is negative.)
How does secondary amyloid affect the kidney?	Chronic inflammatory diseases stimulate amyloid A production in the liver, which is deposited in the kidney as AA.

What is the clinical presentation of amyloidosis and light chain deposition?	Proteinuria, edema, weight loss, and fatigue. The classic signs of amyloidosis (e.g., hepatomegaly, splenomegaly, macroglossia, CHF, and carpal tunnel syndrome) are frequently absent.
How do you diagnose amyloidoisis and light chain deposition?	Abdominal, rectal, skin, kidney, liver, or fat pad biopsy

What is the treatment for the following:

Primary amyloidosis	Melphalan and prednisone
Light chain deposition disease	No effective treatment; poor prognosis
Secondary amyloidosis	Treatment of the primary disease

IgA NEPHROPATHY

What is IgA nephropathy (Berger's disease)?	The most common glomerulonephritis worldwide. It is usually idiopathic and can be associated with advanced liver disease and intestinal and pulmonary diseases.
What is the histopathology of IgA nephropathy?	IgA deposits in the mesangium, mesangial cellularity, and increased matrix.
What is the clinical presentation of IgA nephropathy?	Incidental microscopic hematuria or recurrent episodic gross hematuria and proteinuria Occurrence 3–5 days after an upper respiratory infection or a gastrointestinal infection Rarely nephrotic syndrome
What are clues that lead to diagnosis of IgA nephropathy?	Lack of family history of renal disease or hematuria (e.g., Alport's syndrome), normal complement levels, and lack of systemic illness
What is the clinical course of IgA nephropathy?	Good prognosis overall but ESRD develops in up to 20% of cases

What is the treatment for IgA nephropathy?	None proven

POSTINFECTIOUS GLOMERULONEPHRITIS

What causes postinfectious glomerulonephritis (PSGN)?	Bacterial, viral, or parasitic infections
What is the pathogenesis of PSGN?	Circulating immune complexes deposit in the kidney and cause white blood cell infiltration, which leads to crescent formation and necrosis.
What is the histopathology of PSGN?	Intense glomerular hypercellularity, mesangial proliferation, narrowed capillary lumens, crescents, and necrosis IgG and C3 deposition shown on immunofluorescence Diagnostic immune deposits called "humps" shown on electron microscopy
What is the most common pathogen of PSGN?	Group A beta-hemolytic streptococci (certain strains)
What is the clinical presentation of PSGN?	It follows 10 days after pharyngitis or 21 days after impetigo and is more common in children. (If PSGN occurs after 5 days or less, consider IgA nephropathy.) "Coca-Cola" urine and bilateral flank pain are common.
What are the signs of PSGN?	Gross hematuria, mild hypertension, edema, and oliguria
What are the laboratory findings of PSGN?	Red blood cell and other casts, pyuria, and proteinuria on urinalysis Elevated creatinine, low complement levels, increased rheumatoid factor, cryoglobulins, and elevated plasma ASO titer
What is the treatment for PSGN?	Supportive treatment and antibiotics for infection

What is the prognosis for PSGN?	Almost all patients recover from acute episodes.
What other specific bacterial infections cause identical renal manifestations?	Bacterial endocarditis (*Staphylococcus aureus* or *Streptococcus viridans*) and an infected ventriculoatrial shunt (*S. aureus*)

MEMBRANOPROLIFERATIVE GLOMERULONEPHRITIS

How common is MPGN?	It is an uncommon cause of glomerulonephritis.
For MPGN, what are the associated infections?	Hepatitis B/C, bacterial endocarditis, infected ventriculoatrial shunts, visceral abscesses, and schistosomiasis
What malignancies are associated with MPGN?	Chronic lymphocytic leukemia and malignant melanoma
What drugs are associated with MPGN?	Chlorpropamide and heroin
What deficiency states are associated with MPGN?	Complement deficiencies and alpha$_1$-antitrypsin deficiency
What are the types of idiopathic MPGN and how do they differ?	Type 1—discrete mesangial and subendothelial deposits Type 2—continuous, dense deposits on basement membranes
What is a common histopathologic finding in both MPGN type 1 and MPGN type 2?	Mesangial hypercellularity and thickening of basement membrane with deposition of new basement membrane (tram tracks)
What are the clinical presentations of MPGN types 1 and 2?	Cellular and granular casts with proteinuria in all patients Normal or elevated creatinine Low complement levels Acute hematuria, edema, hypertension (like PSGN) Episodic hematuria (like IgA nephropathy) Incidentally discovered hematuria and proteinuria Nephrotic syndrome

What signs suggest diagnosis of MPGN?	Hypocomplementemia without signs of lupus or PSGN
What is the clinical course of MPGN?	Slow decline in renal function to ESRD
What is the treatment for MPGN?	Uncertain—steroids and antiplatelet agents given in progressive disease; renal transplantation undertaken for ESRD
How common is recurrence of MPGN in the transplant?	Type 1, 30%; type 2, 90%. Loss of transplant secondary to recurrence is rare.

LUPUS NEPHRITIS

What are the types of lupus nephritis (by World Health Organization classification)?	Class I—normal (no deposits) Class II—mesangial (mesangial deposits) Class III—focal proliferative (focal and segmental with mesangial and subendothelial deposits; if crescents and necrosis are present, < 50% of glomeruli are involved) Class IV—diffuse proliferative (diffuse deposits and sclerosis; > 50% of glomeruli are involved) Class V—membranous (thickened basement membrane)
What types of deposits are seen by immunofluorescence?	IgG, C3, C4, IgM, IgA ("full house")
What is the pathogenesis of lupus nephritis?	Autoantibodies deposit in the kidney and cause complement activation. Immune complexes initially form in the mesangium (class II) but may spill over into the subendothelial space (classes III and IV).
What class is most commonly seen at biopsy?	Class IV—diffuse proliferative
What class has the worst prognosis if untreated?	Class IV—diffuse proliferative

Which drugs cause a lupus-like reaction?

Hydralazine, procainamide, quinidine, INH, methyldopa, and β blockers (all are less likely to cause nephritis)

Which classes tend to present as a nephritic syndrome?

Classes III and IV—focal and diffuse proliferative

Which class tends to present as a nephrotic syndrome?

Class V—membranous

What serologic tests suggest the diagnosis of lupus nephritis?

High ANA titer, double-stranded DNA, and low C3 and C4 levels

Which class can present with negative serologic results and precede systemic illness?

Class V—membranous

What is the treatment for the following:
Class I and II?

No treatment. The proteinuria in mesangial deposits can even spontaneously resolve.

Class III and V?

Prednisone or observation

Class IV?

Cyclophosphamide monthly for 6–8 months, then every 3 months for 1–3 years, and prednisone

What percentage of patients with lupus nephritis develop ESRD?

30%

Does lupus nephritis recur in the transplanted kidney?

Rarely. Transplantation and dialysis are associated with a remission of systemic disease.

HEREDITARY NEPHRITIS

What is hereditary nephritis (Alport's syndrome)?

Rare progressive glomerular disease mostly affecting males. It is associated with deafness and lenticular defects.

What is the histopathology of hereditary nephritis?	Longitudinal splitting of basement membranes and absence of normal glomerular basement antigen
What are the inheritance patterns?	X-linked dominant, autosomal dominant (but associated with the X chromosome), and rarely autosomal recessive
What are the symptoms of hereditary nephritis?	High-pitch sensorineural hearing loss, cataracts, and recurrent episodes of gross hematuria
What are the signs of hereditary nephritis?	Normal BP and GFR at presentation, gross or microscopic hematuria, and normal complement levels. Hearing loss and hematuria begin in childhood but may go unnoticed.
What is the clinical course of hereditary nephritis?	Cases in males progress to ESRD; women may have microscopic hematuria but rarely have decreased GFR.
What is treatment for hereditary nephritis?	Renal transplantation
What may happen to a transplanted kidney in patients with hereditary nephritis?	Anti-GBM disease may occur because the native kidneys do not have the glomerular basement antigen and the donor has the normal antigen. The recipient's body recognizes this antigen as foreign and directs antibodies against it.

TUBULOINTERSTITIAL DISEASES

ACUTE INTERSTITIAL NEPHRITIS

What is AIN?	The sudden onset of renal dysfunction characterized by a prominent inflammatory cell infiltrate within the renal interstitium
What are the most common causes of AIN?	Infectious pyelonephritis, drugs, and toxins
What are other causes?	SLE, sarcoidosis, crystal disease, and transplant rejection

Which infectious agents are associated with AIN?

Typical UTI pathogens, *Rickettsia*, *Mycoplasma*, fungus, cytomegalovirus, and *Campylobacter*

What are culprit drugs in AIN?

Antibiotics (1/3), NSAIDs (1/7), contrast media (1/8), and diuretics (1/20)

Which antibiotics are associated with AIN?

Methicillin (one sixth of all drug-induced cases), other penicillin derivatives, sulfa-based drugs, and rifampin

What is the incidence of AIN?

Population statistics unknown
Approximately one eighth of cases of ARF

What are the symptoms and signs of AIN?

Sometimes asymptomatic; otherwise, fever, rash, edema, arthralgias, uremia, and sudden and unexplained decrease in renal function may be seen

What are the urinalysis findings in patients with AIN?

Hematuria, mild to moderate proteinuria, sterile pyuria, WBC casts, eosinophiluria, glucosuria, and low pH

What are the laboratory findings in patients with AIN?

Peripheral eosinophilia, progressively increasing creatinine and decreasing GFR, and elevated ESR

What are the urinary indices in patients with AIN?

They are inconsistent, but FE_{Na} is generally > 1%.

What are the renal ultrasound findings in patients with AIN?

Normal or increased kidney size

What diagnostic tests are ordered for patients suspected of having AIN?

Radioactive gallium citrate scan to demonstrate increased uptake of the isotope by the kidneys

What is the renal histopathology of AIN?

Diffuse or patchy mononuclear cell infiltrate in the interstitium

What is the prognosis for patients with AIN?

Most cases are reversible. The extent of damage correlates with the degree of interstitial infiltration on biopsy and with duration of disease.

What is the treatment for AIN?	Withdrawal of offending drugs, treatment of any infection, and supportive measures, including dialysis if indicated
How often is dialysis required?	In approximately one third of patients
Are steroids useful in AIN?	Steroids have not yet been shown to improve outcomes but they may cause quicker resolution.

ANALGESIC NEPHROPATHY

What is analgesic nephropathy?	Renal papillary necrosis caused by chronic repeated ingestion of analgesic medications
What are the most common causes of analgesic nephropathy?	Aspirin, phenacetin, acetaminophen, aminopyrine, phenazone, and salicylamide
What cumulative dose causes analgesic nephropathy?	> 3 kg
What is the mechanism of action?	Inhibition of renal prostaglandin synthesis Metabolism of analgesics to reactive compounds that are concentrated in the papillae
What are risk factors for analgesic nephropathy?	Advanced age, longer duration of exposure, and use of multiple analgesic agents
What is the incidence of analgesic nephropathy?	15% of cases of ARF 15%–33% of cases of chronic interstitial nephritis 1%–2% of cases of ESRD 5:1 female:male ratio
What are symptoms and signs of analgesic nephropathy?	Notable absence of fever, rash, and eosinophilia; presence of chronic pain for which the analgesic is used, evidence of sodium retention, hyperkalemia, hypertension, and anemia

What acid–base abnormality is seen in analgesic nephropathy?	Nongap acidosis
What are the urinalysis findings for analgesic nephropathy?	< 1 g proteinuria, gross hematuria, and/or sterile pyuria
What are the renal ultrasound findings for analgesic nephropathy?	Small kidneys
What is the renal histopathology in patients with analgesic nephropathy?	Cortical atrophy, necrotic papillae, periglomerular and interstitial fibrosis, and nephrosclerosis
What diagnostic test is used for analgesic nephropathy?	IVP, which demonstrates abnormalities in approximately 90% of cases; predominantly widening of calices with leakage of contrast early in disease; blunted calices and decreased kidney size in advanced disease
What is the treatment for analgesic nephropathy?	Discontinuation of analgesic use may result in improved renal function depending on the degree of scarring.

CHRONIC TUBULOINTERSTITIAL NEPHROPATHY

What is chronic interstitial nephritis?	Progressive disorder affecting the renal tubules and interstitium while sparing the glomeruli and vasculature. It is a less common cause of ESRD.
What are the most common causes of chronic interstitial nephritis?	Drugs or toxins, infection, obstruction, or secondary to hematologic or hereditary disorders (e.g., sickle cell disease)
What are symptoms of chronic interstitial nephritis?	Patients are asymptomatic until late in the disease course when symptoms of impaired renal function manifest.
What electrolyte disturbances are caused by chronic interstitial nephritis?	Depends on the region and extent of disease

When the proximal tubule is affected, what are the laboratory abnormalities in chronic interstitial nephritis?	Proximal RTA (type II) and Fanconi's syndrome with inability to resorb HCO_3^-, with increases in urinary glucose, amino acids, and PO_4
When the distal tubule is affected, what are the laboratory abnormalities in chronic interstitial nephritis?	Distal RTA (type I) with salt-wasting, hyperkalemia, and nongap metabolic acidosis
When multiple sites are affected, what are the laboratory abnormalities in chronic interstitial nephritis?	Combinations of the above abnormalities. In general, there is Na^+ wasting, impaired concentrating ability, and mild proteinuria.
What test suggests tubule damage from chronic interstitial nephritis?	Radioimmunoassay for Tamm-Horsfall protein as a marker for tubule dysfunction
What may be seen on urinalysis that would suggest chronic interstitial nephritis?	Mild proteinuria, tubular casts, and glucosuria $U_{osm} < 600$ mmol/kg = severe damage; > 800 mmol/kg = mild damage
What is the FE_{Na} in chronic interstitial nephritis?	$FE_{Na} > 1\%$
What is the renal histopathology in chronic interstitial nephritis?	Infiltration of the parenchyma with a mononuclear inflammatory cell infiltrate Interstitial fibrosis Tubular atrophy
What is the treatment for chronic interstitial nephritis?	Withdrawal of all offending agents and control systemic diseases that may contribute to further renal failure

CHRONIC URIC ACID NEPHROPATHY

What are risk factors for chronic uric acid nephropathy?	Prolonged hyperuricemia and lead intoxication (e.g., from "moonshine")

What are the symptoms and signs of chronic uric acid nephropathy?	Tophaceous gout, increased creatinine, and slowly progressive renal insufficiency
What are the laboratory findings for chronic uric acid nephropathy?	Increased serum uric acid level that is more than expected for the amount of renal insufficiency and increased urinary lead excretion
What does urinalysis show for chronic uric acid nephropathy?	Results are normal.
What is seen on renal biopsy?	Uric acid crystal deposition in the medullary interstitium
What is the treatment for chronic uric acid nephropathy?	Lead chelation with EDTA for lead intoxication and treatment for gout if present

OTHER CAUSES OF TUBULOINTERSTITIAL NEPHRITIS

What neoplasms can cause tubulointerstitial nephritis?	Multiple myeloma, lymphoma, and leukemia
What other drug that has not been discussed is a cause of tubulointerstitial nephritis?	Lithium
What granulomatous disease is a cause of tubulointerstitial nephritis?	Sarcoidosis

URINARY TRACT INFECTION

Identify the following UTIs:	
Cystitis	Infection of the bladder
Pyelonephritis	Infection of the kidneys
Complicated UTI	Urologic abnormalities or failure to respond to therapy in 72 hours
What is the incidence of UTI?	UTIs are common, with a female predominance in adults and a male predominance in newborns

What are risk factors for UTI?

Female gender (adults), use of an indwelling catheter, DM, obstruction (e.g., benign prostatic hypertrophy), use of a diaphragm and spermicide (alters natural flora), uncircumcision in males, neurogenic bladder, pregnancy (decreased ureteral tone and peristalsis, incompetence of vesicoureteral valves), immunocompromised state, and ESRD

What are the symptoms and signs of UTI?

Cystitis—abdominal or suprapubic pain, dysuria, frequency, urgency, obstructive symptoms possible in men, occasionally suprapubic tenderness, hematuria (30%), and cloudy urine
Pyelonephritis—fever, nausea, vomiting, flank pain, with or without symptoms of cystitis, and CVA tenderness

How can you distinguish upper UTIs from lower UTIs?

Fever is more common in upper UTIs. CVA tenderness is nonspecific.

What is seen on the urinalysis dipstick?

Positive for blood, leukocyte esterase, and nitrites

What is seen on microscopic analysis of urine?

Results are positive for RBC, WBC, and bacteria without epithelial cells. Sterile pyuria is common in hospitalized patients.

What are the laboratory findings for UTI?

1. Greater than 10 WBCs/HPF of centrifuged urine defines pyuria. Combined with dysuria, this has a sensitivity of 95% for UTIs.
2. Urine culture demonstrates greater than or equal to 10^5 bacteria/ml in a voided specimen or > 100 CFU/ml of a single or predominant pathogen in a straight catheter or suprapubic aspiration specimen.
3. Bacteria may be seen on microscopic examination of the unspun urine specimen when > 10^5 CFU/ml are present.

What is the differential diagnosis for UTI?	Vulvovaginitis and sexually transmitted diseases, which have a more gradual onset and less severe symptoms
In which hosptial patients should you consider a UTI?	In those with fever, abdominal pain, proteinuria, incontinence, and mental status changes (elderly patients)
What are the common bacteria involved in UTI?	*Escherichia coli* (80%—serotypes O, K, and H), *Proteus, Serratia, Klebsiella, Enterobacter, Pseudomonas, Staphylococcus,* and *Providencia*
What are settings in which UTIs are typically caused by *Staphylococcus saprophyticus*?	In young women aged 16–25 years with pyuria and symptoms of lower UTIs
What bacteria are associated with instrumentation?	*S. aureus* and enterococci
What viruses are associated with UTI?	Adenovirus associated with acute hemorrhagic cystitis
Why is *S. aureus* worrisome in UTI?	It may indicate bacteremia, pyelonephritis, or endocarditis.
Why is *Proteus* worrisome in UTI?	It produces urease, which can lead to formation of struvite calculi, making bacteria more resistant to antimicrobials. It can also lead to formation of staghorn calculi.
Why is *Klebsiella* worrisome in UTI?	It produces polysaccharides, leading to stone formation.
What is empiric treatment for the following: **Cystitis**	Trimethoprim-sulfamethoxazole, amoxicillin-clavulanate, and flouroquinolones provide reasonable coverage.

Pyelonephritis

Selection of an antibiotic should be based on Gram stain results if possible; however, a third-generation cephalosporin, ampicillin-sulbactam, fluoroquinolone, and aztreonam are reasonable empiric choices.

What is the duration of therapy for:
Cystitis in women?

Single dose, 3 days, or 7–10 days

Pyelonephritis

14 days minimum

What is the treatment if the UTI is catheter-associated?

Remove the catheter and treat as discussed. If the catheter is necessary, give no treatment if the patient is asymptomatic because treatment may not eradicate the bacteria and will breed organisms that are generally more resistant to antibiotic therapy. Consider in–out catheterization instead of an indwelling catheter.

Which bacteria are more likely to recur?

Pseudomonas and enterococci

What is sterile pyuria?

The presence of leukocytes in urine in the absence of positive bacterial cultures

What is the differential diagnosis of sterile pyuria?

Renal tuberculosis, acute urethritis, foreign body or tumor of the urinary tract, and nonbacterial infections in the genital tract

Which patients should have a workup?

Men who do not have acute prostatitis, urethritis, or a history of recent instrumentation
School-aged girls after their first episode of bacteriuria
Women with multiple infections (> 3–4) or UTI associated with stones
Women with pyelonephritis associated with bacteremia or with symptoms that persist for more than 3 days following pyelonephritis
Women with recurrent infections with the same organism

What radiologic studies are useful?

IVP and renal sonography. In certain circumstances, CT scans, cystoscopy, and voiding cystourethrograms are useful.

What is the microbiologic significance of a urinary pH greater than or equal to 7.5 in chronic UTIs?

Signifies urease production, usually by *Proteus* species and occasionally *Klebsiella* or other urease producers

NOSOCOMIAL UTI

What is the incidence of nosocomial UTI?

40% of all nosocomial infections
400,000 to 1 million infections per year

What pathogens are involved in nosocomial UTI?

Enterobacteriaceae are most common (e.g., *E. coli*, *Proteus mirabilis*). If prior antibiotics have been given, *Pseudomonas aeruginosa*, *Serratia*, and *Enterobacter* may be present. Gram-positive pathogens (including enterococcus) and *Candida albicans* also occur.

What are risk factors for nosocomial UTI?

Foley catheterization (> 80% of cases), other genitourinary tract instrumentation, and diarrhea

What laboratory and diagnostic tests are ordered for nosocomial UTI?

CBC, urinalysis, and urine Gram stain and culture

How is the diagnosis made for nosocomial UTI?

Patients with Foley catheters in place may have only fever and cloudy or foul-smelling urine.

What is the treatment for nosocomial UTI?

Treatment is directed against the specific pathogen, if known. Empiric therapy is directed against the most likely pathogen by Gram stain of urine as follows:
Gram-negative bacilli—third-generation cephalosporin (cefotaxime or ceftriaxone). There is no need for ceftazidime unless there is a high likelihood of pseudomonal infection.

Gram-positive cocci—if the pathogen is *Enterococcus*, use ampicillin with or without gentamicin. Consider vancomycin if enterococci are resistant and the patient is very ill.

What is bacteriuria?   Colonization of the urinary tract with bacteria without tissue invasion. Patients are asymptomatic.

VASCULAR DISEASES

WEGENER'S VASCULITIS

What organs are affected in Wegener's vasculitis?   Upper and lower respiratory tract and kidneys

What size vessels are affected?   Small to medium-sized vessels

What are symptoms of Wegener's vasculitis?   Sinus or chest pain, hemoptysis, fever, anorexia, weight loss, arthralgias, and photosensitivity

What are the signs and laboratory findings of Wegener's vasculitis?   Conjunctivitis, uveitis, hematuria, red cell casts, and proteinuria

What is limited Wegener's?   Respiratory pathology without renal pathology or vice versa

What is the renal histopathology in Wegener's vasculitis?   Segmental necrosis, vascular inflammation and necrosis, rarely granulomas, and no immune deposits on immunofluorescence

What is the treatment for Wegener's vasculitis?   Oral cyclophosphamide and prednisone

What is the course of Wegener's vasculitis?   Almost all untreated patients die within 2 months. If treated, renal function is preserved in 75% of patients.

Can patients with Wegener's vasculitis undergo renal transplantation?   Yes. Patients with ESRD can undergo transplantation once remission is established.

POLYARTERITIS NODOSA

What are the types of PAN?
Classic, microscopic, Churg-Strauss, and overlap syndrome

What are the symptoms of all types of PAN?
Fever, weight loss, and anorexia

What are the signs of PAN?
Hypertension, asymmetric polyneuropathy, benign to nephritic urinalysis, and impaired renal function

What size vessels are affected in classic PAN?
Medium-sized vessels

What is the diagnostic procedure for PAN?
Celiac or renal angiogram, which shows constricted segments and tapering of small arteries as well as aneurysms

What is the renal histopathology for classic PAN?
Focal and segmental necrosis similar to Wegener's vasculitis and no immune deposits

What is microscopic PAN?
It is similar to classic PAN except smaller vessels are involved and more segmental glomerular sclerosis is seen on biopsy.

What are the symptoms of Churg-Strauss disease?
Asthma or other allergic symptoms

What are the signs and laboratory findings of Churg-Strauss disease?
Asthma-related signs with peripheral eosinophilia, pulmonary infiltrates on chest radiograph, hypertension, and coronary vasculitis

What is the renal histopathology in Churg-Strauss disease?
Segmental necrosis with interstitial nephritis and eosinophilic infiltrates and granulomas

What percent of patients with PAN have ARF?
10%

What is overlap syndrome?
Features of classic PAN, microscopic PAN, and Churg-Strauss

What is the course of all types of PAN?	Poor prognosis for untreated disease
What is the treatment for PAN?	Prednisone or cyclophosphamide and prednisone Patients can recover function even after being dialysis dependent. Renal transplantation if needed is recommended after remission of PAN.

HYPERSENSITIVITY VASCULITIS

What are the hypersensitivity vasculitides?	Henoch-Schönlein purpura, mixed essential cryoglobulinemia, and serum sickness
What size vessels are involved in hypersensitivity vasculitis?	Arterioles, capillaries, and postcapillary venules
What is a major clinical sign of hypersensitivity vasculitis?	Leukocytoclastic vasculitis with palpable purpura

HENOCH-SCHÖNLEIN PURPURA

What is Henoch-Schönlein purpura?	Vascular IgA deposition disease mainly seen in children
What is the symptom triad?	Abdominal pain, arthritis–arthralgias, and petechiae–purpura
What are the signs of Henoch-Schönlein purpura?	More commonly, microscopic hematuria and cellular casts occur, but there may be nephrotic proteinuria, hypertension, and impaired renal function.
What is the renal histopathology in Henoch-Schönlein purpura?	Mesangial expansion and hypercellularity with IgA deposits (like IgA nephropathy)
What is the clinical course of Henoch-Schönlein purpura?	Resolves spontaneously, with some recurrences. Patients with nephrotic-range proteinuria and > 50% crescents on biopsy have a worse prognosis.

What is the treatment for Henoch-Schönlein purpura?	Immunosuppressive agents in patients with renal disease have not been proven to be effective.
Is there a chance of recurrence in a renal transplant?	Yes

ESSENTIAL MiXED CRYOGLOBULINEMIA

What are cryoglobulins?	Antigen–antibody complexes that precipitate when cooled
What lesion is seen in the skin from cryoglobulin precipitation?	Leukocytoclastic vasculitis without IgA
What are symptoms of essential mixed cryoglobulinemia?	Fatigue, lethargy, arthralgias, and lower extremity rash
What are the signs of essential mixed cryoglobulinemia?	Lower extremity palpable purpura, lymphadenopathy, hepatosplenomegaly, peripheral neuropathy, and Raynaud's phenomenon
What does the urinalysis show for essential mixed cryoglobulinemia?	Mild hematuria, proteinuria, and cellular and granular casts
What do laboratory results show for essential mixed cryoglobulinemia?	Hypocomplementemia, increased liver enzymes, and cryoglobulin titer
What is the renal histopathology in essential mixed cryoglobulinemia?	Mesangial and endothelial proliferation and basement membrane thickening, cryoglobulin-caused thrombi, and deposits of IgG, IgM, and C3 on immunofluorescence
How common is renal involvement?	50% of patients
What is the clinical course of essential mixed cryoglobulinemia?	Slowly progressive renal insufficiency

What is the treatment for essential mixed cryoglobulinemia?	No treatment has been proven effective. Plasmapheresis and prednisone or other immunosuppressives are only used in fulminant cases.

SERUM SICKNESS

What is serum sickness?	An immune response provoked by a drug or protein
What are common drugs associated with serum sickness?	Penicillins, sulfonamides, and phenytoin
What are common symptoms of serum sickness?	Fever, urticaria, and arthralgias occurring 7–10 days after first exposure or 2–7 days after repeat exposure
What are signs of serum sickness?	Lymphadenopathy and edema
What are the urinalysis findings for serum sickness?	Hematuria, proteinuria, and cellular casts
Is ARF common in cases of serum sickness?	No
What are the laboratory findings for serum sickness?	Low complement levels
What is the renal histopathology in serum sickness?	Immunofluorescence reveals IgG and C3 deposition in glomerular capillary walls.
What is the treatment for serum sickness?	Removal of the drug

SCLERODERMA RENAL CRISIS

What is scleroderma renal crisis?	ARF and hypertension, which progress in 1–2 months to ESRD if untreated
What causes the hypertension?	Ischemia-induced renin release

When in the course of the illness does it occur?	Usually in the first 4 years of the systemic illness
What are the urinalysis findings for scleroderma renal crisis?	Normal to only mild proteinuria and casts
What is the treatment for scleroderma renal crisis?	ACE inhibitor to block renin-induced hypertension and to stabilize renal function

CHOLESTEROL EMBOLI

What procedures are associated with cholesterol emboli?	Procedures involving large arteries (e.g., angiography, angioplasty, and vascular surgery) and systemic anticoagulation
What is the renal histopathology in cholesterol emboli?	Clefts in small- to medium-sized arteries Later, intimal proliferation and macrophage infiltration occur with fibrosis.
What causes the arterial clefts?	Cholesterol emboli (crystals), which dissolve with tissue processing
What are the symptoms of cholesterol emboli?	Visual deficits, abdominal pain, myalgias, and pain in the affected areas
What are the signs of cholesterol emboli?	Orange plaques in the retina, livedo reticularis, and gangrene of toes with intact distal pulses
What are the urinalysis findings in the cholesterol emboli syndrome?	Usually few casts or cells but there may be hematuria and RBC casts
What are the laboratory findings in the cholesterol emboli syndrome?	ARF or subacute renal failure, which is irreversible, and peripheral eosinophilia
What is the treatment for the cholesterol emboli syndrome?	None specific, but supportive care for renal abnormalities (e.g., electrolyte correction, medication adjustment, dialysis) may be indicated.
What is the clinical course of the disease?	Progressive renal failure or stabilized renal insufficiency

PREECLAMPSIA

What is preeclampsia?	Development of hypertension, proteinuria, and edema after the 20th week of pregnancy
What is the incidence of preeclampsia?	5%–10% of pregnancies
What are risk factors for preeclampsia?	Age younger than 20 years, primigravida
What is the renal histopathology in preeclampsia?	Swelling of the glomerular endothelium (glomerular endotheliosis)
What are the symptoms of preeclampsia?	Headache, edema, and epigastic pain (hepatic edema)
What are the signs of preeclampsia?	Labile hypertension (BP > 140/90) Edema Rollover test showing a BP difference of > 20 mm Hg from a left lateral decubitus position to a supine position Hyperreflexia
What are the urinalysis findings for preeclampsia?	Few red or white cells and proteinuria, which can be nephrotic
What are the laboratory findings for preeclampsia?	Mildly elevated serum creatinine (except in the HELLP syndrome), serum uric acid > 5 mg/dl, 24-hour urine calcium < 100 mg, and proteinuria
What is the HELLP syndrome?	**H**emolysis **E**levated **l**iver enzymes **L**ow **p**latelets
What is eclampsia?	Development of seizures in preeclampsia
What is the treatment for preeclampsia?	Rapid delivery if possible If fetus < 30 weeks' gestation, bed rest, treatment of hypertension, and close observation In cases of HELLP syndrome, untreatable hypertension, or seizures, immediate delivery to protect the mother

What antihypertensives are used in preeclampsia?

Methyldopa, calcium channel blockers, with or without β blockers, and hydralazine

What antihypertensives must be avoided?

ACE inhibitors and diuretics

5 _____ Gastroenterology

ABBREVIATIONS

5-ASA	5-Aminosalicylic acid
AFP	α-Fetoprotein
AIDS	Acquired immune deficiency syndrome
ALT	Alanine aminotransferase
ARDS	Adult respiratory distress syndrome
AST	Aspartate aminotransferase
AVM	Arteriovenous malformation
BUN	Blood urea nitrogen
CBC	Complete blood count
CD	Crohn's disease
CEA	Carcinoembryonic antigen
CLO	*Campylobacter*-like organism
CMV	Cytomegalovirus
CT	Computed tomography
DIC	Disseminated intravascular coagulation
EGD	Esophagogastroduodenoscopy
ELISA	Enzyme-linked immunosorbent assay
ERCP	Endoscopic retrograde cholangiopancreatography

FPC	Familial polyposis coli
GB	Gallbladder
GERD	Gastroesophageal reflux disease
GI	Gastrointestinal
HAV	Hepatitis A virus
HBcAb	Hepatitis B virus core antibody
HBeAg	Hepatitis B virus e antigen
HBsAb	Hepatitis B virus surface antibody
HBsAg	Hepatitis B virus surface antigen
HBV	Hepatitis B virus
HCC	Hepatocellular carcinoma
HCV	Hepatitis C virus
HDV	Hepatitis D virus
HEV	Hepatitis E virus
HGV	Hepatitis G virus
HIV	Human immunodeficiency virus
Hp	*Helicobacter pylori*
IBD	Inflammatory bowel disease
IBS	Irritable bowel syndrome
IV	Intravenous
IVDA	Intravenous drug abuse
LES	Lower esophageal sphincter
LGI	Lower gastrointestinal
LLQ	Left lower quadrant

MEN	Multiple endocrine neoplasia
NG	Nasogastric
NSAIDs	Nonsteroidal antiinflammatory drugs
OLT	Orthotopic liver transplantation
PABA	Paraaminobenzoic acid
PBC	Primary biliary cirrhosis
PCR	Polymerase chain reaction
PPI	Proton pump inhibitor
PSC	Primary sclerosing cholangitis
PSE	Portal systemic encephalopathy
PT	Prothrombin time
PTT	Partial thromboplastin time
PUD	Peptic ulcer disease
RBC	Red blood cell
RLQ	Right lower quadrant
RUQ	Right upper quadrant
SBP	Spontaneous bacterial peritonitis
$\mathbf{T_{1/2}}$	Half-life
TIPS	Transjugular intrahepatic portosystemic shunt
UC	Ulcerative colitis
UGI	Upper gastrointestinal
VIP	Vasoactive intestinal polypeptide
ZES	Zollinger-Ellison syndrome

HISTORY AND PHYSICAL EXAMINATION

What questions should you ask about abdominal pain?

Abdominal pain is a common, yet nonspecific complaint. When taking a history in patients with abdominal pain, remember **PQRST:**

Presentation—How and where does the pain present?

Quality—Is the pain sharp, dull, burning, or colicky?

Radiation—Does the pain radiate to, for example, the groin, back, or shoulder?

Severity—How bad is the pain? What makes it better or worse?

Timing—When does the pain occur? How long does it last?

What should you look for on abdominal examination?

1. Be organized and focus on the patient's complaints.
2. The patient should lie supine with arms at sides and knees slightly flexed. Inspect the skin for scars, dilated veins, and rashes; inspect the umbilicus; inspect the contour of the abdomen for distention, protuberance, and scaphoid.
3. Auscultate the character and frequency of bowel sounds and other sounds (e.g., arterial bruit, venous hum, friction rub).
4. Percuss the liver (total size along right midaxillary line), the spleen (total size, left costal dullness), other masses, and ascites (shifting dullness, fluid wave).
5. Palpate the liver and spleen (lower border, shape, and consistency), other organs and masses (e.g., aorta and kidney), and areas of abdominal tenderness (rebound, guarding).

Why should you do a rectal examination?

The rectal examination is an imperative part of every examination.

Perianal inspection evaluates for fissures, fistulae, signs of trauma, hemorrhoids, and prolapse.

Digital rectal examination evaluates
sphincter tone, masses, the prostate,
peritoneal irritation, and stool color,
consistency, and guaiac.

**When are the two times
when it is appropriate to
omit the rectal
examination?**

When the patient does not have a
rectum or is neutropenic

NUTRITION

**What is normal energy
metabolism?**

Adults require 25–30 kcal/kg body
weight per day (i.e., 2100 kcal/day in a
70-kg person). A typical American
derives 40%–45% of calories from
carbohydrates, 40%–45% from lipids,
and 10%–15% from protein.

**What nutrients do humans
require?**

Macronutrients, the major part of the
    diet, include proteins, carbohydrates,
    lipids (fats), water, and electrolytes.
Micronutrients, which are often used in
    minute amounts, include trace
    elements and vitamins.

**What are the fat-soluble
vitamins?**

A, D, E, and K

What is malnutrition?

The Latin translation is "bad nutrition,"
    or any disorder of nutrition (e.g.,
    starvation and obesity).
Marasmus is protein–calorie
    malnutrition, which results in growth
    retardation, wasting of subcutaneous
    fat, and diminished maintenance of
    mental status.
Kwashiorkor is severe protein deficiency,
    which results in retarded growth, skin
    changes, mental status changes, and
    hepatic fibrosis.
Obesity and edema may mask true
    malnutrition.

**What is the incidence of
malnutrition?**

Malnutrition is common, especially in
chronically ill medical patients. One
third to one half of patients admitted to
the hospital are undernourished; their

status is usually worse at discharge than on admission.

How do patients become malnourished?

Poor intake (cannot get it). The patient is not being fed (most common) or has limited intake (e.g., in dysphagia after a stroke, anorexia, or a UGI tract malignancy).

Decreased absorption (cannot use it), for example, in celiac sprue, chronic pancreatitis, and short bowel syndrome after massive small bowel resection

Excessive losses (cannot keep it in), for example, in diarrhea, chronic vomiting, and high-output enteric fistula

Increased needs (cannot keep up), for example, in malignancy, pregnancy, and postoperative burns

What are the symptoms and signs of the following deficiencies:

Thiamine (beriberi)

Muscle weakness, tachycardia, and heart failure

Niacin (pellagra)

Glossitis and cheilosis

Vitamin A

Xerophthalmia, hyperkeratosis, and poor wound healing

Vitamin B$_{12}$

Megaloblastic anemia

Vitamin C (scurvy)

Bleeding gums, perifollicular hemorrhage, and poor wound healing

Vitamin E

Cerebellar ataxia and areflexia

Vitamin K

Bleeding due to decreased activity of clotting factors II, VII, IX, and X

Zinc

Hypogeusia and acrodermatitis

Chromium

Glucose intolerance

What are the most common deficiencies with intestinal disease?

Folate, calcium (duodenum and jejunum), and B_{12} (terminal ileum)

How do you assess for malnutrition?

History—more important than anthropometric measurements (e.g., triceps skinfold thickness and mid-upper arm circumference)

Weight change—< 10% or > 10%, acute vs. chronic

Dietary intake—quantity and composition

GI symptoms—nausea, vomiting, anorexia, diarrhea

Functional capacity and stress—postoperative status, burns, and sepsis

Physical signs—loss of subcutaneous fat, muscle wasting, fluid retention, and mucosal lesions

What laboratory tests suggest malnutrition?

Low serum albumin, prealbumin, carotene, transferrin, total lymphocyte count, nitrogen balance, and delayed hypersensitivity skin response to common antigens are useful indices for visceral protein status.

What is the goal of nutrition support?

Positive nitrogen balance. Intake of protein must equal or exceed the breakdown of body protein.

How much should healthy adults be fed?

20–25 kcal/kg calories; 0.8–1.0 g/kg protein

How much should obese adult patients or patients adapted to "starvation" be fed?

20–25 kcal/kg calories; 1.0–1.2 g/kg protein

How much should adult patients experiencing mild to moderate stress be fed?

25–30 kcal/kg calories; 1.3–1.5 g/kg protein

How much should adult patients experiencing moderate to severe stress be fed?

30–35 kcal/kg calories; 1.6–2.5 g/kg protein

What is the general rule of thumb for nutrition?

If the gut works, use it.

What are the three modes of nutrition?

1. Oral supplementation in addition to regular diet
2. Enteral nutrition (tube feeding)
3. Parenteral nutrition (total or partial)

What are the advantages of enteral feeding?

It is simple, safe, cost effective, and maintains mucosal integrity.

When should parenteral feeding be used?

When patients cannot ingest or absorb sufficient calories through the GI tract

What are potential complications of parenteral nutrition?

Hyperglycemia, hypoglycemia, catheter infection, azotemia, elevated transaminases, and acalculous cholecystitis

What are the components of the feeding formula?

Think **FACE MTV**
Fluids
Amino acids and protein
Calories—carbohydrates, fat
Electrolytes
Miscellaneous (anything else that needs to be added)
Trace elements
Vitamins

What is the refeeding syndrome?

Metabolic disarray (hypophosphatemia, hypokalemia, and hypomagnesemia) that may be accompanied by cardiopulmonary and neurologic complications in starved patients being refed enterally or parenterally

How do you follow up nutritional status?

Measure prealbumin, which has a $T_{1/2}$ of 3–4 days and which is a good indication of positive nitrogen balance. Do not measure albumin, which has a long $T_{1/2}$ (19–21 days). Assess weight, intake and output, glucose, electrolytes, and nitrogen balance as needed.

Clinical pearl

Recovery is slow. It is much easier to prevent malnutrition than to treat it.

GASTROINTESTINAL BLEEDING

What is GI bleeding?	Bleeding from any point of the GI tract, from the mouth to the anus. The bleeding can be gross or occult and can range from an insignificant leak to a catastrophic hemorrhage.

DEFINITIONS

Hematemesis	Vomiting of blood. Bright red or "coffee grounds" emesis, usually indicates UGI bleeding, above the ligament of Treitz. The coffee grounds appearance comes from rapid (within minutes) degradation of hemoglobin by gastric acid and pepsin.
Melena	Passage of black, tarry stools from bacterial breakdown of hemoglobin. It usually indicates UGI bleeding above the ligament of Treitz but can occur with slower bleeding from the terminal ileum or right colon. At least 100 ml of blood must be present in the GI tract for melena to occur. Note: Iron, bismuth, and some foods can cause black stools.
Hematochezia	Bright red blood per rectum, usually indicating an LGI source but which can also occur from vigorous UGI bleeding

UPPER AND LOWER GASTROINTESTINAL BLEEDING

What information is important when taking a history for GI bleeding?

1. Duration of bleeding (acute versus chronic)
2. Presence of abdominal pain, dysphagia, dyspepsia, and nausea and vomiting; change in bowel habits; weight loss; anorexia; weakness; fatigue, dizziness; and easy bruisability
3. Past medical history of PUD or bleeding episodes; cirrhosis (previous varices or portal gastropathy); inherited coagulopathy; or aortic bypass graft

4. Use of certain medications, including acetylsalicylic acid, NSAIDs, warfarin, and heparin
5. Social history of alcohol and tobacco use

What are symptoms and signs of bleeding?

Depends on the source and severity of the bleed and on any coexistent diseases

What are symptoms and signs of acute, severe GI bleeding?

Hemodynamic instability (i.e., tachycardia, tachypnea, orthostatic hypotension, angina, mental status change or coma, and cold extremities)

What are symptoms and signs of chronic blood loss?

Signs of anemia (e.g., weakness, fatigue, pallor, angina, and dizziness)

What additional signs may be present in a cirrhotic patient?

Hepatic encephalopathy or hepatorenal syndrome. Look for stigmata of chronic liver disease—spider angiomata, palmar erythema, gynecomastia, testicular atrophy, and Dupuytren's contracture.

What are the most common causes of UGI bleeding?

Peptic ulcer, hemorrhagic gastritis, Mallory-Weiss tear, erosive esophagitis, aortoenteric fistula, varices, neoplasm, and hemobilia. Think **UVA MED:**
Ulcers (PUD)
Varices
AVMs
Mallory-Weiss tear, malignancies
Erosions (stress gastritis), esophagitis
Dieulafoy's lesion

Clinical pearl

In a patient with varices, always investigate other sources of bleeding. One third of patients with varices have other sources.

What are the most common causes of LGI bleeding?

Hemorrhoids and fissures, which rarely require hospitalization, AVMs, diverticulosis, ischemia, neoplasms, IBD, infectious colitis, radiation colitis, and Meckel's diverticulum. Think **NADIR:**
Neoplasia
AVMs
Diverticulosis

IBD and infectious colitis
'**R**hoids (hemorrhoids)

What are the most common causes of LGI bleeding in the following patients?

    Patients older than 60 years

Diverticulosis, ischemic bowel, AVMs, and carcinoma

    Young patients

Hemorrhoids, fissures, colonic polyps, IBD, and infectious colitis

Clinical pearl

The most common cause of an LGI bleed is a UGI bleed.

What is the workup for GI bleeding?

The patient must be stabilized before a diagnostic workup is started. Depending on the clinical presentation, the workup may include NG aspiration, rectal examination, upper endoscopy, lower endoscopy, radionuclide imaging, selective arteriography, and/or barium studies.

Is NG aspiration necessary in LGI bleeding?

Yes, in all patients with GI bleeding, even hematochezia, unless the patient has physician-witnessed hematemesis

How is NG aspiration helpful?

It is helpful in determining the rate of blood loss. Continuous loss of bright red blood demonstrates active, vigorous bleeding. A "coffee grounds" appearance is more consistent with bleeding that is slower or has stopped. There is a 16% false-negative rate for NG lavage (bile visualized) in patients with endoscopically active UGI bleeding.

Is a rectal examination needed for UGI bleeding?

Yes, in any patient with GI bleeding (even apparently obvious UGI bleeding). Character and color of stool can help determine the severity and source of bleeding.

How is upper endoscopy helpful?

EGD is the best tool for diagnosing or potentially treating a UGI bleed.

What therapeutic procedures are possible with EGD?	Thermal coagulation, injection of epinephrine, ethanol, and sclerosing agents, variceal banding, laser photocoagulation, and application of blood-clotting agents or tissue adhesives
When is proctosigmoidoscopy or colonoscopy used?	When diagnosing LGI bleeding, unless active bleeding precludes visualization
How is radionuclide scanning used?	Nuclear medicine labeling of red blood cells may indicate the site of bleeding.
What bleeding rate allows nuclear scans to detect active bleeding?	0.1 ml/min. A positive scan may localize the source of bleeding and assist in directing therapeutic procedures.
How much bleeding allows selective arteriography to localize the source?	0.5–1.0 ml/min. Arteriography is less sensitive than a nuclear medicine bleeding scan.
What interventional procedures are there for GI bleeding?	Injection of gel foam, coils, or vasopressin
Are barium studies helpful for detecting GI bleeding?	They are not recommended because they provide a much lower diagnostic yield than any of the other tests discussed. Barium in the GI tract can hinder endoscopy and render arteriography uninterpretable.
What laboratory tests are used in the workup of GI bleeding?	1. CBC, PT, PTT, blood type and screen 2. Electrolytes, glucose, and BUN are very important. Elevated BUN may occur in up to 75% of patients with acute UGI bleeding due to digestion of blood proteins and absorption of nitrogenous compounds in the small intestine. 3. Possibly arterial blood gas, liver function tests, amylase, and cardiac enzymes 4. Serial hemoglobin and hematocrit
What is the treatment for GI bleeding?	Stability of the patient dictates course of action.

What is the treatment for hemodynamic instability in patients with GI bleeding?

Admit the patient to the intensive care unit, obtain large-bore IV access, commence with vigorous crystalloid and colloid resuscitation. Frequent monitoring of vital signs and urine output is essential. Note: Blood transfusion can lower serum calcium if citrate is used in the stored blood. Give 1 ampule calcium gluconate IV for every 3–4 units of transfused blood. Platelets and clotting factors may also be diluted (give platelet and fresh-frozen plasma infusion).

What is the treatment for coagulopathies in patients with GI bleeding?

Fresh-frozen plasma or vitamin K; platelets for thrombocytopenia

What is the treatment for varices in patients with GI bleeding?

IV octreotide can be used to decrease portal pressure without the significant cardiac and vascular side effects of vasopressin and nitroglycerin.

Endoscopic band ligation or sclerotherapy is usually the initial choice of definitive treatment.

Sengstaken-Blakemore tube, a temporary measure (probably not exceeding 48 hours) to compress gastroesophageal varices by balloon tamponade, should be used by experienced physicians only because serious complications can occur, including perforation, airway occlusion, aspiration, and ischemic necrosis of bowel.

TIPS is used at some institutions to decompress portal venous collaterals to treat acute variceal bleeding.

Surgery with portacaval shunt or esophageal transection may be used.

How are antisecretory agents—H₂ receptor antagonists, PPIs, and antacids—useful in GI bleeding?

They neutralize pathogenic gastric acid following UGI bleeding. Maintaining intragastric pH greater than 4.0 reduces the direct harmful effects of acid and pepsin on the bleeding lesion and allows platelets to aggregate.

What is the role of surgery in GI bleeding?
Acute bleeding frequently stops spontaneously, but there is a high risk of rebleeding in the first 72 hours. Fifteen percent of patients with GI bleeding require surgery because bleeding continues despite medical, endoscopic, or radiographic therapeutic measures.

What are the prognostic factors for GI bleeding?
Severe persistent bleeding (e.g., variceal or arterial bleeding from an ulcer) is associated with a higher mortality rate.
Onset of bleeding after admission or rebleeding in the hospital carries a mortality rate of at least 30%.
The mortality rate from GI bleeding doubles in patients older than 60 years of age.
The mortality rate doubles in patients with concomitant CNS, hepatic, pulmonary, or neoplastic disease. In patients with renal disease, the mortality rate triples. The mortality rate increases several-fold in patients with cardiac or pulmonary disease.
Urgent surgery for UGI bleeding is associated with a 25% mortality rate (versus a 2% rate associated with elective surgery).

What is the mortality rate associated with GI bleeding?
The 5%–10% mortality rate associated with acute GI bleeding has not changed despite improved diagnostic, endoscopic, surgical, and intensive monitoring capabilities.

ESOPHAGUS

DYSPHAGIA, REFLUX, AND MOTILITY

What is dysphagia?
Difficulty in swallowing (the inability to initiate swallowing or the sensation that food "sticks" in the esophagus)

What information is important when taking a history for esophageal dysphagia?
It is important to determine whether the dysphagia occurs equally with solids and liquids.
Solid food > liquid suggests structural abnormality.

gar Land, Texas 77478   713/240-1000

Systems

Sys

S

Systems

Systems

Systems

Solids = liquids suggests neuromuscular (motility) etiology.

What other history is important?

Whether symptoms are intermittent or progressive, whether there is associated heartburn, and whether there are other medical conditions or medications affecting smooth muscle

What are the types of dysphagia?

Oropharyngeal dysphagia and esophageal dysphagia

What is oropharyngeal dysphagia?

Also known as transfer dysphagia, oropharyngeal dysphagia is difficulty propelling food to the hypopharynx.

What are symptoms of oropharyngeal dysphagia?

Dysphagia with liquids worse than solids, nasal regurgitation, cough, and aspiration

What are the causes of oropharyngeal dysphagia?

CNS disease (e.g., stroke and bulbar), disease of striated muscle (e.g., myasthenia gravis, polio, muscular dystrophy, and dermatomyositis), and inflammatory conditions (e.g., infectious pharyngitis, tonsillitis, and esophagitis)

What are symptoms of esophageal dysphagia?

Sensation of food being "stuck" behind the sternum

What are causes of esophageal dysphagia?

Structural disorders (e.g., intrinsic lesion and external compression), tumor (e.g., squamous carcinoma, adenocarcinoma, and leiomyoma), stricture (e.g., peptic, pill-induced esophagitis, and caustic ingestion), rings and webs, and extrinsic compression (e.g., mediastinal tumor, vascular lesions, and esophageal diverticula)

Define the following esophageal motility disorders:
  Achalasia

Incomplete relaxation of the LES with high resting LES pressure and absent peristalsis in esophageal smooth muscle

Diffuse esophageal spasm	High-amplitude, nonperistaltic "spastic" or simultaneous contractions in the esophageal smooth muscle
Nutcracker esophagus	High-amplitude contractions, usually with normal peristalsis and LES function (chest pain greater than dysphagia)
Scleroderma	In 80% of cases, there is decreased amplitude of peristalsis in smooth muscle and decreased LES pressure. Initially, it is a neuromuscular disorder but, later, severe reflux predisposes the patient to stricture.
What diagnostic modalities are used in evaluating dysphagia, reflux, and dysmotility?	Modified barium swallow, cine-esophagogram (usually first study to work up dysphagia), esophageal manometry, EGD, and chest CT
What is the specific use for barium study?	To define anatomy (e.g., intrinsic lesion and external compression), to define dysphagia to thin and thick liquids and solids, and to assess oropharyngeal function, peristalsis, and reflux
What is the specific use for esophageal manometry?	To measure esophageal contraction amplitude and peristalsis with wet and dry swallows and to measure LES pressure and relaxation
What is the specific use for EGD?	To visualize and biopsy intrinsic lesions and to dilate rings, webs, and strictures. It has limited usefulness in defining motility.
What is the specific use for chest CT?	To define extrinsic compression involving the great vessels, the mediastinal structures, and the lung
What is the treatment for oropharyngeal dysphagia?	Mild symptoms often respond to changes in food consistency and positional maneuvers (coordinated treatment with speech pathology). Severe symptoms often preclude further oral intake, necessitating gastrostomy placement.

What is the treatment for esophageal structural lesions?

Strictures, rings, and webs can be dilated endoscopically or radiographically. Tumors can be surgically removed or palliated with laser-treated endoscopic stents or radiation and chemotherapy.

What is the treatment for esophageal dysmotility?

Achalasia can be treated with surgical myotomy or pneumatic balloon dilation of the LES. Other motility disorders are difficult to treat and may respond to calcium channel blockers or nitrates.

What is "steakhouse syndrome"?

Acute obstruction due to a foreign body, which may also be associated with airway obstruction. A food bolus lodged in a narrowed esophagus accompanied by the inability to handle salivary secretions often requires emergent endoscopic removal.

What is GERD?

Gastroesophageal reflux disease is the reflux of gastric contents up into the esophagus.

What are symptoms of GERD?

Heartburn, regurgitation (water brash), chest pain, dysphagia, halitosis, and pulmonary manifestations (e.g., chronic cough, hoarseness, wheezing, asthma)

How common is esophageal reflux?

Common. More than 33% of Americans have intermittent symptoms; 10% have daily heartburn.

What is the cause of GERD?

Most cases are caused by transient LES relaxation (same mechanism that allows belching), whose specific cause is unknown. Fewer cases are due to decreased LES pressure. Delayed gastric emptying may also contribute to GERD.

What is the pathogenesis of GERD?

The extent and severity of esophageal injury depend on the frequency and duration of esophageal exposure to acid and pepsin and the ability of the esophageal mucosa to clear refluxate and heal mucosa.

What risk factors are associated with GERD?

Ingestion of fat, alcohol, chocolate, or mints, as well as smoking, decreases LES pressure.

Hiatal hernia alters gastroesophageal junction anatomy.

Obesity increases intraabdominal pressure.

Medications can reduce LES pressure (e.g., calcium channel blockers, progesterone, anticholinergics, benzodiazepines, narcotics, and nitrates.)

What diagnostic studies are useful in GERD?

EGD with biopsy, barium swallow, acid perfusion (Bernstein) test, pH monitoring, and manometry

How are the following tests helpful:
 EGD with biopsy

Gross findings of esophagitis (e.g., erosion, friability, ulcer stricture, Barrett's esophagus) on EGD provide the most definitive diagnosis of GERD.

Barium swallow

This test is useful in patients who complain of dysphagia to assess for structural abnormality and peristalsis.

Acid perfusion (Bernstein) test

This test is positive if instillation of 0.1 N HCl into the midesophagus produces pyrosis twice and the pyrosis is relieved by saline.

pH monitoring

This test is the gold standard to measure GERD (a pH less than 4 is associated with symptoms). The test measures pH above the LES in conjunction with meals, position, activity, and sleep as recorded in a patient diary. The test assesses percentage of time of esophageal acid exposure, percentage of exposure in various positions, and number and duration of reflux episodes.

Manometry

This test documents esophageal perstaltic function, LES tone, and transient relaxation.

What are the downsides to the following:

EGD with biopsy

A normal EGD does not rule out reflux (histologic examination of biopsies may confirm inflammatory changes).

Barium swallow

The test is insensitive to mild inflammation of the mucosa. Radiographic reflux can be demonstrated in only 40% of patients with severe GERD and in as many as 25% of normal patients.

Acid perfusion (Bernstein) test

This test does not evaluate esophagitis or actually measure reflux. A negative test does not rule out GERD.

pH monitoring

The test may be uncomfortable and the patient must be able to push a button (indicating symptoms) and record the symptoms in a diary.

Manometry

Test has limited usefulness because most patients have transient relaxations in LES pressure, not decreased LES pressure.

What is the nonpharmacologic treatment of GERD?

Lifestyle changes—elevation of the head of the bed (6–8 inches), weight loss, avoidance of tight-fitting clothes, smoking cessation, decreased caffeine and alcohol consumption, avoidance of foods and medications that decrease LES pressure, intake of nothing orally for a few hours before lying supine, and consumption of frequent, small, high-protein meals

What is the pharmacologic treatment of GERD?

H_2 receptor antagonists, PPIs, and prokinetics. Metoclopramide increases LES pressure and improves esophageal and gastric emptying; cisapride augments LES tone.

What is the surgical treatment of GERD?

Open or laparoscopic Nissen fundoplication, which is reserved for patients who have failed medical therapy. Competency of surgical repair may deteriorate over time.

What are complications of GERD?	Esophageal ulceration, peptic stricture, Barrett's esophagus, adenocarcinoma, bleeding, pulmonary problems, and noncardiac chest pain
What is Barrett's esophagus?	Replacement of normal squamous epithelium of the distal esophagus with metaplastic columnar (intestinal type) epithelium
Clinical pearl	Barrett's esophagus rarely develops in blacks.
What are the risk factors for development of Barrett's esophagus?	Recurrent chemical irritation from gastroesophageal reflux disorders (e.g., hiatal hernia), tobacco use, or alcohol abuse
What type of cancer arises in Barrett's esophagus more commonly than in other areas of the esophagus?	Adenocarcinoma. In contrast, 98% of carcinomas of the esophagus are squamous cell in origin.
How frequent is adenocarcinoma with Barrett's esophagus?	Dysplasia and adenocarcinoma have a prevalence of 3%–9%.
How should Barrett's esophagus be followed up?	Periodic endoscopic surveillance biopsies for dysplasia should be performed, but their cost-effectiveness remains controversial.
What is the treatment for severe cases of Barrett's?	Surgical esophagectomy is recommended for severe dysplasia.
What are the most common esophageal causes of noncardiac chest pain?	GERD, nutcracker esophagus, nonspecific esophageal motility disorder, diffuse esophageal spasm, and achalasia
What symptoms suggest an esophageal origin?	Associated dysphagia or heartburn
Clinical pearl	The character of the pain does not help to differentiate cardiac from noncardiac sources. Pain with esophageal origins may radiate to the neck, arm, or jaw and can be aggravated by stress and exercise.

What is odynophagia?	Painful swallowing, most commonly experienced with esophageal mucosal lesions (e.g., from infections, caustic ingestion, and pill esophagitis)
What are symptoms and signs of esophageal infection?	Odynophagia, dysphagia, fever, and occasionally bleeding
What organisms are commonly found in esophageal infection?	*Candida* (most common in immunocompromised patients such as HIV-positive patients, patients undergoing chemotherapy, and post-transplant patients), herpesvirus, CMV, and bacteria (especially in neutropenic patients)
What diagnostic studies are used in esophageal infection?	EGD with biopsy or cytologic brushing is most useful.
What is the typical EGD appearance of esophageal infection with the following:	
Candida	Confluent or nodular white–yellow plaques
Herpesvirus	Vesicles
CMV	Diffuse ulceration or giant esophageal ulcer
What is the symptomatic treatment for esophageal infection?	Viscous lidocaine
What is the treatment for esophageal infection with *Candida*?	Fluconazole, ketoconazole, nystatin, or amphotericin B
What is the treatment for esophageal infection with herpesvirus?	Acyclovir
What is the treatment for esophageal infection with CMV?	Ganciclovir

What medications can cause pill esophagitis?	Doxycycline, tetracycline, NSAIDs, quinidine, iron sulfate, vitamin C, potassium chloride, and alendronate
What is the treatment for pill esophagitis?	As a preventive measure, the patient should be in an upright position to take the pills and a full glass of liquid should be taken with the pills. In symptomatic cases, treatment is with viscous lidocaine and sucralfate.
What is the most common benign tumor of the esophagus?	Leiomyoma

STOMACH

GASTRITIS AND GASTROPARESIS

What are the types of gastritis?	Erosive and nonerosive
What are the causes of erosive gastritis?	Serious illness (e.g., trauma, burns, and sepsis), stress-related mucosal disease, drug ingestion (e.g., NSAIDs), alcohol ingestion, mucosal trauma (e.g., irradiation and caustic ingestion), and ischemia
What part of the stomach is involved?	Any part of the stomach but the fundus is most common
What are symptoms and signs of erosive gastritis?	Dyspepsia and bleeding
What is the treatment for erosive gastritis?	Prevention (consider prophylactic H_2 receptor antagonists), correction of underlying condition, removal of the offending agent (e.g., a drug), and acid suppression for complications
What are the types of nonerosive gastritis?	Type A—fundic gland gastritis Type B—antral gland gastritis
What are symptoms of nonerosive gastritis?	It is usually asymptomatic.

What is the pathogenesis of type A gastritis?

It is associated with decreased acid secretion and increased gastrin from fundic gland atrophy. A small subset of patients may have pernicious anemia.

What is the pathogenesis of type B gastritis?

It is associated with Hp infection (100% of cases) and with healthy aging (50% of cases occur in persons older than age 50 years). Intestinal metaplasia can occur with increased gastric CA risk.

What are some other causes of specific gastritis?

Ménétrier's disease, sarcoidosis, CD, tuberculosis, and syphilis

What is dumping syndrome?

After pyloroplasty or antrectomy and with loss of pyloric regulation of gastric emptying, hyperosmolar food is "dumped" rapidly into the proximal small bowel.

What occurs during early and late phase dumping?

In the early (hyperosmolar) phase within 1 hour after eating, "dumping" of hyperosmolar food pulls water into the small bowel lumen and stimulates motility and release of vasoactive peptides, producing hypotension, dizziness, and tachycardia.

In the late (hypoglycemic) phase 1–3 hours after a meal, rapid absorption of large amounts of glucose stimulates excessive insulin release and hypoglycemia, resulting in tachycardia, light-headedness, and diaphoresis.

What are the most common causes of gastroparesis?

Diabetes, the aftermath of viral infections, disorders of smooth muscle (e.g., scleroderma and dermatomyositis), and idiopathic causes

What are symptoms and signs of gastroparesis?

Nausea, vomiting, bloating, difficulty controlling blood glucose, and bezoar formation

How is the diagnosis of gastroparesis made?

Nuclear medicine gastric emptying studies of solids are difficult to standardize but are the best test to define degree of delayed function. $T_{1/2}$ greater than 90 minutes suggests delayed gastric emptying.

EGD or barium studies can be a useful adjunct to exclude other processes such as gastric outlet obstruction.

What is the treatment for gastroparesis?

Prokinetics (e.g., metoclopramide or cisapride), erythromycin, or domperidone (experimental)

PEPTIC ULCER DISEASE

What is the pathogenesis of PUD?

Mucosal ulceration occurs as a result of imbalance between aggressive factors and mucosal protective (defensive) factors.

What are the aggressive factors?

Hp, acid, pepsin, NSAIDs, alcohol, and smoking. Stress is not associated.

What are the defensive factors?

Mucosal mucus layer, bicarbonate, prostaglandins, blood flow, growth factors, and epithelial regeneration

What are symptoms of PUD?

Dyspepsia (epigastric burning pain), nausea, ill-defined abdominal distress, bloating, and belching

How is the diagnosis of PUD made?

EGD or barium UGI series, plus the establishment of Hp status

What if a gastric ulcer is found by EGD?

Gastric ulcers (but not duodenal ulcers) should be assessed with a repeat EGD after 8 weeks of therapy because nonhealing gastric ulcers may be malignant.

What is Hp?

Helicobacter pylori is a spiral gram-negative rod with 6–7 flagella and potent urease enzyme.

Is Hp commonly found with ulcers?

Yes, Hp is associated with 100% of type B antral gastritis, more than 90% of duodenal ulcers, and 70% of gastric ulcers.

How does Hp cause ulcers?

Hp resides below the mucous layer just above the gastric epithelium (it does not invade the mucosa). It causes ulceration by the following:

1. Causing a local and systemic inflammatory response with cytokine release
2. Increasing gastrin and acid via interference with somatostatin release from antral D cells, thus impairing the feedback inhibition to antral G cells
3. Producing direct cytopathic effects to the mucosa (urease, cytotoxins), thus producing toxic ammonia from enzymatic cleavage of urea

What are diagnostic tests for Hp?

Hp serology (ELISA), flexsure, CLO test (rapid urease test), histology, breath tests (^{13}C, ^{14}C), and Hp culture

What are the uses and advantages of the following:
    Hp serology (ELISA)

IgG antibody against Hp is detected. The test is noninvasive and inexpensive.

    Flexsure

Flexsure is an office-based rapid serum test that tests for IgG.

    CLO test (rapid urease test)

An antral mucosal biopsy specimen is placed in a gel that contains urea and pH indicator. If Hp (and thus urease) is present, urea is broken down to CO_2 and NH_3, resulting in increased pH and a color change from yellow to red. Results are available within hours.

    Histologic study

Giemsa or Warthin-Starry stains provide direct microscopic visualization of Hp.

    Breath tests (^{13}C, ^{14}C)

Radiolabeled urea is ingested and, if Hp (and thus urease) is present in the stomach, NH_3 and radiolabeled CO_2 are generated, absorbed into the bloodstream, and measured in exhaled air. It is safe, noninvasive, and has

	very low radiation exposure. It is the test of choice to document eradication of Hp.
Hp culture	The test is useful only when resistance is suspected.

What are the disadvantages of the following:

Hp serology (ELISA)	Titers remain high for a year or more so it cannot accurately confirm Hp eradication.
CLO test	Requires EGD
Histologic study	Requires EGD
Breath tests (^{13}C, ^{14}C)	Require minimal amounts of radiation exposure
Hp culture	Requires a technically complex research tool with limited availability
What is triple therapy for Hp?	The gold standard is bismuth (Pepto-Bismol), metronidazole, and tetracycline. Noncompliance is an issue because of the side effects and the number of pills that must be taken.
What other therapy is there for Hp?	New combinations and shorter courses of therapy are constantly being tried. Metronidazole, PPIs, and clarithromycin (or amoxicillin) twice daily for 7 days is currently recommended.
What is the treatment for PUD?	Eradication of Hp if present (eradication means cure)
	Discontinuation of NSAIDs, tobacco, and alcohol (consider prostaglandin E_2 analogs if NSAIDs must be continued)
	Acid inhibition (H_2 receptor antagonists or PPIs)
	Surgery (vagotomy with or without pyloroplasty) reserved for medically refractory PUD or for complications from PUD
	No dietary restrictions other than those that relieve symptoms

What are the complications of PUD?	Bleeding, perforation, pyloric stenosis, and gastric outlet obstruction
What are the causes of elevated gastrin?	Hypochlorhydric and achlorhydric conditions (e.g., pernicious anemia, Hp infection, and gastric atrophy) Hypersecretory conditions (e.g., ZES, retained antrum syndrome, antral G cell hyperplasia, gastric outlet obstruction, short bowel syndrome, systemic mastocytosis, and basophilic granulocytic leukemia) Decreased clearance (e.g., renal failure)
What is ZES?	Think **GUT:** **G**astrin elevation (acid hypersecretion) **U**lcer disease (severe and often in multiple sites) **T**umor (gastrinoma)
What is the epidemiology of ZES?	Mean age of onset 50 years old Occurs in men more frequently than women
Is ZES a common cause of PUD?	No. ZES accounts for < 1% of all PUD.
What conditions are associated with ZES?	25% percent of cases are associated with MEN-I, 75% are sporadic, and 50% are solitary (40% pancreatic, 15% duodenal, and 10% lymph node).
How is the diagnosis of ZES made?	Elevated fasting gastrin (98% of cases) Elevated basal acid output (98% of cases) Positive secretin test (> 90% of cases). After IV administration of 2 U/kg of secretin, there is an increase of gastrin to more than 200 pg/ml above the basal gastrin level.
How is the tumor localized?	EGD, endoscopic ultrasound, nuclear medicine octreoscan, CT scan of the abdomen, or selective vascular sampling via abdominal angiography
Are gastrinomas frequently found in ZES?	In 35% of cases, no tumor can be located.

What are common metastatic sites?	Bone and lung
What is the treatment of ZES?	Decrease gastric acid hypersecretion (PPIs , total gastrectomy with vagotomy) and surgical excision of primary gastrinoma
What is the prognosis for ZES following surgical excision?	5%–20% cure rate

SMALL AND LARGE INTESTINE

DIARRHEA

What vital information should be obtained from the history in cases of diarrhea?	1. Duration (acute versus chronic) 2. Frequency (number of bowel movements per day) 3. Volume and consistency of each bowel movement (e.g., measured in cups or squirts) 4. Relation of bowel movements to meals 5. Episodes of nocturnal diarrhea or incontinence 6. Associated symptoms (e.g., fever, abdominal pain, nausea and vomiting, blood or mucus in stool, tenesmus, orthostasis, and weight loss) 7. History of diarrhea-causing illness (e.g., hyperthyroidism, ZES) 8. Past medical history, sexual history, HIV status, travel history, and contact with animals 9. Medications (e.g., laxatives and magnesium-containing antacids) 10. Recent possible ingestion of contaminated food or water
What is the average content of stool?	100 ml water, 40 mEq/L Na^+, 90 mEq/L K^+, 16 mEq/L Cl^-, and organic anions from bacterial fermentation of carbohydrates
What is diarrhea?	Volume of > 200–250 g stool/day (not frequency, liquidity, or incontinence)

What are the major types of diarrhea?

Secretory, osmotic, motility disorder, and exudative

What is the pathophysiology of secretory diarrhea?

Increased secretion of water and electrolytes into the gut lumen and, in most cases, associated partial inhibition of intestinal absorption

What are features of secretory diarrhea?

1. Large stool volume (> 1 L/day)
2. Watery stool
3. No pus, blood, or mucus in stools
4. Persistent diarrhea, despite 24- to 48-hour fast (except with bile salt and laxative-induced diarrhea when fats and laxatives are not ingested)
5. Stool osmolality equal to plasma osmolality, with no anion gap

What are causes of secretory diarrhea?

Enterotoxins—cholera and infection with *Escherichia coli, Staphylococcus aureus, Bacillus cereus*

Hormonal secretagogues—VIP, calcitonin, serotonin, prostaglandins

Gastric acid hypersecretion—ZES, short bowel syndrome, mastocytosis

Laxative abuse—castor oil, bisacodyl, senna, phenolphthalein

Bile salts—terminal ileal resection or disease, bile duct obstruction

Fatty acids—pancreatic insufficiency, small bowel mucosal disease

What is the pathophysiology of osmotic diarrhea?

Increased amounts of poorly absorbable, osmotically active solutes into the bowel lumen

What are features of osmotic diarrhea?

1. Diarrhea typically stops when the patient fasts.
2. Measured stool osmolality is greater than calculated stool osmolality. Calculated stool osmolality = $2([stool\ Na^+] + [stool\ K^+])$.
3. Anion gap is greater than 50 mg/dl.
4. Stool pH may be helpful in identifying osmolar substances as follows:
   acid pH—carbohydrates

Alkaline pH—milk of magnesia
Neutral pH—poorly absorbable
salts of Mg^{2+} or SO_4^{2-}

What are causes of osmotic diarrhea?

Carbohydrate malabsorption (e.g., lactose intolerance, aftermath of infectious gastroenteritis with mucosal inflammation, ingestion of mannitol or sorbitol, lactulose deficiency, or primary disaccharidase deficiency)

Generalized malabsorption (e.g., sprue, radiation enteritis, or ischemia)

Ingestion of osmotically acting substances (e.g., sodium sulfate, sodium phosphate, magnesium sulfate, milk of magnesia, and magnesium-containing antacids)

What is the pathophysiology of motility disorders?

Increased or decreased contact between the luminal contents and the mucosa

What motility disorders cause diarrhea?

Increased small-bowel motility, resulting in decreased contact time (e.g., hyperthyroidism, carcinoid, and dumping syndrome)

Decreased small-bowel motility, resulting in small-bowel overgrowth (e.g., hypothyroidism, scleroderma, and amyloid)

Increased colonic motility, such as in IBS

Anal sphincter dysfunction, which may cause incontinence (e.g., aftermath of surgery, neuromuscular disease, and inflammation)

What is the pathophysiology of exudative diarrhea?

Active inflammation can decrease absorption, cause secretory diarrhea via prostaglandin generation, or increase osmotic load by exudation of mucus, blood, pus, or protein into the gut lumen

What inflammatory states cause diarrhea?

Idiopathic states (e.g., CD and UC)

Infectious states (e.g., infection with *Shigella, Salmonella,* and *Clostridium difficile*)

Ischemia and vasculitic states
Postradiation therapy

Define acute diarrhea.

Abrupt onset of diarrhea lasting 2–3 weeks

List the common causes of acute diarrhea.

Infection, drugs, miscellaneous

Which is the most common cause of acute diarrhea?

Infection

What are the infectious causes of diarrhea?

Food poisoning; viral, bacterial, and parasitic infection

What are features of food poisoning?

Preformed toxins, no mucosal invasion, watery stools, and no inflammation

What are the causes of food poisoning?

S. aureus (dairy products), *B. cereus* (fried rice), *Clostridium perfringens* (reheated meat), and *Vibrio parahaemolyticus* (seafood)

What are features of viral infections?

No mucosal invasion, watery stools, and no inflammation

What are the causes of viral infections?

Rotavirus, Norwalk virus, enteric adenovirus

What are features of bacterial infections of the small bowel?

No inflammation and watery diarrhea

What are causes of bacterial infections in the small bowel?

Vibrio cholerae and toxigenic *E. coli*

What are features of bacterial infections of the colon?

Inflammation, mucosal invasion, and blood and fecal leukocytes

What are causes of bacterial infections in the colon?

Campylobacter (most common), *Salmonella* (poultry), *Shigella* (day care centers), *Yersinia,* invasive *E. coli,* and *C. difficile* (antibiotic-associated diarrhea)

What are features of parasitic infections of the small bowel?	No inflammation and watery diarrhea
What are causes of parasitic infections of the small bowel?	*Giardia* (well water) and *Cryptosporidium*
What are features of parasitic infections of the colon?	Inflammation, mucosal invasion, and blood and fecal leukocytes
What organism causes parasitic infections of the colon?	*Entamoeba histolytica*
What drugs cause acute diarrhea?	Laxatives, antacids, lactulose, theophylline, NSAIDs, PGE$_2$ derivatives, colchicine, quinidine, diuretics, propranolol, and antibiotics, among others
What are miscellaneous causes of acute diarrhea?	Fecal impaction and ischemic bowel disease
What are common causes of traveler's diarrhea?	*E. coli, Salmonella, Giardia,* and *E. histolytica*
Define chronic diarrhea.	Any diarrheal illness lasting longer than 3 weeks
List the common causes of chronic diarrhea.	Infection, inflammation, malabsorption, drugs, endocrine disorders, and motility disorders
What are the infectious causes of chronic diarrhea?	*Giardia, E. histolytica* (institutions), *Mycobacterium tuberculosis, Cryptosporidia* (AIDS), and *C. difficile* (pseudomembranous colitis)
What are the inflammatory causes of chronic diarrhea?	UC, CD, collagenous colitis, ischemia, and solitary rectal ulcer
What are the malabsorptive causes of chronic diarrhea?	Small bowel mucosal disease, disaccharidase deficiency (lactose intolerance), pancreatic insufficiency, radiation enteritis, and bacterial overgrowth

What drugs cause chronic diarrhea?

Surreptitious laxative use, antibiotics, diuretics, NSAIDs, and theophylline

What are the endocrinologic causes of chronic diarrhea?

ZES, hyperthyroidism, carcinoid, VIPoma, villous adenoma, adrenal insufficiency, hyperparathyroidism, and diabetes

Which motility disorders cause chronic diarrhea?

IBS, narcotic bowel, and dumping syndrome

What characterizes small-bowel diarrhea?

Large-volume, watery, greasy stools with occasional food particles; intermittent crampy abdominal pain

What characterizes left colon and rectal diarrhea?

Small-volume stool with possible mucus, blood, or pus, tenesmus, and pelvic or sacral pain relieved by passing stool

Which infectious agents are a common cause of bloody stool?

Think **CHESS:**
Campylobacter
Hemorrhagic *E. coli*, serotype 0157:H7
Entamoeba histolytica
Salmonella
Shigella

Which infections cause WBCs or lactoferrin in stool?

CHESS plus cytotoxic *C. difficile*

What laboratory tests should be ordered for diarrhea?

Initial evaluation should include CBC with differential, serum electrolytes, BUN, creatinine, and chemistry profile

What should you look for in stool?

Blood (gross or occult), fecal leukocytes or lactoferrin, fat (Sudan stain), trophozoites, and phenolphthalein (to rule out laxative abuse)

What tests are available for stool samples?

Bacterial culture (*Salmonella, Shigella,* and *Campylobacter*), stool osmolality and electrolytes, *C. difficile* toxin assay (not culture), and acid-fast stain (cryptosporidiosis, *Isospora belli*). *E. histolytica* is frequently diagnosed by serology.

Clinical pearl	The absence of fecal leukocytes does not rule out an inflammatory state because false-negative results do occur (especially in samples that sit too long in the laboratory, resulting in lysis of WBCs).
What diagnostic tests are ordered for diarrhea?	1. Proctosigmoidoscopy and colonoscopy, especially for bloody diarrhea and to rule out IBD and pseudomembranous colitis 2. 72-hour quantitative fecal fat test if fat malabsorption is suspected 3. Cortrosyn stimulation test 4. Duodenal aspirate for *Giardia* 5. Small-bowel biopsy if malabsorption is suspected 6. Breath tests to diagnose lactose intolerance or small-bowel bacterial overgrowth
What is the treatment for diarrhea?	1. Direct treatment of the underlying cause 2. For acute diarrhea, correction of fluid and electrolyte abnormalities and reduction of symptoms of diarrhea (with adsorbents, antisecretory drugs, opiate derivatives, anticholinergic agents, and antimicrobial agents)
Clinical pearls	Avoid antibiotic therapy in enteric *Salmonella* infection because a prolonged carrier state may be induced. Antimotility agents must be used with caution in patients with inflammatory diarrhea (e.g., IBD and pseudomembranous colitis)

MALABSORPTION

What is malabsorption?	Impaired ability of the bowel to absorb or digest nutrients
What causes impaired absorption?	Abnormal epithelium-instrinsic small-bowel disease

What are the causes of intrinsic small-bowel disease?	Lactase deficiency, celiac sprue, tropical sprue, Whipple's disease, collagenous colitis, amyloidosis, impaired lymphatic drainage from the gut, and decreased gut absorptive surface area
What is lactase deficiency?	Diminished amounts of the brush border enzyme, lactase, result in a decreased ability to break down lactose
Who is affected by lactase deficiency?	Most common in blacks, Orientals, Eskimos, and Central and South Americans
What is celiac sprue?	Gluten intolerance (wheat, barley, rye, and oats)
What dermatologic manifestation is associated with celiac sprue?	Dermatitis herpetiformis
What does small-bowel biopsy show in celiac sprue?	Findings are characteristic but not diagnostic, showing blunt, flattened villi and an inflammatory infiltrate in the lamina propria.
How is the diagnosis of celiac sprue made?	By response to a gluten-free diet and positive anti-gliadin, anti-endomysial antibodies
What other risks are associated with celiac sprue?	Lymphoma and carcinoma
What is tropical sprue?	An acquired form of sprue infrequently encountered in America that improves with antibiotic therapy
What is Whipple's disease?	Systemic disorder with fever and myalgia
What does small-bowel biopsy show in Whipple's disease?	PAS-positive macrophages that contain the bacillus *Tropheryma whippelii*

What is collagenous colitis?

Collagenous colitis is a variant of IBD diagnosed pathologically by finding a thickened collagen basement membrane in the colonic epithelium. It has a variable response to treatment (similar to IBD).

How is the diagnosis of amyloidosis made?

By Congo red stain of a rectal, gastric, or fat pad biopsy

What are other causes of instrinsic small-bowel disease that result in malabsorption?

CD, lymphoma, parasitic infection, radiation enteritis, abetalipoproteinemia, and ischemia

What causes impaired lymphatic drainage from the gut?

Congenital and idiopathic lymphangiectasia, lymphoma, in association with congestive heart failure, right heart valvular disease, or lymphatic obstruction (e.g., retroperitoneal fibrosis and metastatic cancer)

What can reduce the absorptive surface area of the gut?

Intestinal resection (e.g., for CD, bowel infarction, or volvulus)

What is malabsorbed after proximal small-bowel resection?

Calcium, folic acid, and iron

What is malabsorbed after distal (ileum) resection?

Bile acids and vitamin B_{12}

What causes impaired digestion?

Pancreatic exocrine insufficiency, bile acid insufficiency, small-bowel bacterial overgrowth, and inadequate mixing of gastric acid, bile salts, and pancreatic enzymes

What are the causes of pancreatic exocrine insufficiency?

Chronic pancreatitis, pancreatic cancer, and cystic fibrosis result in a decreased amount of the pancreatic enzymes necessary for digestion of fat, protein, and carbohydrates.

What are the causes of bile acid insufficiency?	Any disorder of bile acid enterohepatic circulation (e.g., severe intrinsic liver disease, biliary obstruction, and disorders of the terminal ileum)
How does malabsorption occur in bile acid insufficiency?	Insufficient bile acids impair the formation of intraluminal micelles resulting in fat and fat-soluble vitamin (A, D, E, and K) malabsorption. Carbohydrate and protein absorption are normal. Bile acids stimulate colonic secretion.
When is small-bowel bacterial overgrowth seen?	Commonly seen in blind loops after Billroth II resection and in states of altered intestinal motility (e.g., scleroderma and diabetes).
What are clinical problems with bacterial overgrowth?	Bile salt deconjugation and fat malabsorption
When does inadequate mixing of gastric acid, bile salts, and pancreatic enzymes occur?	After gastric surgery, especially after Billroth II procedures
Clinical pearl	Always consider malabsorption with the triad of anemia, weight loss, and diarrhea.

What are symptoms and signs of malabsorption?

1. Diarrhea
2. Steatorrhea—greasy, foul-smelling stools that float
3. Weight loss
4. Bone pain or tetany—calcium deficiency
5. Glossitis and stomatitis—iron and riboflavin deficiency
6. Edema—hypoalbuminemia
7. Bleeding and easy bruisability—vitamin K deficiency
8. Night blindness—vitamin A deficiency

What are the laboratory findings in malabsorption?

1. Anemia—iron, folate, or B_{12} deficiency
2. Decreased calcium, magnesium, carotene, albumin, and cholesterol
3. Elevated prothrombin time

What diagnostic tests can be performed to determine the cause of malabsorption?

Fecal fat determination, plain films of the abdomen, small-bowel biopsy and aspirate, stool examination, pancreatitis function tests, bile acid breath tests, the D-xylose test, breath hydrogen test, and the Schilling test

What is qualitative fecal fat testing?

Sudan staining of stool. More than 80 g of fat/day should be ingested for testing.

How is qualitative testing useful?

As a screening test. Results are reliable when they are positive, but negative results do not rule out fat malabsorption.

What problem is associated with quantitative (72-hour fecal fat determination) testing of stool?

The collection of stool (without urine) is a cumbersome 3-day process.

What criterion renders a quantitative test positive?

Stool fat > 5 g/24 hours on a 100-g fat diet

What should you look for on plain films of the abdomen in cases of malabsorption?

Possible pancreatic calcification in chronic pancreatitis

What is the purpose of small-bowel biopsy and aspirate in cases of malabsorption?

Several mucosal diseases can be diagnosed by characteristic histologic features. Jejunal aspirate for bacterial quantitation can assess for bacterial overgrowth.

What clues for malabsorption are seen on examination of stool?

Undigested food material

What is the bentiromide test?

A test of pancreatic exocrine function. Oral bentiromide is ingested and normally cleaved by pancreatic chymotrypsin, releasing PABA, which is absorbed and excreted in the urine.

What test result is suggestive of pancreatic enzyme deficiency?

< 60% excretion of PABA

What might false-positive test results signify?

Small-bowel mucosal disease or renal insufficiency

What is the bile acid breath test used for?

To establish the presence of small-bowel bacterial overgrowth

How is the test performed?

^{14}C-glycocholate is ingested. Normally, 95% is absorbed in the terminal ileum and 5% enters the colon and is deconjugated by bacteria to $^{14}CO_2$, which is absorbed and exhaled in expired air.

How is a positive test determined?

With bacterial overgrowth, earlier bacterial deconjugation occurs and a larger amount of $^{14}CO_2$ is measured.

What is the d-xylose test used for?

To test for carbohydrate malabsorption

How is the test performed?

d-Xylose is normally absorbed intact across the intestinal mucosa. Xylose is ingested and measured in the serum and in the urine in a 5-hour collection.

What results constitute a positive test?

Less than 5 g of xylose in 5 hours suggests small-bowel mucosal disease.

What might false-positive results signify?

Ascites, bacterial overgrowth, or renal insufficiency

What is the breath hydrogen test used for?

To test for lactose intolerance

How is it performed?

If orally administered lactose is not absorbed in the small bowel, it reaches the colon where bacterial fermentation occurs.

How is a positive test determined?

Bacterial fermentation results in production of excessive amounts of radiolabeled hydrogen, which is absorbed and exhaled from the lungs.

What does the Schilling test evaluate?	Terminal ileal and pancreatic function
How is the test performed?	Dietary B_{12} is bound to gastric R protein and cleaved by pancreatic enzymes. In the small bowel, B_{12} is rapidly transferred to intrinsic factor, which is absorbed in the terminal ileum.
How is a positive test determined?	Less than 10% urinary excretion of cobalt-labeled B_{12} (ingested with intrinsic factor) over 24 hours is suggestive of terminal ileal or pancreatic dysfunction.
What is the treatment for malabsorption?	Therapy is directed at the specific cause of malabsorption. Dietary modification is frequently necessary—low-fat diets (restriction of long-chain fatty acids) or medium-chain triglycerides (which do not require bile acids for absorption) may also be used. Pancreatic enzyme replacement can be given orally with meals and snacks. Bile acid binders (cholestyramine) may improve bile salt diarrhea but can significantly worsen steatorrhea. Antibiotics can be used to treat Whipple's disease, tropical sprue, and bacterial overgrowth. Abnormal electrolytes and vitamin deficiencies should be corrected.

IRRITABLE BOWEL SYNDROME

What is IBS?	The most common digestive disorder, accounting for up to 50% of patients referred to gastroenterologists. It is a group of chronic functional bowel disorders with a variety of symptoms.
What are symptoms and signs of IBS?	Abdominal pain, constipation, diarrhea, alternating constipation and diarrhea, gas, bloating, incomplete evacuation, tenesmus, rectal pain, or mucus in stool

What is the epidemiology of IBS?

Female patients outnumber male patients 2:1, and there is a higher incidence among whites than among other races.

What is the pathophysiology of IBS?

Unknown. It is probably a disorder of bowel motility with abnormalities in myoelectric activity of colon and intestinal motor activity.

How is the diagnosis of IBS made?

Identification of typical symptoms with a normal examination and exclusion of organic diseases

What clues suggest the diagnosis of IBS?

The patient appears healthy.
Symptoms are related to stress.
Weight is stable or increasing.
Symptoms are chronic.

What diagnostic tests rule out organic disease?

Test for occult blood in stool
If diarrheal, test for ova and parasites, culture, and fecal leukocytes
Sigmoidoscopy
Serum chemistry, hematocrit, and thyroid function tests
In selected patients, consider EGD, colonoscopy, small-bowel aspirate and biopsy, breath hydrogen testing for lactose intolerance, GB ultrasound, pancreatic function tests, and abdominal CT scanning

What is the treatment for IBS?

1. Emotional support and reassurance as well as stress reduction
2. Diet and fiber therapy—avoidance of foods that cause symptoms (e.g., lactose and gas-producing foods), high-fiber diets in some patients, and supplemental fiber (e.g., psyllium)
3. Medication—antispasmodics when abdominal pain and constipation predominate, antidiarrheals when diarrhea predominates, laxatives when constipation predominates, and antidepressants

Clinical pearl	Some cases of IBS have been associated with a past history of physical and sexual abuse.

ISCHEMIC BOWEL

What is ischemic bowel?	Insufficient arterial blood flow to or insufficient venous blood flow away from the gut
What are the general causes of ischemic bowel?	Vascular occlusion (arterial or venous) or non-occlusive vascular disease (low flow states)
What are common causes of occlusive vascular disease?	Thrombolic and embolic disease of the celiac axis, superior and inferior mesenteric arteries, or their branches, and dissecting aortic aneurysm
What are the risk factors for occlusive vascular disease?	Hypercholesterolemia, atrial fibrillation, endocarditis, myocardial infarction, atrial myxoma, rheumatic heart disease, polycythemia, hypercoagulable state, and some hemoglobinopathies
What are symptoms and signs of acute vascular occlusion?	1. Severe, diffuse abdominal pain in the face of a relatively benign physical examination (pain > tenderness; 20%–30% are painless) 2. Decreased or absent bowel sounds 3. Occult blood that rapidly progresses to frankly bloody stool 4. Hypotension, tachycardia, fever, elevated white blood cell count, and acidosis develop as transmural infarction and peritonitis develop.
What is the treatment of acute vascular occlusion?	Immediate reestablishment of blood flow is necessary to save the bowel. Angiography is used to localize the occlusion, followed by embolectomy. Frequently, transmural necrosis has already occurred and surgical resection is indicated.
What are the two types of non-occlusive vascular disease?	Abdominal angina and ischemic colitis

What are risk factors for non-occlusive vascular disease?

Low flow states—atherosclerosis involving at least two of the three major visceral arteries, cardiovascular conditions predisposing the patient to transient reductions in bowel perfusion (e.g., congestive heart failure and arrhythmia), and shock

What is abdominal angina?

An uncommon entity with severe, incapacitating midabdominal pain that occurs several minutes after eating due to insufficient postprandial mucosal blood flow

What symptoms are often associated with abdominal angina?

Weight loss—commonly, 5–15 kg
Sitophobia—fear of eating due to pain
Malabsorption—a result of ischemic mucosa
Occasional nausea, vomiting, or postprandial diarrhea

What do diagnostic tests show in patients with abdominal angina?

Abdominal angiography demonstrates complete or near complete occlusion of at least two of the three major splanchnic arteries.

What is the treatment for abdominal angina?

Surgical arterial bypass or endarterectomy

What is ischemic colitis?

Mucosal ischemia as a result of transient low blood flow through atherosclerotic splanchnic vasculature

Where does ischemic colitis most commonly occur?

In watershed areas (i.e., areas that fall between major supply vessels)—the splenic flexure and sigmoid colon

What is the clinical presentation of ischemic colitis?

Abrupt onset of lower abdominal pain and bloody stool

How is the diagnosis of ischemic colitis made?

Plain abdominal radiographs. "Thumbprinting" is indicative of submucosal edema.
Flexible sigmoidoscopy. Erythema, ulceration, and edema are suggestive of colitis and may reveal blue–black necrotic mucosa.

Angiography is rarely useful because ischemic colitis is due to low flow, not occlusion.

What is the treatment for ischemic colitis?

In most patients, the disease course is self-limited with spontaneous recovery.
Initial treatment includes intravenous fluids and nothing by mouth, with frequent abdominal examinations.
Antibiotics are generally unnecessary.
In a minority of patients, peritoneal signs and absent bowel sounds indicate infarction. Treatment consists of segmental resection of affected bowel. Strictures in areas of necrosis may develop and should be evaluated with a follow-up barium enema 6–8 weeks after recovery.

DIVERTICULAR DISEASE

What is diverticular disease?

Congenital diverticula are outpouchings of the entire thickness of the intestinal wall.
Acquired diverticula are outpouchings of the mucosa and submucosa through the muscular layer of the intestinal wall, occurring anywhere in the small bowel or colon but most commonly at the site of a nutrient artery.

What is the incidence of diverticular disease?

Congenital Meckel's diverticulum occurs in approximately 2% of the population.
Acquired colonic diverticula are common, occurring in approximately 50% of patients older than 60 years of age.

Where do small-bowel diverticula most commonly arise?

In the proximal duodenum, near the ampulla of Vater. They are common, occurring in approximately 20% of the population.

What is the significance of small-bowel diverticula?

Most are asymptomatic, but they can cause common bile duct obstruction.

What is Meckel's diverticulum?	Persistent omphalomesenteric duct—the most common congenital abnormality of the GI tract
What are the complications of a Meckel's diverticulum?	Approximately one third of cases contain functional gastric mucosa, which can ulcerate, bleed, or perforate, necessitating surgical intervention.
What is the rule of 2's?	Meckel's diverticulum occurs in 2% of the population, it is found 2 feet from the ileocecal valve, and it is approximately 2 cm long.
Where do most colonic diverticula commonly arise?	Sigmoid colon
What are the risk factors for the development of colonic diverticula?	A low-fiber, high-fat diet causes slower bowel transit time, decreased stool bulk, and increased colonic segmentation. The latter forms high-pressure zones, resulting in pulsion diverticula from herniation of mucosa and submucosa through the bowel wall at the point where blood vessels penetrate.
Clinical pearl	Ninety percent of patients with colonic diverticula are asymptomatic.

DIVERTICULITIS*

What is diverticulitis?	Obstruction of a diverticulum causing acute inflammation
What is the most common location for diverticulitis to occur?	Sigmoid colon secondary to increased intraluminal pressures
What is the cause of diverticulitis?	It is probably secondary to mechanical blockage of diverticula by undigested food particles and bacteria. This decreases the blood supply to the diverticulum and renders it susceptible to invasion by colonic bacteria.

---

* In collaboration with V. Shami, N. Thielman, and C. Sable

How common is diverticulitis?	Occurs in 10% of patients with diverticular disease Occurs with a recurrence rate of 50% Occurs with increasing age
What are the symptoms and signs of diverticulitis?	Fever, constipation, LLQ pain, muscle spasm, guarding, rebound tenderness, and occult rectal bleeding (in 25% of cases)
What are the laboratory findings in cases of diverticulitis?	Leukocytosis
How is the diagnosis of diverticulitis made?	Abdominal CT scan may be useful. Invasive diagnostic studies such as colonoscopy should be avoided.
What is the treatment for diverticulitis?	In patients with nonperforated bowels, bowel rest, stool softeners, liquid diet, and broad-spectrum antibiotic coverage (including coverage for anaerobes) are indicated. In patients with perforated bowels or who suffer repeated attacks, surgical resection is needed.
What are the complications of diverticulitis?	Perforation can result in peritonitis with fever, leukocytosis, and peritoneal signs. Rarely, sepsis and shock can occur. Fistulae to the bladder, skin, or vagina Ureteral obstruction Bowel obstruction Retroperitoneal fibrosis Septic thromboembolus Hepatic abscess
What are other complications of colonic diverticula?	1. Spastic diverticular disease—episodic or constant constipation, crampy lower quadrant abdominal pain, and postprandial abdominal distention. Pain is often relieved by defecation. 2. Bleeding—erosion into a branch arteriole causing significant bleeding manifested as hematochezia or maroon stools. Bleeding is usually painless. Seventy percent of diverticular bleeds are localized in the

right colon. Bleeding stops
spontaneously in 80% of cases.
3. Strictures—secondary to chronic
inflammation

INFLAMMATORY BOWEL DISEASE

What is IBD?

Idiopathic IBD is comprised of CD and
UC and is characterized by chronic
bowel inflammation. There is significant
overlap between CD and UC, but each
has characteristic clinical, endoscopic,
and histologic features.

**What is the epidemiology
of IBD?**

Incidence of IBD is approximately
    30,000 new cases per year.
The highest incidence is in developed
    countries.
Persons of Jewish ancestry are affected
    more than whites, who are affected
    more than blacks.
Peak incidence occurs in persons
    between 15 and 40 years old and in
    men and women equally.

What are the differences between CD and UC?

Table 5–1

	Crohn's Disease	Ulcerative Colitis
Gastrointestinal tract involvement	Mouth to anus	Colon
Gross inflammation	Skip lesions	Continuous from rectum
Rectal involvement	Rectal sparing	99%
Histologic inflammation	Transmural	Mucosal/submucosa
Histology	Focal inflammation and granulomas	Diffuse inflammation
Fistulas	Common	Rare
Ulcers	Linear/transverse	Diffuse/superficial
Bleeding	20%	98%
Abdominal pain	Common	Uncommon
Perianal disease	80%	25%
Abdominal mass	Common	Uncommon
Carcinoma	Uncommon	Common
Toxic megacolon	Rare	More likely
Post-surgical recurrence	Frequent (70%)	Rare
Smoking	Exacerbates CD	May be protective

What are the extraintestinal manifestations of IBD?	Manifestations that occur concurrently with intestinal disease activity, or Unpleasant Entities that Parallel "Entestinal" Activity: Uveitis Episcleritis Pyoderma gangrenosum Erythema nodosum Arthritis (peripheral) Manifestations that occur independently of intestinal disease activity: Ankylosing spondylitis Sacroiliitis PSC

CROHN'S DISEASE

What is the anatomic distribution of disease in CD?	Gastroduodenitis: 10% Jejunoileitis–ileitis: 33% Ileocolitis: 50% Colitis: 15%

What are the clinical features of CD?

1. Stricture formation, primarily in the terminal ileum, with symptoms of partial obstruction (colicky pain, distention, anorexia, nausea, vomiting, and weight loss)
2. Palpable right lower quadrant inflammatory mass (25% of cases)
3. Fistulas to bowel, skin, vagina, or bladder. Infection and abscess may occur, and there is perianal involvement in 20%–40% of patients.
4. "Cobblestone" appearance, a deep linear and transverse ulceration with heaped-up mucosa in the terminal ileum or colon, often causing abdominal pain
5. Diarrhea due to many factors, including fat malabsorption with jejunal inflammation, bile salt malabsorption from terminal ileum involvement, decreased absorptive surface area with significant small-bowel involvement or fistula formation, bacterial overgrowth, and decreased absorption of fluid and electrolytes in diseased colon
6. Malnutrition, specifically, hypoalbuminemia, hypocholesterolemia, and iron or B_{12} deficiency anemias
7. Growth retardation and delayed sexual maturation in adolescents
8. Gallstone development, due to impaired ileal reabsorption of bile salts

How is the diagnosis of CD made?

The clinical symptoms and signs, combined with radiographic evidence of ulcerations, strictures, and skip areas, suggest CD. A biopsy demonstrating noncaseating granulomas is also helpful.

What is medical treatment for CD?

Therapy of CD depends on the severity of inflammation and the site of involved bowel. The medications used to treat IBD include 5-ASA derivatives, corticosteroids, antibiotics, and immunosuppressives. Supportive therapy is used as well.

How are the 5-ASA derivatives used?

To treat acute disease and maintain remission. Sulfasalazine is available to the colon; other oral 5-ASA derivatives (e.g., olsalazine and mesalamine) have varied availability from the pylorus through the colon. Topical 5-ASA in enema or suppository form is available to the left colon and rectum.

Should corticosteroids be used to treat CD?

Only in cases of acute disease. Corticosteroids come in oral, topical (e.g., enema and foam), and intravenous forms.

How should antibiotics be used in treatment of CD?

For fistulous and perianal disease. Antibiotics used include ciprofloxacin and metronidazole.

How should immunosuppressive therapy be used in treatment of CD?

With caution. Immunosuppressive therapy may be used for steroid sparing and maintenance of remission, but has limited usefulness in treating severe, acute disease. Drugs include azathioprine, 6-mercaptopurine, cyclosporine, and methotrexate.

What is important supportive therapy?

Nutrition, antidiarrheal agents, and vitamins

When is surgical treatment used?

Surgery may be required in symptomatic obstructive or fistulous disease that is unresponsive to medical therapy. The goal is palliation and to preserve as much bowel as possible. Postoperative recurrence is high (approximately 70%).

ULCERATIVE COLITIS

What is the anatomic distribution of disease in UC?

Proctitis (up to 12 cm): 30%
Left-sided colitis (up to splenic flexure):
   50%
Pancolitis: 20%

What are the clinical features of proctitis or left-sided colitis?

Rectal bleeding and tenesmus. Systemic symptoms are absent and diarrhea is variably present. Extension of disease can occur but is uncommon. Few cases progress to fulminant colitis and there is little or no malignant potential.

What are the clinical features of moderate disease?

Patients have frequent (4–6) bouts of bloody diarrhea per day, accompanied by abdominal pain and low-grade fever. A moderate number of cases progress to fulminant colitis.

What are the clinical features of fulminant colitis?

Severe bloody diarrhea (at least 10 episodes per day). Fever, hypovolemia, and anemia are common.

What are complications of UC?

Toxic megacolon, colonic perforation, and colon cancer

Why does toxic megacolon develop?

As inflammation progresses, the colon loses tone and begins to dilate.

What findings are associated with toxic megacolon?

Peritonitis, hypoalbuminemia, hypokalemia, marked leukocytosis, and high fever

What are possible precipitating factors for toxic megacolon?

Barium enema, colonoscopy, antidiarrheal agents, and opiates

What is the medical treatment for toxic megacolon?

Serial abdominal films and aggressive medical therapy with steroids, antibiotics, fluid–electrolyte replacement, and blood transfusion

When is surgery required?

If resolution does not occur within 24–72 hours

In whom does colonic perforation occur?

Most commonly in patients with toxic megacolon; also in patients with fulminant colitis without bowel dilatation. Colonoscopy and barium enema increase the risk of perforation.

What determines the risk of colon cancer?

Risk correlates with the duration and extent of the illness. Risk is negligible during the first 10 years of disease activity but begins to increase sharply after 20 years. Patients with pancolitis are especially susceptible.

How should patients with UC be followed up?

Surveillance colonoscopy with biopsies for dysplasia or prophylactic colectomy are recommended after 10 years.

How do colon cancers present in patients with UC?

They are typically intramural and multicentric.

What is the surgical treatment for UC?

The goal of surgery in UC is cure. The recommended procedure is total proctocolectomy with Brooke ileostomy or ileoanal anastomosis.

When is surgery indicated in UC?

1. When the disease is intractable to medical therapy
2. When there is fulminant colitis with or without toxic megacolon
3. When there is severe hemorrhage
4. When there is colonic perforation
5. When cancer or high-grade dysplasia develops

APPENDICITIS*

What age-group has the highest incidence of appendicitis?

20- to 30-year-old age-group

What is the cause of appendicitis?

Obstruction of the appendiceal lumen is identified in 30% of cases. Appendicitis is thought to result in bacterial multiplication, necrosis, and, ultimately, perforation.

What causes obstruction?

Fecalith, enlarged lymphoid follicles, neoplasms, foreign body, and worms

---

* In collaboration with V. Shami, N. Thielman, and C. Sable

What are symptoms and signs of appendicitis?	Poorly localized periumbilical pain (secondary to visceral irritation) is followed several hours later by a more steady, localized RLQ pain (secondary to parietal peritoneal irritation). Anorexia, nausea, and vomiting usually follow. Psoas, obturator, and Rovsing's signs are frequently found with advanced appendicitis.
What is the psoas sign?	Elicitation of pain when the hip and knee are fully extended
What is the obturator sign?	Elicitation of pain when the leg is internally rotated with the hip and knee flexed
What is Rovsing's sign?	Elicitation of pain in the RLQ while the LLQ is palpated
How is the diagnosis of appendicitis made?	History and physical examination
What is the treatment for appendicitis?	Appendectomy as soon as possible
When is immediate surgery not indicated and what is the treatment in those cases?	1. Several days after the onset of symptoms when a phlegmon has most likely developed. Treatment is with broad-spectrum antimicrobial agents, intravenous fluids, and rest, followed later by elective appendectomy. 2. In cases of appendiceal abscess. Treatment is with drainage and elective appendectomy several weeks later.
What is the risk of perforation in appendicitis?	25% by 24 hours after the onset of symptoms, 50% by 36 hours, and 75% by 72 hours

COLONIC POLYPOSIS SYNDROMES AND NEOPLASIA*

What is a polyp?	A benign or malignant protrusion into the lumen of the GI tract. Polyps are

---

* In collaboration with D. Woytowitz and S. Miesfeldt

commonly classified as sessile (broad-based protuberance) and pedunculated (attached to the bowel by a stalk).

Name the types of polyps.

Adenomatous (tubular, villous, or tubulovillous), hamartomatous, hyperplastic, and inflammatory

What are symptoms of polyposis?

1. Most cases are asymptomatic.
2. The bleeding risk increases with increased polyp size.
3. Abdominal discomfort is rare.
4. Obstruction and intussusception are manifestations.

How is the diagnosis of polyps made?

Polyps can be diagnosed by barium studies or endoscopically. The latter is preferred because it allows for polypectomy and histologic identification.

Clinical pearl

If a polyp is found at flexible sigmoidoscopy, there is a 10%–15% chance of finding a more proximal synchronous polyp; therefore, colonoscopy is recommended.

What is the treatment for colon polyps?

Endoscopic polypectomy or surgical resection with careful histologic evaluation

What attributes affect the risk of carcinoma in an adenomatous polyp?

Size, degree of villous architecture, and severity of dysplasia

What is the treatment if a resected polyp is benign?

No further treatment is necessary.

What treatment is required if there is extension of cancer into the bowel mucosa?

Colon resection. No further treatment is necessary if invasive cancer does not extend through the stalk into the bowel submucosa.

What are the hereditary polyposis syndromes?

FPC, Gardner's syndrome, Turcot syndrome, Peutz-Jeghers syndrome, juvenile polyposis, neurofibromatosis, and Cronkhite-Canada syndrome

What are the genetics for FPC?	Autosomal dominant; situated on the long arm of chromosome 5
What type of polyps are found in FPC?	Adenomas of the colon, stomach, and small bowel
What is the age of onset of FPC?	Puberty
What is the risk of cancer with FPC?	100% (adenocarcinoma)
What is the treatment for FPC?	Prophylactic proctocolectomy recommended by age 20–25 years
What are the genetics for Gardner's syndrome?	Autosomal dominant
What type of polyps are found in Gardner's syndrome?	Adenomas
What findings are associated with Gardner's syndrome?	Osteomas of the mandible, skull, and long bones, desmoid tumors, epidermoid and sebaceous cysts, supernumerary teeth, thyroid and adrenal tumors, and hypertrophy of pigmented retinal epithelium
What is the risk of cancer with Gardner's syndrome?	100% (adenocarcinoma)
What is the treatment for Gardner's syndrome?	Prophylactic proctocolectomy recommended by age 20–25 years
What are the genetics for Turcot's syndrome?	Autosomal dominant
What type of polyps are found in Turcot's syndrome?	Adenomas of the colon
What findings are associated with Turcot's syndrome?	Brain tumors

What is the risk of cancer with Turcot's syndrome?

100% (adenocarcinoma)

What is the treatment for Turcot's syndrome?

Prophylactic proctocolectomy recommended by age 20–25 years

What are the genetics for Peutz-Jeghers syndrome?

Autosomal dominant with variable, incomplete penetrance

What type of polyps are found in Peutz-Jeghers syndrome?

Hamartomatous polyps (mostly small bowel, also colon and stomach)

What complications are associated with Peutz-Jeghers syndrome?

Polyps can cause intussusception or obstruction, or they can infarct, causing bleeding and abdominal pain.

What findings are associated with Peutz-Jeghers syndrome?

Pigmentation of buccal mucosa, hands, feet, and perianal skin; bladder and nasal polyposis

What is the risk of cancer with Peutz-Jeghers syndrome?

< 3%

What type of polyps are found in juvenile polyposis?

Hamartomas and adenomas (mostly colonic, also stomach and small bowel)

What is the risk of cancer with juvenile polyposis?

Synchronous adenomatous polyps may become malignant.

What type of polyps are found in neurofibromatosis?

Neurofibromas of the stomach and small bowel

What findings are associated with neurofibromatosis?

Neurofibromas of skin

What is the risk of cancer with neurofibromatosis?

No malignant potential

What are the genetics for Cronkhite-Canada syndrome?

Acquired, nonfamilial syndrome

What type of polyps are found in Cronkhite-Canada syndrome?

Hamartomas and adenomas (mostly small bowel, also stomach and colon)

What findings are associated with Cronkhite-Canada syndrome?

Alopecia, cutaneous hyperpigmentation, dystrophic nails, diarrhea, weight loss, abdominal pain, and malnutrition in middle-aged (average 62 years) patients.

What is the risk of cancer in Cronkhite-Canada syndrome?

Rare risk of malignancy in synchronous adenomas

How common is colon cancer?

It is the second most common cancer overall in the United States, with a 5% lifetime risk in the general population. Age-specific incidence increases from the 2nd to the 9th decade of life.

Who is at risk for colon cancer?

Older people. The incidence doubles every decade from after age 40 years to age 80 years.

What risk factors are associated with colon cancer?

1. Low-fiber, high-fat diet
2. Age older than 40 years
3. Personal history of colorectal adenomas (synchronous or metachronous) or colon cancer
4. Family history of polyposis syndromes (e.g., FPC, Gardner's syndrome, and Turcot's syndrome), cancer family syndrome, first-degree relatives with colon cancer (> 15% risk compared with 5% risk in general population)
5. IBD (CD or UC)
6. Genital tract cancers in women

What colorectal syndromes have an associated genetic basis?

Several genes have recently been identified that are directly related to the development of colorectal cancer. Inherited colorectal cancer susceptibility syndromes include the following:

FPC, the most prevalent of which is the familial adenomatous polyposis syndrome associated with the APC gene

Hereditary nonpolyposis cancer syndrome associated with the mismatch repair genes

What are general presenting symptoms of colorectal cancer?

1. Bleeding (gross or occult)
2. Change in bowel habit, decreased caliber of stool, or constipation or diarrhea
3. Anemia, weight loss, anorexia, and malaise

How do right-sided lesions present in colorectal cancer?

Generally with fatigue, weakness, and occult blood loss. A palpable mass is sometimes present. Because of the increased compliance of the right colon and because its contents are liquid, obstruction usually occurs late.

How do left-sided lesions present in colorectal cancer?

Apple-core lesions usually encircle the bowel and cause bleeding and early obstruction. Diarrhea can develop around partially obstructing lesions.

What are the laboratory findings in colorectal cancer?

CEA is a nonspecific tumor antigen associated with colon cancer. It is not diagnostic and is useful only to monitor for recurrence or metastatic spread.

How is the diagnosis of colorectal cancer made?

The most effective procedure is fiberoptic endoscopy with biopsy.

What is the most common location for colorectal cancer?

Left side of the colon. Approximately two thirds of all colon cancers are within reach of the flexible sigmoidoscope.

How is colonoscopy helpful?

Localization of the lesion, biopsy of the tumor, and visualization of the entire colon (for synchronous neoplasia)

What is the disadvantage of barium enema?

It is frequently used for the initial diagnosis of polyps or mass lesions; however, approximately one third of tumors and polyps are missed.

What are the major histologic subtypes of colorectal cancer?

Adenocarcinoma accounts for 90%–95% of all colorectal cancers. Additional rare epithelial tumors include squamous cell carcinoma, adenosquamous cancer, and undifferentiated carcinoma. Carcinoids and sarcomas rarely involve the large intestine.

What staging systems are used for colorectal cancers?

The two most commonly used staging systems for colorectal cancers are the TNM/UICC (tumor, nodes, metastasis/ Union Internationale Contra le Cancer) system and the modified Astler-Coller Dukes' classification based on the depth of invasion and lymph node metastasis.

What is the extent of malignancy penetration for the following:
    Dukes' A

Tumor invades to the muscularis propria but not through it

    Dukes' B

Tumor penetrates through the bowel wall but does not involve the nodes as follows:
        B1—tumor penetration into but not through the muscularis propria
        B2—tumor penetration through the bowel wall, with negative lymph nodes

    Dukes' C

There is nodal involvement as follows:
        C1—tumor penetration limited to the bowel wall with positive lymph nodes
        C2—tumor invasion through the bowel wall with positive lymph nodes

    Dukes' D

Distant metastatic spread

What is the prognosis of colon cancer by Dukes' staging?

5-year survival rate for Dukes' staging: A, 80%; B1, 65%; B2, 43%; C1, 53%; C2, 15%; D, 0%. Survival rates have changed little in the last 20 years.

What are other negative prognostic factors?

High-grade tumor and the presence of obstruction or perforation

Do colorectal cancers have the same survival rate based on stage?

Individuals with tumors involving the rectum or the rectosigmoid have a lower 5-year survival rate than those with cancers detected elsewhere in the large bowel.

What is the presurgical evaluation of colorectal cancer patients with potentially resectable disease?

The presurgical evaluation of colorectal cancer patients includes the following:
1. Detailed history (including family history)
2. Physical examination, including breast and pelvic examinations in women to rule out synchronous cancers involving the breast, endometrium, or ovary
3. Laboratory evaluation to include a CBC, liver profile, and CEA
4. Colonoscopy
5. Radiographs including a chest study and liver CT scan

How is surgical resection used in treatment of colorectal cancer?

For "cure" in Dukes' A, B, and C; for palliation in Dukes' D

What is adjuvant chemotherapy used for in treatment of colorectal cancer?

Use of 5-fluorouracil–levamisole prolongs survival after surgical resection of Dukes' C disease.

In which patients is adjuvant chemoradiotherapy used?

Generally in patients with Dukes' stage B2 or C disease

How is an isolated hepatic metastasis treated in colorectal cancer?

Surgical resection (synchronous or after primary resection) may improve long-term survival.

What is the role of chemotherapy in metastatic or unresectable colorectal cancer?

Chemotherapy is considered palliative in the management of patients with metastatic colorectal cancer.

Clinical pearl

The incidence of metachronous colon cancer is 1%–5%.

How should patients be screened for colon cancer?	1. They should be given annual rectal examinations after age 40 years. 2. They should undergo annual fecal occult blood testing after age 50 years. To prepare for such a test, the patient's diet should exclude red meat, NSAIDs, peroxidase-containing foods (e.g., horseradish, parsnips), vitamin C, citrus juices, and iron-containing drugs. 3. They should undergo sigmoidoscopy every 3–5 years after age 50 years.

PANCREAS

EXOCRINE AND ENDOCRINE FUNCTION

What is the exocrine function of the pancreas?	The pancreas produces and secretes digestive enzymes, zymogens, and bicarbonate to provide an alkaline pH for optimal enzyme function.
How extensive is the exocrine reserve?	Approximately 90% of the parenchyma must be destroyed before the clinical manifestations of pancreatic insufficiency become apparent.
What is the hormonal regulation of exocrine function?	Secretin—gastric acid stimulates the release of secretin from the duodenum; secretin stimulates the release of water and electrolytes (bicarbonate). Cholecystokinin—long-chain fatty acids, amino acids, and gastric juice stimulate cholecystokinin release, resulting in release of pancreatic enzymes (e.g., trypsinogen and chymotrypsinogen).
What is the neural control of exocrine function?	Parasympathetic nervous system, via the vagus, exerts some control over secretion; its influence, however, is minor compared to hormonal mechanisms.
What is the endocrine function of the pancreas?	In the islets of Langerhans, alpha cells secrete glucagon, beta cells secrete insulin and comprise two thirds of all

islet cells, delta cells produce
somatostatin and VIP, and
enterochromaffin cells synthesize
serotonin and motilin.

ACUTE PANCREATITIS

What is acute pancreatitis?

A discrete episode of acute inflammation
of the pancreas resulting from
intrapancreatic activation of digestive
enzymes and autodigestion. There is a
wide spectrum of causes, severity,
complications, and outcome.

**What are the causes of
acute pancreatitis?**

Think **"IT HURTS BADLY"**:
Infection—viruses (e.g., mumps,
  coxsackie virus), *Mycoplasma*, and
  other organisms
Trauma—including postsurgical status
  and ERCP
Hypercalcemia—hyperparathyroidism
Ulcer—perforated peptic ulcer
Renal—uremia, postrenal transplant
Tumor—ampullary or pancreatic tumor
  with localized obstruction
Structure—pancreas divisum, annular
  pancreas, duodenal diverticulum
Biliary—gallstones
Alcohol ingestion
Drug that **"DEFEATS"** the pancreas:
  Didanosine
  Estrogen
  Furosemide
  Erythromycin
  Azathioprine
  Tetracycline and thiazides
  Sulfas
Lipids—types I, IV, and V
  hyperlipidemia
Y—idiopathic

**What are the most
common causes of acute
pancreatitis?**

Alcohol use and gallstones cause more
than two thirds of all cases.

**What factors suggest
gallstone pancreatitis?**

There is a 90% predictive value with
three or more of the following criteria:
age older than 50 years, female gender,

amylase > 4000 IU/L, AST > 100 IU/L, and alkaline phosphatase > 300 IU/L

What are Ranson's criteria?

Prognostic indicators determined at presentation and within 48 hours of admission. An increased risk of mortality occurs when three or more of the following risk factors are present:
At presentation:
Age > 55 years
WBC > 16,000/μl
Glucose > 200 mg/dl
AST > 250 IU/L
Lactate dehydrogenase > 350 IU/L
Within 48 hours:
Base deficit > 4 mEq/L
BUN increase > 5 mg/dl
Fluid sequestration > 6 L
Serum calcium < 8 mg/dl
Hematocrit decrease > 10%
PO_2 < 60 mm Hg
Note: Amylase measurement is not one of Ranson's criteria.

What is the mortality rate based on the following criteria?

1–2 risk factors—< 1%
3–5 risk factors—10%–20%
6–7 risk factors—100%
Patients at high risk should be admitted to an intensive care unit and may require surgical intervention.

What are symptoms and signs of acute pancreatitis?

Severe epigastric or periumbilical pain of a constant, boring quality that radiates to the back; nausea and vomiting; decreased bowel sounds and tenderness to palpation but usually no rebound or guarding. Tetany, due to hypocalcemia, is rare.

Characterize the following signs:
  Cullen's sign

Bluish discoloration around the umbilicus (suggests hemoperitoneum)

  Turner's sign

Bluish discoloration at the flanks and costovertebral angles

Which signs are alarming?   Shock (e.g., hypotension and
tachycardia), respiratory failure, renal
failure, and hypocalcemia

**What are the laboratory
findings in pancreatitis?**

Elevated serum amylase
  Most sensitive indicator of
    pancreatitis; present in 75% of
    patients with acute pancreatitis
  No correlation between degree of
    amylase elevation and severity of
    pancreatitis
  Elevated within 24 hours and
    resolves in 3–5 days
  May be falsely low with
    hypertriglyceridemia
Elevated serum lipase
  Most specific indicator of
    pancreatitis; elevated in 70% of
    patients with acute pancreatitis
  Remains elevated longer than
    amylase
Leukocytosis—10,000–20,000/μl is
  frequent
Hyperglycemia—occurs from decreased
  insulin and increased glucagon
  release
Hypocalcemia—occurs in 25% of cases
  from calcium sequestration in fat
  soaps and elevated glucagon and
  calcitonin
Arterial hypoxemia—occurs in 25% of
  cases

**What are other causes of
hyperamylasemia?**

Pancreatic—trauma, pseudocyst, ascites,
  abscess, cancer, and ERCP
Biliary—acute cholecystitis, common bile
  duct obstruction, and cholangitis
Intestinal—perforated peptic ulcer,
  intestinal obstruction, and ischemia or
  infarction
Other—peritonitis, ruptured ectopic
  pregnancy, dissecting aortic aneurysm,
  cancer of lung, esophagus, or ovary,
  renal insufficiency, burns, salivary
  gland disease, diabetic ketoacidosis,
  cerebral trauma, and
  macroamylasemia

What are the radiographic findings on plain films in acute pancreatitis?

A "sentinel loop" of small bowel or a "colon cut-off" sign suggest acute pancreatitis. Findings of bowel perforation, ileus, and ascites are nonspecific.

How is abdominal CT helpful in acute pancreatitis?

It can be used to determine size and appearance of the pancreas, spread of inflammation, and condition of the biliary tree. CT is far superior to ultrasound in visualizing the pancreas. CT can be useful in draining fluid collections and obtaining samples to assess for infected fluid collections.

What is seen by dynamic CT in acute pancreatitis?

Patchy enhancement or lack of enhancement of the pancreas is diagnostic of pancreatic necrosis. (Bolus IV contrast establishes whether pancreatic microcirculation is disrupted.)

How is ERCP used in acute pancreatitis?

ERCP is generally contraindicated during the acute phase of pancreatitis unless there is an impacted common bile duct stone. Endoscopic sphincterotomy is indicated in severe gallstone pancreatitis with clinical suspicion of biliary obstruction or sepsis.

What is the treatment for acute pancreatitis?

Treat the illness, not the laboratory tests:
Supportive care—85%–90% of patients have self-limited disease with resolution in 3–10 days.
Analgesia (avoid morphine, it may cause sphincter of Oddi spasm)
Maintenance of intravascular volume and electrolyte replacement
Frequent monitoring of vital signs
Treatment of complications
Nutritional support—oral, nasojejunal, or IV as tolerated
Note: If the patient is not improving or clinically deteriorates, look for complications.

Which medications or treatment has been shown to improve the course of acute pancreatitis?	None (including anticholinergics, H$_2$-receptor antagonists, prophylactic antibiotics, and NG suction)
What are potential complications of acute pancreatitis?	Spread of the inflammatory process, pancreatic abscess, pseudocysts, hemorrhage, necrosis, polyserositis, ARDS, DIC, and cardiovascular shock
Why does the inflammatory process spread in acute pancreatitis?	Activated pancreatic enzymes dissect through tissue planes.
What structures are potentially affected in the inflammatory process?	Bile duct, duodenum, mesenteric vessels, spleen, posterior mediastinum, and diaphragm. Pancreatic ascites, sterile pleural effusion, and pneumonitis may be seen.
What accompanies hemorrhagic pancreatitis?	Retroperitoneal hemorrhage and extensive parenchymal necrosis
What are pseudocysts?	Accumulations of necrotic tissue, pancreatic juice, blood, and fat within or near the pancreas which occur approximately 1–4 weeks after the onset of acute pancreatitis. These accumulations do not have a true capsule with an epithelial lining.
Where are pseudocysts commonly located?	Ninety percent are solitary and located in the body and tail of the pancreas.
What is the treatment for pseudocysts?	Pseudocysts larger than 5 cm or those not resolving in 6–8 weeks should be considered for drainage to prevent infection, rupture, and hemorrhage.
What are pancreatic abscesses?	Secondary infection of pancreatic inflammatory tissue or pseudocyst
What is the treatment for pancreatic abscesses?	Antibiotics are required and drainage may be necessary.

How is the diagnosis of pancreatic necrosis made?	By dynamic CT
When is pancreatic necrosis seen?	In association with severe pancreatitis
What is the prognosis for pancreatic necrosis?	Mortality rate is 10% (versus < 1% for interstitial pancreatitis). Infected pancreatic necrosis has a 30% mortality rate and always requires surgical intervention.
Why do polyserositis and ARDS occur in acute pancreatitis?	Activated pancreatic enzymes enter the circulation and attack distant sites.
What sites are involved in polyserositis and ARDS in association with pancreatitis?	Pericardium, pleura, and synovial surfaces. Alveolar–capillary membranes may also be disrupted, leading to noncardiogenic pulmonary edema or ARDS.
What is the cause of pancreatic-induced DIC?	Circulating pancreatic enzymes
What causes cardiovascular shock in pancreatitis?	It is usually due to hypovolemia or circulating vasodilators.

CHRONIC PANCREATITIS

What is chronic pancreatitis?	Progressive, destructive inflammation resulting in permanent parenchymal loss and pancreatic endocrine–exocrine insufficiency
What is the most common cause of chronic pancreatitis in the United States?	Chronic alcohol abuse (> 2/3 of cases), usually after 10–20 years of ingesting > 60 g/day.
What are other causes of chronic pancreatitis?	Hypercalcemia, hyperlipidemia, trauma, and hereditary causes (e.g., pancreas divisum and cystic fibrosis). Note: Repeated attacks of gallstone pancreatitis probably do not lead to chronic pancreatitis.

What is the classic triad of chronic pancreatitis?

Steatorrhea, calcification, and diabetes ($< 25\%$ of cases)

What are symptoms and signs of chronic pancreatitis?

Abdominal pain, malabsorption, diabetes, and jaundice

Characterize the abdominal pain associated with chronic pancreatitis.

Steady, boring, achy pain in the midepigastrium, upper quadrants, or periumbilical area, radiating to the back, worse when supine, better when sitting up and leaning forward. The pain is the worst in the first 5 years after diagnosis and then may diminish or resolve in two thirds of patients.

What types of malabsorption occur in chronic pancreatitis?

Fat and protein—loss of 90% of pancreatic exocrine function results in fat and protein loss, leading to steatorrhea and malnutrition
Carbohydrate—rare, but due to loss of amylase secretion
Vitamin B_{12}—due to loss of trypsin-induced cleavage of R protein from B_{12}

What complications from diabetes mellitus affect the patient with chronic pancreatitis?

Microangiopathy and nephropathy rarely occur.

Why does jaundice occur in chronic pancreatitis?

Common bile duct obstruction from pancreatic scarring. Pancreatic malignancy must be ruled out.

What are the laboratory findings in chronic pancreatitis?

Normal or slightly elevated amylase and lipase, elevated liver function tests (suggest concomitant liver disease), elevated glucose (diabetes mellitus), elevated alkaline phosphatase (osteomalacia), and elevated prothrombin time (vitamin K malabsorption)

What radiographic finding is seen on plain films in chronic pancreatitis?

One third show diffuse pancreatic calcification.

What does abdominal CT show in chronic pancreatitis?

CT is a more sensitive detection of calcification than plain films. Pseudocysts, ductal dilation, and tumors can also be visualized.

What does ERCP demonstrate in chronic pancreatitis?

ERCP is the gold standard to demonstrate pancreatic ductal anatomy. Ductal dilatation, cystic changes, stricture, and calculi may be visualized and treated (e.g., by stent placement, dilation, and stone removal). Brushings to rule out pancreatic carcinoma can also be done.

What diagnostic studies may be ordered for chronic pancreatitis?

If clinical presentation and imaging studies are inconclusive, tests of pancreatic exocrine function may be useful (e.g., 72-hour quantitative fecal-fat collection and bentiromide test)

What are local complications of chronic pancreatitis?

Pancreatic—pseudocyst, abscess, ascites
Common bile duct obstruction
Duodenal obstruction
Portal and splenic vein thrombosis
Increased risk of pancreatic cancer

What is the treatment for chronic pancreatitis?

Supportive and directed at disease manifestations

What measures are taken to manage pain in chronic pancreatitis?

Abstinence from alcohol, pancreatic enzyme replacement, use of narcotics (addiction is common), celiac ganglion blockade, ERCP stone removal, stricture dilation, duct drainage, and surgical drainage or resection

What measures are taken to manage malabsorption in chronic pancreatitis?

Pancreatic enzyme supplementation, ingestion of low-fat, frequent small meals, and replacement of fat-soluble vitamins and B_{12}

How is diabetes mellitus managed in chronic pancreatitis?

Glucose control. Insulin and glucagon deficiency result in susceptibility to hypoglycemia.

PANCREATIC NEOPLASIA

What are the types of pancreatic neoplasia?	Ductal adenocarcinoma—90% of all pancreatic malignancies Acinar cell, giant cell, epidermoid, adenoacanthoma, sarcoma, and cystadenocarcinoma account for < 10%. Islet cell tumors—5% of pancreatic tumors

LIVER AND BILIARY TRACT

When is jaundice detectable on physical examination?	When total bilirubin is greater than 2.5 mg/dl
Why does jaundice occur?	Because of abnormal processing of bilirubin
What is the normal bilirubin metabolism?	1. Bilirubin is formed from the breakdown of heme proteins that are tightly bound to albumin in a 1:1 ratio. 2. Hepatic uptake of unbound bilirubin is rapid through a saturable protein carrier in the plasma membrane. 3. Cytosolic binding of bilirubin to ligandin and Z protein occurs. 4. Conjugation via UDP-glucuronyl transferase to bilirubin diglucuronide occurs, rendering bilirubin more water soluble. 5. Secretion to the bile canaliculi involves a specific carrier. 6. Bilirubin is excreted in bile to the small bowel. 7. Colonic bacteria degrade bilirubin to urobilinogens, which are mostly excreted in the stool (enterohepatic circulation of bilirubin is minor). 8. Bilirubin only is excreted in the urine as the conjugated glucuronide. Albumin-bound and unconjugated bilirubin are not excreted.
What does jaundice with bilirubinuria suggest?	Hepatobiliary disease

What does jaundice without bilirubinuria suggest?	Unconjugated hyperbilirubinemia
What are the causes of unconjugated hyperbilirubinemia?	Increased bilirubin production— hemolytic anemia (e.g., DIC, hemoglobinopathy, enzyme deficiency, and autoimmune disease), ineffective erythropoiesis (e.g., pernicious anemia, thalassemia, iron deficiency anemia, sideroblastic anemia, and lead poisoning), blood transfusion, and resolving hematoma Hereditary disorders (Gilbert's syndrome, Crigler-Najjar types I and II) Drugs
What is Gilbert's syndrome?	Partial deficiency in bilirubin glucuronyl transferase, a benign, common cause of mild unconjugated hyperbilirubinemia, often incidentally diagnosed. Serum bilirubin is 1.3–3.0 mg/dl (rarely > 5 mg/dl).
What are the genetics of Gilbert's syndrome?	Autosomal dominant with incomplete penetrance
What causes increases in bilirubin?	Fasting, surgery, fever, infection, excessive alcohol ingestion, and intravenous glucose
What is the treatment for Gilbert's syndrome?	No therapy is required.
What are specific causes of conjugated hyperbilirubinemia?	Hereditary disorders (e.g., Dubin-Johnson syndrome, Rotor's syndrome) Hepatocellular disease (e.g., viral and alcoholic hepatitis, cirrhosis, and medication-induced hepatitis) Infiltrative diseases (e.g., sarcoidosis, Hodgkin's lymphoma, tumor, infection, tuberculosis, and abscess) Drug-induced cholestasis (e.g., oral contraceptives, sulfa drugs, thiazides, NSAIDs, and phenothiazines)

Extrahepatic cholestasis (e.g., gallstones, biliary stricture or tumor, and pancreatic disease)
Sepsis
Postoperative jaundice
PBC
PSC
Recurrent jaundice of pregnancy

What do bilirubin levels of 10–30 mg/dl suggest?

Biliary obstruction

What do bilirubin levels > 30 mg/dl suggest?

Hepatocellular disease

CHOLELITHIASIS

What is the epidemiology of cholelithiasis?

1 million new cases annually; 500,000 cholecystectomies performed each year

What types of stones are found in cholelithiasis?

Cholesterol gallstones (75%) and pigment gallstones (25%)

What is the pathogenesis of cholesterol gallstones?

They are formed when the GB becomes supersaturated with cholesterol (from increased biliary cholesterol secretion or decreased biliary bile salt or lecithin secretion) leading to nucleation and stone formation.

What are the characteristics of cholesterol gallstones?

Pure or mixed (> 70% cholesterol), small or large (> 2.5 cm), solitary or multiple, smooth or faceted. A thin rim of calcification may occur.

What is the pathogenesis of pigmented stones?

Unclear, but increased insoluble, unconjugated bilirubin, abnormal GB motor function, reduced bile salt concentration, and biliary tract infection may contribute.

Who is at risk for pigmented gallstones?

Elderly patients, patients in hemolytic states, and cirrhotic patients

What are the characteristics of pigmented gallstones?

Multiple, irregular, and contain < 25% cholesterol, calcium, bilirubinate, phosphate, and carbonate. Central calcification is typical.

What are risk factors for cholesterol gallstones?	Think **four F's:**
	    Female
	    Fat
	    Fertile
	    Forty
	Diabetes
	Diet—high-calorie, cholesterol-lowering diets
	Drugs—estrogen, oral contraceptives, clofibrate
	Hyperlipidemia
	Heredity—especially Pima Indian women
	Bile salt malabsorption—pancreatic insufficiency, cystic fibrosis, ileal disease, ileal bypass, ileal resection

ACUTE CHOLECYSTITIS*

What is acute cholecystitis?	Inflammation of the GB
What causes acute cholecystitis?	Acute inflammation of the GB, usually secondary to biliary tract obstruction by a stone
What are symptoms of acute cholecystitis?	Biliary colic. Approximately 70% of patients have experienced prior attacks that spontaneously resolved. With progression of the inflammation, the pain becomes more consistent and localized to the RUQ, sometimes radiating to the right scapula and shoulder. Fever, chills, rigors, anorexia, nausea, and vomiting are common.
What are signs of acute cholecystitis?	An enlarged GB is palpable in one third of patients. Other physical examination findings include Murphy's sign, abdominal distention, and hypoactive bowel sounds.
What is Murphy's sign?	Inspiratory arrest and increased pain during deep inspiration while palpating the RUQ
How is the diagnosis of acute cholecystitis made?	History and physical examination. The triad of sudden onset of RUQ tenderness, fever, and leukocytosis is

---

° In collaboration with V. Shami, N. Thielman, and C. Sable

highly suggestive. An ultrasound reveals a stone in greater than 90% of cases.

How is the diagnosis of cholelithiasis made?

Typical symptoms with demonstration of gallstones by ultrasound (sensitivity 95%, specificity 98%)

Nuclear medicine (iminodiacetic acid) scans and oral cholecystograms demonstrating acute cystic duct obstruction

ERCP may be useful in diagnosing and treating cholelithiasis.

What does microbiologic study show in acute cholecystitis?

Enteric gram-negative bacilli, enterococci, anaerobes including *Bacteroides, Clostridia,* and *Fusobacterium* species

What is the treatment for acute cholecystitis?

Conservative therapy includes giving nothing by mouth, NG tube placement if the patient has been vomiting, meperidine for analgesia, and intravenous antimicrobial agents.

Cholecystectomy—open or laparoscopic

Cholecystostomy—in severe cases where laparotomy is contraindicated

Bile salt dissolution therapy—best for a limited number of small cholesterol stones

What are complications of cholecystitis?

Empyema, hydrops, gangrene, perforation, fistula formation, and gallstone ileus

What is hydrops?

The obstructed GB fills with a clear transudate produced and secreted by the mucosal epithelial cells. This results in an enlarged, nontender, often asymptomatic, palpable GB. Cholecystectomy is indicated because perforation can occur.

What are complications of gallstones?

Cystic duct obstruction and choledocholithiasis

What are consequences of cystic duct obstruction?

Biliary colic, acute cholecystitis, cholangitis, sepsis, common bile duct obstruction (Merizzi's syndrome), perforation, peritonitis, fistulization, and gallstone ileus

What are consequences of choledocholithiasis?

Obstructive jaundice, cholangitis, sepsis, acute pancreatitis, and stricture formation

What is gallstone ileus?

Mechanical intestinal obstruction by a large, impacted gallstone that has fistulized from the GB to the bowel

What is acalculous cholecystitis?

Severe inflammation of the GB in the absence of gallstones. It is associated with a high incidence of complications (e.g., necrosis, gangrene, and GB perforation).

When is acalculous cholecystitis seen?

In serious trauma, burns, prolonged parenteral hyperalimentation, GB adenocarcinoma, diabetes mellitus, torsion of the GB, and bacterial and parasitic infection

What is the mortality rate of acalculous cholecystitis?

50%. The majority of affected patients are elderly or debilitated with coexisting disease or trauma. It is also seen in intensive care patients postoperatively or on total parenteral nutrition.

How is the diagnosis of acalculous cholecystitis made?

Requires a high index of suspicion because symptoms (e.g., abdominal pain, nausea, and fever) and laboratory results (e.g., leukocytosis and elevated liver function tests) are nonspecific

What is the treatment for acalculous cholecystitis?

Antibiotics and cholecystectomy

What is emphysematous cholecystitis?

Infection of the GB by gas-producing organisms including anaerobes such as *Clostridium welchii* (i.e., *C. perfringens*). Diabetes is a predisposing factor. Diagnosis is made by identifying gas within the GB lumen or wall via abdominal film or ultrasound.

CHOLANGITIS

What is Charcot's triad?	Biliary pain, jaundice, and chills, rigors, or fever
What bacteria cause cholangitis?	*E. coli, Klebsiella, Proteus, Enterobacter, Pseudomonas, Streptococcus fecalis*, and *Clostridium*
What are complications of cholangitis?	Sepsis, hepatic abscess, biliary strictures, pigment gallstones, secondary biliary cirrhosis, and portal hypertension
What is the treatment for cholangitis?	Prompt diagnosis Relief of obstruction is essential (ERCP, percutaneous tranhepatic cholangiography, or surgery). Intravenous antibiotics against enteric organisms

PRIMARY SCLEROSING CHOLANGITIS

What is the pathophysiology of PSC?	PSC is an idiopathic, chronic, diffuse, progressive fibrosing inflammation of the intrahepatic and extrahepatic bile ducts, resulting in cholestasis, bile duct obliteration, and cirrhosis of the liver.
What is the prevalence of PSC and who is most likely to develop the disorder?	Prevalence 5/100,000; men aged 25–45 years. It is associated with HLA-B8 and HLA-DR3.
What is the clinical presentation of PSC?	Jaundice, pruritus, fatigue, weight loss, and RUQ pain. There is asymptomatic elevation in alkaline phosphatase in patients with UC.
What are the laboratory findings in PSC?	Elevated alkaline phosphatase (> 2 times normal), elevated serum transaminases (2–5 times normal), and variable bilirubin Elevated serum IgM in 50% of cases Possible positive antineutrophil cytoplasmic antibody (perinuclear staining pattern) in patients with UC

How is the diagnosis of PSC made?

ERCP demonstrates multifocal stricturing or "beading" of extrahepatic and intrahepatic bile ducts. Pancreatic ducts are abnormal in 10% of cases.

Liver biopsy is usually nonspecific, but characteristic "onion skinning" around bile ducts may be seen. It is very useful in staging PSC.

What diseases are associated with PSC?

UC (50%–75% of cases)

CD, Sjögren's syndrome, retroperitoneal and mediastinal fibrosis, thyroiditis, Peyronie's disease, rheumatoid arthritis, and sarcoidosis

What are complications of PSC?

Progressive cholestasis (resulting in fat malabsorption, steatorrhea, fat-soluble vitamin deficiency, and hepatic osteodystrophy)

Cirrhosis and portal hypertension

Cholangitis

Cholelithiasis and choledocholithiasis

Cholangiocarcinoma

What is the prevalence of cholangiocarcinoma in patients with PSC?

0.5%. It is usually multicentric and can involve intrahepatic or extrahepatic bile ducts.

What is the medical therapy for PSC?

Antibiotics (for ascending cholangitis)

Cholestyramine or charcoal (for pruritus)

Fat-soluble vitamin replacement

Ursodeoxycholic acid (for pruritus)

How is ERCP used in the treatment of PSC?

Biliary balloon dilation, stone removal, and drainage

What is surgical therapy used for in PSC?

Biliary drainage procedures (if ERCP is unsuccessful)

Liver transplantation (the third most common indication in adults)

What are secondary causes of sclerosing cholangitis?

Bacterial infection, immunodeficiency-related opportunistic infections, graft versus host disease, and ischemia

Clinical pearl	PSC can precede UC symptoms by several years, so colon evaluation (e.g., colonoscopy or barium enema) should be performed despite the absence of bowel symptoms.

PRIMARY BILIARY CIRRHOSIS

What is PBC?	Idiopathic, chronic inflammation of medium-sized intrahepatic bile ducts leading to chronic cholestasis and cirrhosis. It may be in the spectrum of autoimmune liver disease.
Who gets PBC?	Middle-aged women (90% of cases)
What conditions are associated with PBC?	Sjögren's syndrome, scleroderma, CREST syndrome, and thyroiditis. Sicca complex is found in 75% of patients.
What is the clinical presentation of PBC?	Insidious fatigue and pruritus with jaundice developing months or years later (50%–60% of cases) Hyperpigmentation, hirsutism, steatorrhea, weight loss, and xanthomata
What are the laboratory findings in PBC?	Alkaline phosphatase is markedly elevated (2–20 times), transaminases are slightly elevated (1–5 times), bilirubin increases with progression of disease (a prognostic indicator), cholesterol and triglycerides are elevated
What other laboratory findings are seen in PBC?	Elevated serum IgM (4–5 times normal) and 90% of patients have antimitochondrial antibody. Other autoantibodies may also be present.
What is seen on liver biopsy in PBC?	Granulomas are classic, but, more commonly, there is inflammatory destruction of bile ducts with lymphocytes and plasma cells, paucity of bile ducts, and portal fibrosis.
What is the treatment for PBC?	Supportive care. PBC is a common indication for transplantation in adults.

How is pruritus in PBC treated?	With cholestyramine, phenobarbital, and terfenadine
How is hyperlipidemia in PBC treated?	With cholestyramine and plasmapheresis
How are gallstones, which are present in 40% of PBC cases, treated?	With cholecystectomy and ERCP
How is fat malabsorption in PBC treated?	With fat-soluble vitamin replacement and medium-chain triglycerides
How is hepatic osteodystrophy in PBC treated?	With calcium and vitamin D replacement
What specific drug is used in the treatment of PBC?	Ursodeoxycholic acid has been shown to decrease symptoms, and preliminary studies suggest lower mortality or an increased time to transplantation.
What is the prognosis for PBC?	Course is variable and unpredictable. Symptoms and elevated bilirubin are poor prognostic indicators (bilirubin > 6 mg/dl portends a poor 2-year survival).

ACUTE HEPATITIS*

What is acute hepatitis?	Hepatic inflammation and hepatocyte necrosis due to an acute insult, most commonly from viruses, toxins, and alcohol
What are symptoms of acute hepatitis?	Acute illness with malaise, fever, anorexia, nausea, abdominal pain, jaundice, pruritus, dark urine, and light-colored stools

VIRAL HEPATITIS*

What are symptoms and signs of viral hepatitis?	The symptoms of acute hepatitis A, B, and C are indistinguishable—anorexia, fatigue, myalgia, and nausea 1 to 2 weeks prior to onset of jaundice. Less commonly, cough, pharyngitis, rash, arthritis, and glomerulonephritis may occur in addition to jaundice, hepatomegaly, and/or splenomegaly.

---

* In collaboration with V. Shami, N. Thielman, and C. Sable

Hepatitis A

What type of virus is HAV?

RNA picornavirus

What is the mode of transmission for HAV?

Fecal–oral, person-to-person contact (e.g., homosexual contact and in day care centers), contaminated food or water (e.g., undercooked seafood). HAV is endemic in underdeveloped countries.

What is the usual clinical presentation of HAV infection?

Incubation period is 2–7 weeks. Mild, asymptomatic disease occurs in children; short-lived (< 1 month), benign acute hepatitis occurs in adults.

How common is jaundice in HAV infection?

Occurs in < 50% of cases

What is the course of HAV infection?

Usually self-limited and does not result in a chronic carrier state. Fulminant hepatic failure resulting in encephalopathy or death is rare.

What are potential complications of HAV infection?

Cholestatic HAV may mimic obstructive jaundice.
Relapse may occur months after initial recovery.

How is the diagnosis of HAV infection made?

Transaminitis and the presence of IgM anti-HAV in serum during acute illness.

What does serologic testing demonstrate in HAV infection?

HAV IgM is present with the development of symptoms and confirms the diagnosis of acute HAV. It disappears within months.
HAV IgG denotes previous infection and recovery or vaccination with HAV vaccine. It is present in all patients after 3 weeks of disease and persists indefinitely.

Why is parenteral transmission of HAV rare?

Because the viremic phase is short, lasting 2 weeks before and up to 1 week after the development of jaundice

What is the treatment for HAV infection?

Purely supportive (good nutrition, avoidance of alcohol ingestion and hepatotoxic agents, and enteric precautions). More than 99% of cases resolve without serious sequelae. Most patients do not require hospitalization. Transplantation is done if fulminant hepatitis occurs (very rare).

How is HAV infection prevented?

Avoidance of unsanitary conditions or undercooked foods, passive immunization with immunoglobulin, or active immunization with hepatitis A vaccine, which is considered for travelers to endemic areas and for persons at high risk, such as day care and health care workers.

What is used as prophylaxis after exposure?

0.02 mg/kg of serum immunoglobulin for household and sexual contacts within 2 weeks of exposure

Hepatitis B

What type of virus is HBV?

Partially double-stranded, circular DNA retrovirus of the Hepadnaviridae family

What are the three possible clinical states that may occur after infection with HBV?

1. Acute hepatitis
2. Chronic hepatitis
3. Asymptomatic carrier

What happens to hepatocytes after infection with HBV?

HBV infects hepatocytes, producing complete viral particles and excess HBsAg. The virus is not cytopathic but generates a host immune response, resulting in lysis of infected hepatocytes.

What is the mode of transmission for HBV?

Parenteral (e.g., IVDA and blood transfusions), sexual contact, and perinatal

What are symptoms and signs of HBV infection?

Most infected individuals are asymptomatic. Rarely, the infection progresses to fulminant hepatic failure or chronic infection and cirrhosis.

How common is a subclinical infection with HBV?

A transient subclinical infection occurs in two thirds of patients infected with HBV.

What is the course for subclinical HBV infections?

Rapid clearance of the virus with a strong immune response and high titers of HBsAb, which confers immunity. HBcAb is also produced but it neither confers nor suggests immunity.

How common is acute HBV infection?

Occurs in 25% of cases

What is the incubation period for acute HBV infection (time from exposure to jaundice)?

1–6 months

What happens serologically during acute HBV infection?

HBcAb IgM is present when jaundice appears, establishing acute HBV infection. HBcAb IgG reaches high titers at recovery. Serum becomes positive for HBsAg, HBV DNA, DNA polymerase, and HBeAg. HBeAg is detected in patients with high circulating levels of HBV; it is found only in HBsAg-positive serum and signals active, ongoing infection and infectivity.

What are the extrahepatic manifestations of acute HBV infection?

Circulating antigen–antibody complexes can result in rash, neuralgia, arthralgia, arthritis, glomerulonephritis, vasculitis, mixed cryoglobulinemia, and aplastic anemia.

What are other laboratory findings in HBV infection?

Increase in transaminases (5–20 times) and bilirubin (may be very high, > 30 mg/dl) with modest elevations in alkaline phosphatase (2–10 times), reflecting hepatocellular damage.

What is the clinical course for acute HBV infection?

In patients who can mount a vigorous immune response, HBV is cleared and patients recover in 1–6 months. Fulminant hepatic failure develops in 1%–5% of patients, necessitating liver transplantation.

How is the diagnosis of HBV infection made?	The presence of HBsAg and anti-HBc IgM in serum. Anti-HBc IgG indicates prior infection.

In cases of acute HBV infection, what happens to the following?

HBV DNA and DNA polymerase	Become undetectable within 1–8 weeks
HBsAg	Clears in months
HBcAb IgM	Clears in weeks
HBcAb IgG	Reaches high titers at recovery and persists for life
HBeAb	Appears when HBeAg declines and often disappears within a few months or years
HBsAb	Increases during recovery after HbsAg has cleared. There is usually a "window" period before HBsAb develops. Of patients who clear HBV, HBsAB never develops in 5%–15% but most have positive HBcAb IgM denoting recent acute HBV infection.
What is the treatment for HBV infection?	Most cases resolve spontaneously with supportive therapy. Transplantation should be considered in cases of fulminant hepatic failure. In chronic disease, interferon alpha-2b may be used; 30% of patients respond.
In what percent of HBV-infected individuals does chronic infection develop?	Approximately 10%
What happens to the serologic markers in chronic HBV infection?	HBsAg, HBeAg, HBV DNA, and DNA polymerase persist for > 6 months. Over time, HBcAg IgM wanes and HBcAb develops. Continued replication may occur in some patients with continuous presence of HBeAg. This is more common in Asia and with infection acquired at a young age.

How commonly does a transition from a replicative to a nonreplicative stage occur?	Decreased viral replication may occur in approximately 50% of cases with disappearance of HBeAg and appearance of HBeAb.
What happens during this phase of decreased viral replication?	A flare of hepatitis and loss of HBV DNA and DNA polymerase from the serum. This phase is marked by an increased immune response to clear viral replication and is followed by marked improvement in liver histology.
When does reactivation of hepatitis occur in HBV-infected individuals?	Reactivation of quiescent HBV with an acute-type hepatitis occurs spontaneously or after withdrawal of immunosuppressive drugs or therapy (e.g., chemotherapy, steroids, and organ transplantation).
What happens to HBV in healthy carriers with no evidence of viral replication?	Integration of HBV into the host hepatocyte, increasing the risk for HCC.
What is superinfection in individuals infected with HBV?	Infection with other hepatotrophic viruses (e.g., HAV, hepatitis C and D viruses, and cytomegalovirus). It can occur in chronic carriers with increased transaminases.
What may happen to HBsAg titers with superinfection?	May decrease due to viral interference
How common is viral clearance in individuals with chronic HBV infection?	Occurs in 1% with clearance of HBsAg and development of HBsAb, especially if the infection was acquired during adulthood
How common is cirrhosis in individuals with chronic HBV?	Develops in 10%–30% of such individuals
How is infection with HBV prevented?	A protective antibody develops in more than 90% of persons vaccinated with hepatitis B vaccine and remains positive 5 years after initial vaccination. Timing and consideration of a booster remain

controversial. After sexual exposure to HBV, both HBIg and the first of three hepatitis vaccines should be administered within 14 days of exposure. Follow-up doses are given at 1 and 6 months. Note: Ig and vaccine should be given at different sites.

Who should be given hepatitis B vaccine?

Persons with occupational risk (e.g., health care workers), all infants, persons with multiple sexual partners, IVDAs, household and sexual contacts of HBV carriers, and travelers at risk

Hepatitis C

What type of virus is HCV?

Single-stranded RNA virus similar to flaviviruses. It is the cause of most cases of non-A, non-B hepatitis.

Is there more than one genotype of HCV?

Six major genotypes have been identified worldwide. Subtypes 1a and 1b are most common in the United States and western Europe.

How is HCV transmitted?

By blood and body fluids. Major risk factors include blood transfusion, IV drug abuse, hemodialysis, household exposure (e.g., sharing of razors and toothbrushes), and occupational exposure (e.g., by needle stick). In 40% of cases, no source of infection can be identified.

What are symptoms and signs of acute hepatitis in HCV infection?

Similar to those of HAV and HBV infection, but most cases (70%–80%) are subclinical and asymptomatic.

What is the incubation period for HCV infection?

5–12 weeks after exposure

How common is fulminant HCV infection?

Very rare (< 1% of cases)

How common is chronic HCV?

60%–90% of cases. Ultimately, 40% of chronic cases progress to cirrhosis. As with HBV infection, chronic HCV infection can lead to end-stage liver disease or HCC.

After infection with HCV, what is the mean time to clinical presentation of chronic hepatitis?

5–15 years. Clinical cirrhosis occurs in 10–20 years.

What increases the risk and shortens the time to development of HCV chronic liver disease?

Current and remote alcohol use

How is the diagnosis of HCV infection made?

Anti-HCV antibody detection. Repeat testing may be necessary to document acute HCV infection (prolonged window). PCR-based methods for detection of viral RNA can also be used.

What are ELISA II and RIBA II?

Antibody tests against HCV antigens c100-3, c200, c22, and c33c. Both tests usually are positive within 20 weeks of infection.

What does a positive ELISA II or RIBA II mean?

Current infection or a past (resolved) infection. The majority of cases with positive antibody are viremic. The presence of antibody does not confer immunity.

What is reverse transcriptase PCR?

Qualitative measure of HCV RNA in the serum; results are positive or negative only. The virus can be detected as early as 2 weeks after infection.

How is reverse transcriptase PCR helpful?

To confirm viremia in an antibody-positive patient

How is quantitative PCR helpful?

As a quantitative measure of HCV RNA. Currently the gold standard to measure viral load, quantitative PCR is used to assess efficacy of treatment for HCV.

What are the extrahepatic manifestations of HCV infection?

Mixed cryoglobulinemia, porphyria cutanea tarda, and membranous glomerulonephritis

What is the treatment for acute HCV hepatitis?

Supportive care

What is the treatment for chronic HCV hepatitis?

Alpha interferon, 3 million units subcutaneously three times weekly for 12 months. Normalization of AST and ALT occurs in 40% of cases. Relapse occurs in 50%–70% of cases after therapy is discontinued (therapy probably suppresses HCV in the majority of cases rather than eradicating it).

Is there effective postexposure prophylaxis?

No. Immunoglobulin is not effective.

Is there a vaccine?

Not available. Major efforts are underway to develop a vaccine; however, because of the large number of genotypic subtypes and efficient escape mutation by the virus, prospects for development of a vaccine seem tenuous at best.

Hepatitis D

What type of virus is HDV?

A defective RNA virus that requires coinfection with HBV (specifically HBsAg) for replication

What is the mode of transmission for HDV?

Primarily parenteral, less often by sexual contact, and rarely perinatal

What is the mechanism of HDV hepatic injury?

Damage is by direct cytopathic effect rather than by immune-mediated damage.

What is the usual course of HBV/HDV coinfection?

Self-limited disease similar to acute HBV infection

What are clinical manifestations of HDV infection?

They are indistinguishable from those of HBV alone, but there is a higher risk for fulminant hepatic failure. Cirrhosis develops in up to 70% of cases.

What are the usual laboratory findings in HDV infection?

Concurrent HBV and HDV infection. Findings are positive for HBsAg, HBcAb IgM, and IgM antibody to HDV.

What is HDV superinfection?

Acute HDV infection in the setting of chronic HBV infection

What are the serologic findings in HDV superinfection?	Findings are positive for HBsAg and IgM antibody to HDV; findings are negative for HBcAb IgM.
Who should be tested for HDV?	Patients with HBV infection who have rapidly progressing disease
What is the prognosis for HDV infection?	HDV has a high mortality rate; 2% of cases of acute HDV infection result in fulminant hepatic failure.
What percent of HDV infections result in cirrhosis?	> 50%
What is the mortality rate of HDV infection?	15% 3-year mortality rate
What is the treatment for HDV infection?	Experimental therapy with alpha interferon has proven beneficial, but withdrawing the drug often results in recurrence. Control of infection depends on prevention. HBV vaccination prevents both HBV and HDV infection.

Hepatitis E

What type of virus is HEV?	RNA virus of the Caliciviridae family
How is HEV transmitted?	Fecal–oral transmission (similar to HAV infection); epidemics in southeast and central Asia, India, and Nepal
What is the clinical presentation of HEV infection?	Acute hepatitis only; no chronic hepatitis or carrier states
What is the clinical course of HEV infection?	Similar to that of HAV infection, with mild to moderate acute hepatitis being more common in adults than in children
What is the mortality rate in pregnant women with HEV infection?	High (10%)
What does serologic testing demonstrate in HEV infection?	HEV IgM, which is diagnostic of acute infection

Is there a vaccine for HEV infection?	It is under development.

Hepatitis G

What type of virus is HGV?	An RNA virus currently being studied. The virus family is not yet established.
How is HGV transmitted?	Parenteral transmission (e.g., blood transfusion)
What is the clinical presentation of HGV infection?	Asymptomatic carrier, chronic hepatitis or "cryptogenic" non-A, B, C, D, E cirrhosis
What does serologic testing demonstrate in HGV infection?	HGV RNA PCR is being used as a research tool.

DRUG-INDUCED LIVER DISEASE

What is the epidemiology of drug-induced liver disease?	Accounts for 2% of all patients hospitalized with jaundice. Twenty-five percent of all cases of fulminant hepatic failure in the United States are drug related.
What is the pathophysiology of drug-induced liver disease?	The liver controls metabolism (e.g., by activation and detoxification) of many drugs via conjugation reactions or via the cytochrome p450 system. Acute hepatic drug injury can mimic all patterns of liver injury, that is, hepatocellular necrosis, cholestasis, macrovesicular and microvesicular fat deposition, and tumor formation.
How is the diagnosis of drug-induced liver disease made?	A good history is vital, and other causes (e.g., viral) must be excluded.
Is liver biopsy helpful in the diagnosis of drug-induced liver disease?	Liver biopsy obtained early can be helpful in identifying the type and extent of injury.

What common offenders cause drug-induced liver disease?	Alcohol, acetaminophen, Dilantin, isoniazid, amiodarone, methotrexate, ketoconazole, halothane, occupational exposures (e.g., carbon tetrachloride), and amanita mushrooms

ACETAMINOPHEN HEPATOTOXICITY

What happens to acetaminophen when it is ingested?	Approximately 4% of therapeutic doses of acetaminophen are metabolized by the cytochrome p450 system to a toxic intermediate, which is rapidly conjugated to glutathione and detoxified for renal excretion. Large ingestions result in toxic metabolite in excess of glutathione and hepatocyte death.
What determines hepatotoxicity with acetaminophen?	Toxicity depends on total quantity ingested, blood level achieved, rate of disposition, activity of p450 system, and adequacy of glutathione stores. Toxicity is increased with concomitant alcohol use, preexisting liver disease, and malnutrition.
Why treat acetaminophen toxicity with N-acetylcysteine?	Such treatment is aimed at enhancing glutathione stores.

CHRONIC LIVER DISEASE

Autoimmune Hepatitis

What is autoimmune hepatitis?	Idiopathic, autoimmune liver inflammation due to abnormal suppressor T cells, characterized by autoantibodies against hepatocyte surface antigens
Who gets autoimmune hepatitis?	Predominantly young to middle-aged females
What are symptoms and signs of autoimmune hepatitis?	Fatigue, malaise, anorexia, weight loss; less commonly, jaundice, hepatomegaly, and a picture of acute hepatitis

What conditions are associated with autoimmune hepatitis?

Glomerulonephritis, fibrosing alveolitis, pulmonary hypertension, pericarditis, thyroiditis, colitis, positive Coombs test, hemolytic anemia, skin rash, fever, and arthropathy

What are the serologic findings in autoimmune hepatitis?

Anti–smooth muscle antibody (70% of cases)
High titer antinuclear antibody (80% of cases)
Anti–double-stranded DNA (40% of cases)
Anti–mitochondrial antibody (30% of cases)
Elevated IgG levels (majority of cases)

What is seen on liver biopsy in autoimmune hepatitis?

Liver biopsy shows portal inflammation with lymphocytes and plasma cells with erosion of the limiting plate, piecemeal necrosis, and rosette formation.

What is the treatment for autoimmune hepatitis?

Prednisone with or without azathioprine for many years

What is the prognosis for autoimmune hepatitis?

There is a 50%–90% relapse rate upon withdrawal of steroids, usually within months after stopping therapy. Overall prognosis is good with more than 50% of patients being alive 15 years after diagnosis.

Wilson's Disease

What is Wilson's disease?

Rare, autosomal recessive disorder of progressive copper accumulation due to decreased biliary copper excretion. Copper accumulates and can cause irreversible damage to the liver, brain, cornea, and kidneys.

What is the clinical presentation of the following:
　Liver disease

Occurs in children older than 6 years old and young adults and can present as chronic hepatitis, fulminant hepatitis, or cirrhosis

Neurologic disease	Incoordination, tremor, dysarthria, excessive salivation, and dysphagia
Kayser-Fleischer rings	Corneal copper deposits in Descemet's membrane
Psychiatric disease	Adjustment disorder, anxiety, hysteria, bipolar affective disorder, and schizophrenia
Hematologic disease	Coombs' negative hemolytic anemia
Renal disease	Renal insufficiency, Fanconi's syndrome, renal tubular acidosis, microscopic hematuria, and proteinuria
How is the diagnosis of Wilson's disease made?	Low serum copper, ceruloplasmin < 20 mg/dl (95%), elevated 24-hour urinary copper (> 100 µg/day), and liver biopsy with quantitative copper analysis
What is the treatment for Wilson's disease?	Decreased dietary copper (e.g., that found in organ meats, shellfish, peas, whole wheat, and chocolate) and therapy with D-penicillamine to chelate copper

Hemochromatosis

What is hemochromatosis?	Relatively common autosomal recessive disorder of iron accumulation resulting from increased intestinal mucosal absorption of dietary iron. Iron is deposited in the liver, heart, pancreas, synovium, skin, pituitary, thyroid, and adrenal glands.
What is the clinical presentation of hemochromatosis?	Liver disease with hepatomegaly (95% of cases), progressing to cirrhosis and an increased risk of HCC (30% of cases) Hyperpigmentation due to iron and melanin deposition Diabetes mellitus in 30%–60% of cases due to iron toxicity to beta cells in the pancreas Hypogonadism with loss of libido and testicular atrophy Increased frequency of other endocrine disorders (e.g., Addison's disease, hypothyroidism, and hypoparathyroidism)

Arthropathy (e.g., osteoarthritis and
pseudogout)
Cardiomyopathy and arrhythmias in
15%–20% of patients

**How is the diagnosis of
hemochromatosis made?**

Elevated serum iron and percent
saturation of transferrin, elevated serum
ferritin, and liver biopsy with iron
staining and quantitative iron
determination

**What is the treatment for
hemochromatosis?**

Phlebotomy is usually done weekly for
2–3 years, then every 3–4 months for
life.
With desferoxamine chelation, it is
difficult to achieve negative iron
balance.

Cirrhosis

What is cirrhosis?

Diffuse hepatic parenchymal destruction
replaced with scar tissue and
regenerating nodules that disrupt the
normal hepatic architecture

**What are the most
common causes of
cirrhosis?**

Alcohol use and viral hepatitis

**What are characteristic
physical findings of
cirrhosis?**

Palmar erythema, spider angiomata,
gynecomastia, testicular atrophy,
Dupuytren's contractures, Terry's nails,
parotid enlargement, splenomegaly,
ascites, prominent abdominal wall
superficial veins, and prominent left lobe
of the liver

What is Child's classification?

A classification of cirrhosis (based on nutritional status, ascites, PSE, bilirubin, albumin, and prothrombin time) that predicts overall prognosis.

Score	1	2	3
Albumin	> 3.5 gm/dl	2.8–3.4	< 2.8
Ascites	Nil	Slight	Mod
Bilirubin	< 2 mg/dl	2–3	> 3
PSE	Nil	Slight	Moderate–severe
Protime	< 14 sec	15–17	> 18
Child's class	A = score 5–7		
	B = 7–10		
	C = 10–15		

What are complications of cirrhosis?

Varices, ascites, SBP, hepatorenal syndrome, encephalopathy, and hypersplenism

VARICES

Why do varices form?

To decompress the high pressures in the portal system

Where do varices form?

Esophageal and gastric varices are most common, but small bowel, colonic, hemorrhoidal, intercostal, diaphragmatic, retroperitoneal, lumbar, and omental varices can occur.

How are varices diagnosed?

Best by EGD

What is the prognosis for varices?

Risk of bleeding is increased with variceal size and worsening liver function. Overall mortality rate from bleeding varices is 70%–80%.

What is the treatment for varices?

Prophylactic β blockers in doses to reduce the resting pulse by 25% can decrease the incidence of variceal bleeding. Treatment of bleeding varices includes IV octreotide, endoscopic band ligation or sclerotherapy, TIPS, and surgical portacaval shunts or Blakemore tube.

ASCITES

What is ascites?	Accumulation of fluid in the peritoneal cavity
Why does ascites occur?	Portal hypertension increasing total splanchnic volume, increased renal sodium and water retention, and decreased lymphatic drainage in the peritoneum
What are symptoms and signs of ascites?	Patients present with increased abdominal girth, umbilical herniation, scrotal edema, pleural effusion, and peripheral edema.
What are complications of ascites?	Dyspnea, anorexia, esophageal reflux, ventral hernia, and leaking umbilical hernia
How is the diagnosis of ascites made?	Physical examination can easily detect > 2 L of fluid, or ultrasound can detect as little as 30 ml. Paracentesis should be performed to characterize the fluid.
After paracentesis, what should the fluid be sent for?	Fluid should be sent for four C's as follows: Cell count (WBC plus differential) Culture (aerobic and anaerobic in blood culture bottles) Chemistry (protein, albumin, glucose, amylase, triglycerides, pH) Cytology
What is the serum ascites–albumin gradient?	Gradient = serum albumin – ascites albumin (g/dl)

How is the ascites–albumin gradient helpful?

≥ 1.1	< 1.1
Portal hypertension	Peritoneal carcinomatosis
Cardiac ascites	Tuberculous peritonitis
"Mixed" ascites	Pancreatic ascites
Massive liver metastases	Bowel obstruction/infarct
Fulminant hepatic failure	Nephrotic syndrome
Portal vein thrombosis	Postoperative lymph leak
Budd-Chiari	Serositis in rheumatic disease
Myxedema	

What is the treatment for ascites?	Abstinence from alcohol, 2 g/day sodium diet, water restriction only if hyponatremia is present, diuretics (Aldactone and Lasix), and repeated large-volume paracentesis with albumin replacement.
What invasive treatments are available for ascites?	TIPS and peritoneovenous shunting

SPONTANEOUS BACTERIAL PERITONITIS

How common is SBP?	Occurs in 8%–10% of alcoholic cirrhotic patients
What are symptoms and signs of SBP?	Symptoms may be nonspecific. Patients may be asymptomatic or have worsening PSE or mild abdominal discomfort, and many do not have fever.
What is the pathogenesis of SBP?	Hematogenous spread of bacteria from the GI tract (most commonly) and low opsonic activity in ascitic fluid
What are the most common organisms involved in SBP?	Most commonly aerobic gut flora (e.g., *E. coli* and *Klebsiella*). Anaerobic infection is rare. Organisms average one per milliliter of ascitic fluid so inoculation into blood culture bottles is necessary and Gram staining of fluid is almost always negative for organisms.

What if multiple organisms are cultured?	Consider secondary peritonitis (e.g., bowel perforation, abscess)
How is the diagnosis of SBP made?	Ascitic fluid neutrophil count > 250 or positive culture
What is the treatment for SBP?	Third-generation cephalosporin (avoid aminoglycosides due to renal toxicity). Untreated SBP has a very high mortality rate.

HEPATORENAL SYNDROME

What is hepatorenal syndrome?	Progressive, functional renal failure accompanying severe, decompensated liver disease (usually associated with cirrhosis and tense ascites)
What is the pathogenesis of hepatorenal syndrome?	Unclear, but selective renal vasoconstriction of cortical arterioles with shunting to the medulla results in decreased glomerular filtration rate.
How is the diagnosis of hepatorenal syndrome made?	Progressive azotemia with creatinine > 2.5 mg/dl, urine volume < 500 ml/day, urine sodium < 10 mEq/L, and normal urinalysis. Hepatorenal syndrome is often difficult to distinguish from prerenal azotemia.
What is the prognosis of hepatorenal syndrome?	Poor. Mortality rate is greater than 90%.
What is the treatment for hepatorenal syndrome?	Avoidance of nephrotoxins (especially aminoglycosides and NSAIDs), dehydration and excessive diuresis (should try a fluid challenge to rule out prerenal azotemia), and hemodialysis

ENCEPHALOPATHY

What is encephalopathy?	Alteration in mental status and behavior with pyramidal and extrapyramidal neurologic abnormalities

What is the pathogenesis of encephalopathy?

Poorly understood, but probably involves shunting of blood from the gut directly to the systemic circulation with systemic accumulation of "toxins" (e.g., gamma-aminobutyric acid and false neurotransmitters)

What are common precipitants of encephalopathy?

GI bleeding, electrolyte abnormalities (hypokalemia), hypoxia, azotemia, infection, and drug use (e.g., benzodiazepines)

What are symptoms and signs of encephalopathy?

Patients have mental status changes, fetor hepaticus (feculent–fruity odor to breath), and asterixis (flapping motion of hands due to intermittent loss of extensor tone)

What are the four stages of PSE?

I—inappropriate behavior, altered sleep pattern, asterixis
II—confusion, disorientation, asterixis
III—stuporous with marked confusion, somnolent but arousable, hyperreflexia, rigidity, and clonus can be elicited
IV—deep coma with no response to stimuli, flaccid limbs

What are the laboratory findings in PSE?

Increased arterial ammonia (90% of cases), but level of elevation does not correlate with stage of PSE

What is the treatment for PSE?

Correction of precipitating causes, improvement in hepatic function, and intestinal cleansing (e.g., with use of lactulose and neomycin)

HYPERSPLENISM

Why does hypersplenism occur with cirrhosis?

An enlarged or engorged spleen results from portal hypertension, which causes sequestration and destruction of blood cells.

What are the laboratory findings in hypersplenism?

Commonly, mild to moderate neutropenia, thrombocytopenia, and decreased RBC survival

Should patients with hypersplenism undergo splenectomy?

Surgical splenectomy is not routinely recommended.

TUMORS OF THE LIVER

What are the most common primary benign liver tumors?

Hemangioma and adenoma

How common are hemangiomas?

The most common hepatic tumor (5% of all autopsies)

What is the treatment for hemangiomas?

The patient is usually asymptomatic, and no treatment is required.

How are hemangiomas recognized?

Characteristic enhancement on CT scan with contrast

What are adenomas?

Smooth, solitary tumors of hepatocytes and bile ducts

What associations or conditions are linked with adenomas?

Oral contraceptives use and pregnancy

What is the clinical presentation of adenoma?

The patient may be asymptomatic or may present with abdominal pain or rupture and intraperitoneal bleeding.

What is the characteristic imaging finding in adenomas?

Adenomas are seen as very vascular with a characteristic capillary blush on arteriography, and they are seen as "cold" on nuclear medicine liver–spleen scans.

What is the most common involvement of the liver by malignancies?

Metastases from other sources. The liver is involved in one third of all cancers regardless of their source.

What is the most common primary malignancy affecting the liver?

HCC (i.e., hepatoma). Worldwide it is the most common cause of death from cancer.

What are predisposing factors for HCC?

Cirrhosis of any cause, race (e.g., Asian and Eskimo), environmental carcinogens (e.g., alcohol, tobacco, and aflatoxin), viral infection (especially HBV, HCV, and HDV), hemochromatosis, and clonorchis

What are symptoms and signs of HCC?

HCC should be considered when a previously stable cirrhotic patient decompensates with worsening encephalopathy, new onset ascites (often due to portal vein thrombosis), or RUQ abdominal pain.

How is the diagnosis of HCC made?

Diagnosis and localization of tumor can be accomplished with abdominal CT, magnetic resonance imaging, or angiography. High-risk patients should be screened with AFP testing and ultrasound. Erythrocytosis from tumor-derived erythropoietin occurs in 1% of cases, and elevation of serum AFP is characteristic, especially with levels greater than 1000 ng/dl.

What is the treatment for HCC?

Only 1% of HCCs are surgically resectable (local spread and vascular invasion preclude surgery). Operative mortality rate is 10% in these patients who often have underlying cirrhosis.

What are palliative measures for HCC?

Systemic chemotherapy, radiation therapy, chemoembolization, and absolute ethanol infusion

What is the prognosis for transplantation for HCC?

Prognosis is good only if a small tumor is discovered incidentally at the time of OLT; however, studies using adjuvant chemotherapy or chemoembolization are underway.

ORTHOTOPIC LIVER TRANSPLANTATION

Clinical pearl

The first human liver transplantation was performed by Starzl in 1963.

What is OLT?

The diseased liver is removed and replaced with a donor liver. In heterotopic transplantation, an extra liver is inserted at another site.

What are indications for OLT?

Chronic, irreversible liver disease or fulminant liver failure for which no acceptable alternative therapy is available. Diseases include the following:
Congenital or acquired cirrhosis (e.g., PBC, PSC, and viral, alcoholic, or cryptogenic cirrhosis)
Metabolic disorders (e.g., Wilson's disease, hemochromatosis, and glycogen storage disease)
Vascular disorders (e.g., Budd-Chiari disease)
Fulminant hepatic failure
Biliary atresia, neonatal hepatitis, and congenital hepatic fibrosis

What are contraindications to OLT?

Advanced cardiopulmonary or renal disease, sepsis, malignancy, active alcohol or drug abuse, and inability of the patient to understand or accept the procedure

What is the selection of transplantation recipients based on?

ABO compatibility and status of the patient

What is the average operating room time and blood use?

8 hours and 17 units of packed RBCs

What is the postoperative medical therapy for OLT?

Immunosuppressive regimens to prevent rejection vary but usually include cyclosporine or tacrolimus, corticosteroids, and azathioprine.

What are postoperative complications of OLT at the following times:
   Immediate postoperative period

Harvest injury (graft dysfunction due to inadequate preservation), thrombosis and stenosis of vascular anastomosis, bile leak, and hyperacute rejection (usually due to preformed antibodies)

Early postoperative period

Acute cellular rejection (usually after the 5th day postoperatively); bacterial, viral, fungal infection; renal insufficiency

Later postoperative period

Chronic rejection ("vanishing bile duct syndrome") and recurrence of primary disease (e.g., infection with HBV, HCV, PSC, and HCC)

What is the prognosis for patients who undergo OLT?

1-year survival, 70%–90% depending on disease

5-year survival, 70% for PBC, PSC

Twenty percent to 25% of patients will require retransplantation, usually due to primary graft failure, hepatic arterial thrombosis, and chronic rejection.

Survivors usually have a good quality of life; 85% return to their previous occupation, and women have had subsequent normal pregnancies.

6   Hematology

ABBREVIATIONS

ABO	Blood types
aPTT	Activated partial thromboplastin time
AT III	Antithrombin III
BMT	Bone marrow transplantation
BUN	Blood urea nitrogen
CBC	Complete blood count
CML	Chronic myelogenous leukemia
CMML	Chronic myelomonocytic leukemia
CVA	Cerebrovascular accident
DDAVP	1-desamino-8-D-arginine vasopressin (desmopressin acetate)
DIC	Disseminated intravascular coagulation
DVT	Deep vein thrombosis
Fe	Iron
G-CSF	Granulocyte colony stimulating factor
G6PD	Glucose-6-phosphate dehydrogenase
HELLP	Hemolysis, elevated liver enzymes, and low platelets
HIV	Human immunodeficiency virus
HUS	Hemolytic uremic syndrome

INR	International normalized ratio
ITP	Idiopathic (immune) thrombocytopenic purpura
LAP	Leukocyte alkaline phosphatase
LDH	Lactate dehydrogenase
MCV	Mean corpuscular volume
MDS	Myelodysplastic syndrome
MI	Myocardial infarction
PNH	Paroxysmal nocturnal hemoglobinuria
PT	Prothrombin time
RA	Refractory anemia
RAEB	Refractory anemia with excess blasts
RAEB-T	Refractory anemia with excess blasts in transformation
RARS	Refractory anemia with ring sideroblasts
RBC	Red blood cell
RDW	Red cell distribution width
SLE	Systemic lupus erythematosus
TIBC	Total iron binding capacity
TTP	Thrombotic thrombocytopenic purpura
vWD	von Willebrand's disease
vWF	von Willebrand factor
WBC	White blood cell

RED BLOOD CELL

What is the shape of a normal RBC?	The RBC is a biconcave disc. This shape allows for a large surface area to volume ratio, which permits marked deformability and enables the red cell to squeeze through capillaries.
What is the average life span of an RBC?	120 days
What is the ratio of hemoglobin to hematocrit?	Approximately 1 to 3
What is hemoglobin?	Hemoglobin functions as an oxygen-transporting protein. It is a tetrameric protein of two pairs of unlike globin chains. Each chain is paired with a heme molecule. Heme is a porphyrin ring with iron in the middle, which reversibly binds oxygen.
What is normal adult type hemoglobin?	Hemoglobin A. Hemoglobin A is a tetramer of two alpha chains and two beta chains.
What is hemoglobin A2?	Hemoglobin A2 is a tetramer of two alpha chains and two delta chains. Hemoglobin A2 comprises approximately 2% of normal adult hemoglobin.
What is hemoglobin F?	Fetal hemoglobin is a tetramer of two alpha chains and two gamma chains. Hemoglobin F disappears early in life. Less than 0.5% of hemoglobin in adult life is hemoglobin F.
What is the MCV?	Mean corpuscular volume. Normal range is approximately 80–100 fl.
What is anisocytosis?	Variability in RBC size
What is poikilocytosis?	Variability in RBC shape

What is hypochromia?

Hypochromia is pallor of the RBC secondary to decreased quantity of hemoglobin. RBCs are considered hypochromic when the central pallor is greater than one third the diameter of the RBC.

What is polychromasia?

A bluish or grayish hue to the RBCs, secondary to residual RNA and incomplete hemoglobinization. Polychromatophilic cells are usually large and correspond with reticulocytes.

When are teardrop cells seen?

In myelophthisic disorders (e.g., cancer cell infiltration of the bone marrow, myeloproliferative disorders, especially myeloid metaplasia with myelofibrosis, and infection, such as in tuberculosis). Myelophthisic disorders are commonly associated with a leukoerythroblastic blood smear.

What is a leukoerythroblastic blood smear?

The presence of nucleated RBCs, early myeloid precursors (metamyelocyte and younger), and giant platelets

What is a schistocyte?

Fragmented RBC caused by physical fragmentation of the red cell in the circulation

When are schistocytes seen?

With mechanical heart valves, TTP, DIC, and vasculitides

What is basophilic stippling?

Multiple punctate dark spots seen within the RBC and representing residual RNA

When is basophilic stippling seen?

Fine basophilic stippling is seen in red cells that have been prematurely released from the bone marrow (e.g., reticulocytes, thalassemias, and hemoglobinopathies) and in lead poisoning.
Coarse basophilic stippling is seen in states of abnormal marrow hematopoiesis, such as in MDS.

What is an acanthocyte?

An RBC with a few irregular spiny projections unevenly distributed on the membrane of a cell with a reduced volume

When are acanthocytes seen?

In spur cell anemia, severe liver disease, and abetalipoproteinemia

What is a burr cell?

Also called an echinocyte, burr cells are characterized by numerous regular scalloped projections that are evenly distributed on the red cell surface.

When are echinocytes seen?

In patients with severe renal disease

What is a sickle cell?

Red cells that are shaped like a crescent or sickle

When are sickle cells seen?

In sickle cell anemia

What is a target cell?

An RBC with a bulls-eye appearance with hemoglobin color in the center and periphery of the cell

When are target cells seen?

In thalassemia or liver disease

What is a stomatocyte?

An RBC with a slit-like central pale area. These cells are also referred to as fish-mouth cells.

When are stomatocytes seen?

In ethanol abuse and in an inherited disorder called hereditary stomatocytosis

What is a spherocyte?

An RBC with little or no central pallor. The cell is no longer biconcave but has become more spherical. A spherocyte has the smallest possible surface area to volume ratio, rendering the cell less deformable and prone to premature destruction, predominantly within the spleen.

When are spherocytes seen?

In autoimmune hemolytic anemia and hereditary spherocytosis

What are Heinz bodies?	The precipitation of denatured proteins, mostly hemoglobin, usually secondary to an oxidative chemical insult within the red cell. Finding bite cells or ghost cells on the peripheral blood smear is suggestive of a Heinz body hemolytic anemia. Heinz bodies cannot be seen using the standard Wright stain and require staining with either crystal violet or cresyl blue to be seen.
In what disorders are Heinz bodies seen?	Unstable hemoglobinopathies, methemoglobinemia, G6PD deficiency, and other inherited enzyme deficiencies
What are Howell-Jolly bodies?	Howell-Jolly bodies are single circular black dots seen in the periphery of RBCs. They represent large DNA fragments.
When are Howell-Jolly bodies seen?	After splenectomy or with hyposplenism and in hemolytic anemias when the spleen becomes overwhelmed

ANEMIAS

What is anemia?	A decreased hematocrit or hemoglobin
What are symptoms of anemia?	Fatigue, light-headedness, dyspnea, and headache
What are physical examination findings in anemia?	Pallor, tachycardia, and tachypnea
Is acute or chronic anemia more likely to produce symptoms?	Acute. The rapidity of developing anemia and the patient's underlying cardiopulmonary reserve are the chief determinants of symptoms from anemia. Note: Red cell transfusions should not be given at a specific hematocrit or hemoglobin; rather they should be given for symptoms or the anticipation that

the rapidity of blood loss will require blood transfusions in the near future.

What tests should be ordered in the initial workup of anemia?

The MCV can be used to categorize the anemia as microcytic, normocytic, or macrocytic. Measuring the reticulocyte count and reviewing the peripheral smear are also integral parts of the initial workup.

What is a normal reticulocyte count?

The normal reticulocyte count, which is expressed as a percentage of all red cells, in patients without anemia is 0.5%–1.5%.

What is the corrected reticulocyte count?

Less than or equal to 5%, which can be determined by the following methods:
1. The percent reticulocytes are multiplied by the patient's hematocrit and divided by 45 (normal hematocrit).
2. The absolute reticulocyte count equals the reticulocyte count expressed as a percentage multiplied by the RBC count. An absolute reticulocyte count $> 100,000/\mu L$ suggests an adequate bone marrow response to blood loss or hemolysis.

How does an abnormal reticulocyte count help in the diagnosis of anemia?

The reticulocyte count distinguishes marrow production abnormalities from blood loss or RBC destructive disorders. An elevated reticulocyte count suggests that the anemia is secondary to acute blood loss or a hemolytic process. A low reticulocyte count suggests that the process is due to decreased bone marrow production.

MICROCYTIC ANEMIAS

What is microcytic anemia?

Anemia with an MCV < 80 fl

What are the causes of microcytic anemia?

Iron deficiency, thalassemia, anemia of renal failure, sideroblastic anemia, and anemia of chronic disease

In a patient with an elevated reticulocyte count and microcytic anemia, what diagnosis is suggested?	Thalassemia. To confirm this suspicion, the peripheral smear should be reviewed and a hemoglobin electrophoresis ordered.
In a patient with a microcytic anemia and a low reticulocyte count, what tests should be ordered?	A serum ferritin test. If the ferritin is low, the patient suffers from iron deficiency anemia. There is no need to order any further blood tests. Note: A cause of blood loss needs to be identified.
In a patient with an elevated RDW and microcytic anemia, what diagnosis is suggested?	Iron deficiency
If the ferritin is normal with a low reticulocyte count, what tests should be ordered next?	BUN and creatinine. If the patient has an elevated BUN and creatinine with a normal ferritin, the likely cause of anemia is renal failure. In patients with minor abnormalities of renal function, it is useful to check the erythropoietin level for confirmation.
In a patient with a low reticulocyte count, normal ferritin, and normal renal function, what blood test should be done?	TIBC. A low TIBC suggests a diagnosis of anemia of chronic disease.
What is the most common cause of significant microcytosis without anemia?	Thalassemia

Iron Deficiency

What are the causes of iron deficiency anemia?	Blood loss (gastrointestinal, menstrual, hemoptysis, or hematuria) or impaired absorption (e.g., after gastrectomy).
What is the most common cause of iron deficiency in men and postmenopausal women?	Gastrointestinal bleeding. All patients with iron deficiency should be evaluated for the cause of iron deficiency. In men and postmenopausal women, this usually involves examination of the gastrointestinal tract.

Does a normal serum ferritin rule out iron deficiency anemia?

No. Inflammatory states and liver disease can artificially elevate the serum ferritin level (ferritin is an acute phase reactant).

What is the gold standard for the diagnosis of iron deficiency?

Prussian blue stain for iron stores in a bone marrow aspirate

How is iron stored?

Iron is stored in tissues as ferritin and hemosiderin. Iron is transported between tissues by transferrin.

How is iron deficiency treated?

Ferrous sulfate, 325 mg by mouth, three times daily, between meals. Ferrous sulfate is best absorbed away from meals; however, it is better tolerated with food. Simultaneous administration of vitamin C facilitates iron absorption.

What are some of the side effects of oral iron therapy?

Gastrointestinal upset, constipation, and nausea

How long does it take for oral iron to begin to increase the reticulocyte count?

The reticulocyte count peaks in 5 to 10 days. It usually takes 2 to 3 months of continuous iron therapy to reestablish the body's iron stores.

Anemia of Renal Failure

What is the cause of anemia in patients with renal insufficiency?

Erythropoietin deficiency

What kidney disease can cause end-stage renal disease without leading to significant anemia?

Polycystic kidney disease. In this disorder, erythropoietin production is usually normal.

Thalassemias

What is thalassemia?

Thalassemias are one of the most common genetic disorders known. They are a heterogeneous group of inherited anemias characterized by defects in the synthesis of one or more of the globin chains of the hemoglobin tetramer.

What populations are affected?

Most frequently, peoples of the Mediterranean basin, equatorial Asia, and Africa

What is the pathophysiology of the thalassemias?

Decreased synthesis of one of the globin chains results in an imbalance of either the alpha or beta chain, which results in a decreased quantity of the normal hemoglobin tetramer and may result in polymerization of the excess normal globin chain. Polymerization may result in the production of RBCs with unusual shapes, decreased deformability, and shortened life span.

What is alpha thalassemia?

Alpha thalassemia is a defect in the synthesis of the alpha chain. There are four genes for alpha chains in the human genome. If only one of the genes is affected, the only finding is a low MCV without anemia. If the patient has two genes affected, then mild anemia with a low MCV results.

What is the hemoglobin electrophoresis pattern with alpha thalassemia trait?

Normal. A low MCV with normal ferritin without evidence for beta thalassemia or a hemoglobinopathy may be the only clue to the diagnosis.

What is hydrops fetalis?

Deletion of all four alpha globin genes. This is incompatible with life and the fetus usually dies in utero.

What is hemoglobin H disease?

Three of the four loci of the alpha globin gene are affected. Hemoglobin H is a tetramer of beta chains. This is the most severe form of alpha thalassemia that is compatible with life.

How does hemoglobin H disease present?

As significant anemia in early childhood

What are the major medical problems of hemoglobin H disease attributable to?

Iron overload secondary to massive transfusion requirements

What is beta thalassemia?

Decreased synthesis of beta globin. There are two beta globin genes, whereas there are four alpha globin genes.

What is beta thalassemia minor?

One of the beta globin genes is missing or dysfunctional. This type of beta thalassemia is also referred to as beta thalassemia trait.

How is the diagnosis of beta thalassemia minor made?

By demonstration of microcytic anemia with target cells and ovalocytes, moderate poikilocytosis, basophilic stippling, and reticulocytosis. Hemoglobin electrophoresis shows an elevated percentage of hemoglobin A2.

What is beta thalassemia major?

Abnormalities of both beta globin genes with markedly reduced to absent beta chain synthesis. This disorder is also referred to as Cooley's anemia.

How does beta thalassemia major present?

With severe anemia within the first 6 months of life. The predominant medical problems are attributable to iron overload secondary to massive transfusion requirements.

What is beta thalassemia intermediate?

Both beta globin genes are abnormal, but a small amount of normal beta globin chain can still be synthesized.

What are the symptoms and signs of beta thalassemia intermediate?

Usually, patients do not require transfusion and have mild splenomegaly. However, cardiomegaly and osteoporotic fractures can develop.

Sideroblastic Anemia

What is sideroblastic anemia?

Microcytic hypoproliferative anemia with ringed sideroblasts seen on bone marrow aspirate

What is a sideroblast?

An erythroid precursor with iron granules

What are ringed sideroblasts?

Erythroid precursors with large iron granules within mitochondria ringing the nucleus. Normal erythroid precursors have a few small punctate iron granules scattered throughout the cytoplasm.

What is the defect that results in the accumulation of iron within the mitochondria in ring sideroblasts?

An enzymatic defect of heme synthesis does not allow iron to be incorporated into the heme molecule. When this is a lifelong process, it is referred to as primary sideroblastic anemia.

What are the secondary, or acquired, causes of sideroblastic anemia?

MDSs, lead poisoning, and drug use (e.g., use of isoniazid, hydralazine, chloramphenicol, and ethanol)

What is the treatment for sideroblastic anemia?

Pyridoxine (vitamin B_6) may lead to an increase in the hematocrit in some patients. Supportive care is the mainstay in the MDS variety.

Hemoglobinopathies

What is a hemoglobinopathy?

A molecular abnormality of the hemoglobin molecule

Which is the most clinically significant hemoglobinopathy in the United States?

Hemoglobin S disease (sickle cell anemia)

What is the defect in hemoglobin S?

A mutation in the beta chain gene that results in a change in amino acid number 6 from glutamic acid to valine

What is the pathophysiology of hemoglobin S disease?

On deoxygenation, hemoglobin S becomes relatively insoluble and aggregates into long strands or fibers, resulting in a characteristic RBC shape (sickle cell), which is markedly less deformable. Because the sickle cells can no longer deform to squeeze through the capillaries, they clog up the microvasculature and result in ischemia.

What are the complications of sickle cell anemia?

Painful crises, aplastic crises, infections (e.g., sepsis, cholecystitis, and osteomyelitis), and ischemia or infarction of any organ system (e.g., CVA, MI, pulmonary vascular occlusion, renal medullary infarction, lower extremity ulcers, avascular necrosis of the hip, proliferative retinopathy, and priapism)

Why are sickle cell anemia patients thought to be particularly prone to sepsis?

They become functionally asplenic early in life secondary to vasoocclusive ischemia of the spleen and thus susceptible to infection with encapsulated bacteria such as *Haemophilus influenzae* and *Streptococcus pneumoniae.*

How do you make the diagnosis of sickle cell anemia?

Hemoglobin electrophoresis shows the presence of hemoglobin S. The peripheral smear shows characteristic sickle RBCs.

Is prophylaxis against infection useful in sickle cell anemia?

Early in the patient's life, oral penicillin helps prevent pneumococcal sepsis. All patients should receive the multivalent pneumococcal vaccine.

What is the treatment for patients with sickle cell and fever?

A high index of suspicion for sepsis needs to be maintained. Hospitalization, blood cultures, and treatment with broad-spectrum antibiotics until blood cultures are negative for 48 hours is the safest approach.

What is the management of sickle cell painful crises?

Hydration and pain medication. Occasionally, red cell exchange is used in patients with severe complications of sickle cell anemia or refractory sickle cell pain crises. Recently, long-term treatment with hydroxyurea has been shown to decrease the frequency of emergency room visits for painful crises in patients with sickle cell anemia who have frequent painful crises.

What is hemoglobin SC disease?

A heterozygous condition in which one allele for the beta chain is hemoglobin S and the other allele is hemoglobin C.

How is hemoglobin SC disease different from sickle cell anemia?

Usually, patients with hemoglobin SC disease have fewer symptoms, but they may be equally affected. Patients with SC disease have a higher frequency of avascular necrosis of the femoral head and proliferative retinopathy.

What is sickle beta thalassemia disease?

One of the beta chain alleles has hemoglobin S and the other allele has dysfunctional beta chain synthesis. Even though the disease is usually less severe than sickle cell anemia, the clinical course can be identical. The amount of normal hemoglobin A present usually correlates with the severity of the disease.

NORMOCYTIC ANEMIAS

What are the causes of normocytic anemia?

Anemia of chronic disease, recent blood loss, hemolytic anemias, endocrinopathies, and anemia of renal failure

Anemia of Chronic Disease

What is anemia of chronic disease?

A hypoproliferative anemia secondary to poor uptake and utilization of iron by red cell precursors. Inflammatory cytokines are thought to play a role in inhibiting erythropoiesis.

What is seen on bone marrow staining in anemia of chronic disease?

Staining the bone marrow reveals normal iron stores, but iron within the erythroblasts is decreased to absent.

Anemia of chronic disease is associated with what disorders?

Malignancies, connective tissue diseases (e.g., rheumatoid arthritis and SLE), and chronic infections (e.g., osteomyelitis)

How is the diagnosis of anemia of chronic disease made?

The diagnosis should be considered in a patient with a systemic illness, a hypoproliferative anemia, and normal iron stores. A low TIBC is highly suggestive of anemia of chronic disease.

How do you differentiate iron deficiency from anemia of chronic disease?

In iron deficiency anemia, the RDW is high, the ferritin is low (unless there is a concomitant inflammatory process or hepatitis), and the TIBC is elevated. In patients with anemia of chronic disease, the RDW is normal, the serum ferritin level is usually normal, and the TIBC is decreased. In some situations an iron stain of the bone marrow is required to differentiate these disorders.

How do you treat anemia of chronic disease?

Ideally, the underlying disorder is treated and the anemia resolves. Patients rarely need red cell transfusions for anemia; if a patient requires transfusions, alternative causes for the anemia should be considered. Erythropoietin injections can increase the hematocrit in many patients, if necessary.

Hemolytic Anemias

What is hemolysis?

Premature RBC destruction

What is hemolytic anemia?

Anemia in which the destruction of RBCs exceeds the ability of the marrow to increase red cell production

What are the broad categories of hemolytic anemias?

Thalassemias, hemoglobinopathies, autoimmune hemolytic anemia, red cell membrane disorders, microangiopathic hemolytic anemias, and enzyme deficiencies of the hexose monophosphate shunt, and the Embden-Meyerhof pathway

How do you distinguish autoimmune hemolytic anemias from all the other types of hemolytic anemias?

The direct Coombs' test is usually positive in autoimmune hemolytic anemia, indicating the presence of antibodies attached to the patient's red cells.

Is the reticulocyte count usually elevated in hemolytic anemia?

Yes, unless the bone marrow is simultaneously affected by a hypoproliferative process such as iron deficiency, vitamin B_{12} deficiency, or anemia of chronic disease

What chemical abnormalities suggest a hemolytic anemia?

Elevated LDH and unconjugated bilirubin with a decreased haptoglobin and positive urine hemosiderin test

What are the early laboratory findings in intravascular and extravascular hemolysis?

	Intravascular	Extravascular
LDH	Increases	Increases
Reticulocyte count	Increases	Increases
Bilirubin	Increases	Increases
Haptoglobins (24 hours)	Decreases	Normal
Serum/urine hemoglobin (6 hours)	Present	Absent
Methemalbumin (36 hours)	Increases	Normal
Urine hemosiderin (1 week)	Positive	Negative

What disorders are associated with cold antibody autoimmune hemolytic anemia?

Lymphoproliferative disorders, *Mycoplasma pneumoniae*, infectious mononucleosis, and syphilis

What physical finding is often present in autoimmune hemolytic anemia?

Splenomegaly

What is the treatment of autoimmune hemolytic anemia?

Steroids are the mainstay of treatment. In refractory cases, splenectomy may be successful. Transfusion of red cells is imperative in patients with circulatory collapse and symptoms associated with heart disease.

What is the difficulty in transfusing these patients?

Finding compatible blood. It is important to work closely with the blood bank to obtain units of blood that are the least incompatible.

What are the common RBC membrane disorders associated with hemolysis?

Paroxysmal nocturnal hemoglobinuria, hereditary spherocytosis, hereditary elliptocytosis, and spur cell anemia of severe liver disease

What is the most common red cell membrane defect to cause hemolysis in whites?

Hereditary spherocytosis, an autosomal dominant disorder

How does hereditary spherocytosis present?

Patients usually have a family history of mild anemia, a peripheral smear showing spherocytes, and a negative Coombs' test. The diagnosis can be confirmed with an osmotic fragility test.

What is the most common molecular defect identified as a cause of hereditary spherocytosis?

Defective or deficient ankyrin, a protein linking the red cell membrane to the skeleton of the red cell

What infection can worsen the anemia in patients with hereditary spherocytosis?

Parvovirus infection can lead to an aplastic crisis.

What is the most common red cell enzyme deficiency associated with hemolytic anemia?

G6PD deficiency

What is the biochemical consequence of G6PD deficiency?

G6PD is an enzyme in the hexose monophosphate shunt that helps maintain oxidative reduction power in the red cell. In the absence of reduction power, hydrogen peroxide accumulates within red cells. Hydrogen peroxide destroys lipids within the red cell membrane, leading eventually to hemolysis. This enzyme deficiency is usually found in the heterozygous state, so, on average, the red cells contain 50% of the normal enzyme level. Under normal conditions, these cells can handle routine oxidative stresses, but, in circumstances of greatly increased stress, such as infections or certain drug exposures, oxidation leads to hemolysis.

What conditions can precipitate hemolytic episodes in patients with G6PD deficiency?

The most common cause is drug use (the most common culprits are anticonvulsants, Pyridium, phenylhydrazine, and sulfa drugs); fever and infection are also associated with hemolysis.

How is the diagnosis of G6PD deficiency made?

Red cell G6PD levels can be measured. Note: The level should not be measured during or shortly after a hemolytic episode because the older red cells containing decreased amounts of G6PD will have lysed, leaving only the younger cells containing higher levels of G6PD. A falsely normal level could then be measured and the diagnosis missed.

How is methemoglobin formed?

Oxidation of the iron in heme from Fe^{2+} to Fe^{3+}

What is the earliest clinical sign of methemoglobinemia?

The patient appears blue, yet has a normal arterial PO_2.

What are the causes of microangiopathic hemolytic anemia?

Mechanical heart valves, infected heart valves, TTP, malignant hypertension, DIC, preeclampsia, HELLP, connective tissue diseases, and malignancy

What is the pathophysiologic process in microangiopathic hemolytic anemia?

Mechanical heart valves may directly shear the RBCs. In other disorders, fibrin strand formation in the microcirculation traps and shears the red cells.

Macrocytic Anemias

What is macrocytosis?

MCV > 100 fl

What are the causes of macrocytic anemia?

Vitamin B_{12} deficiency, folate deficiency, chemotherapy, hemolysis, liver disease, MDSs, and hypothyroidism

What is megaloblastic anemia?

Macrocytic anemia associated with delayed nuclear maturation, with normal to increased cytoplasmic maturation, producing large cells. This type of anemia is caused by disorders affecting the nucleus.

What are the causes of megaloblastic anemia?

Vitamin B_{12} and folate deficiency, chemotherapy exposure, and MDS

What should be the first test ordered for the evaluation of a patient with macrocytic anemia?

Reticulocyte count and peripheral blood smear

A patient with an elevated reticulocyte count and macrocytic anemia suggests what diagnosis?

Hemolytic anemia

Why is the MCV elevated in patients with hemolytic anemia?

There is an increase in the percentage of reticulocytes, which are large cells.

What are the causes of anemia associated with liver disease?

Anemia of chronic disease, iron deficiency secondary to gastrointestinal blood loss, vitamin B_{12} and folate deficiency, hypersplenism with pooling, and mild hemolysis

What peripheral smear findings suggest liver disease?

Macrocytosis with target cells. In severe end-stage liver disease, markedly abnormal red cell shapes (spur cells) can be seen. These abnormalities appear to be caused by cholesterol synthesis abnormalities in the liver.

What peripheral smear findings suggest an MDS?

Pancytopenia. The red cells are usually large with macroovalocytes. Coarse basophilic stippling can be seen. Hypogranulation and hyposegmentation of the nucleus of the neutrophils are highly suggestive.

What test is done to confirm the diagnosis of an MDS?

Examination of the bone marrow aspirate and biopsy are required to make a definitive diagnosis of an MDS. Dysplastic changes of the hematopoietic precursors, an increased percentage of blasts, pathologic and ringed sideroblasts, and clonal cytogenetic abnormalities are all suggestive of an MDS.

What are the causes of anemia in a patient who abuses alcohol?

Poor nutrition with resultant deficiency of iron, vitamin B_{12}, and folic acid. Iron deficiency may be a result of gastrointestinal hemorrhage. Alcohol abuse can lead to liver disease, which can cause anemia by several different mechanisms.

Does excessive alcohol use cause macrocytosis in the absence of liver disease, vitamin B_{12} deficiency, and folate deficiency?

Yes

What is the most common cause of folate deficiency?

Decreased dietary intake. Deficiency can develop after 3–4 months of decreased intake. Folate deficiency is often seen in alcoholics.

What are some common causes of vitamin B_{12} deficiency?

Pernicious anemia, gastric surgery, ileal surgery, or a malabsorption syndrome, such as tropical sprue

What is the pathophysiology of pernicious anemia?

Pernicious anemia is essentially synonymous with intrinsic factor deficiency. Patients may have an autoantibody to intrinsic factor or to parietal cells, which produce intrinsic factor. Intrinsic factor is needed for optimal absorption of vitamin B_{12} in the ileum.

What physical findings suggest the diagnosis of vitamin B_{12} deficiency?

Peripheral neuropathy, pallor, jaundice, and splenomegaly

How is vitamin B_{12} absorbed?

Parietal cells within the stomach produce intrinsic factor, which binds vitamin B_{12} and transports it to the ileum where it is absorbed.

What diagnostic tests are used to aid in the diagnosis of pernicious anemia?

Serum vitamin B_{12} level
Intrinsic factor antibody—positive in 60% of patients
Antiparietal cell antibody—found in 90% of patients with pernicious anemia, but specificity is low
Schilling's test

What is a Schilling's test?

A nuclear medicine test that measures vitamin B_{12} absorption. A radioactive dose of vitamin B_{12} is ingested and simultaneously an intramuscular injection of nonradioactive B_{12} is given. The quantity of radioactive vitamin B_{12} excreted in the urine is measured. If radioactivity is measured in the urine, then the vitamin B_{12} taken orally was absorbed and the patient does not have pernicious anemia. If no radioactivity is measured in the urine, then part 2 of the Schilling's test is performed to confirm the diagnosis. In part 2, radioactive vitamin B_{12} is ingested with intrinsic factor. If radioactivity is then detected in the urine, then the patient has pernicious anemia.

ERYTHROCYTOSIS

What is erythrocytosis?

Erythrocytosis is synonymous with polycythemia; that is, the number of red cells is increased.

What is relative erythrocytosis?

The RBC mass is normal, but the plasma volume is decreased.

What conditions cause relative erythrocytosis?

Hemoconcentration secondary to volume depletion, hypertension, preeclampsia, cigarette use, and stress erythrocytosis (Gaisböck's syndrome)

What is absolute erythrocytosis?

The RBC mass is increased.

What are the three mechanisms that can lead to absolute erythrocytosis?

1. Autonomous RBC production, primary erythrocytosis, or polycythemia vera
2. Secondary erythrocytosis from tissue hypoxia
3. Inappropriate erythropoietin production

What is the most common cause of an elevated red cell mass?

Tissue hypoxia

What are the causes of erythrocytosis secondary to tissue hypoxia?

The most common cause is lung disease. Other causes include sleep apnea, chronic exposure to high altitudes, cyanotic congenital heart disease, chronic carbon monoxide intoxication (e.g., from cigarette use), and abnormal hemoglobins.

What are the causes of erythropoietin excess?

Tumors—renal cell carcinoma, hepatoma, cerebellar hemangioblastoma, adrenal tumor, uterine tumor, pheochromocytoma, and tumors associated with von Hippel-Lindau disease
Renal disease—renal cysts, glomerulonephritis, and nephrotic syndrome

Who exhibits the classic situation in which stress erythrocytosis (Gaisböck's syndrome) is seen?

Hypertensive, obese, middle-aged men who smoke

What is the mechanism by which tissue hypoxia results in absolute erythrocytosis?

Peritubular interstitial cells of the inner cortex of the kidney sense hypoxia and increase their secretion of erythropoietin.

What three mechanisms produce the increased hematocrit seen in cigarette smokers?

1. Decreased plasma volume (unknown mechanism)
2. Commonly, underlying lung disease
3. Lower oxygen delivery to tissues. Carbon monoxide from smoke has a higher affinity for hemoglobin than oxygen, resulting in the lower oxygen delivery.

PANCYTOPENIA

What is pancytopenia?

The combination of leukopenia, anemia, and thrombocytopenia

What are the causes of pancytopenia?

Disorders involving infiltration of the bone marrow, hypersplenism, vitamin B_{12} or folate deficiency, MDSs, and aplastic anemia

What are some of the infiltrative disorders of the bone marrow that are associated with pancytopenia?	Metastatic cancer, multiple myeloma, myelofibrosis, lymphoproliferative disorders, and acute leukemia
What is the characteristic finding on peripheral smear in infiltrative disorders of bone marrow?	Leukoerythroblastosis
What are the disorders of the spleen that result in pancytopenia?	Congestive splenomegaly (e.g., cirrhosis and portal vein thrombosis), lymphomas, Gaucher's disease, Niemann-Pick disease, Letterer-Siwe disease, and infectious diseases (e.g., kala-azar, miliary tuberculosis, and syphilis)

APLASTIC ANEMIA

What is aplastic anemia?	Pancytopenia caused by bone marrow hematopoietic failure
What is the most common cause of aplastic anemia?	Idiopathic cause
What are some other common causes of aplastic anemia?	Infections (e.g., hepatitis), radiation, chemicals (e.g., benzene), drugs (e.g., chloramphenicol), and autoimmune causes
What is Fanconi's anemia?	Aplastic anemia caused by an inherited defect in DNA repair, often associated with congenital anomalies
Pure red cell aplasia may be caused by what infectious agent?	Parvovirus B19
What tumor may be associated with pure red cell aplasia?	Thymoma
What are treatment options for aplastic anemia?	Immunosuppression with antithymocyte globulin or cyclosporine plus steroids, or BMT

What is the differential diagnosis of aplastic anemia?	Toxins, viral infection, hypoplastic MDS, hypoplastic acute leukemia, paroxysmal nocturnal hemoglobinuria, and myelofibrosis

LEUKOCYTES

What are the five major types of leukocytes in peripheral blood?	Neutrophils (granulocytes), monocytes, lymphocytes, eosinophils, and basophils
What is the average life span of a granulocyte?	6–12 hours
What is chronic granulomatous disease?	A rare inherited disorder in which granulocytes and monocytes are unable to make superoxide anion and are thereby unable to kill phagocytosed microorganisms
How does chronic granulomatous disease present?	As recurrent lymphadenitis, hepatic abscesses, or osteomyelitis, with a positive family history of frequent infections
How is the diagnosis of chronic granulomatous disease made?	Nitroblue tetrazolium test. Superoxide from normal phagocytes converts yellow tetrazolium dye to blue.
What is Chédiak-Higashi syndrome?	A rare autosomal recessive disorder with neutrophil dysfunction and large cytoplasmic granules in the granulocytes, monocytes, and lymphocytes
How does Chédiak-Higashi syndrome present?	Normally, it presents in infants. Patients have an increased susceptibility to infection with neutropenia and a platelet function defect.

LEUKOPENIA

What is neutropenia?	$< 2 \times 10^9$ neutrophils/L ($< 1.5 \times 10^9$/L in blacks)

Below what neutrophil count is the patient at significantly increased risk of serious bacterial infection?

$0.5 \times 10^9/L$

What are the common sites of infection in neutropenic patients?

Lungs, skin, urinary tract, and oropharynx

What are some common causes of neutropenia?

Drugs (e.g., phenytoin, chemotherapy, phenothiazines, procainamide, and beta-lactams), bone marrow disorders (e.g., tumor infiltration and fibrosis), megaloblastic disorders, sepsis, autoimmune neutropenia, collagen vascular diseases, and hypersplenism

What is agranulocytosis?

Complete absence of granulocytes. The disease is most often caused by the use of certain drugs. Patients are at increased risk of infection and sepsis. Bone marrow examination shows no myeloid activity.

What is the treatment for agranulocytosis?

Immediate discontinuation of all drugs associated with agranulocytosis, administration of antibiotics and G-CSF, and, occasionally, granulocyte transfusions if there is evidence of infection.

What is Felty's syndrome?

Neutropenia caused by hypersplenism and antineutrophil antibodies in a patient with rheumatoid arthritis

What is lymphopenia?

Lymphocyte count $< 1.5 \times 10^9/L$

What is the most common cause of lymphopenia worldwide?

Protein–calorie malnutrition

What are some other common causes of lymphopenia?

Viruses (e.g., varicella zoster, measles, HIV), Hodgkin's disease, and corticosteroids

LEUKOCYTOSIS

What is leukocytosis?

WBC count > 11×10^9/L

What is a leukemoid reaction?

An increase in the WBC count to > 25 $\times 10^9$/L, secondary to another condition

In a patient with leukocytosis, what is the most important test to order?

A differential to determine the type of leukocytes responsible for the elevation. The peripheral smear should be reviewed if the elevated cell type does not fit the clinical picture. For example, an asymptomatic patient should not have an elevated WBC count, whereas a patient with pneumonia usually has an elevated neutrophil count.

What are causes of leukocytosis?

Leukemia and reactive states, such as infection and cancer

NEUTROPHILIA

What are the causes of neutrophilia?

Inflammatory processes—infection, malignancy, burns, ischemic necrosis, postoperative states, gout, collagen vascular diseases, and hypersensitivity reactions
Malignant hematologic disorders—CML and other myeloproliferative disorders, acute myeloid leukemia, and, occasionally, MDSs
Intoxications—uremia and diabetic ketoacidosis
Miscellaneous—hemorrhage, eclampsia, hemolysis, exercise, post-ictal state, and corticosteroids

What is the most common cause of neutrophilia?

Acute infection

What are toxic granulations?

An increase in intensity of staining and number of myeloperoxidase granules within neutrophils

In whom are toxic granulations seen?

In patients with active infection

| How can a leukemoid reaction be differentiated from CML? | In contrast to a leukemoid reaction, in CML, the spleen is usually enlarged, the leukocyte alkaline phosphatase level is very low, and there is often basophilia and the presence of the Philadelphia chromosome or breakpoint cluster region rearrangement. |

LYMPHOCYTOSIS

What is lymphocytosis?	Lymphocyte count $> 5 \times 10^9$/L
What is the most common cause of mild to moderate lymphocytosis?	Viral infections (e.g., Epstein-Barr virus, cytomegalovirus, and hepatitis)
What are the causes of marked lymphocytosis ($> 15 \times 10^9$/L)?	Infectious mononucleosis, pertussis infection, chronic lymphocytic leukemia, and acute lymphocytic leukemia

EOSINOPHILS

What are some common causes of eosinophilia?	Think **NAACP**: **N**eoplasm **A**ddison's disease **A**llergy (includes drug reactions) and **A**sthma **C**ollagen vascular diseases **P**arasites
What is the hypereosinophilic syndrome?	Persistent eosinophilia ($> 1.5 \times 10^9$/L for more than 6 months) in the absence of an identifiable underlying cause and with organ involvement
What organs are commonly involved in the hypereosinophilic syndrome?	Heart (endomyocardial fibrosis), liver, skin, lungs, and central nervous system
What is the standard first-line therapy for hypereosinophilic syndrome?	Corticosteroids

PLATELETS

What is the average life span of a platelet?	7–10 days
Where are platelets made?	In the bone marrow from megakaryocytes
What are some of the platelet dense granule contents?	Calcium, serotonin, and adenosine diphosphate
What are some of the platelet alpha granule contents?	Platelet factor 4, β-thromboglobulin, factor V, vWF, and transforming growth factor-β

THROMBOCYTOPENIA

What is thrombocytopenia?	Platelet count < 150 × 10⁹/L
What are the symptoms associated with thrombocytopenia?	Mild to severe hemorrhage. Epistaxis, hematuria, easy and spontaneous bruising, menorrhagia, and gingival bleeding are common sites of bleeding associated with thrombocytopenia.
What physical signs point to thrombocytopenia?	Petechiae and numerous small ecchymoses
What do petechiae look like?	Minute red to purplish flat spots on the skin that do not blanch with pressure. Petechiae are usually seen in areas of vascular congestion (e.g., areas below a tourniquet site or blood pressure cuff), dependent areas, areas exposed to constriction (tight clothing), and bony prominences.
At what platelet count is there a significantly increased risk of bleeding from trauma or surgery?	Platelet counts > 50 × 10⁹/L are usually sufficient to prevent major bleeding from surgical procedures and trauma. The more severe the trauma and the larger the operation, the greater the risk of bleeding; brain surgery usually requires a platelet count closer to 100 × 10⁹/L.

At what platelet count does spontaneous hemorrhage become a risk?

Ecchymoses and petechiae usually do not occur until the platelet count is < 50 × 10⁹/L.

At what platelet count does spontaneous life-threatening hemorrhage become a distinct possibility?

< 5 × 10⁹/L

When should platelets be transfused?

At a platelet count of < 100 × 10⁹/L when there is life-threatening or clinically significant bleeding. Prophylactic platelet transfusion is routinely given to patients with platelet counts < 10 × 10⁹/L when they have decreased platelet production (< 20 × 10⁹/L if there is concomitant infection, fever, uremia, or other additional bleeding risk).

What are the three basic processes that result in thrombocytopenia?

Decreased production, increased destruction, and splenic sequestration

What is the differential diagnosis of decreased platelet production?

Myelophthisic disorders, acute leukemia, MDSs, aplastic anemia, viral infection, AIDS, drug use, vitamin B_{12} deficiency, and folate deficiency

What are the causes of increased destruction or consumption?

Idiopathic thrombocytopenic purpura, TTP, and DIC

What are the causes of splenic sequestration?

Splenomegaly, as seen in myeloproliferative disorders, lymphoma, cirrhosis, portal vein thrombosis, splenic vein thrombosis, hepatic vein thrombosis, Felty's syndrome, SLE, sarcoid, and hemolytic anemia

How is thrombocytopenia as a result of decreased production distinguished from increased destruction or consumptive process or splenic sequestration?

The gold standard is the bone marrow aspirate. A normal to increased number of megakaryocytes suggests a peripheral destructive or consumptive process or splenic sequestration.

IMMUNE THROMBOCYTOPENIC PURPURA

What is ITP?

Autoantibodies are directed against platelet surface antigens, leading to premature platelet destruction and thrombocytopenia.

What are symptoms of ITP?

Symptoms are attributable to thrombocytopenia. Some patients complain of a viral syndrome several weeks before onset of the disease.

What are physical signs of ITP?

Ecchymoses and petechiae. There are no other specific findings.

How is the diagnosis of ITP made?

ITP is a diagnosis of exclusion. The combination of isolated thrombocytopenia without any intercurrent illnesses, normal kidney function, normal red cell morphology on peripheral smear, normal PT/aPTT, and increased megakaryocytes on a bone marrow aspirate is highly suggestive.

What diseases are associated with ITP?

Chronic lymphocytic leukemia, Hodgkin's disease, non-Hodgkin's lymphoma, SLE, rheumatoid arthritis, and HIV infection

Should all patients with ITP receive treatment?

No, only if there is significant bleeding history or a platelet count $< 30 \times 10^9$/L. Occasionally, the disease spontaneously regresses, especially in childhood.

Do platelet transfusions increase the platelet count in ITP?

No; however, if severe uncontrollable bleeding occurs, then platelet transfusion is indicated.

What is the mainstay of initial treatment of severe ITP in adults without bleeding?

Corticosteroids

What are some alternative treatments for steroid-refractory patients with ITP?

Intravenous immunoglobulin, which gives the most rapid increase in platelet count, but generally the effect is transient and expensive, anti–D immunoglobulin, splenectomy, and danazol

THROMBOTIC THROMBOCYTOPENIC PURPURA AND HEMOLYTIC UREMIC SYNDROME

What is TTP?

Thrombotic thrombocytopenic purpura

What is the clinical diagnostic pentad of TTP?

Fever, microangiopathic hemolytic anemia with schistocytes, thrombocytopenia, neurologic changes, and renal dysfunction

What is HUS?

A triad of thrombocytopenia, hemolytic anemia, and renal failure. Some investigators think that TTP and HUS are the same disease.

What are the differences between TTP and HUS?

HUS is associated with a greater degree of renal failure and, less often, with other end organ damage (e.g., heart, brain, lungs, gastrointestinal tract, and retinal vessels). Thrombocytopenia and hemolysis are more profound in TTP than in HUS. HUS is more frequent in children.

What is the differential diagnosis of TTP and HUS (thrombocytopenia, hemolysis, and schistocytes)?

DIC, preeclampsia and eclampsia, HELLP syndrome, malignant hypertension, and severe vasculitis

What are some inciting factors for TTP and HUS?

Infection, pregnancy, immune disorders, and chemotherapy

What are the two drugs that have been associated with TTP and HUS?

Cyclosporine and mitomycin C

What is the treatment for TTP?

Daily plasma exchange of 3–4 L leads to improvement in many patients within 1 week. Before the institution of plasma exchange therapy, TTP was nearly universally fatal.

What peripheral blood smear findings are essential for the diagnosis of TTP?

Schistocytes and thrombocytopenia

THROMBOCYTOSIS

What is thrombocytosis?

Platelet count > 450 × 10^9/L.

What are the two major categories of thrombocytosis?

1. Essential thrombocythemia (primary; one of the myeloproliferative disorders)
2. Secondary (reactive) thrombocytosis

What two laboratory tests may help differentiate reactive thrombocytosis from essential thrombocythemia?

Fibrinogen and C-reactive protein levels, which are often elevated with reactive thrombocytosis because many of the reactive disorders cause elevation of acute-phase reactant protein levels

What are some of the causes of reactive thrombocytosis?

Acute infection, inflammatory states, malignancy, iron deficiency, and post-splenectomy

MYELOPROLIFERATIVE DISORDERS

What are the myeloproliferative disorders?

A diverse group of clonal, neoplastic hematologic disorders that have abnormal proliferation of hematopoietic precursors

What are the four myeloproliferative disorders?

Polycythemia vera, essential thrombocythemia, CML, and myelofibrosis with myeloid metaplasia

Is splenomegaly common in myeloproliferative disorders?

Yes. A normal-sized spleen is unusual.

POLYCYTHEMIA VERA

Is only the hematocrit elevated in polycythemia vera?

No. Polycythemia vera is characterized by an excessive proliferation of myeloid, erythroid, and megakaryocytic elements in the bone marrow, increased cell counts in peripheral blood specimens, and increased erythrocyte mass. The leukocyte count is elevated in two thirds of patients and the platelet count is elevated in 50%.

What are the presenting symptoms in patients with polycythemia vera?

Headache, blurred vision, dizziness, vertigo, paresthesias, focal weakness, and erythromelalgia. Many patients with polycythemia vera have intense pruritus after bathing. Patients may have an acute arterial ischemic event such as stroke or MI, or a venous thrombosis (e.g., DVT or portal vein thrombosis). Additional symptoms include sweats and weight loss.

What physical findings are common in patients with polycythemia vera?

Splenomegaly, plethora, and macroglossia

How is the diagnosis of polycythemia made?

Major criteria—elevated red cell mass, oxygen saturation > 92%, splenomegaly

Minor criteria—leukocytosis, thrombocytosis, elevated leukocyte alkaline phosphatase, and elevated B_{12} binding proteins

Diagnosis is made if all three major criteria are present or with an elevated red cell mass with an O_2 saturation > 92% and two of the minor criteria.

What is the median survival of patients with polycythemia vera?

10 years, with phlebotomy

What is the major cause of death in polycythemia vera?

Thrombosis; less often, hemorrhage

Is there an increased risk for development of acute leukemia in polycythemia vera?

Yes. This risk is not nearly as high as that seen with the MDSs, and it is often associated with an alkylating agent or radioactive phosphorus treatment.

What is the treatment for polycythemia vera?

Phlebotomy to a hematocrit of less than or equal to 42%. In the case of marked splenomegaly or thrombocytosis, hydroxyurea is effective. There is an investigational agent, anagrelide, which shows excellent promise in reducing elevated platelet counts without the leukemogenic potential of hydroxyurea.

What is the "spent phase" of polycythemia?

The development of myelofibrosis with metaplasia. This state is indistinguishable from agnogenic myeloid metaplasia. The onset averages 10 years from diagnosis and occurs in approximately 15% of patients with polycythemia vera. This phase is marked by increasing splenomegaly, anemia, and bone marrow fibrosis with associated leukoerythroblastic blood smear. Acute leukemia eventually develops in 25%–50% of patients with this complication.

ESSENTIAL THROMBOCYTHEMIA

What is essential thrombocythemia?

A myeloproliferative disorder with persistent thrombocytosis (platelet count $> 600 \times 10^9$/L) that is not reactive to another disorder and is not caused by another myeloproliferative disorder. Bone marrow shows megakaryocte hyperplasia and clustering.

What are symptoms and signs of essential thrombocythemia?

Headache, transient ischemic attacks, paresthesias, erythromelalgia, digital pain, bleeding, weight loss, sweating, fevers, and pruritus. Thrombocytosis is found on a routine blood test.

What are some of the common clinical problems patients with essential thrombocythemia encounter?

Thrombosis and hemorrhage (CVA, MI, digital ulceration, DVT, epistaxis, and gastrointestinal bleeding)

What abnormalities are seen in the peripheral blood in essential thrombocythemia?

Thrombocytosis, often with very large platelets, leukocytosis (30% of cases), leukoerythroblastic blood smear (25% of cases), eosinophilia, and basophilia

What is the differential diagnosis for essential thrombocythemia?

Other myeloproliferative disorders, MDSs (e.g., 5q-), and reactive thrombocytosis

What is the typical age of onset of essential thrombocythemia?

It is usually not seen until the 6th or 7th decade of life, but a second peak occurs in young women in the 3rd and 4th decades of life.

What is the treatment for essential thrombocythemia?

It is somewhat controversial for asymptomatic patients. For patients with acute thrombosis, plateletpheresis is followed by administration of platelet-lowering drugs (e.g., hydroxyurea). For patients with hemorrhage, normal platelets should be given, then platelet-lowering drugs.

What is the chronic treatment for essential thrombocythemia?

In patients at high risk for thrombosis or who have had a previous thrombotic event, the platelet count should be lowered into the normal range with an alkylating agent such as hydroxyurea. A new drug, anagrelide, which specifically blocks platelet production and does not have the leukemogenic potential of alkylating agent chemotherapy, seems promising. Antiplatelet drugs, such as aspirin, may also be helpful in patients with thrombosis.

CHRONIC MYELOGENOUS LEUKEMIA

What cells are characteristically elevated in patients with CML?

Mature, normal-appearing neutrophils. At the time of diagnosis, the WBC count is often between 100 and 300×10^9/L, with a mild normochromic normocytic anemia and moderate splenomegaly.

How is a leukemoid reaction distinguished from early CML?

The leukocyte alkaline phosphatase is characteristically very low in CML and is markedly elevated in a leukemoid reaction.

What chromosomal abnormality is highly associated with CML?

The Philadelphia chromosome is usually found; this is a balanced translocation between chromosome 9 and 22. This results in a fusion protein (bcr-abl) with transforming properties.

What are symptoms of CML?

Lethargy, weight loss, increasing abdominal girth, sweating, and easy bruising and bleeding, as well as symptoms attributable to anemia and splenomegaly

What are physical findings of CML?	Splenomegaly and hepatomegaly
What are the three phases of CML?	Chronic phase, accelerated phase, and blast phase
What is the usual length of the chronic phase of CML?	3–5 years. During this period, patients can perform many of their usual activities and the disease is easily controlled with oral chemotherapy.
What is the treatment of CML in the chronic phase?	Young patients in good health with an HLA-matched sibling should probably proceed to allogeneic BMT. A recent study demonstrated that the use of alpha-interferon while the patient is in the chronic phase can induce cytogenetic complete remissions and prolong survival.
What brings about the progression from the chronic phase to the accelerated phase to the blast phase in CML?	New nonrandom cytogenetic abnormalities have been found in up to 80% of patients in the blast phase.
What changes occur at the onset of the accelerated phase of CML?	An elevated leukocyte count, which is difficult to control with oral chemotherapy, persistent thrombocytosis, increase in percent blasts and promyelocytes in blood and bone marrow, increased splenomegaly, development of myelofibrosis, and development of chloromas
What is the clinical course of the accelerated phase of CML?	Usually, over a several month period, transformation into the blast phase occurs.
What indicates the onset of the blast phase of CML?	> 30% blasts in the peripheral blood or bone marrow
What is the usual phenotype of the CML blasts?	Usually myeloid but occasionally lymphoid. Treatment for each phenotype is different.

What is treatment of the blast phase of CML?

The treatment is essentially no different than for de novo acute leukemia. With chemotherapy, some patients can be converted back into the chronic phase. The duration of partial or complete remission is usually short.

MYELOFIBROSIS WITH MYELOID METAPLASIA

What is myelofibrosis with myeloid metaplasia?

A neoplastic hematopoietic stem cell disorder characterized by bone marrow fibrosis, marked splenomegaly, extramedullary hematopoiesis, pancytopenia, and a leukoerythroblastic blood smear

How does myelofibrosis with myeloid metaplasia typically present?

With symptoms attributable to splenomegaly (left upper quadrant abdominal pain and early satiety) or anemia, fever, night sweats, anorexia, weight loss, and diarrhea

What are common physical findings in myelofibrosis with myeloid metaplasia?

Splenomegaly and hepatomegaly. Ectopic myeloid metaplasias are localized collections of immature myeloid precursors, which can appear in the lungs, brain, gastrointestinal tract, spinal cord, and urinary tract and thus can be associated with signs and symptoms attributable to the affected organ.

What are findings on peripheral smear in myelofibrosis with myeloid metaplasia?

Teardrop RBCs with nucleated RBCs, early myeloid forms, including blasts, and large platelets

What is the differential diagnosis for myelofibrosis with myeloid metaplasia?

Other myeloproliferative disorders, metastatic carcinoma, lymphoma, hairy cell leukemia, MDSs, disseminated tuberculosis, and histoplasmosis

What is the treatment for myelofibrosis with myeloid metaplasia?

Supportive care with transfusions, growth factors, and antibiotics as needed. Hydroxyurea, splenectomy, and radiation therapy can palliate symptomatic splenomegaly.

What is the median survival for patients with myelofibrosis with myeloid metaplasia?	5 years
What are the common causes of death attributable to agnogenic myeloid metaplasia?	Myocardial infarction or heart failure (30%), hemorrhage (25%), acute leukemia (20%), and infection (10%)

MYELODYSPLASTIC SYNDROMES

What are the MDSs?	A diverse group of clonal, neoplastic hematologic disorders affecting pluripotent hematopoietic stem cells and resulting in peripheral blood cytopenias
How does MDS commonly present?	Symptoms are attributable to cytopenias. Anemia results in weakness and congestive heart failure, for example; neutropenia results in infection; and thrombocytopenia results in bleeding.
What are some of the risk factors for development of MDS?	Prior cytotoxic chemotherapy, especially alkylating agents, and exposure to benzene and possibly other organic solvents
How is the diagnosis of MDS made?	Dysplastic features of hematopoietic precursors are found on examination of bone marrow. The presence of dysplastic granulocytes on peripheral smear with the exclusion of nutritional deficiencies is highly suggestive of an MDS and, in certain clinical circumstances, does not need to be confirmed by a bone marrow procedure.
What is the classification of MDS?	There are five categories: RA, RARS, RAEB, RAEB-T, and CMML
What is the median survival of patients with MDS?	RA, 3–4 years; RARS, 4–7 years; RAEB, 10–15 months; RAEB-T, 6 months; CMML, 12–18 months

What are the causes of death in patients with MDS?

Acute leukemia in 30% and cytopenias in 30%. The remaining die of comorbid conditions because MDS is a disease of the elderly.

What are the most important prognostic factors for MDS?

Percentage of blasts in the bone marrow, presence of particular clonal cytogenetic abnormalities, and presence of pancytopenia are the strongest predictors of a poor prognosis.

What clonal cytogenetic abnormality can portend a good prognosis for MDS?

The 5q- syndrome is classically seen in elderly women with transfusion-dependent anemia, thrombocytosis, and a normal leukocyte count. Some cytogenetic abnormalities, especially -5 and -7, are associated with a poor prognosis.

What is the treatment of MDS?

Supportive care with transfusions, growth factors, and antibiotics, as needed. In patients younger than 45 years old, allogeneic BMT may have a role. Young patients requiring frequent transfusions or with excess blasts should be considered for leukemia induction chemotherapy or allogeneic BMT. At the time of transformation to acute leukemia, induction chemotherapy may be considered, but complete response rates are considerably less than in de novo acute leukemia.

SPLEEN AND LYMPH NODES

What is the role of the spleen?

The spleen plays important roles in the function of both the humoral and cellular immune systems. It also acts as a filter for the blood (filtering microorganisms and defective or aged blood cells).

What fraction of the body's platelets are normally found in the spleen?

30%

With splenomegaly, this percent of platelets can increase to up to what percent?	90%
When is a palpable spleen pathologic?	In any adult. It may be a normal finding in early childhood.
What infections commonly cause splenomegaly?	Epstein-Barr virus–mediated mononucleosis, viral hepatitis, malaria, and rickettsial infections
What storage disorders are associated with splenomegaly?	Gaucher's disease, Niemann-Pick disease, and sea-blue histiocytosis
What is hypersplenism?	Increased splenic function associated with splenomegaly, including sequestration of blood cells, leading to neutropenia, thrombocytopenia, and anemia
What are the common causes of lymphadenopathy?	Reactive causes—viral infection (e.g., Epstein-Barr virus and HIV) and bacterial infection (e.g., syphilis) Direct infiltration by infectious agents— tuberculosis, histoplasmosis, staphylococcal infections Neoplastic causes—lymphomas, leukemias, metastatic cancer

TRANSFUSION MEDICINE

What is the hematocrit of a unit of packed RBCs?	Approximately 55% in a volume of approximately 300 ml
Transfusion of 1 unit of packed red cells should increase the patient's hematocrit by how much?	Approximately 3% per unit transfused
What two naturally occurring antibodies are responsible for severe hemolysis after transfusion of mismatched blood?	Anti-A and anti-B. Patients with type B blood have anti-A antibodies without ever having been exposed to transfused type A blood and those with type A blood have anti-B antibodies. Patients with type AB blood have no antibodies, whereas those with type O blood have both anti-A and anti-B antibodies.

What subclass of antibodies are anti-A and anti-B?

IgM. Reaction of these antibodies with mismatched RBCs is the cause of immediate-type transfusion reactions.

What are symptoms and signs of acute transfusion reaction?

Fever, nausea, and back or chest pains. Patients may also have wheezing, vomiting, hemoglobinuria, and hypotension.

What is the mortality rate for transfusion of ABO mismatched blood?

5%–10%

When after the transfusion do delayed transfusion reactions usually occur?

3–10 days

What is the cause of delayed transfusion reactions?

An amnestic increase in antibodies or the formation of new antibodies to antigens on the red cells transfused

What types of antibodies cause delayed transfusion reactions?

IgG. These antibodies are directed against blood group antigens other than the A and B antigens. These reactions are predominantly seen in individuals who were previously transfused.

What kind of hemolysis occurs in a delayed transfusion reaction?

Extravascular. The decrement in hematocrit is generally less than in an immediate transfusion reaction mediated by ABO incompatibility, which is intravascular.

What is a febrile nonhemolytic transfusion reaction?

A temperature increase of more than 1 degree Celsius when no other cause can be found. The reaction is often accompanied by shaking chills and is mediated by cytotoxic or agglutinating antibodies in the patient's plasma directed against antigens present on transfused donor leukocytes.

What is the importance of the Rh red cell antigen system?

All units of blood used for transfusion are characterized with regard to their Rh type. Rh-positive patients have an immunogenic D antigen on their red cells. After exposure to Rh-positive

RBCs, approximately 50% of Rh-negative individuals produce anti-D antibodies with resultant delayed transfusion reaction on subsequent transfusion of Rh-positive (D-antigen–positive) blood. In addition, hydrops fetalis (i.e., hemolytic disease of the newborn) results from maternal IgG anti-D antibodies crossing the placenta and causing hemolysis of the D-antigen–positive fetal RBCs in a mother who is Rh negative.

How is the Rh system–induced hemolytic disease of the newborn prevented?

Rh immune globulin is administered to Rh-negative mothers shortly after delivery to prevent immunization of the mother by exposure to Rh-positive fetal RBCs at the time of delivery. This prevents the development of hemolytic disease of the newborn with the subsequent pregnancy, because no maternal anti-D IgG is formed.

What viruses may be transmitted by administration of a routine unit of packed RBCs?

Hepatitis C (less commonly A and B), HIV, human T-cell lymphotrophic virus types I and II, and cytomegalovirus

HEMOSTASIS AND THROMBOSIS

What are the three phases of response to vascular damage that lead to cessation of bleeding?

1. Vasoconstriction
2. Primary hemostasis—platelet adhesion and aggregation
3. Secondary hemostasis—fibrin clot formation

What is the key trigger for blood coagulation?

Exposure of tissue factor to circulating blood

What is platelet-type bleeding?

Bleeding at mucocutaneous sites, multiple small bruises, and immediate bleeding after trauma or surgery

What is coagulation factor–type bleeding?

Soft-tissue bleeding with occasional large bruises or hematomas and delayed bleeding after trauma or surgery

What does the bleeding time measure?	Platelet number, platelet adhesion and aggregation, and connective tissue integrity; therefore the bleeding time is a test of platelet function, vWF function, and connective tissue integrity
What is the PT?	Prothrombin time
What factors are assessed by the PT?	Fibrinogen and factors II, V, VII, and X (extrinsic and common pathways)
What is the INR?	International normalized ratio. It is a method for standardizing the degree of anticoagulation using different laboratory systems for patients on oral anticoagulants.
What is the aPTT?	Activated partial thromboplastin time
What factors are assessed by the aPTT?	Fibrinogen, factors II, V, VIII, IX, X, XI, and XII, prekallikrein, and high–molecular-weight kininogen (intrinsic and common pathways)
What factors are measured by the PT and aPTT?	Fibrinogen and factors II, V, and X
What are the vitamin K–dependent coagulation factors?	Factors II, VII, IX, and X
What are the vitamin K–dependent anticoagulants?	Protein C and protein S
What enzyme is directly responsible for the conversion of fibrinogen to fibrin?	Thrombin

APPROACH TO BLEEDING DISORDERS

What are the four broad categories of bleeding disorders?	Platelet related, coagulation factor related, fibrinolysis, and connective tissue abnormalities
What disorders are associated with platelet-related bleeding?	Thrombocytopenia, platelet function defects, and vWD

What are the causes of coagulation factor–type bleeding?

Hemophilia A (factor VIII deficiency), hemophilia B (factor IX deficiency), hemophilia C (factor XI deficiency), and other rare deficiencies of factors II, V, VII, and X, and fibrinogen

What factor deficiency is associated with delayed bleeding and poor wound healing?

Factor XIII

How is bleeding associated with factor XIII deficiency treated?

Fresh-frozen plasma or cryoprecipitate

What abnormalities of connective tissue are associated with abnormal bleeding?

Amyloidosis, Osler-Weber-Rendu disease, ataxia telangiectasia, scurvy, Ehlers-Danlos syndrome, and Cushing's syndrome

What history and physical examination findings distinguish platelet-related bleeding from coagulation factor deficiency bleeding?

Platelet-related bleeding is usually mucocutaneous and immediate in relation to trauma or surgery. Coagulation factor deficiency bleeding is associated with soft tissue and joint bleeding and is delayed in relation to trauma or surgery.

What historical factors point to a bleeding diathesis?

Frequent and severe epistaxis requiring nasal packing or transfusion, hemarthroses, menorrhagia, excessive bleeding after tooth extraction, surgical procedures, circumcision, or childbirth, easy bruisability, and excessive gingival bleeding

What suggests the presence of a true bleeding disorder in patients with easy bruisability?

Spontaneous bruising (i.e., bruising that is not associated with trauma), location of bruising on the trunk or in other areas not typically prone to daily trauma, large size of bruises, and long period of time for bruising to resolve

What four screening tests are most useful in the initial evaluation of patients with suspected bleeding disorders?

PT, aPTT, CBC with platelet count, and bleeding time

What bleeding disorders may be associated with an isolated prolonged PT?

Factor VII deficiency, vitamin K deficiency, Coumadin use, and liver dysfunction. Deficiencies of factor II, V, X, and fibrinogen are usually associated with prolongation of both the PT and APTT.

What bleeding disorders may be associated with an isolated prolongation of the aPTT?

Deficiencies of factors VIII, IX, and XI, either acquired or inherited, and vWD

What bleeding disorders may be associated with a prolongation of the PT and aPTT?

Simultaneous deficiency of multiple factors, as seen with liver disease and DIC. Rarer causes include isolated deficiencies of or acquired inhibitors of factors II, V, and X, or fibrinogen.

What bleeding disorders are associated with thrombocytopenia?

Idiopathic thrombocytopenic purpura, TTP, leukemia, and many others discussed under Thrombocytopenia

What bleeding disorders prolong the bleeding time?

vWD, platelet function defects (e.g., Bernard-Soulier syndrome), paraproteinemia, myeloproliferative disorders, DIC, uremia, and afibrinogenemia

Can patients have a significant bleeding diathesis with a normal bleeding time, normal platelet count, and normal PT and aPTT?

Yes. The most common bleeding disorder, vWD, may present in this fashion. Other causes include factor XIII deficiency, hyperfibrinolysis, mild factor deficiencies, and disorders of connective tissue.

What is hemophilia A?

An X-linked inherited deficiency of factor VIII associated with coagulation factor–type bleeding

What is hemophilia B?

An X-linked inherited deficiency of factor IX associated with coagulation factor–type bleeding

What is hemophilia C?

An autosomal inherited deficiency of factor XI associated with variably penetrant coagulation factor–type bleeding

How is severe bleeding into a joint of a hemophilia A patient stopped?	Administration of factor VIII concentrate (intermediate purity, monoclonal, or recombinant). Rarely, cryoprecipitate is appropriate. Other important measures include rest, application of ice, and elevation.
Before recombinant factor VIII concentrate and more effective viral inactivation methods became available, what viral diseases did many patients with severe hemophilia A routinely acquire after treatment with factor VIII concentrates?	HIV, hepatitis C, and hepatitis B
What is the most common inherited bleeding disorder?	vWD
What is the most common genetic reason for an elevated PTT?	Factor XII deficiency
What is the treatment for patients with factor XII deficiency?	None. Factor XII deficiency does not cause bleeding.
What is the treatment for acute bleeding in a patient with factor XI deficiency?	Fresh-frozen plasma
What is the treatment for severe joint bleeding in a patient with hemophilia B?	Factor IX concentrate
What are the common causes of bleeding in patients with cirrhosis?	Thrombocytopenia, platelet dysfunction, coagulation factor deficiencies, DIC, primary fibrinolysis, and vitamin K deficiency

von Willebrand's Disease

What is vWD?	An inherited disorder with deficient or defective vWF associated with a bleeding tendency

What is the function of vWF?

vWF mediates adhesion of platelets to the vessel wall basement membrane after vascular injury.

Where is vWF synthesized?

Endothelial cells and megakaryocytes

What laboratory tests are used in testing for vWD?

Ristocetin cofactor activity, vWF antigen, factor VIII activity levels, bleeding time, multimer testing, and platelet function studies

What does the ristocetin cofactor activity measure?

It is an approximation of vWF function.

Can a patient with mild vWD have a normal amount and function of vWF?

Yes. vWF behaves as an acute phase reactant; thus the levels may be increased in times of stress, pregnancy, and with estrogen replacement.

What are the subtypes of vWD?

Type 1—quantitative decrease in levels of functionally normal vWF. This subtype is the most common, comprising 70%–80% of cases.

Type 2—qualitative abnormalities of vWF. This subtype comprises 15%–30% of vWD cases. There are several subtypes of type 2, of which 2A and 2B are the most common. It is important to distinguish type 2B from all other types of vWD because administration of DDAVP can cause thrombocytopenia in patients with this subtype.

Type 3—absence of vWF. This is a rare form and may be associated with profound bleeding problems.

Platelet type—the platelet receptor for vWF (glycoprotein Ib) has increased affinity for vWF, resulting in increased clearance of plasma vWF.

How is vWD inherited?

Usually autosomal dominant, but patients with type 3 may be autosomal recessive or doubly heterozygous. In contrast, hemophilia A and B are X-linked recessive.

What is the treatment of bleeding in patients with vWD?	It is important to establish the subtype of vWD, because DDAVP is the treatment of choice for type 1 patients, but DDAVP can be deleterious if given to type 2B or platelet-type patients. Some patients with type 2 and all with type 3 do not respond to DDAVP. Virally inactivated intermediate purity factor VIII concentrates should then be used. For major operations or life-threatening hemorrhage, these concentrates should be given to all subtypes.
When should cryoprecipitate be used to treat vWD?	In an emergency when no virally inactivated intermediate purity factor VIII product is available.
What are the adverse effects of DDAVP?	DDAVP may be contraindicated in certain subtypes of vWD. In addition, DDAVP can cause hyponatremia, resulting in seizures. Common adverse effects include facial flushing, minor alterations in blood pressure, nausea, and headache.
What is the most common cause of aPTT prolongation in severe vWD?	Factor VIII deficiency. Factor VIII circulates attached to vWF. In the absence of vWF, the half-life of factor VIII is shortened.
What are the most common bleeding problems in patients with vWD?	Epistaxis, easy bruising, and menorrhagia

Platelet Function Disorders

What is Glanzmann's thrombasthenia?	An autosomal recessive inherited defect in the platelet glycoprotein IIb/IIIa receptor, the receptor for fibrinogen on platelets, which is essential for platelet aggregation. Patients have long bleeding times and platelet-type bleeding.
What is Bernard-Soulier syndrome?	An autosomal recessive inherited defect in platelet glycoprotein Ib receptor, the receptor for vWF, which is essential for platelet adhesion. Patients have

prolonged bleeding times and platelet-type bleeding.

What is the gray platelet syndrome?

An inherited deficiency of platelet alpha granules, which is associated with a prolonged bleeding time and mild platelet-type bleeding. Platelets appear gray (pale) on routine peripheral smear examination.

Vascular Bleeding Disorders

What is Osler-Weber-Rendu syndrome?

Hereditary hemorrhagic telangiectasia. It is an autosomal dominant disorder of the microvasculature associated with mucocutaneous telangiectasias, which causes mucosal surfaces to bleed.

How does Osler-Weber-Rendu syndrome present?

Patients frequently have epistaxis and gastrointestinal bleeding; often, arteriovenous malformations develop in the lung, gastrointestinal tract, and central nervous system.

What is Kasabach-Merritt syndrome?

A syndrome of large congenital hemangiomas (also called cavernous hemangiomas) associated with thrombocytopenia and, often, DIC.

THROMBOTIC DISORDERS

What is a hypercoagulable state?

The maintenance of blood in a fluid state is a fine balance between anticoagulant forces and prothrombotic forces. A hypercoagulable state is when the balance is shifted toward a prothrombotic state.

Under what circumstances should a hypercoagulable state be suspected?

Thrombosis without a precipitating risk factor, thrombosis at a young age, recurrent thromboses, thrombosis in an unusual location (e.g., upper extremity, portal vein, mesenteric vein, cerebral vein), family history of thrombosis, and resistance to anticoagulation with heparin or warfarin

What conditions predispose a patient to venous thrombosis?

Sedentary lifestyle, postoperative state, obesity, congestive heart failure, nephrotic syndrome, protein-losing enteropathy, oral contraceptive use, and pregnancy

What conditions predispose a patient to arterial embolism?

Left-sided valvular heart disease, atherosclerosis, and atrial fibrillation

What are the known inherited hypercoagulable states?

Activated protein C resistance (factor V Leiden mutation), protein C deficiency, protein S deficiency, AT III deficiency, dysfibrinogenemia, and hyperhomocysteinemia. There are several others, but they are rare. More than 50% of patients who clinically appear to have an inherited hypercoagulable state currently have no identifiable abnormality.

What is the most common inherited disorder associated with an increased risk of venous thrombosis?

Activated protein C resistance (factor V Leiden mutation)

What is the relationship between activated protein C resistance and factor V Leiden mutation?

A specific mutation in the factor V gene (factor V Leiden) renders the factor V protein resistant to degradation by activated protein C.

What acquired conditions are associated with a hypercoagulable state?

Malignancy, myeloproliferative disorders, paroxysmal nocturnal hemoglobinuria, connective tissue diseases (e.g., SLE, Behçet's syndrome, and thromboangiitis obliterans), antiphospholipid antibody syndrome, hyperviscosity states (e.g., paraproteinemia and polycythemia vera), TTP, and DIC

What is the specific name of the hypercoagulable state associated with malignancy?

Trousseau's syndrome (migratory thrombophlebitis)

How is protein C activated?

Thrombin binds to endothelial cell thrombomodulin, which, when bound, converts protein C to activated protein C.

What does activated protein C do?

Degrades the cofactors of coagulation, factors Va and VIIIa

What is activated protein C resistance?

An inherited disorder associated with an increased risk of thrombosis. Patient plasma demonstrates less prolongation of the aPTT (compared with that of normal subjects) after the addition of activated protein C.

What is the primary inhibitor of thrombin?

AT III

What enzyme is responsible for the degradation of fibrin?

Plasmin, which is activated from plasminogen by tissue-type plasminogen activator or urokinase

Antiphospholipid Antibody Syndrome

What is the antiphospholipid antibody syndrome?

A disorder in which the patient has autoantibodies to a complex of phospholipids and protein. It is associated with an increased risk of recurrent spontaneous abortions and arterial and venous thromboses.

What are the two categories of autoantibodies assessed when this disorder is suspected?

Lupus anticoagulant and anticardiolipin antibodies

What is a lupus anticoagulant?

An autoantibody against phospholipid and protein. It interferes with and prolongs phospholipid-dependent clotting tests (e.g., aPTT).

What are anticardiolipin antibodies?

Antibodies measured in serum with specificity toward a specific phospholipid, cardiolipin

In what conditions are anticardiolipin antibodies and lupus anticoagulants found?	Connective tissue disorders, malignancies, drug use, and acute infections
Do all patients with anticardiolipin antibodies or lupus anticoagulants have an increased risk of thrombosis?	No. Many of these autoantibodies are transient and appear to carry little or no risk of thrombosis. Many more patients do not have clots than do have clots.
When are antiphospholipid antibodies clinically meaningful?	In the setting of an acute thrombosis, they are suggestive of a hypercoagulable state; if the antiphospholipid antibody persists, then long-term anticoagulation should be considered.

Disseminated Intravascular Coagulation

What is DIC?	DIC is a syndrome that develops in the presence of a variety of clinical conditions in which diffuse activation of coagulation overwhelms the body's normal anticoagulant defense systems, leading to excessive fibrin formation and platelet activation. This leads to diffuse microvascular clot formation with organ damage and dysfunction. Secondarily, the fibrinolytic system becomes activated, producing consumption of coagulation factors and lysis of thrombi, leading to clinical hemorrhage.
What are the common causes of DIC?	Sepsis, head trauma, cancer, abruptio placentae, eclampsia, snake bites, viral infections, rickettsial infections, and collagen vascular diseases
How is the diagnosis of DIC made?	In a patient with an appropriate potential underlying illness or predisposing condition, prolongation of the PT, elevation of the D-dimer titer with thrombocytopenia, and hypofibrinogenemia support the diagnosis of DIC. Serial measurements of the parameters listed are usually helpful.

What are the predominant adverse consequences of DIC?

Bleeding and thrombosis. In acute DIC, microvascular thrombosis appears first, resulting in organ dysfunction; later, consumption and degradation of clotting factors combined with thrombocytopenia, platelet dysfunction, and hyperfibrinolysis lead to hemorrhage.

What is the treatment of DIC?

Treatment of the underlying disease and supportive measures. Interruption of the procoagulant cascade with concentrates of the endogenous anticoagulants, AT III, or protein C or treatment with heparin remains controversial. For severe hemorrhage, correction of the prolonged PT, thrombocytopenia, and hypofibrinogenemia with plasma, platelets, and cryoprecipitate may be necessary.

ANTICOAGULATION

What are the two most commonly used anticoagulants in the United States?

Heparin and warfarin (Coumadin).

What does heparin do?

Heparin is a cofactor for AT III, the primary inhibitor of factor IIa (thrombin), Xa, IXa, and XIa. It downregulates coagulation.

How is low–molecular-weight heparin different from standard heparin?

Smaller fragments of heparin interact with AT III to have greater inhibition of factor Xa and lesser inhibition of thrombin.

How is intravenous heparin therapy currently monitored?

By aPTT

How is warfarin therapy monitored?

By PT with conversion to the INR

How is the effect of heparin reversed in a bleeding patient?

Administration of protamine

How is the effect of warfarin reversed in a bleeding patient?

Administration of vitamin K. For severe bleeding, plasma or a concentrate of vitamin K–dependent clotting factors must be given.

7

Oncology

ABBREVIATIONS

5-FU	5-Fluorouracil
ACS	American Cancer Society
AFP	Alpha-fetoprotein
AIDS	Acquired immune deficiency syndrome
ALL	Acute lymphocytic leukemia
AML	Acute myeloid leukemia
β-HCG	β-Human chorionic gonadotropin
CBC	Complete blood count
CLL	Chronic lymphocytic leukemia
CNS	Central nervous system
CT	Computed tomography
DCIS	Ductal carcinoma in situ
DIC	Disseminated intravascular coagulation
EBV	Epstein-Barr virus
EGGCT	Extragonadal germ cell tumor
ERCP	Endoscopic retrograde cholangiopancreatography
GCT	Germ cell tumor
GRFoma	Gastrin-releasing factor–producing tumor

H&P	History and physical examination
HPV	Human papilloma virus
HTLV I	Human T-cell lymphotrophic virus type 1
IMA	Inferior mesenteric artery
ITP	Idiopathic thrombocytopenic purpura
LCIS	Lobular carcinoma in situ
LGL	Large granular lymphocyte
MGUS	Monoclonal gammopathy of undetermined significance
MRI	Magnetic resonance imaging
NHL	Non-Hodgkin's lymphoma
NK	Natural killer
NSCLC	Non–small cell lung cancer
NSGCT	Nonseminomatous germ cell tumor
PDA	Poorly differentiated adenocarcinoma
PDC	Poorly differentiated carcinoma
PP	Pancreatic polypeptide
PPoma	Pancreatic polypeptide–producing tumor
PSA	Prostate specific antigen
PSC	Primary sclerosing cholangitis
PT	Prothrombin time
PTC	Percutaneous transhepatic cholangiogram
PTT	Partial thromboplastin time

RPLN	Retroperitoneal lymph node
RPLND	Retroperitoneal lymph node dissection
RTIO	Radical transinguinal orchiectomy
SCLC	Small cell lung cancer
SMA	Superior mesenteric artery
SVC	Superior vena cava
TNM	Tumor, node, metastasis
VIPoma	Vasoactive intestinal polypeptide–producing tumor
WBC	White blood cell
WDLL	Well-differentiated lymphocytic lymphoma

CANCER SCREENING

What is cancer screening used for?

Detecting cancer at an earlier stage

What are the advantages of cancer screening?

The major advantage of cancer screening is detecting cancers at an earlier "curable" stage. Additional advantages include the following:
1. Less aggressive therapy may be needed for earlier cancers.
2. It is less expensive to treat earlier malignancies.
3. The patient is reassured if the test is negative.

What are the disadvantages of cancer screening?

The major disadvantage is increased costs. Additional disadvantages include the following:
1. The risk of morbidity and potential mortality associated with screening procedures
2. The need for unnecessary evaluation of false-positive tests
3. False-negative results

What factors contribute to an effective screening test?

1. The disease has a detectable, curable stage.
2. The malignancy is a major health problem.
3. The screening test is low cost and low risk.
4. The test is effective in detecting the tumor.
5. The cancer is treatable.

For which tumors do effective screening tests exist?

Cancers of the cervix, breast, prostate, colon, and rectum

Is there a consensus among the U.S. health care policy organizations regarding the recommended tests and testing intervals for those cancers with effective screening tests?

No. There is considerable variability in screening guidelines, but those of the ACS are the most widely quoted and followed.

Do the same recommendations pertain to all patients?

No. Individuals with either a personal or family history that puts them at increased risk for cancer are offered more aggressive screening.

According to the ACS, who, at what age, and how often should self-examination begin for the following:

Skin

Women and men age 20 years and older on a monthly basis

Testicles

Men aged 20 years and older on a monthly basis

Breasts

Women aged 20 years and older on a monthly basis

According to the ACS, who, at what age, and how often should the following examinations be given by a clinician?

Breast examination

Women aged 20 to 40 years every 3 years, then every year thereafter

| Digital rectal examination | Men and women aged 40 years and older on a yearly basis |

According to the ACS, who, at what age, and how often should the following tests be obtained?

PSA	Men aged 50 years and older on a yearly basis
Stool Hemoccult	Men and women aged 50 years and older on a yearly basis
Papanicolaou smear and pelvic examination	Women aged 18 years and older every year for 3 years, then less often
Sigmoidoscopy	Men and women aged 50 years and older every 3–5 years
Mammogram	Women aged 40 years and older every 1–2 years

| According to the ACS, when and how often should general cancer checkups be obtained? | At age 20 or older, then every 3 years |

ONCOLOGIC EMERGENCIES

SPINAL CORD COMPRESSION

| How common is spinal cord compression? | Approximately 18,000 cases per year in the United States |

| How many patients are ambulatory when they are first seen with spinal cord compression? | As many as 80% of patients are no longer ambulatory at the time of presentation. Patients with a history of cancer must be advised that the development of back pain is a potentially threatening symptom that should be promptly evaluated by their physician. |

| What are symptoms of spinal cord compression? | More than 90% of patients complain of back pain. Symptoms of neurologic compromise include numbness, paresthesias, muscular weakness, and urinary and fecal incontinence. |

What is the character of spinal cord compression pain?

Pain is localized to the spine and exacerbated by movement, recumbency, cough, sneezing, or strain. The pain can be radicular in nature, that is, sharp and electric shock–like, radiating in the distribution of a spinal nerve root.

What is the duration of pain in most patients with spinal cord compression?

Most patients have pain for weeks before the onset of neurologic symptoms; however, neurologic compromise usually is more rapid, typically occurring in hours to days.

What are the physical findings in patients with spinal cord compression?

Tenderness to percussion at the involved spine. Neck flexion, or straight leg raise precipitates pain at the level of the problem. Neurologic findings are decreased sensation and motor strength, positive Babinski's sign, and hyperreflexia.

What are the most common malignancies involved in spinal cord compression?

Lung, breast, prostate, lymphoma, and multiple myeloma. Other more unusual cancer causes are colorectal, melanoma, sarcoma, and renal cell carcinoma.

In a cancer patient with back pain and no neurologic symptoms, what is the first study that should be done?

Plain radiographs of the affected area. If the plain films show evidence of metastatic cancer, then an MRI should be done on an outpatient basis. If the plain films are negative, then a bone scan should be done.

Can a patient have spinal cord compression with normal plain radiographs?

Yes; therefore, if neurologic symptoms are present, then an MRI of the spine to rule out cord compression should be done.

What is the radiographic study of choice to rule out spinal cord compression?

A CT myelogram is probably the most specific and sensitive study. However, an MRI has virtually supplanted the myelogram as the initial study because it is nearly as accurate, it is noninvasive, and it is quicker.

What is the prognosis for regaining lost neurologic function?

Poor. Few patients with paraplegia regain neurologic function. Most patients (80%) who are ambulatory at the time of treatment are ambulatory after treatment. As many as one third of patients with mild to moderate neurologic dysfunction have improvement of symptoms with treatment.

How does metastatic cancer cause loss of neurologic function in the spinal cord?

The tumor restricts the vascular supply to the spinal cord with resultant spinal cord infarction.

What is the treatment of acute spinal cord compression?

High-dose dexamethasone followed by radiation therapy and/or surgery. Occasionally, chemotherapy can be used alone or in combination with radiotherapy.

Who should receive radiotherapy for the treatment of spinal cord compression?

Patients with known radiation-sensitive tumor and no spinal instability or patients with spinal involvement without spinal instability or neurologic deficit

Who should receive surgery followed by radiation in treatment of spinal cord compression?

Patients with a pathologic fracture with spinal instability or compression of the spinal cord by bone, patients with radiation-resistant tumors with neurologic deficits, and patients with an unknown tissue diagnosis.

Who should receive surgery alone in treatment of spinal cord compression?

Patients whose tumors relapse or fail to respond to radiation

Who should receive chemotherapy alone in treatment of spinal cord compression?

Pediatric patients with responsive tumors, adults with responsive tumors (as adjuvant therapy), and patients whose tumors relapse at a site of radiation and surgery

INCREASED INTRACRANIAL PRESSURE

What are the malignant causes of increased intracranial pressure?

Carcinomatous meningitis and intracranial metastases

What are symptoms and signs of intracranial metastatic disease?	Headache, altered mental status, seizures, visual loss, focal neurologic deficits, papilledema, and coma
How are intracranial metastases diagnosed?	CT scan or MRI of the head
What is the treatment for acutely symptomatic intracranial metastases?	Treatment options include: High-dose steroids Anticonvulsants Mannitol Hyperventilation (if the patient is intubated) Radiation therapy (if the diagnosis is known or if there are multiple metastases)
When is surgery indicated in cases of increased intracranial pressure presumed to be related to cancer?	1. To make a diagnosis 2. If symptoms are refractory or progressive after medical or radiation therapy 3. If the patient has had good performance status with a single metastasis and a long disease-free interval
What are the symptoms of carcinomatous meningitis?	Headache, altered mental status, diplopia, and blurred vision
How is the diagnosis of carcinomatous meningitis made?	Lumbar puncture for cytology. The glucose level is usually less than 45 mg/dl, the protein level is generally increased, and pleocytosis is often present. Three lumbar punctures are usually performed to rule out carcinomatous meningitis.
What are the physical signs of carcinomatous meningitis?	Cranial nerve palsies, other focal neurologic defects, and papilledema
What is the treatment for carcinomatous meningitis?	Whole brain radiation therapy. Intrathecal chemotherapy is occasionally successful for a short time.

SUPERIOR VENA CAVA SYNDROME

What is SVC syndrome?	The clinical expression of the obstruction of blood flow through the SVC
What are common signs of SVC syndrome?	Superficial thoracic vein collaterals, neck vein distention, facial edema, and tachypnea are the most common signs of SVC syndrome. Occasionally, facial plethora, cyanosis, upper extremity edema, Horner's syndrome, and vocal cord paralysis are also present.
What are the chest radiographic findings in the SVC syndrome?	A right mediastinal mass
What are the causes of SVC syndrome?	Malignant causes (80%–90% of cases)— most commonly, lung cancer, lymphoma, thymoma, GCTs, and breast cancer Nonmalignant causes (10%–20% of cases)—histoplasmosis with mediastinal fibrosis, syphilis, tuberculosis, and thrombosis, usually as a result of an indwelling central venous catheter
Is SVC syndrome usually acutely life threatening?	Not usually. In the past, patients underwent emergent radiation therapy.
What is the treatment for SVC syndrome?	First, a biopsy sample is obtained for a definitive diagnosis because there are some nonmalignant causes. In malignant cases, both chemotherapy and radiation may be used depending on the type of cancer.

HYPERCALCEMIA (SEE ALSO CHAPTER 4)

What is the treatment for hypercalcemia?	Aggressive hydration is the mainstay. Diuretics following aggressive intravenous hydration can enhance calciuresis. In myeloma, lymphoma, leukemia, and occasionally breast cancer, steroids can be helpful. Bisphosphonates are effective and are commonly used

after rehydration. Calcitonin has a rapid onset of action, but it is a weak hypocalcemic agent and its effect is short lived. Plicamycin is used in refractory cases.

HYPERURICEMIA

What problems are associated with hyperuricemia?	Renal insufficiency (urine becomes supersaturated with urate and crystals of uric acid) and uric acid arthropathy
What malignancies are commonly associated with hyperuricemia?	AML, high-grade lymphoma, myeloproliferative disorder, and high WBC count with chronic leukemia
What is the management of hyperuricemia?	Prophylactic measures need to be undertaken before cytotoxic chemotherapy. Medications that lead to an elevated serum uric acid or that acidify urine are discontinued. Allopurinol is started, intravenous hydration is begun to maintain good urine output, and urine is alkalinized with sodium bicarbonate to a pH of 7.0.

TUMOR LYSIS SYNDROME AND NEUTROPENIC FEVER

Which malignancies are the most common cause of the tumor lysis syndrome?	Large bulky tumors that are responsive to chemotherapy (e.g., ALL, AML, high-grade lymphomas such as Burkitt's lymphoma)
What are the electrolyte and metabolic abnormalities that occur with tumor lysis syndrome?	Hyperuricemia, hypocalcemia, hyperkalemia, hyperphosphatemia, and metabolic acidosis
What causes renal failure in patients with tumor lysis syndrome?	Precipitation of urate crystals in the tubules
How is tumor lysis syndrome treated?	Hydration and alkalinization of the urine (the urinary pH is maintained at 7.0 or higher)

What prophylactic therapy should be used in patients with a large tumor burden who are at risk for this syndrome?

Allopurinol

At what WBC count is the patient at significant risk for infection?

An absolute neutrophil count that is below 1000/mm^3 places the patient at risk for infection. Patients with absolute neutrophil counts below 500/mm^3 are at the greatest risk.

Which patients with neutropenia are at greatest risk for infection?

Those with prolonged neutropenia and those with immunodeficiencies as a result of their primary disease or therapy (e.g., leukemias and lymphomas)

What is the management of patients with significant neutropenia, fever, and no obvious source of infection?

Panculture and broad-spectrum antibiotics (e.g., a penicillinase-resistant β lactam or third-generation cephalosporin + an aminoglycoside). The choice of antibiotic depends on the flora and sensitivities at the hospital. If fevers continue, then agents that are effective against fungi and gram-positive organisms should be considered (especially in patients with indwelling lines).

What other treatment options are considered for patients with neutropenic fever?

G-CSF

ACUTE LEUKEMIA

What is the definition of acute leukemia?

A neoplastic disorder characterized by the proliferation and accumulation in blood and bone marrow of immature hematopoietic precursors

What is the prognosis if acute leukemia is left untreated?

Death in weeks to months

What are common presenting symptoms of acute leukemia?

Fatigue, dyspnea, malaise, bleeding (e.g., epistaxis, easy bruising, and bleeding from the gums or tooth extraction), infection, fever, and headache

What are common physical findings in patients with acute leukemia?

Pallor, petechiae, ecchymoses, splenomegaly, lymphadenopathy, gingival hyperplasia, cranial nerve palsies, papilledema, subcutaneous masses (i.e., chloromas), and skin changes (i.e., leukemia cutis, or violaceous, nontender plaques or nodules)

What are urgent clinical findings in acute leukemia?

Neurologic findings including altered mental status, seizures, headache, and cranial nerve palsies or other focal neurologic signs, suggesting leukemic meningitis, leukostasis, or bacterial meningitis
Pulmonary edema secondary to leukostasis
Tumor lysis
Hemorrhage (CNS, visceral, or gastrointestinal)
Infection or fever with or without neutropenia

What are the treatment options for leukemic meningitis or leukostasis with neurologic findings?

Leukopheresis, emergent cranial irradiation, and hydroxyurea

How do you manage tumor lysis in acute leukemia?

Hydration, alkalinization of the urine, and allopurinol

How do you manage fever with or without neutropenia in acute leukemia?

Panculture and broad-spectrum antibiotics

How do you manage hemorrhage in acute leukemia?

Red cell and platelet transfusion to maintain platelet count > 20,000/mm^3 and hematocrit > 25–30 mg/dl. Check for evidence of DIC with PT, PTT, fibrinogen, and D-dimer.

How is the diagnosis of leukemia made?	Presence of leukemic blasts on peripheral smear, bone marrow aspirate, and biopsy. Auer rods suggest AML. Histochemical stains, flow cytometry, and cytogenetics are useful in subtyping leukemias and determining treatment options.
What congenital disorders are associated with an increased incidence of leukemia?	Down syndrome, Bloom's syndrome, Fanconi's anemia, and ataxia telangiectasia
What acquired disorders are associated with an increased incidence of leukemia?	Myeloproliferative diseases, myelodysplastic syndromes, and aplastic anemia
What environmental exposures are associated with an increased incidence of leukemia?	Exposure to alkylating agents, radiation, cigarette smoke, benzene, and other organic solvents
What are the subtypes of acute leukemia?	Lymphoid (ALL) and myeloid (AML)

ACUTE LYMPHOID LEUKEMIA

How many cases of ALL occur in adults each year in the United States?	Approximately 1000. ALL comprises < 20% of adult acute leukemia. In children, ALL accounts for two thirds of acute leukemia.
What are the subtypes of ALL?	L1—Blasts are small with scanty cytoplasm and inconspicuous nucleoli. This subtype accounts for 85% of childhood ALL. L2—Blasts are larger with abundant cytoplasm and prominent nucleoli. The majority of adult ALL patients have this type. L3—Burkitt's leukemia or lymphoma. Blasts are large with deeply basophilic cytoplasm and prominent cytoplasmic vacuoles. This type comprises < 5% of ALL.

What other way can ALL be subtyped?

With flow cytometry and immunohistochemical stains, ALL can be subtyped into four additional categories with prognostic significance: T-cell, B-cell, pre B-cell, and pro B-cell.

What is the long-term disease-free survival rate in adults?

20%–35% is stated in the literature, but, with all patients considered, the rate is probably significantly less. In contrast, two thirds of children are long-term disease-free survivors at 5 years.

What is the peak age of incidence for ALL in adults?

Older than age 65 years

What physical findings are more common in ALL than AML?

Lymphadenopathy occurs in more than half of patients with ALL and is relatively uncommon in AML. Hepatosplenomegaly occurs in more than two thirds of patients with ALL. Hepatomegaly is uncommon in AML although splenomegaly occurs in approximately half of patients with AML.

What are sanctuary sites in ALL?

Common sites of solitary relapse include the CNS and testes. To protect the CNS, all patients with ALL undergo prophylactic cranial irradiation or intrathecal chemotherapy along with induction chemotherapy.

What is Burkitt's leukemia or lymphoma?

Burkitt's leukemia or lymphoma cells are B cells because they usually express surface immunoglobulin. A specific translocation t(8;14) is universally seen in this subtype.

What molecular genetic event occurs with the translocation seen in Burkitt's leukemia or lymphoma?

The heavy chain promoter region is juxtaposed next to the c-*myc* oncogene. This leads to the aberrant expression of the c-*myc* protein, which is intricately involved in cellular proliferation. Occasionally, the promoters of the lambda light chain or kappa light chain are juxtaposed to the c-*myc* gene and lead to the same phenotype.

**What is the standard
induction regimen for
ALL?**

Vincristine, prednisone, L-asparaginase,
and an anthracycline. The complete
remission rate in adults is 60%–80%.

**What are the good and
bad prognostic factors for
ALL?**

Good prognostic factors include L1
morphology, pro–B-cell phenotype,
hyperdiploidy, and complete response
to induction chemotherapy.

Bad prognostic factors include B-cell
phenotype, L3 morphology, presence
of the Philadelphia chromosome
[t(9;22)], hypoploidy, pseudodiploidy,
lymphadenopathy,
hepatosplenomegaly, WBC > 50,000,
t(4;11), demonstration of myeloid
markers by flow cytometry, age older
than 10 years, African-American
descent, association with HTLV I, and
non–T-cell phenotype.

**How do you differentiate
ALL from AML?**

Flow cytometry is the gold standard.
Periodic acid–Schiff histochemical stain
is positive in ALL. Myeloperoxidase
histochemical stain is positive in myeloid
leukemias.

ACUTE MYELOID LEUKEMIA

**What is the most common
type of acute leukemia in
adults?**

Myeloid leukemia comprises > 80% of
all cases of acute leukemia in adults.

**What is the age
distribution for AML?**

Most patients are older than age 65
years.

**What are the subtypes of
AML?**

M1—myeloblastic without differentiation
(15%–20% of cases)
M2—myeloblastic with differentiation
(25%–30% of cases)
M3—promyelocytic (10%–15% of cases)
M4—myelomonocytic (25%–30% of
cases)
M5—monocytic (10%–15% of cases)
M6—erythroleukemia [Di Guglielmo's
disease (5% of cases)]
M7—megakaryocytic (5% of cases)

Which subtype of AML is commonly associated with DIC?

Promyelocytic (M3)

Promyelocytic leukemia is associated with what chromosomal translocation?

A translocation between chromosomes 15 and 17, commonly abbreviated as t(15;17)

What molecular genetic event occurs in this translocation, which is thought to play a role in the pathogenesis of promyelocytic leukemia?

The promyelocytic leukemia gene is juxtaposed next to the retinoic acid receptor alpha gene, yielding a fusion protein.

What vitamin induces a complete remission in 90% of patients with promyelocytic leukemia?

Transretinoic acid

What percent of AML patients achieve complete remission with induction chemotherapy?

50%–70%

What is the standard induction regimen for AML patients?

Cytarabine (100 mg/m^2) by continuous infusion over 24 hours for 7 days and daunorubicin (45 mg/m^2) intravenously for 3 days (commonly abbreviated as 7 + 3)

How many patients are cured if they go into complete remission?

None. They all need some form of consolidation chemotherapy.

What is the 5-year survival rate in patients who undergo treatment for AML?

10%–35%. For all patients with AML, 5%–10% survive more than 5 years. For young patients who are candidates for intensive chemotherapy and bone marrow transplant, then 20%–35% is the more accurate number.

What is consolidation chemotherapy?

Consolidation chemotherapy is usually referred to as equipotent chemotherapy to induction and is given for 1–4 cycles after attainment of a complete remission.

How long is a patient usually hospitalized after initiation of induction chemotherapy?	4–6 weeks. Patients commonly need several courses of intravenous antibiotics as well as multiple red blood cell and platelet transfusions.
What are good prognostic factors for AML?	De novo leukemia (i.e., leukemia that is not preceded by a myelodysplastic syndrome), young age, and presence of specific cytogenetic abnormalities, including t(15;17), t(8;21), and Inv 16
What are poor prognostic factors for AML?	Leukemia evolving out of a prior myelodysplastic syndrome or associated with prior alkylating chemotherapy, advanced age, high peripheral WBC count, and the presence of the following cytogenetic abnormalities: -5, 5q-, -7, +8

LYMPHOPROLIFERATIVE DISORDERS

What is a lymphoproliferative disorder?	A clonal neoplastic proliferation of lymphocytes
What are the lymphoproliferative disorders?	CLL, hairy cell leukemia, LGL leukemia, lymphoma (e.g., Hodgkin's disease, and NHL), and plasma cell dyscrasias (e.g., multiple myeloma and Waldenström's macroglobulinemia)

CHRONIC LYMPHOCYTIC LEUKEMIA

What is the most common form of leukemia in western civilization?	CLL comprises 30% of all cases of leukemia, with an annual incidence of 2 in 100,000 persons
What is CLL?	A neoplastic proliferation with accumulation of immune-incompetent lymphocytes within the bone marrow, peripheral blood, and lymphoid organs
What are the morphologic characteristics of CLL?	Small, mature lymphocytes with clumped chromatin and scant cytoplasm
What is the median age of onset of CLL?	65 years

What are the symptoms of CLL?

As many as 70% of persons with CLL are asymptomatic at diagnosis. Generalized lymphadenopathy, fever, night sweats, weight loss, easy fatigability, weakness, and increased bleeding are common complaints. Frequent infections and exaggerated responses to insect bites are occasionally noted.

Patients with CLL are susceptible to what types of infections?

Both bacterial and viral infections secondary to hypogammaglobulinemia and defects in cell-mediated immunity

Do patients with CLL have an increased incidence of autoimmune diseases?

Yes. Autoimmune hemolytic anemia occurs in 10%–25% of cases. ITP and pure red cell aplasia are more common in CLL.

How is the diagnosis of CLL made?

An increase in the absolute number of lymphocytes in the peripheral blood, which, on the peripheral smear, appear morphologically as small, mature lymphocytes. Flow cytometry shows a monoclonal population that coexpresses CD 19 and CD 5. Frequently, there is lymphadenopathy, splenomegaly, and bone marrow infiltration, making it difficult to distinguish CLL from its lymphomatous counterpart, WDLL.

What is the differential diagnosis for CLL?

Lymphoproliferative disorders such as the leukemic phase of follicular lymphoma, monocytoid B-cell lymphoma, mantle cell lymphoma, WDLL, LGL syndrome, lymphoplasmacytic lymphoma, Sézary cell lymphoma, hairy cell leukemia, splenic lymphoma with villous lymphocytes, and Waldenström's macroglobulinemia. A few of the nonmalignant causes of lymphocytosis include tuberculosis, mononucleosis, and pertussis infection.

What is the median survival expectation for a person with CLL?

8 years

What is the staging system for CLL?	The Rai system is the one most commonly used: Stage 0—lymphocytosis alone Stage I—lymphocytosis with lymphadenopathy Stage II—lymphocytosis with spleen or liver involvement Stage III—lymphocytosis with anemia Stage IV—lymphocytosis with anemia and thrombocytopenia
What are the median survival times for the following: **Stage 0**	> 15 years
Stage I	9 years
Stage II	5 years
Stage III	2 years
Stage IV	2 years
What is the treatment for CLL?	Observation if the patient is asymptomatic. Oral alkylating agent chemotherapy with or without prednisone is the standard if the patient is symptomatic with fever, night sweats, fatigue, or massive splenomegaly. Other indications for initiating treatment include the presence of autoimmune hemolytic anemia, autoimmune thrombocytopenia, bulky lymphadenopathy, progressive hyperlymphocytosis, and frequent bacterial infections.

HAIRY CELL LEUKEMIA

What is hairy cell leukemia?	A chronic lymphoproliferative disorder with a clonal neoplastic proliferation of a lymphocyte that is related to memory B-cells, activated B-cells, and preplasma cells

What is the morphologic appearance of hairy cell leukemia?	A large lymphocyte with an eccentric nucleus, with delicate, lacy chromatin and small nucleoli as well as abundant grayish-blue cytoplasm with fine irregular filamentous projections
What is the median age of onset of hairy cell leukemia?	52 years of age. Half of the cases occur between the ages of 40 and 60 years. There is a male to female ratio of 3–5:1.
What are the presenting symptoms of hairy cell leukemia?	Weakness, weight loss, recent pyogenic infection, or symptoms attributable to splenomegaly
What are the physical findings of hairy cell leukemia?	Splenomegaly occurs in 80% of cases. Rarely, patients have lymphadenopathy or hepatomegaly.
Do patients with hairy cell leukemia have an elevated WBC count?	Not usually; 80% of patients have leukopenia. Pancytopenia is a common presentation.
How is the diagnosis of hairy cell leukemia made?	By the appropriate clinical scenario and by "hairy cells" seen on peripheral smear or bone marrow examination. A special stain called TRAP is confirmatory as is flow cytometric data.
What is the treatment for hairy cell leukemia?	2-Chlorodeoxyadenosine is the treatment of choice and induces a prolonged complete remission in more than 85% of patients.

LARGE GRANULAR LYMPHOCYTE SYNDROME

What is an LGL?	On peripheral smear, an LGL appears as a large lymphocyte with abundant pale cytoplasm with prominent azurophilic granules.
What are the two types of LGL syndromes?	T-cell and NK cell
How is the diagnosis of LGL made?	Increase in LGLs on peripheral smear, which, by flow cytometry, shows clonality with the appropriate phenotype

What is the presentation of T-cell LGL?

Chronic, sometimes severe, neutropenia with frequent bacterial infections. Infiltration of the spleen, bone marrow, and liver are not uncommon. Interestingly, 25% of cases are associated with rheumatoid arthritis, making it difficult to distinguish from Felty's syndrome.

What is the presentation of NK-cell LGL?

Usually, an acute clinical course involving fever and B symptoms (e.g., fever, drenching night sweats, anorexia, weight loss). Anemia and thrombocytopenia are more common than with T-cell LGL. Massive hepatomegaly, lymph node involvement, and gastrointestinal symptoms are common.

LYMPHOMA

What is lymphoma?

A heterogenous group of malignancies of lymphocytes that usually arise in lymph nodes but may originate in any organ

What are the two broad categories of lymphomas?

Hodgkin's disease and NHL

How do NHL and Hodgkin's disease differ in their natural history?

NHL commonly presents with diffuse disease, whereas Hodgkin's disease presents more commonly with localized disease.

What are typical presenting symptoms of lymphoma?

Persistent painless adenopathy and B symptoms. Generalized pruritus with unexplained lymphadenopathy and pain in lymph nodes following alcohol ingestion are highly suggestive of Hodgkin's disease. Lymphomas can present with symptoms attributable to enlarged lymph nodes anywhere in the body.

What are typical presenting symptoms for CNS lymphoma?

Headache, altered mental status, and focal neurologic findings

What are typical presenting symptoms involving Waldeyer's ring?	Sinusitis and earaches
What are typical presenting symptoms of mediastinal lymphomas?	Cough, shortness of breath, chest pain, and hemoptysis
What are typical presenting symptoms of abdominal lymphomas?	Abdominal pain, nausea, vomiting, and back pain
What are B symptoms?	Fever, drenching night sweats, anorexia, and weight loss
What are typical physical findings in lymphoma?	Lymphadenopathy and hepatosplenomegaly are the most predominant findings.

HODGKIN'S DISEASE

What are the histologic subtypes of Hodgkin's disease?	Lymphocyte predominant, nodular sclerosing, and mixed cellularity. The lymphocyte-depleted subtype usually appears only at the end stage of disease.
What is the name of the pathologic cell in Hodgkin's disease?	Reed-Sternberg cell
What is the incidence of Hodgkin's disease?	8000 new cases per year in the United States
What is the age distribution of Hodgkin's disease?	There is a bimodal age distribution with a young adult form peaking in persons aged 16–34 years and an older adult form peaking in persons aged 55–74 years.
How is Hodgkin's disease staged?	Stage I—involvement of a single lymph node region or single extralymphatic site Stage II—involvement of two or more lymph node regions on the same side of the diaphragm Stage III—involvement of lymph node regions on both sides of the diaphragm

Stage IV—diffuse or disseminated involvement of one or more extralymphatic organs or tissues with or without associated lymph node involvement

What are the common sites of extranodal Hodgkin's disease?

Liver, lung, bone marrow, bone, and skin

What are the standard tests used to work up Hodgkin's disease?

H & P, CBC, Chem 17, CT scan of the chest, abdomen, and pelvis, and bilateral bone marrow biopsies. Occasionally, lymphangiograms, exploratory laparotomies, and bone scans are used. Gallium scans are used in certain scenarios, before initiating therapy and after completing therapy.

What are the dominant factors that determine therapy in Hodgkin's disease?

Stage, presence of extranodal disease, bulk of disease, and the presence of B symptoms. Histologic subtype has little or no bearing on choice of therapy. Bulky disease within the chest is defined as lymphadenopathy greater than one third the diameter of the chest. Bulky disease elsewhere is defined as lymphadenopathy > 10 cm.

What is the treatment for Hodgkin's disease?

Nonbulky stage I and IIA—radiotherapy alone
Bulky stage I and IIA—chemotherapy plus radiotherapy
Nonbulky stage IIB, III, and IV— combination chemotherapy
Bulky stage IIB, III, and IV— combination chemotherapy with radiotherapy to areas of bulky disease

What is the 5-year survival rate of Hodgkin's disease for the following:

   Stage I

> 90%

   Stage II

80%–90%

   Stage III

60%–85%

Stage IV	50%–60%
What are late complications of treatment of Hodgkin's disease?	Acute leukemia and myelodysplasia as a result of alkylating agent chemotherapy Solid tumors within and adjacent to the radiation port Cardiac disease as a result of radiation and Adriamycin exposure Sterility and hypothyroidism

NON-HODGKIN'S LYMPHOMA

What is the incidence of NHL?	50,000 new cases per year and increasing
What risk factors are associated with the development of NHL?	Exposure to herbicides by agricultural workers, autoimmune diseases, congenital immunodeficiency states, AIDS, EBV, and HTLV I
What are the histologic subgroups of NHL?	The histologic classification of NHL is complex and controversial. The most commonly used system is the working formulation. It is useful to subcategorize NHL into three broad categories: low grade, intermediate grade, and high grade.
What is the clinical behavior of low-grade NHL?	Typically indolent and not curative. Median survival is 7 years.
What is the typical clinical behavior of intermediate and high-grade NHL?	Rapid progression and death, if not treated. However, these entities are curable. Cure is achieved in one third of patients treated with standard combination chemotherapy regimens.
What is the staging system for NHL?	Ann Arbor staging is the most commonly used: Stage I—one lymph node–bearing area Stage II—two or more areas of nodal involvement on one side of the diaphragm Stage III—lymphatic involvement on both sides of the diaphragm Stage IV—liver, bone marrow, or other extranodal disease

What factor is crucial for choosing therapy for NHL?	Histologic grade. Most cases of NHL (especially low-grade cases) are disseminated at the time of presentation.
Are B symptoms common in NHL?	Yes
What is the treatment for low-grade NHL?	Observation if the patient is asymptomatic. Oral chemotherapy can be effective as initial treatment for symptomatic disease. Localized symptomatic NHL can be effectively palliated with radiation therapy. Combination chemotherapy and single-agent nucleoside analogs are effective but not proven to be better than oral regimens as initial treatment.
What is the treatment for intermediate and high-grade NHL?	Combination chemotherapy carries a 60%–70% complete response rate, but recurrence occurs in approximately half of patients within 1–2 years.

PLASMA CELL DYSCRASIAS

What is a plasma cell dyscrasia?	An abnormal proliferation of plasma cells that usually secrete a monoclonal immunoglobulin
What is the monoclonal protein associated with plasma cell dyscrasias?	An immunoglobulin. The most common is IgG, with IgA being a close second. All of the following may be present: IgM, kappa light chains, lambda light chains, IgD, and IgE monoclonal proteins.
What are the major plasma cell dyscrasias?	MGUS, multiple myeloma, Waldenström's macroglobulinemia, cryoglobulinemia, and primary amyloidosis
What is the definition of an MGUS?	The presence of an M protein (monoclonal protein) without evidence of multiple myeloma, amyloidosis, cryoglobulinemia, Waldenström's macroglobulinemia, or other lymphoproliferative disorder

How is an MGUS distinguished from multiple myeloma?	An MGUS must have serum M protein < 3 g/dl, < 5% plasma cells in the bone marrow, no or a small number of light chains in the urine, no lytic bone lesions, no anemia, no renal insufficiency, and no hypercalcemia.
What is the incidence of MGUS?	In persons aged 50 to 80 years old, the incidence increases from 1% to 10%.
Does an MGUS transform into a plasma cell dyscrasia?	Yes. In 10 years, 20% of MGUSs and, in 20 years, 33% transform into a plasma cell dyscrasia. Two thirds of the transformations are into multiple myeloma.

MULTIPLE MYELOMA

What is multiple myeloma?	A malignant proliferation of terminally differentiated B lymphocytes (plasma cells) resluting in end-organ damage
What is the incidence of multiple myeloma?	1% of all cancers and 10% of all hematologic malignances
What are the risk factors for development of multiple myeloma?	The median age for development of multiple myeloma is the 7th decade. The disease is much more common in blacks. Exposures to radiation, alkylating agents, asbestos, and pesticides have been implicated as risk factors.
Do all patients with multiple myeloma have a monoclonal protein in the serum?	No. Only 80% of patients have an M protein in serum; 20% have only light chains, which are not measurable in the serum and must be measured in a 24-hour urine collection. Approximately 1% of patients with multiple myeloma are termed nonsecretors and have no identifiable monoclonal protein.
In nonsecretors, where is the immunoglobulin?	On staining of the plasma cells, the protein is shown to be within the cytoplasm but the plasma cells cannot excrete the immunoglobulin molecule.

What are the clinical manifestations of multiple myeloma?

Osteolytic bone lesions with an associated risk of pathologic fractures of the long bones, vertebrae, pelvis, and ribs

Anemia and pancytopenia

Hypercalcemia

Renal insufficiency

Recurrent bacterial and viral infections

Hyperviscosity

Peripheral neuropathies

Spinal cord compression

Myelomatous meningitis

What are the causes of renal insufficiency or failure in patients with multiple myeloma?

Amyloidosis, light chain deposition disease, hypercalcemia, hyperuricemia with uric acid crystallization within the collecting ducts and tubules, and plasma cell infiltration

How is the diagnosis of multiple myeloma made?

An increased percentage of plasma cells on bone marrow aspirate (minimum of 15%–30%) with osteolytic bone lesions. Some patients have diffuse osteoporosis with no clear lytic bone lesions. Bone marrow plasmacytosis with unexplained anemia or pancytopenia, renal insufficiency, and hypercalcemia without osteolytic bone lesions are suggestive of multiple myeloma.

What tests should be done in the workup of a patient suspected to have multiple myeloma?

CBC, chemistry panel to include uric acid, serum protein electrophoresis, 24-hour urine collection for protein electrophoresis, and beta-2-microglobulin, total body skeletal survey, and bone marrow aspirate and biopsy

What is the treatment for multiple myeloma?

Alkylating agent chemotherapy with corticosteroids is the mainstay. Oral melphalan with prednisone is the least toxic and least expensive regimen. Randomized trials do not conclusively show that more intensive chemotherapy is more effective. Allogeneic bone marrow transplantation can cure the disease, but its use is limited because multiple myeloma is a disease of the elderly. High-dose chemotherapy with peripheral stem cell rescue is promising but still experimental.

What is the median survival?

Untreated 6 months, treated 2–3 years. 5 year survival is < 10%.

What is a plasmacytoma?

A tumor mass consisting of plasma cells. A solitary plasmacytoma can generally be treated with localized radiation therapy for cure; however, 80% recur with multiple myeloma.

Where are plasmacytomas typically found?

Within bone, but they can arise outside of the bone marrow

WALDENSTRÖM'S MACROGLOBULINEMIA

What is the characteristic cell type in Waldenström's macroglobulinemia?

Lymphocyte with plasma cell features. The disease is commonly referred to as a lymphoplasmacytic disorder.

What are the differences between Waldenström's macroglobulinemia and multiple myeloma in respect to the following?
    Physical findings

Patients with Waldenström's macroglobulinemia commonly have lymphadenopathy with hepatosplenomegaly and rarely have bone lesions.

    Paraproteins

By definition, Waldenström's macroglobulinemia must involve a monoclonal IgM paraprotein, whereas, in multiple myeloma, IgG and IgA are the most common immunoglobulins involved.

    Neoplastic cells

Waldenström's macroglobulinemia shows lymphoplasmacytic morphology and the neoplastic cell in multiple myeloma is a plasma cell.

    Symptom complex

Hyperviscosity is a more common problem in Waldenström's macroglobulinemia.

What are common presenting symptoms of Waldenström's macroglobulinemia?
Weakness, fatigue, oral and nasal mucocutaneous bleeding, symptoms attributable to splenomegaly, and symptoms attributable to hyperviscosity

What are symptoms attributable to hyperviscosity?
Headache, blurred vision, paresthesias, focal or diffuse weakness, deafness, and symptoms secondary to congestive heart failure

What are important physical findings of Waldenström's macroglobulinemia?
Hepatosplenomegaly and lymphadenopathy

What is the treatment for Waldenström's macroglobulinemia?
Similar to that for low-grade lymphomas and multiple myeloma (i.e., oral alkylating agents)

What is the median survival for patients with Waldenström's macroglobulinemia?
3–5 years

HEAD AND NECK CANCER

What is the incidence of head and neck cancer, and how many deaths are attributable to head and neck cancer annually?
43,000 cases per year with 11,600 deaths per year

Does local disease or metastatic disease cause the major morbidity in head and neck cancers?
Local disease, which invades the vital structures of the head and neck. Metastases occur but usually are not as problematic.

What are risk factors for head and neck cancer?
Tobacco smoking and use of smokeless tobacco. Ethanol use potentiates tobacco risk and is a risk factor independent of tobacco. Nickel refining, woodworking, and exposure to textiles have all been implicated as occupational risks. Infections with HPV and EBV are important risk factors worldwide, with EBV infection being a particular risk factor in China.

What are the presenting signs and symptoms for malignancies in the following:

Oral cavity

Pain, ulcers, change in denture fit

Oropharynx, hypopharynx, and supraglottic larynx

Sore throat, hoarseness, dysphagia, ear pain, and adenopathy

Larynx

Hoarseness

Nasopharynx

Otitis media, cranial neuropathies, and adenopathy

Paranasal sinuses

Swelling of the cheeks, proptosis, sinusitis, loose teeth, epistaxis, and pain

Are there identifiable premalignant lesions in the upper aerodigestive tract?

Erythroplakia and leukoplakia

What is the most common histologic occurrence of head and neck cancer?

Squamous cell carcinoma

What percent of patients present with localized disease?

30%, but this amount varies with tumor location

When a patient is first seen, at which anatomic locations is disease more commonly advanced?

Supraglottic larynx, oropharynx, and hypopharynx

What are the staging criteria for head and neck cancer?

Each site has its own specifics. The four general stages are (1) local, (2) locally advanced but resectable, (3) locally advanced but unresectable, and (4) metastatic.

To what locations does head and neck cancer usually metastasize?

First to localized lymph nodes, then to lungs, bones, and liver

What is the diagnostic workup for head and neck cancer?	Careful H & P, CBC, chemistry panel, chest radiograph, thorough panendoscopy of the entire head and neck region, and CT scan of the head and neck
What is the general treatment approach for head and neck cancer?	Local disease—radiation or surgery Resectable locally advanced disease— surgery followed by radiation Unresectable locally advanced disease— radiation followed by surgery Metastatic disease—palliative chemotherapy In advanced laryngeal cancer and advanced nasopharyngeal cancer, chemotherapy and radiation are commonly used in lieu of surgery.
What is the surgical procedure for head and neck cancer?	Wide local excision with ipsilateral radical neck dissection. Contralateral radical neck dissection is performed if clinical or radiologic evidence of disease is present within the contralateral neck.
What is the 5-year survival rate for the following: **Local disease?**	60%–90%
Locally advanced disease?	30%
Metastatic disease?	< 5%
What is the incidence of new aerodigestive cancers arising in a patient previously rendered disease-free from a head and neck cancer?	Each year, a new cancer of the aerodigestive epithelium develops in 3%–7% of patients. This effect is referred to as field cancerization.

BREAST CANCER

What is the yearly incidence of breast cancer in the United States, and how many women die of this disease?	Breast cancer is the most common cancer and the second most common cause of cancer death among women in the United States. In 1996, over 180,000 new cases occurred, and over 44,000 women died of this disease.

What are the risk factors for the development of breast cancer?

Increasing age, family history, personal history of breast cancer, biopsy-confirmed benign breast disease (e.g., atypical hyperplasia), and hormonal factors (e.g., early age at menarche or late menopause, late age at first pregnancy, few pregnancies, oral contraceptive pill use, and prolonged postmenopausal estrogen use)

How can the mortality rate associated with breast cancer be controlled?

Early detection with mammography can reduce the breast cancer mortality rate by at least 30% in women aged 50 years and older.

What inherited genetic abnormalities are associated with breast cancer?

It is estimated that 5%–10% of all cases of breast cancer in the United States are related to inherited genetic abnormalities. Genes involved include BRCA1, BRCA2, p53 (associated with Li-Fraumeni syndrome), and ATM (associated with ataxia telangiectasia).

What are the most common presenting symptoms of breast cancer?

Most breast cancer patients present with a painless breast mass, although 10% of patients have pain and no mass. Others have breast thickening, swelling, or nipple discharge, tenderness or inversion.

What percentage of patients with breast cancer present with metastatic disease?

6% of breast cancer patients present with metastatic disease.

What symptoms are most often associated with metastatic breast cancer?

The symptoms are attributable to the site of metastases and include the following:

CNS—headache, visual changes, altered mental status, paresthesias, weakness, incontinence

Intrathoracic—chest pain, shortness of breath

Intraabdominal—nausea, vomiting, anorexia, weight loss, abdominal pain

Skeletal—bony pain, neurologic symptoms (if the spine is involved)

What are the most common sites involved by metastases from breast cancer?	The lung, liver, and bone are the three most common sites of metastatic involvement.
What are the histologic subtypes of in situ breast carcinomas?	DCIS and LCIS
What is the most common histologic subtype of invasive breast cancer?	Infiltrating ductal carcinomas make up approximately 70% of all histopathologic diagnoses, followed by infiltrating lobular carcinoma, accounting for 5%–10% of invasive breast cancers. Medullary, mucinous, and tubular histologic subtypes are less common.
What is the staging system for invasive cancer of the breast?	Stage I—primary tumor less than or equal to 2 cm, with no nodal involvement Stage IIA—primary tumor less than or equal to 2 cm with ipsilateral mobile axillary nodal involvement, or tumor greater than 2 cm but less than or equal to 5 cm with no nodal involvement Stage IIB—primary tumor greater than 2 cm but less than or equal to 5 cm with ipsilateral mobile axillary nodal involvement Stage IIIA—primary tumor greater than 5 cm with ipsilateral nodes fixed to one another or other structures, or primary tumor greater than 5 cm with ipsilateral mobile axillary nodal involvement Stage IIIB—primary tumor of any size involving skin or chest wall; includes peau d'orange ("skin of orange") changes Stage IV—metastatic disease
What is the treatment for in situ cancer of the breast?	DCIS is treated with local excision plus radiation versus simple mastectomy. LCIS is managed with careful bilateral breast observation.

Women with LCIS who are unable to comply with screening recommendations or are unable to accept a 20%–30% risk of development of invasive breast cancer may be offered bilateral simple mastectomy.

What is the surgical treatment for invasive cancer of the breast?

Modified radical mastectomy with axillary lymph node dissection versus lumpectomy with axillary lymph node dissection followed by local radiation

Is lumpectomy plus radiation equivalent to mastectomy in the primary management of breast cancer?

Yes. This has been confirmed by seven studies.

What adjuvant (postsurgical) treatments improve the survival rate in women with invasive breast cancer?

Compared with surgery alone, the use of adjuvant drug therapy in breast cancer can decrease the risk of systemic recurrence by approximately one third. The choice of treatment depends on the health and menopausal status of the patient, the receptor status of the tumor, and the stage of disease. Adjuvant pharmacologic treatments include cytotoxic chemotherapy, hormonal therapy, or a combination of the two. Local adjuvant radiotherapy improves local control of disease in certain circumstances.

What is the role of bone marrow transplantation in the management of breast cancer?

Bone marrow transplantation is still experimental in the management of breast cancer. It is a treatment option in young, otherwise healthy women with locally advanced or metastatic disease.

What is the management of metastatic breast cancer?

Metastatic breast cancer is not curable (except, possibly, when bone marrow transplantation is successful). Treatment is based on the clinical status of the patient and involves either cytotoxic chemotherapy or hormonal therapy.

What is the 5-year survival rate for women with breast cancer?	Roughly 80%–85% for all stages. For women with cancers localized to the breast, the 5-year survival rate is 96%. Women with regional metastases (positive axillary node involvement) have a 75% 5-year survival rate. Those with distant metastases have a 20% 5-year survival rate.

LUNG CANCER*

What is the incidence of lung cancer?	It is the most common malignancy in the United States with 170,000 new cases and 150,000 deaths per year.
Does this malignancy usually present at an early stage?	No, lung cancer commonly presents with advanced disease.
What are the risk factors for lung cancer?	Exposure to cigarette smoke, asbestos, uranium, radon, arsenic, chromium methyl ethers, nickel, chloromethyl, and polycyclic aromatic hydrocarbons. Risk factors that are more rarely involved include preexisting scars from old granulomatous disease, diffuse interstitial fibrosis, and scleroderma.
Does passive exposure to cigarette smoke increase cancer risk?	Yes
What percentage of lung cancer cases are related to smoking?	85%
What are symptoms of lung cancer?	Local disease—shortness of breath, chest pain, hemoptysis Metastatic disease—headache, confusion, focal neurologic findings, anorexia, weight loss, abdominal pain, bony pain
What are paraneoplastic syndromes?	A group of disorders associated with malignant diseases that are not related to the physical effects of the tumor itself

---

* In collaboration with V. Shami, S. Koenig and M. Robbins

What are the most frequent initial symptoms and signs of lung cancer?	Cough (75%) Dyspnea (60%) Chest pain (45%) Hemoptysis (35%) Other pain (25%) Clubbing (21%)

What physical findings can be seen secondary to the following:

Intrathoracic disease	Rales, pleural effusion, symptoms suggestive of SVC syndrome, and symptoms suggestive of pericardial tamponade—distended neck veins, hypotension, pulsus paradoxus, pericardial knock, diminished heart sounds
Extrathoracic disease	Altered mental status, focal neurologic findings, papilledema, hepatomegaly, intraabdominal mass, subcutaneous mass, bony tenderness
What is the first thing that should be done when a chest radiograph shows a solitary pulmonary nodule?	Check an old radiograph.
What diagnostic tests should be performed for lung cancer?	Initial evaluation should include a chest radiograph and sputum cytologic testing; bronchoscopy with biopsy or percutaneous biopsy can be done if cytologic results are negative.
What is the differential diagnosis for a solitary nodule?	Malignant causes—lung cancer, metastasis, carcinoid tumor, sarcoma Benign causes—infectious granulomas (histoplasmosis, tuberculosis), hamartoma, abscess, rheumatoid nodule, lipoma, fibroma, infarct, arteriovenous malformation
What radiographic finding is pathognomonic of a benign nodule?	Calcification of a "popcorn" variety
What is the most common benign tumor of the lung?	Hamartoma

What is found on chest radiograph for lung malignancies?

Squamous cell carcinoma—a central lesion with hilar involvement and frequent cavitation

Adenocarcinoma—a peripheral lesion, which can also cavitate

Bronchoalveolar carcinoma—peripheral, sometimes multifocal, pneumonic-like infiltrates

Large cell carcinoma—usually a peripheral lesion, which can cavitate

Small cell carcinoma—a central lesion with hilar mass and early mediastinal involvement, which does not cavitate

What are the two broad categories of lung cancer?

NSCLC and SCLC

What histologic entities comprise NSCLC?

Squamous cell carcinoma, adenocarcinoma, and large cell carcinoma

What are the most common types of lung cancers?

Squamous cell carcinoma (35%)
Adenocarcinoma (25%)
Small cell carcinoma (25%)
Large cell undifferentiated carcinoma (14%)

Which cell types are most associated with smokers?

Squamous cell and small cell

Which cell type is most often associated with paraneoplastic syndromes?

Small cell

Which cell type is most often asociated with hypercalcemia?

Squamous cell

Which type of lung cancer is not associated with smoking?

Adenocarcinoma

From what normal cell does SCLC arise from?

Neuroendocrine

What is a Pancoast's tumor?	An apical tumor that involves the inferior cervical ganglion, causing Horner's syndrome (i.e., unilateral miosis, ptosis, exophthalmos, and anhydrosis), arm and shoulder pain, bone destruction, and atrophy of the hand muscles
Pancoast's tumor is most commonly associated with which cell type?	Squamous
What are the most common pulmonary complications of lung cancer?	Atelectasis, postobstructive pneumonia, hemoptysis, pleural effusion, and respiratory failure
What are common sites of lung cancer metastases?	Hilar and mediastinal lymph nodes, pleura, opposite lung, liver, adrenal glands, bone, and CNS
How can extrathoracic spread of cancer be monitored?	By performing liver function tests and measuring serum calcium and alkaline phosphatase levels
Why is it important to differentiate NSCLC from SCLC?	SCLC usually presents with widespread disease and thus rarely can be cured by surgery. SCLC is far more sensitive than NSCLC to chemotherapy.
At which stage are most small cell cancer patients first seen?	Extensive disease is seen in 70% of patients; 30% have limited disease.
How is SCLC staged?	Limited and extensive. In limited-stage SCLC, all disease is within a single radiation port within the chest and supraclavicular fossa. There is a 15%–20% cure rate in limited SCLC with combined radiation and chemotherapy. Extensive-stage SCLC extends outside a single radiation port within the chest.
What is the treatment of extensive disease SCLC?	Combination chemotherapy offers a 50%–70% response rate with a median survival for all patients of 6–9 months. In untreated disease, the median survival is 2–3 months, and responders to

chemotherapy can live up to 2 years with a rare cure (< 2%).

What is the current chemotherapy standard for SCLC?

Cisplatin and etoposide. Oral etoposide is less toxic and thus might be the best choice for elderly patients with SCLC.

What is the staging of NSCLC?

Stage I—negative nodal involvement and an easily resectable tumor

Stage II—easily resectable tumor with ipsilateral peribronchial or hilar node involvement

Stage IIIA—easily resectable tumor with positive ipsilateral mediastinal and subcarinal lymph node involvement, or a marginally resectable tumor with or without ipsilateral lymph node metastases

Stage IIIB—any tumor with contralateral lymph node or supraclavicular lymph node metastases. Any tumor, regardless of lymph node status, that invades the mediastinum, heart, great vessels, trachea, esophagus, vertebral body, or carina or has a malignant pleural effusion

Stage IV—distant metastases

What is the treatment of NSCLC?

Stage I and II—surgical resection

Stage IIIA—surgery alone and radiation with or without chemotherapy. Other combined modality approaches are being investigated.

Stage IIIB—radiation with or without chemotherapy

Stage IV—supportive care versus combination chemotherapy. In patients with a good performance status, chemotherapy offers a 25%–30% response rate, perhaps with a slight improvement in quality of life and survival.

What are the commonly used chemotherapy drugs for NSCLC?

Cisplatin and etoposide is the current standard. Paclitaxel, vinorelbine, and gemcitabine are newer agents that show promise in treatment of NSCLC. A combination of carboplatin with paclitaxel was recently found to have a 60% response rate.

What is the approximate 5-year survival rate of NSCLC for the following:

Stage I   50%

Stage II   .   30%

Stage IIIA   15%

Stage IIIB   5%

Stage IV   < 2%

What are the 5-year survival rates for the different types of cancer?

Squamous—25%
Adenocarcinoma—12%
Large cell carcinoma—13%
Small cell carcinoma—1%

Why do small cell carcinomas have the poorest prognosis?

They have the greatest tendency to metastasize and are almost always disseminated by the time the patient is first seen.

Should patients with surgically resectable disease undergo a mediastinal lymph node sampling?

Yes. In 20%–40% of cases, normal lymph nodes identified by CT scan are positive for cancer, and 20%–40% of enlarged lymph nodes identified by CT scan do not contain cancer.

What are complications of chemotherapy and radiotherapy?

Acute—tumor lysis syndrome, infection and bleeding, myelosuppression, hemorrhagic cystitis (cyclophosphamide), cardiotoxicity (Adriamycin), renal toxicity (cisplatin), peripheral neuropathy (vincristine)
Chronic—neurologic damage (confusion, episodic hemiparesis, ataxia), leukemia, second primary neoplasms

GASTROINTESTINAL CANCER

ESOPHAGEAL CANCER*

How common is esophageal cancer?	Squamous carcinoma and adenocarcinoma account for 1%–2% of all cancers in the United States. Blacks have a three-fold higher risk than whites. The incidence in some areas of China, Puerto Rico, and Singapore is 140 in 100,000 per year.
What factors predispose an individual to an increased risk of esophageal cancer?	Smoking and alcohol abuse are individually associated as well as synergistic. Other predisposing factors include caustic injury (e.g., lye stricture), betel nut chewing, smoking, drinking maize-brewed beverages, thermal injuries (such as from drinking hot liquids), eating foods high in nitrosamines (see Gastric Cancer), ear-nose-throat cancer, Barrett's esophagus (adenocarcinoma), exposure to ionizing radiation and asbestos, Plummer-Vinson syndrome, celiac sprue, and achalasia.
What is the epidemiology for the following:	
Squamous cell carcinoma	Accounts for 90% of esophageal cancer A 4- to 5-fold increased risk for blacks relative to whites Poor prognosis—5-year survival < 10%
Adenocarcinoma	Incidence is increasing (unknown as to why) Usually seen in setting of Barrett's epithelium Predominantly affects whites
What acquired and inherited disorders predispose a person to esophageal cancer?	Tylosis—an autosomal dominant disorder characterized by hyperkeratosis of the skin of the palms and papillomata of the esophagus

* In collaboration with C. Yoshida, G. Goldin, and C. Matthews

Achalasia—occurs 1–2 decades after onset
Barrett's esophagus

What is the concept of field cancerization?

In patients who abuse tobacco or alcohol, carcinomas can develop anywhere in the aerodigestive tract. Esophageal cancer develops in one third of patients with head and neck cancer. Cancers of the tonsil and tongue are the most common offenders. A second new primary tumor arises in the aerodigestive tract at a rate of 4% per year.

What is the classic presentation of esophageal cancer?

A 55- to 65-year-old man with a long history of tobacco and alcohol abuse complaining of dysphagia and weight loss. Other symptoms include food sticking, odynophagia (50%), substernal chest pain, regurgitation of undigested food, cough, shortness of breath, aspiration pneumonia, hemoptysis (suggests a tracheoesophageal fistula), hematemesis, and hoarseness (paralysis of recurrent laryngeal nerve).

What are common physical findings of esophageal cancer?

Cachexia, lymphadenopathy (supraclavicular, cervical, and axillary), ascites, evidence of pleural fluid or infiltrate, and SVC syndrome

How is the diagnosis of esophageal cancer made?

Upper gastrointestinal endoscopy allows direct localization of tumor with biopsy; chest CT and endoscopic ultrasound assist in staging.

What is the most common location of cancer of the esophagus?

The middle third (55%). The esophagus is divided into three portions: upper third, cervical (15%); middle third, upper and midthoracic (55%); lower third, lower thoracic (35%).

What is the natural history of esophageal cancer?

In most tumors, symptoms occur late because the esophagus is distensible. Typically, the tumor has extensive local growth, followed by lymph node metastases, invasion of local structures, and finally distal spread.

What is the treatment of localized esophageal cancer?

For tumors within the muscularis with local lymph nodes, the treatment of choice is surgery.

What is the treatment of choice for locally advanced esophageal cancer?

Palliation of dysphagia is the primary objective. In the event that surgery is not curative, a palliative surgical bypass is not unreasonable. Radiation therapy alone can palliate symptoms in 75% of patients for a median period of 8 months. Combined modality approaches of surgery, radiation, and chemotherapy can offer 10%–20% long-term disease-free survival in select patients. In patients who are not candidates for surgical or combined modality approaches, esophageal stents and dilatations offer a less invasive, less toxic palliative intervention.

What treatments are available for advanced esophageal cancer?

Combination chemotherapy with cisplatin and 5-FU has been reported to give a response rate as high as 40%, but, in most patients, these results are short-lived.

GASTRIC CANCER*

What is the leading cause of cancer death worldwide?

Gastric cancer

Is the incidence of gastric cancer changing in the United States?

Yes. Although one of the most common cancers worldwide, the incidence of gastric cancer in the United States has been steadily decreasing over the past 60 years for unclear reasons. There has been an alarming increase in the incidence of proximal and distal esophageal cancer in the past 20 years in the United States.

What is the usual age, sex, and racial distribution of gastric cancer?

Begins in the 4th decade and peaks in the 7th decade
Twice as common in males than females

---

* In collaboration with C. Yoshida, G. Goldin, and C. Matthews

1.5-fold higher incidence in blacks than in whites

More common in the Far East, South America, and Eastern Europe

What environmental situations and exposures are thought to increase the risk of gastric cancer?

Smoking, long-term early ingestion of foods high in nitrosamines (e.g., dried, smoked, and salted meat and fish), lower socioeconomic status, and *Helicobacter pylori* infection

Is *H. pylori* associated with gastric cancer?

It has been implicated in both adenocarcinoma and lymphoma, but especially in MALT (mucosal associated lymphoid tissue) lymphoma.

What are the two most common types of gastric cancer?

Adenocarcinoma and lymphoma

What are risk factors for gastric adenocarcinoma?

Nation of origin (Japan, Chile, Finland), diet (smoked foods, aflatoxin), achlorhydria, postgastrectomy status (usually > 15 years postoperatively), gastric adenomatous polyps, Menetrier's disease, and blood type A

What types of diets are thought to be protective against gastric cancer?

Diets that include raw uncooked vegetables, fruit, and high-fiber bread; diets low in animal and vegetable fat and protein; diets high in vitamin A and C intake

What medical conditions increase the risk for gastric cancer?

Pernicious anemia, prior gastric surgery, atrophic gastritis, gastric ulcers, Menetrier's disease, and blood type A

What are common presenting symptoms of gastric cancer?

Most patients have advanced disease characterized by weight loss, anorexia, epigastric discomfort, dysphagia, nausea, vomiting, and early satiety. Gastrointestinal bleeding is uncommon.

What are common physical findings in gastric cancer?

Ascites, jaundice, large bowel obstruction secondary to invasion of the gastrocolic ligament, palpable abdominal mass, ovarian mass (Krukenberg tumor), left supraclavicular lymph node

(Virchow's node), left axillary lymph node (Irish's node), umbilical node (Sister Mary Joseph node), and palpable pelvic mass secondary to intraperitoneal spread (Blumer's shelf)

What are the diagnostic and staging tests used in gastric cancer?

H&P, CBC, Chem 17, upper endoscopy or upper gastrointestinal series, and CT scan of the chest, abdomen, and pelvis

What histologic entities other than adenocarcinoma occur in the stomach?

Adenocarcinoma comprises 90%–95% of all stomach cancers. Primary gastric lymphoma is increasing in incidence. Carcinoid tumors, small cell tumors, and sarcomas can also arise in the stomach. Furthermore, other tumors can metastasize to the stomach.

What are the two histologic presentations of gastric adenocarcinoma?

Intestinal and diffuse. Intestinal manifestations arise from precancerous lesions, such as gastric atrophy or intestinal metaplasia. Intestinal gastric cancer is found in epidemic areas (e.g., the Far East). There is a male predominance. Diffuse manifestations occur as symptoms of early satiety secondary to the diffuse involvement of the stomach wall. The term commonly given to this histologic subtype is linitis plastica, which refers to poor distensibility of the stomach as seen on an upper gastrointestinal series.

Where does gastric adenocarcinoma metastasize?

Local nodal metastases within the wall of the stomach extending to the duodenum and esophagus and direct extension to adjacent organs are the most common areas of involvement. As many as 75% of lesions have spread in this fashion by the time of diagnosis. The liver is the most common site of distant metastases. At autopsy, disease involves the liver in 50% of patients, the peritoneum in 25%, the omentum in 20%, and the lungs in 15%.

What is the prognosis for gastric adenocarcinoma?

Because most diagnoses are made late, the prognosis is poor: the 5-year survival rate is approximately 10%. Early gastric cancer confined to mucosa and submucosa with no metastases or lymph node involvement has a 90% 5-year survival rate.

What is the only curative treatment modality for localized gastric carcinoma?

Surgery, but only one third of patients can undergo a curative resection at the time of presentation

What percent of patients are alive at 5 years after undergoing resection for gastric cancer?

25%—in patients with negative nodal involvement, > 50%; in patients with positive nodal involvement, 15%. Many of the recurrences are local.

Does adjuvant chemotherapy improve survival in locally resected gastric cancer?

No. Despite 30 years of trials, no definitive data suggest an improvement.

Is there evidence that adjuvant chemoradiotherapy improves survival in completely resected gastric cancer?

No randomized trials have been done; however, the use of 5-FU with concomitant radiotherapy has resulted in a 10%–15% 5-year survival rate in several series of patients with locally advanced gastric cancer. This information advances the theory that 5-FU and radiation therapy to the gastric bed might improve survival in patients who have undergone resection for gastric cancer.

What is the treatment for advanced gastric cancer?

Palliation of symptoms. Gastric bypass and debulking procedures are sometimes useful. Combination chemotherapy can produce response in 30% of patients, but many of those responses are of short duration. Drugs used include 5-FU, leucovorin, Adriamycin, methotrexate, cisplatin, and etoposide.

SMALL BOWEL NEOPLASM

What is the incidence of small bowel neoplasm?

Rare

What are risk factors for small bowel neoplasm?

Celiac sprue, Crohn's disease, and AIDS

What are the benign small bowel tumors in order of frequency?

Carcinoid, adenoma, leiomyoma, lipoma, and hamartoma

What are the malignant small bowel tumors in order of frequency?

Adenocarcinoma, malignant lymphoma, and carcinoid

What is the most common tumor location in the small bowel?

Proximal small bowel

What are symptoms and signs of small bowel neoplasm?

Pain, partial or total obstruction, anemia, and biliary obstruction (with ampullary tumors)

What is a carcinoid tumor?

Tumors of neuroendocrine cells—90% are located in the gastrointestinal tract. Midgut carcinoid tumors are most common.

Where are carcinoid tumors located?

Appendix—35%–45%
Ileum—10%–15%
Right colon—5%
Other gastrointestinal locations include the rectum (10%–15%), duodenum, stomach, gallbladder, pancreas, esophagus, biliary tract, and Meckel's diverticulum

How are benign tumors distinguised from malignant tumors?

Tumors are distinguished by size rather than histology (with an 80% risk of metastases in tumors > 2 cm).

What is the carcinoid syndrome?

A syndrome characterized by facial flushing, tachycardia, hypotension, watery stools, and wheezing, which occurs in 5%–15% of all gastrointestinal carcinoids metastatic to the liver. Facial cyanosis, telangiectasis, brawny edema, and right heart endocardial fibrosis can occur with advanced tumors.

What is the treatment and prognosis for carcinoid tumors of the small bowel?	Surgical resection can cure small carcinoids, but cure is not possible with metastatic disease. Somatostatin analog controls the vasomotor symptoms and diarrhea.

COLORECTAL CANCER (SEE CHAPTER 5)

PANCREATIC CANCER*

What is the incidence of pancreatic cancer?	Increasing. It is the fifth most common cause of cancer-related death. It is more common in older (> 55 years) persons, blacks, and males. Very few cancers evoke a more dismal prognosis.
What are the risk factors for the development of pancreatic cancer?	Cigarette abuse (increases risk fourfold), lower socioeconomic status, organic solvents, possibly chronic pancreatitis and partial gastrectomy, diabetes, and a high-fat diet. Drinking coffee is probably not related to an increased risk. Neither, probably, is ethanol abuse.
What is the most common histologic subtype of pancreatic carcinoma?	Ductal adenocarcinoma comprises > 80% of pancreatic carcinoma, with 70% arising in the head of the pancreas (possibly resulting in biliary obstruction). Many other histologic subtypes are seen and have a better prognosis. These include carcinoid, lymphoma, sarcoma, nonfunctioning islet cell carcinomas, malignant and benign insulinomas, gastrinomas, and glucagonomas.
What are common presenting symptoms of pancreatic cancer?	Symptoms are insidious, occurring late in the course of the disease, They include anorexia, weight loss, and gnawing, postprandial epigastric pain. More than 50% of patients have jaundice, pruritus, claylike stools, and darkening of the urine. Depression is common (more strongly associated with pancreatic cancer than any other malignancy). Up to 80% of patients may have diabetes or glucose intolerance.

---

* In collaboration with C. Yoshida, G. Goldin, and C. Matthews

Rarely, patients have acute pancreatitis, cholecystitis, gastrointestinal bleeding, polyarthritis, and skin nodules.

What is a common presentation of pancreatic cancer?

Painless jaundice and weight loss

What are common physical findings of pancreatic cancer?

Migratory thrombophlebitis (Trousseau's sign), palpable gallbladder (Courvoisier's sign), hepatomegaly, icterus, abdominal mass, and ascites

What laboratory tests are useful in establishing pancreatic cancer?

There is no specific laboratory test for early detection of pancreatic cancer.

What tumor markers are used in pancreatic cancer?

Gastrin, carcinoembryonic antigen, AFP, beta-2-microglobulin, CA-125, and CA 19-9. None of these, however, are sensitive or specific enough to be used routinely.

How are the following imaging studies helpful?
    Abdominal CT

Determines presence of a mass, biliary and pancreatic ductal dilation, local invasion, and nodal or distant metastases

    ERCP

90% sensitivity in demonstrating pancreatic ductal stenosis or obstruction by tumor. ERCP allows biopsy, brushing, and aspiration of pancreatic juice. Common bile duct obstruction can also be diagnosed and treated.

    Angiography

Celiac and SMA angiography determines resectability of tumor before surgery. Arterial encasement, venous occlusion, and tumor vascularity can be visualized.

How is the diagnosis of pancreatic cancer made?

Cytologic, percutaneous fine-needle aspiration is useful.

At what stage of disease are patients usually first seen?

At presentation, 40% of patients have metastatic disease, 40% have locally advanced disease, and < 20% have disease confined to the pancreas.

What are the most common sites of metastatic disease in pancreatic cancer?

Porta hepatis, liver, peritoneum with malignant ascites, penetration into the splanchnic nerves, and local lymph nodes. Less commonly, lung and bone are affected.

Pancreatic carcinomas at what location and/or of what size are generally unresectable?

Tumors arising in the tail of the pancreas and those > 4 cm are rarely resectable.

What is the treatment for pancreatic cancer?

At presentation, 10%–15% are potentially curable by Whipple resection. Lesions in only one third of patients who are scheduled for resection are actually resectable at the time of the procedure. ERCP with stent placement or palliative bypass surgery may be done for biliary obstruction. Celiac plexus block may be useful for debilitating pain.

What does a Whipple resection involve?

Resection of the distal stomach, common bile duct, gallbladder, and entire duodenum with the first part of the small bowel and head of the pancreas removed en bloc. Next performed are a choledochojejunostomy, pancreaticojejunostomy, and gastrojejunostomy. This procedure is also called a pancreaticoduodenectomy.

What is the overall 5-year survival rate for pancreatic cancer?

3%

What percent of patients who undergo a resection are alive at 5 years?

< 20%

What favorable findings at surgery increase the likelihood of a long-term cure?

Tumor < 2 cm, lymph nodes without evidence of metastatic disease, and no major vessel involvement

Why is it important to make a tissue diagnosis of a pancreatic mass?

A small percentage of different histologic entities have a more favorable prognosis.

Are there any proven adjuvant treatments that improve survival in resectable pancreatic cancer?

One prospective, controlled study demonstrated an improvement in survival (21 months vs. 11 months) with use of postoperative 5-FU and radiation therapy versus surgery alone.

What surgical approaches should be considered for locally unresectable disease?

Palliative and prophylactic biliary bypass surgery. Biliary stent placement either transhepatically or via ERCP is an alternative. Relief of gastric outlet obstruction and duodenal obstruction can be useful. Prophylactic gastric bypass procedures are useful in some scenarios. Splanchnic and celiac ganglion nerve blocks may relieve pain.

Are radiation and chemotherapy useful in the treatment of locally advanced pancreatic cancer?

Radiation therapy alone can improve pain and possibly prolong survival. Combined modality therapy with 5-FU and radiation therapy in one study showed an improvement in survival from 5 to 10 months.

What treatments are there for metastatic pancreatic cancer?

Palliation of symptoms is the most important treatment. 5-FU is associated with a response rate of less than 20% and does not improve the survival rate. A new drug, gemcitabine, has shown moderate promise when used to treat patients with pancreatic cancer.

PANCREATIC ISLET CELL TUMORS*

What is the epidemiology of pancreatic islet cell tumors?

Uncommon—prevalence < 10 per million population (insulinoma > gastrinoma > remainder)

What are the types of pancreatic islet cell tumors?

Endocrine tumors of the pancreas are classified according to the type of clinical syndrome present: insulinoma, gastrinoma (Zollinger-Ellison syndrome), somatostatinoma, VIPoma (e.g., pancreatic cholera, Verner-Morrison syndrome), glucagonoma, PPoma, GRFoma, and nonfunctioning tumors.

---

* In collaboration with C. Yoshida, G. Goldin, and C. Matthews

What are symptoms and signs of an insulinoma?	Hypoglycemia (e.g., tachycardia, diaphoresis, confusion)
Where are insulinomas located?	Pancreas
What are symptoms and signs of gastrinoma (Zollinger-Ellison syndrome)?	Numerous peptic ulcers in unusual locations (e.g., the jejunum), abdominal pain, and diarrhea
Where are gastrinomas located?	Pancreas (60%), duodenum (30%), and other locations (10%)
What clinical entity is associated with gastrinoma?	Frequently, multiple endocrine neoplasia (MEN) type I, characterized by multiple adenomas of the pituitary, parathyroid, and pancreas
What are symptoms and signs of glucagonoma?	Think **DRAW**: **D**iabetes mellitus **R**ash—migratory neurolytic erythema **A**nemia **W**eight loss
Where are glucagonomas located?	Pancreas
What are symptoms and signs of somatostatinoma?	Think the big **S** tumor: **S**ugar (diabetes mellitus) **S**teatorrhea **S**tones (gallstones)
Where are somatostatinomas located?	Pancreas (60%) and small bowel (40%)
What are symptoms and signs of VIPoma (Verner-Morrison syndrome, pancreatic cholera)	Think **WDHA** syndrome: **W**atery **D**iarrhea **H**ypokalemia **A**chlorhydria
Where are VIPomas located?	Pancreas (90%) and other locations (10%)
What are the symptoms and signs of GRFoma?	Acromegaly

Where are GRFomas located?	Pancreas
What are the symptoms and signs of PPoma and nonfunctioning tumors?	Weight loss, abdominal mass, and hepatomegaly (PP is released but there are no known symptoms due to hypersecretion)
Where are PPoma and nonfunctioning tumors located?	Pancreas
How is the diagnosis of pancreatic islet cell tumor made?	Tumor localization

What is the sensitivity of the following tests in localizing islet cell tumors?

Ultrasound	10%–20%
Abdominal CT	20%–40%
Selective angiography	80%–90%
Intraoperative ultrasound	90%
Octreoscan	40%–100% (octreoscan is indium-labeled pentoctreotide used in a nuclear medicine study that is noninvasive; results depend on tumor type)
What is the malignant potential of pancreatic islet cell tumors?	Only 10% of insulinomas are malignant; at least 50% of all other histologic subtypes are considered malignant.
What is the treatment for pancreatic islet cell tumors?	All patients should be considered for possible surgical resection of the tumor. Medical treatment may be useful in unresectable or incompletely resectable tumors.

What is the specific medical treatment for the following:

Insulinoma	Diazoxide and frequent small meals

Gastrinoma	Omeprazole
Glucagonoma	Streptozocin chemotherapy
Somatostatinoma	Streptozocin has worked in a few cases.
VIPoma, glucagonoma, GRFoma, insulinoma, Zollinger-Ellison syndrome	Octreotide

What is the prognosis for pancreatic islet cell tumors?

Islet cell tumors have a far more favorable prognosis than ductal adenocarcinomas because they grow slowly and cause physical symptoms early. Survival is directly related to tumor extent: if no tumor is found at surgery, the 5- to 10-year survival rate is 90%–100%; if there is complete tumor resection, the 5- to 10-year survival rate is 90%–100%; if there is incomplete resection, the 5-year survival rate is 15%–75%; in unresectable cases, the 5-year survival rate is 20%–75%.

CHOLANGIOCARCINOMA*

What is cholangiocarcinoma?

Adenocarcinomas arising from small bile ducts in the liver, from larger hilar ducts, or from the extrahepatic biliary tree

Who is susceptible to cholangiocarcinoma?

Patients with PSC, ulcerative colitis (with or without PSC), choledochal cysts, and liver fluke infestation

What is a Klatskin tumor?

Cholangiocarcinoma arising at the bifurcation of the right and left hepatic ducts

How is the diagnosis of cholangiocarcinoma made?

Ultrasound, abdominal CT, ERCP, and angiography may be useful in localizing the tumor and staging the disease.

° In collaboration with C. Yoshida, G. Goldin, and C. Matthews

Are serum AFP levels elevated in patients with cholangiocarcinoma?	No.
What is the treatment for cholangiocarcinoma?	Surgery is the only definitive therapy. Resectable tumors of the distal bile duct are associated with a 60% 1-year survival rate. Arterial or portal vein involvement precludes resection. ERCP with stent placement and PTC with drainage may be useful palliative procedures to relieve biliary obstruction.
What is the prognosis for cholangiocarcinoma?	Poor with unresectable tumors, with an overall 6- to 12-month survival expectation.

GENITOURINARY CANCER

RENAL CELL CARCINOMA*

In the United States, what are the yearly incidence and mortality rate of renal cell carcinoma?	29,000 new cases with 12,000 deaths per year.
What are risk factors for renal cell carcinoma?	Smoking history, family history, obesity, phenacetin-induced nephropathy, acquired cystic disease in hemodialysis patients, male gender (male to female incidence is 2:1), age 50–70 years, occupational exposure to asbestos, cadmium, leather tannery, and petroleum products
What cytogenetic abnormalities are frequently associated with renal cell carcinomas?	Deletion of 3p, and t(3;8) and t(3;11)
What autosomal dominant disorder is associated with the development of renal cell carcinoma?	von Hippel-Lindau disease, which is associated with the development of multiple tumors, including renal cell carcinoma. This disorder is thought to be secondary to the loss of a tumor suppressor gene on 3p.

---

* In collaboration with C. Gadebeku, S. Koenig, S. Warren, S. Schmidt, and C. Shen

What is the most common presenting symptom in renal cell carcinoma?

Hematuria

Renal cell carcinoma is sometimes referred to as the internist's tumor. Why?

Many patients with renal cell carcinoma can secrete substances that produce signs of systemic disease. Some of the more common findings are pyrexia, cachexia, anemia, nonmetastatic liver dysfunction, amyloidosis, polycythemia, and hypercalcemia.

What is the classic triad associated with renal cell carcinoma?

Flank pain, abdominal mass, and hematuria occur in < 20% of cases.

What percent of patients at presentation have metastatic disease?

30%. Locally advanced disease is seen in 25% of patients at presentation and local disease in 45%. The average size of tumors at presentation is 7 cm.

What are the common sites of metastases in renal cell carcinoma?

Lung (75%), soft tissue (35%), bone (20%), skin (11%), liver (20%), and brain (8%)

What is the most common histopathologic subtype of renal cell carcinoma?

Clear cell carcinoma comprises 75% of the histopathologic diagnoses.

What cell type does renal cell carcinoma arise from?

Proximal renal tubular epithelium

How is renal cell carcinoma staged?

Stage I—within kidney
Stage II—within Gerota's fascia
Stage IIIA—involvement of the renal vein or inferior vena cava
Stage IIIB—involvement of hilar lymph nodes
Stage IV—metastatic disease

What is the treatment of localized renal cell carcinoma?

Radical nephrectomy with lymphadenectomy. Two thirds of patients with stage I and stage II disease survive 5 years.

In addition to surgical resection, what cytotoxic chemotherapy or radiation therapy improves the survival rate?

No adjuvant chemotherapy or radiation treatment has demonstrated benefit in postoperative treatment of renal cell carcinoma.

In patients with metastatic renal cell carcinoma, should a nephrectomy be performed?

Yes. Nephrectomy is indicated to relieve pain, hemorrhage, and paraneoplastic syndromes in patients. Some argue that prophylactic nephrectomy is the standard of practice.

Can patients with metastatic renal cell carcinoma be cured?

Yes. Occasionally, patients with isolated pulmonary or brain metastasis can be cured with surgical resection of the metastatic foci.

What biological therapies are used in renal cell carcinoma?

Interleukin-2 and interferon have 15%–20% response rates in metastatic renal cell carcinoma, with a few responses lasting many years.

Why does cytotoxic chemotherapy have little or no effect in renal cell carcinoma?

Renal cell carcinoma expresses high levels of the multidrug-resistant P-glycoprotein, which detoxifies many of the chemotherapy drugs.

PROSTATE CANCER

What is the incidence of prostate cancer in the United States?

It is estimated that more than 134,000 men will be diagnosed with prostate cancer and approximately 32,000 will die from this disease yearly, making it the most common cause of cancer and the second leading cause of cancer death among men in the United States.

What are the risk factors for clinically evident prostate cancer?

The incidence of clinically evident prostate cancer varies significantly with geographic location, with developed countries carrying the highest risk of disease. Dietary factors (high-fat diet) are presumed to play a role in this geographic variation. In the United States, blacks are at greater risk for prostate cancer than whites, as are individuals with a family history of this malignancy.

What is the natural history of prostate cancer?

More than 30% of men older than 50 years of age have latent foci of prostate cancer detected at the time of autopsy, although only 1% of men with cancer are diagnosed with clinically evident prostate cancer and only 0.3% of this same group die of the disease. An important distinction is that most cancers detected at the time of autopsy are small and of low grade, whereas clinically evident tumors tend to be large and of higher grade. This supports a multistep process in the development of life-threatening prostate cancer.

What are the presenting symptoms of prostate cancer?

Most cases of prostate cancer are clinically silent. Occasionally, patients have symptoms of obstruction. Less often, patients have symptoms related to metastatic disease.

How are prostate cancers diagnosed?

Digital rectal examination, transrectal ultrasonography and biopsy, and PSA measurements are all useful procedures in the diagnosis of prostate cancer.

What are the histologic subtypes of prostate cancer?

The proximal ducts of the prostate give rise to 98% of all prostate cancers, of which the most common histologic subtype is adenocarcinoma. Additional histologic subtypes arising from the proximal ducts include mucinous carcinoma, adenoid cystic carcinoma, carcinoid tumors, and undifferentiated cancers. The distal ducts give rise to 2% of cancers of the prostate including the following histologic subgroups: transitional cell carcinoma, squamous cell carcinoma, papillary carcinoma, and ductal cancer.

How are prostate cancers graded?

The Gleason system is the most widely accepted method of grading prostate cancers. It uses five histologic patterns, which are assigned grade numbers, and combines primary and secondary grade numbers into a single histologic number.

The higher the grade number, the more aggressive the histologic makeup.

How is prostate cancer staged?

Stage A1—focal microscopic disease
Stage A2—diffuse microscopic disease
Stage B—microscopic disease confined to the prostate
Stage C—extracapsular extension
Stage D—metastatic disease

How is prostate cancer treated?

Radiation therapy, radical prostatectomy, and watching and waiting are the three treatment approaches for early stage disease (stages A and B). Patients with no significant comorbid medical problems and a life expectancy of > 10 years are usually offered either surgery or radiation therapy. In late stage disease (stage C or D), anti-testosterone hormonal treatment is effective as initial treatment. Chemotherapy for hormone-refractory metastatic prostate cancer is not very effective, with response rates of 20%–50%, and responses are usually of short duration.

What are potential complications of radical prostatectomy?

Thrombophlebitis, lymphocele, incontinence (permanent incontinence is rare), and impotence

What are potential complications of prostate radiotherapy?

Impotence, urinary frequency, dysuria, temporary tenesmus, diarrhea, bleeding, rectal wall fibrosis, impaired function of the rectal ampulla, and ureteral stenosis

What test is effective in following up prostate cancer patients after treatment?

Serial measurement of PSA

What is the stage-specific 5-year actuarial survival (treated) for the following stages of prostate cancer:
    Stage A

85%

    Stage B

75%

Stage C	65%
Stage D	25%

TESTICULAR CANCER

What is the incidence of testicular cancer?
Testicular cancer makes up only 1% of all male malignancies, but it is the most common neoplasm in the 15- to 35-year-old age-group.

What is the cure rate for testicular cancer?
85%

What are risk factors for testicular cancer?
Cryptorchidism

What are symptoms of testicular cancer?
Testicular swelling is the most common symptom. However, testicular pain occurs in 20%–50% of cases. It is a common misconception that a painful testicular mass excludes malignancy. Other symptoms include swelling of breasts (gynecomastia) or pain in the breasts. Back or flank pain occurs in association with retroperitoneal lymph node metastases. Chest pain, cough, and shortness of breath are seen in mediastinal or lung metastases.

What is the differential diagnosis of a testicular mass?
Epididymitis, hydrocele, varicocele, spermatocele, and testicular torsion

What characteristics suggest testicular carcinoma?
A firm, hard, nontender mass, which has appeared gradually over a period of weeks to months. A mass that has been present for a long time (i.e., years) is not likely to be a cancer. As discussed, a painful mass does not exclude cancer.

What test is used as the initial workup of a testicular mass?
Ultrasound. Any suspicious testicular mass in a young male warrants an ultrasound. It is not unreasonable for treatment to include a course of antibiotics for epididymitis without an ultrasound as long as there is close and reliable follow-up.

What procedure should be done to biopsy a suspicious testicular mass?

Trans-scrotal orchiectomy and needle biopsy are contraindicated in testicular cancer because the lymphatic drainage of the scrotum is different than that of the testicle. Contamination of the scrotum with cancer occurs in 25% of trans-scrotal orchiectomies and requires inclusion of inguinal lymph nodes in addition to the retroperitoneal lymph nodes in the radiation port.

What tests are used in the workup of testicular cancer?

CT scan of the chest, abdomen, and pelvis
Bilateral testicular ultrasound
CBC and chemistry panel, which includes evaluation of liver and renal function, lactate dehydrogenase, β-HCG, and AFP

What are the histologic subtypes of testicular cancer and GCT?

Seminoma, embryonal carcinoma, choriocarcinoma, yolk sac, and teratoma

What chromosome mutation occurs in 90% of GCTs?

Isochromosome 12

Do all GCTs arise within the testicle?

No. As many as 5% of GCTs are termed extragonadal. Extragonadal GCTs arise as a result of malignant transformation of residual midline germinal elements, usually in the mediastinum and retroperitoneum, but occasionally within the pineal gland and sacrococcygeal area.

What is the most common GCT?

Seminoma comprises 40% of GCTs. The other histologic subtypes are referred to as NSGCTs.

What is the natural history of GCT?

GCTs classically spread to retroperitoneal lymph nodes then to mediastinal lymph nodes, liver, and lung.

What are the common sites of metastases for GCTs?

Retroperitoneal and mediastinal lymph nodes, lung, and liver. Bone and brain metastases are rare.

What percent of seminomas are confined to the testicle at presentation?	70%
What percent of NSGCTs are confined to the testicle at presentation?	30%–40%
Which GCT typically results in elevation of β-HCG?	Choriocarcinoma. Seminomas can have an elevated β-HCG, but it is usually < 100. Embryonal carcinoma can also have an elevated β-HCG.
Which GCT typically has an elevated AFP?	Yolk sac and embryonal carcinoma. Pure choriocarcinoma and seminoma do not have an elevated AFP.
What other conditions can elevate β-HCG?	Cancer of prostate, bladder, kidney, and ureter, marijuana use, and pregnancy
What other conditions can elevate the AFP?	Pregnancy, hepatocellular carcinoma, and gastric cancer
How are GCTs staged?	Stage I (A)—tumor confined to the testicle Stage IIA (B1)—minimally bulky RPLNs Stage IIB (B2)—moderately bulky RPLNs Stage IIC (B3)—bulky RPLN Stage III (C)—supradiaphragmatic disease (mediastinal, lung, or liver) Stage IV—extranodal spread (some authors do not use stage IV; rather, they combine mediastinal lymphadenopathy with visceral metastases)
How is stage I seminoma managed?	Radical transinguinal orchiectomy with 25- to 35-Gy radiation therapy to retroperitoneal lymph nodes. Radical transinguinal orchiectomy followed by close observation is a reasonable alternative, probably with an equivalent 5-year survival rate.

How is stage I NSGCT managed?	Radical inguinal orchiectomy with RPLND. Surveillance and adjuvant chemotherapy in lieu of RPLND is an alternative but is not standard.
What is the management of stage II seminoma?	Radiation therapy
What is the management of stage II NSGCT?	Stage IIA and B—RPLND and chemotherapy Stage IIC—chemotherapy
What is the management of all stage III GCTs?	Chemotherapy
What chemotherapy is used?	Cisplatin, etoposide, and bleomycin
What is the 5-year survival rate of seminoma for the following:	
Stage I	> 95%
Stage II	> 95%
Stage III	80%
What is the 5-year survival of NSGCT for the following:	
Stage I	> 95%
Stage II	90%–95%
Stage III	70%
What is the treatment of EGGCT?	Chemotherapy

OVARIAN CANCER

How common is ovarian cancer?	It is the fourth leading cause of cancer death in women, with 22,000 cases reported per year.

When and at what stage does ovarian cancer present?	The peak incidence is in the 6th decade of life; at the time of diagnosis, 70% of women have advanced disease.
What are the risk factors for ovarian cancer?	Uninterrupted ovulation (nulliparity and late age of first pregnancy), Peutz-Jeghers syndrome, gonadal dysgenesis, Lynch II cancer syndrome, hereditary breast-ovarian cancer syndrome (BRCA1), and hereditary breast cancer syndrome (BRCA2). Use of oral contraceptives is protective.
What are symptoms of ovarian cancer?	Increased abdominal girth, abdominal pain, and dysfunctional uterine bleeding are the most common presenting symptoms.
What are the physical findings of ovarian cancer?	Ovarian cancer localizes predominantly to the abdomen and pelvis. Ascites, an ovarian mass, and a palpable intraabdominal mass are the most common physical findings. An umbilical lymph node (Sister Mary Joseph node), as well as axillary and inguinal adenopathy and pleural effusions are occasionally seen.
What is the workup for patients with suspected ovarian cancer?	H & P with a careful pelvic examination, CBC, biochemical profile, CA125, chest radiograph, and pelvic ultrasound. Some patients need a more extensive evaluation to include a CT scan of the abdomen, intravenous pyelography, cystoscopy, proctoscopy, barium enema, or upper gastrointestinal evaluation.
Under what circumstances should a patient with an adnexal mass warrant consideration for surgical exploration?	The patient is premenarchal or postmenopausal. The mass > 8 cm. Complex cysts are shown on ultrasound. There is an increase in size or persistence of the cyst through 2–3 menstrual cycles. The masses are solid and irregular, fixed, or bilateral. There is pain associated with the mass. There is ascites.

Do all patients with ovarian cancer have elevated CA125 levels?	No. However, 80% of patients with advanced disease and 50% of patients with early stage disease have elevated CA125 levels.
What are the most common sites of metastases for ovarian cancer?	Serosal surfaces of intraabdominal tissues and retroperitoneal lymph nodes are the most common sites of metastases. Pelvic lymph nodes, liver, lung, bone, and brain metastases can occur.
What is the staging for ovarian cancer?	Stage I—tumor limited to the ovaries Stage IA—one ovary, intact capsule, no ascites Stage IB—both ovaries, intact capsule, no ascites Stage IC—ruptured capsule, capsular involvement, positive peritoneal washings, or malignant ascites Stage II—ovarian tumor with pelvic involvement Stage IIA—pelvic extension to the uterus or tubes Stage IIB—pelvic extension to other pelvic organs (bladder, rectum, or vagina) Stage IIC—pelvic extension and positive findings in stage IC Stage III—tumor outside the pelvis or positive nodal involvement Stage IIIA—microscopic seeding outside the pelvis Stage IIIB—gross deposits less than or equal to 2 cm Stage IIIC—gross deposits > 2 cm or positive nodal involvement Stage IV—distant organ involvement including the liver or pleural space
What are the histologic subtypes of ovarian cancer?	Epithelial carcinomas comprise 85% of cases and all are approached in essentially the same way. GCTs and sex cord stromal tumors are the predominant nonepithelial tumors and are managed differently.

What is the surgical treatment for ovarian cancer?	Bilateral salpingo-oophorectomy, omentectomy with careful examination of all serosal surfaces, biopsy of suspicious and grossly involved areas, collection of ascites and peritoneal washings, and debulking of all gross disease. If the disease is limited to the ovary, then an RPLND is performed for additional staging.
What paraneoplastic syndromes are seen in ovarian carcinoma?	Hypercalcemia, cerebellar degeneration (pancerebellar dysfunction associated with extensive Purkinje cell loss), sign of Leser-Trélat (sudden increase in the size and number of seborrheic keratosis), and Trousseau's sign (migratory thrombophlebitis)
What is the postoperative management of stage I and II patients?	For stage IA and IB good-risk patients (well or moderately well differentiated histologic grade), no further treatment is indicated. In poor-risk stage I and II, postoperative adjuvant chemotherapy with a cisplatin-based regimen is the standard.
What is the management of stage III and IV (advanced) ovarian cancer?	Following an optimal surgical procedure, adjuvant chemotherapy is with cisplatin or carboplatin and paclitaxel or cyclophosphamide for six cycles. Intraperitoneal chemotherapy is a consideration in optimally debulked stage IIIA and IIIB patients.
What are the survival rates for the following:	
Stage IA and IB with good prognostic factors	> 90% cure rate with surgery alone
Stage II patients or stage I patients with poor prognostic factors and stage IC	60% cure rate with surgery plus adjuvant chemotherapy
Stage IIIA and IIIB	25%–40% cure rate with surgery and adjuvant chemotherapy

Stage IIIC and IV   < 10% cure rate with surgery and adjuvant chemotherapy

CARCINOMA OF UNKNOWN PRIMARY SITE

What is the median survival for persons with carcinoma of unknown primary site?

3–4 months. However, certain subsets of patients can achieve significant palliative benefit and a few can be cured. Few diagnoses in medicine evoke such dismal pessimism as carcinoma of unknown primary site.

What is the workup of a patient suspected to have carcinoma of unknown primary site?

A careful and thorough H & P with pelvic and rectal examination, CBC, chemistry profile, chest radiograph, and CT scan of the abdomen. Biopsy of the most accessible suspected lesion must be done to confirm the diagnosis of a cancer.

Should anyone suspected of having metastatic cancer ever be treated for cancer without a tissue diagnosis?

No. Only under the most unusual circumstances should a patient be given a diagnosis of cancer without a tissue diagnosis, much less be treated.

Should patients with a diagnosis of cancer of unknown primary site undergo an extensive endoscopic and radiographic evaluation to look for a primary site?

No. Endoscopic and radiographic evaluation should be directed toward symptoms and identifying treatable malignancies.

What are the potential histologic diagnoses?

Adenocarcinoma (60%), PDC or PDA (30%), poorly differentiated malignant neoplasm (5%), and squamous cell carcinoma (5%)

What are the treatable forms of adenocarcinoma of unknown primary site?

Breast and ovarian cancer in women and prostate cancer in men. A mammogram and a complete pelvic examination should be done in women, and PSA and rectal examination should be done in men.

What are the treatable forms of PDC and PDA of unknown primary site?	NHL, GCT variants, and malignancies with neuroendocrine features. A small percentage (3%–5%) of these cases are NHL and are therefore potentially curable.
In whom should a GCT variant be suspected?	In a young patient with predominantly midline disease (mediastinal and retroperitoneal lymphadenopathy). However, in any patient with a good performance status with the diagnosis of PDA or PDC, it is not unreasonable to obtain an AFP and β-HCG and treat with chemotherapy for an extragonadal GCT.
Can PDC and PDA with neuroendocrine features be cured with chemotherapy?	No. However, in a patient with a good performance status, a chemotherapy regimen for SCLC may provide significant palliative benefit.
What percent of poorly differentiated malignant neoplasms are NHL?	30%–70% (found by special stain)
What is the management of squamous cell carcinoma in an isolated cervical lymph node?	Squamous cell carcinoma involving a solitary cervical lymph node is usually the result of a head and neck primary and can be cured with a radical neck dissection, radiation therapy, or both. A careful head and neck examination should be undertaken, including inspection of the oropharynx, nasopharynx, hypopharynx, larynx, and upper esophagus.
What is the management of squamous cell carcinoma in an inguinal lymph node?	Careful evaluation of the anorectum, vagina, cervix, and penis. These malignancies are potentially curable with surgery, chemoradiotherapy, or both.
What is the management of adenocarcinoma in an isolated axillary lymph node in a woman?	A mammogram should be performed, followed by a modified radical mastectomy with axillary node dissection. Adjuvant chemotherapy, radiotherapy, or both should be offered according to the final pathologic stage. The survival rate is no different than that for a patient

whose initial presentation of disease is with a breast mass and involved axillary nodes.

What is the management of peritoneal carcinomatosis and pathologic findings demonstrating adenocarcinoma in a woman?

Laparotomy with consideration of a debulking procedure as in patients with ovarian carcinoma. Postoperative chemotherapy is recommended if, after the debulking procedure, ovarian cancer is suspected.

8

Infectious Disease

ABBREVIATIONS

AIDS	Acquired immune deficiency syndrome
ALT	Alanine aminotransferase
APH	Acute pulmonary histoplasmosis
AST	Aspartate aminotransferase
BSI	Bloodstream infection
CBC	Complete blood count
CMV	Cytomegalovirus
CNS	Central nervous system
CPH	Chronic pulmonary histoplasmosis
CSF	Cerebrospinal fluid
CPK	Creatine phosphokinase
CT	Computed tomography
DEET	Diethyltoluamide
EBV	Epstein-Barr virus
ESR	Erythrocyte sedimentation rate
FTA-ABS	Fluorescent treponemal antibody, absorbed
FUO	Fever of unknown origin
GC	Gonococcus

GU	Gonococcal urethritis
HIV	Human immunodeficiency virus
HPF	High-power field
HSV	Herpes simplex virus
Ig	Immunoglobulin
IVDA	Intravenous drug abuse
KOH	Potassium hydroxide
LFT	Liver function test
MAC	*Mycobacterium avium* complex
MHA-TP	Microhemagglutination-*Treponema pallidum*
MRI	Magnetic resonance imaging
MRSA	Methicillin-resistant *Staphylococcus aureus*
NGU	Nongonococcal urethritis
NK	Natural killer
PCP	*Pneumocystis carinii* pneumonia
PCR	Polymerase chain reaction
PDH	Progressive disseminated histoplasmosis
PID	Pelvic inflammatory disease
PMN	Polymorphonuclear neutrophil
PZA	Pyrazinamide
RPR	Rapid plasma reagin
SBP	Spontaneous bacterial peritonitis

SIRS	Systemic inflammatory response syndrome
STD	Sexually transmitted disease
TSS	Toxic shock syndrome
UTI	Urinary tract infection
VDRL	Venereal Disease Research Laboratory
VZV	Varicella zoster virus
WBC	White blood cell

DIAGNOSTIC METHODS

What methods are used to identify a pathogen?	1. Microscopic examination 2. Growth or biochemical characteristics in culture 3. Immunologic techniques to identify antigens or antibodies 4. DNA probes
What types of stains are used to identify pathogens?	Gram stain, acid-fast stain, Ziehl-Neelsen, Kinyoun, Wright's, KOH, India ink, Gomori's methenamine silver, Tzanck
How is the Gram stain performed?	Crystal violet binds to the cell wall after treatment with a weak iodine solution. Some bacteria retain the crystal violet, even after a decolorizer is added. The organisms that retain dye are called gram positive (stain purple) and those with a high lipid content lose the purple color and pick up the counterstain (safranin). These are called gram negative.
How is the acid-fast stain performed?	Mycobacteria have a high lipid and wax content in the cell wall that resists staining; but, once stained, it is not decolorized, even by acid alcohol (called acid fast). The acid-fast organisms are red against a blue-green background.

What is different about the Ziehl-Neelsen stain?	Heat is used to pretreat the organisms so the primary stain can penetrate the cell wall.
What temperature method is used for the Kinyoun stain?	A cold method in which detergent is used to pretreat the organisms
What is the Wright's stain used for?	To identify WBCs in stool wet mount
What is the KOH prep used for?	To identify candida or other fungal elements
How is an India ink stain used?	Cytocentrifuge of CSF with a drop of India ink on a slide is used to identify the capsule of cryptococcus.
What organisms is the Gomori's methenamine silver stain used to identify?	PCP and fungi
How is the Tzanck stain performed and what is it used for?	A vesicle suspected of being caused by a virus is unroofed, its base is scraped, and the material is placed on a glass slide. The material is treated with Wright's stain or methylene blue. The presence of multinucleated giant cells indicate herpesvirus infection.
Name the types of cultures that can be obtained.	1. Throat—90% sensitive for streptococcal pharyngitis
	2. Lower respiratory—fewer than 10 epithelial cells and more than 25 PMNs per low-power field are needed for adequate sputum specimen.
	3. Urine—need "clean catch" midstream urine specimen. If a catheter is in place, disinfect the tubing and collect directly with a sterile needle and syringe. Do not collect the specimen from the bag.
	4. Blood cultures—avoid femoral veins and areas of indwelling catheters, for which there is a higher rate of contamination. In general, draw two

sets to avoid obtaining one positive culture with a potential contaminant.
5. Body fluids—collect in a sterile fashion.
6. CSF—collect serum simultaneously for glucose determination.
7. Viral—use special transport media if the specimen is from throat or skin; buffy coat for HSV and CMV.

What is direct immunofluorescence?

Antigens or antibodies are directly labeled and detected by fluorescent microscopy.

What is PCR?

Polymerase chain reaction. It uses the enzyme DNA polymerase to increase the number of copies (amplify) of DNA or RNA in a sample. PCR is very sensitive because only a few copies of genetic material (and not whole organisms) need to be present. It is useful for organisms that are difficult to culture (including HIV).

What is serologic testing used for?

To diagnose infection when the pathogen cannot be cultured. Measure acute and convalescent sera to detect a fourfold increase in titer (synonymous with recent infection). Diagnosis can only be made retrospectively.

ANTIMICROBIAL THERAPY

GENERAL PRINCIPLES

In which diseases is bactericidal therapy mandatory?

Meningitis, endocarditis, brain abscess, osteomyelitis, and neutropenia

What are reasons for antimicrobial treatment failure?

Development of resistance in vivo, superinfection, decreased activity at the site of infection (e.g., necrotic tissue, foreign body, and lack of penetration into abscess), impaired immune host defenses, improper dosing, and altered pharmacokinetics secondary to drug interactions

What are reasons for combination therapy?

1. To prevent resistance
2. To treat polymicrobial infections
3. To treat single infections with uncertain susceptibility
4. To create synergy
5. To "protect" the antibiotic (e.g., by adding a β-lactamase such as sulbactam to ampicillin)

What is synergy?

Antimicrobial agents are synergistic when their combined effect is greater than the sum of their independent effects.

What is antagonism?

Agents are antagonistic when the activity of the combination is less than the sum of their independent activities.

ANTIBACTERIAL AGENTS

What are the major classifications of penicillins?

Natural penicillins—penicillin G, penicillin V
Penicillinase-resistant—methicillin, nafcillin, dicloxacillin, oxacillin
Aminopenicillins—ampicillin, amoxicillin
Antipseudomonal penicillins—piperacillin, mezlocillin, ticarcillin

What is the antimicrobial spectrum of penicillins?

Penicillin G and penicillin V—most aerobic gram-positive organisms
Aminopenicillins—added activity against some gram-negative rods
Antipseudomonal penicillins—extended activity against gram-negative organisms

Do penicillins cover anaerobes?

The natural penicillins, aminopenicillins, and pseudomonal penicillins are effective for many anaerobes, but not *Bacteroides fragilis.*

What is the incidence of hypersensitivity reactions with penicillins?

0.7%–4%

Name the four types of penicillin hypersensitivity reactions.

Type 1 (IgE)—urticaria, angioedema, anaphylaxis. Frequency is 0.02%; mortality rate is 10%.

Type 2 (IgG)—hemolytic anemia

Type 3 (immune complexes)—serum sickness

Type 4 (cell mediated)—contact dermatitis, idiopathic maculopapular rash, interstitial nephritis, drug fever, eosinophilia, exfoliative dermatitis, Stevens-Johnson syndrome

What is the best way to exclude a Type 1 IgE-mediated reaction?

Negative skin testing excludes an IgE-mediated response with > 97% assurance.

What is the incidence of cross-reactivity of allergy between penicillins and cephalosporins?

Approximately 5%–10%. It is recommended that patients with a history of immediate hypersensitivity reaction to penicillin should not receive a cephalosporin.

What is the antimicrobial spectrum of first-generation cephalosporins?

Most gram-positive cocci (except enterococci, MRSA, and coagulase-negative staphylococci), *Escherichia coli*, *Klebsiella pneumoniae*, and *Proteus mirabilis*

What is the antimicrobial spectrum of second-generation cephalosporins?

Less active against gram-positive cocci than first-generation cephalosporins; more active against some gram-negative organisms such as *Haemophilus influenzae*, *Enterobacter* species and some *Proteus* species

What is the antimicrobial spectrum of third-generation cephalosporins?

Expanded activity against gram-negative rods. Cefotaxime and ceftriaxone have slightly less activity against gram-positive cocci than first-generation cephalosporins. Ceftazidime and cefoperazone have even less activity against gram-positive cocci, but are excellent antipseudomonal agents.

What is the antimicrobial spectrum of imipenem?

Most gram-positive and gram-negative aerobic and anaerobic pathogens except for *Pseudomonas cepacia*,

Stenotrophomonas maltophilia, and MRSA

What serious adverse reactions can imipenem cause?

In addition to allergic reactions and leukopenia, imipenem may cause seizures, particularly in patients with underlying CNS disease or impaired renal function.

What is the antimicrobial spectrum of aztreonam?

Activity against aerobic gram-negative rods (similar to that of aminoglycosides)

What are the three β-lactamase inhibitors?

Clavulanate, sulbactam, and tazobactam

The addition of clavulanate to amoxicillin enhances the antimicrobial activity against which organisms?

Activity is increased substantially against β-lactamase producing *H. influenzae, Moraxella catarrhalis*, staphylococci, *Neisseria gonorrhoeae, E. coli, K. pneumoniae, Proteus* species, and *B. fragilis*.

What is the antimicrobial spectrum of aminoglycosides?

Primarily, activity is against aerobic and facultative gram-negative rods.

What are the most commonly used aminoglycosides?

Gentamicin, tobramycin, amikacin, and streptomycin

What are major adverse effects of aminoglycosides?

Nephrotoxicity in 5%–25% of patients and ototoxicity (vestibular or auditory) in 0.5%–3% of patients. Renal toxicity is usually reversible; ototoxicity is frequently irreversible.

How can aminoglycoside toxicity be avoided?

Careful monitoring of blood levels, serial measurements of serum creatinine, and monitoring for ototoxicity

What is the antimicrobial spectrum of tetracyclines?

Tetracyclines are the drug of choice for Rocky Mountain spotted fever, ehrlichiosis, and *Chlamydia* infections; *Borrelia burgdorferi* and *Mycoplasmas* are also susceptible. Although there may be broad activity against gram-positive cocci and *E. coli*, resistance in hospital-acquired strains is common.

What are major toxicities of tetracyclines?

Discoloration of teeth and bones in children younger than 8 years of age; photosensitivity

What is the antimicrobial spectrum of chloramphenicol?

Broad-spectrum activity against bacteria, many spirochetes, *Rickettsia*, *Chlamydia*, and *Mycoplasmas*. It does not reliably cover *Ehrlichia*.

What toxicities are associated with chloramphenicol?

Reversible bone marrow depression in adults receiving 4 g or more per day and aplastic anemia in approximately 1 in 30,000

What is the antimicrobial spectrum of rifampin?

Staphylococcus aureus, *Staphylococcus epidermidis*, *Neisseria meningitidis*, *N. gonorrhoeae*, *H. influenzae*, *Legionella*, and several mycobacterium species. However, rifampin resistance emerges rapidly with monotherapy. Practically, this drug is most useful (1) as one of several agents for mycobacterial infections, (2) as part of combination therapy with erythromycin in severely ill patients with legionellosis, and (3) occasionally as combination therapy for severe gram-positive infections.

What is the antimicrobial spectrum of metronidazole?

Anaerobes (strict anaerobes)

Through what routes is metronidazole absorbed?

Oral and intravenous dosing results in equivalent blood levels.

What are the macrolides?

Erythromycin, clarithromycin, and azithromycin

What is the antimicrobial spectrum of erythromycin?

Most gram-positive pathogens (including *Streptococcus pneumoniae*, *Streptococcus pyogenes*, *Corynebacterium diphtheriae*), *Bordetella pertussis*, *Legionella pneumophila*, *Mycoplasmas*, and *Chlamydia*

What are significant adverse effects of erythromycin?

Gastrointestinal complaints, transient hearing loss (especially at high doses), and possible cardiac toxicity (torsades de pointes) when given with terfenadine or astemizole

What is the antimicrobial spectrum of clarithromycin?

That of erythromycin plus activity against atypical mycobacteria and some *H. influenzae.* It has better activity against staphylococci and streptococci than erythromycin (2–4 times more active).

What is the antimicrobial spectrum of azithromycin?

Similar to erythromycin. It is 2–4 times less active than erythromycin against staphylococci and streptococci, and it is more active against *H. influenzae.* Single-dose therapy is effective for chlamydial infections.

What is the antimicrobial activity of clindamycin?

Gram-positive cocci and most anaerobes

What is the antimicrobial activity of vancomycin?

S. aureus, S. epidermidis, S. pyogenes, other streptococci, pneumococci, enterococci, *Corynebacterium,* and *Clostridium difficile*

Through what routes is vancomycin absorbed?

Vancomycin is effective in systemic infections only if given intravenously. The oral form is effective only against *C. difficile.*

What is the antimicrobial spectrum of trimethoprim–sulfamethoxazole?

S. aureus, S. pyogenes, S. pneumoniae, E. coli, Proteus mirabilis, Shigella, Salmonella, Pseudomonas cepacia, Pseudomonas pseudomallei, Yersinia, Pneumocystis carinii

What is the antimicrobial activity of quinolones?

Aerobic gram-negative rods, *Haemophilus,* gram-negative cocci (including *Neisseria* and *M. catarrhalis*), *Legionella, Mycoplasma, Chlamydia,* and mycobacteria. Quinolones are not the therapy of choice for infections with staphylococci and streptococci.

ANTIMYCOBACTERIAL AGENTS

What are first-line antimycobacterial agents?

Isoniazid (INH), rifampin, pyrazinamide, ethambutol, and streptomycin

What are major adverse effects of INH?

AST and ALT levels increase in 10%–20% of patients, particularly early in treatment. Severe liver damage is more frequent in patients older than 35 years.

What are major adverse effects of rifampin?

Rifampin may cause hepatotoxicity (particularly cholestatic changes) and gastrointestinal disturbances; it turns urine, tears, and other body fluids orange (contact lens wearers should be cautioned); and it increases metabolism of certain other drugs (e.g., it may reduce the effectiveness of oral contraceptives).

What are major adverse effects of ethambutol?

Optic neuritis and skin rash

What are major adverse effects of streptomycin?

Ototoxicity (particularly vestibular disturbances); less commonly, renal toxicity

What is the management of antimycobacterial drug-induced hepatotoxicity?

If transaminase levels increase to more than five times upper limits of normal, INH, rifampin, and PZA should be discontinued in favor of an alternative regimen. Possible hepatotoxic drugs are reintroduced one at a time to identify the offending agent.

What are second-line antimycobacterial agents?

Capreomycin, kanamycin, amikacin, cycloserine, ethionamide, ciprofloxacin, ofloxacin, and aminosalicylic acid (PAS)

ANTIFUNGAL AGENTS

What is the spectrum of activity of amphotericin B?

Most yeasts (including *Candida, Cryptococcus neoformans*), dimorphic fungi (including *Blastomyces dermatitidis, Histoplasma capsulatum, Coccidioides, Sporothrix*), and other fungi

What toxicities are associated with amphotericin B?	Dose-dependent decrease in glomerular filtration rate, potassium and bicarbonate wasting, decreased erythropoietin production, nausea, vomiting, phlebitis, and acute reactions
What acute reactions are associated with amphotericin B infusions?	Chills, fever, tachypnea, hypoxemia, and hypotension may occur 30 minutes after beginning infusion. Premedication with acetaminophen, hydrocortisone, or meperidine may diminish reactions.
What is the antimicrobial spectrum of fluconazole?	Most *Candida* species, *C. neoformans*, and coccidioidomycoses
Through what routes is fluconazole absorbed?	Fluconazole is well absorbed from the gastrointestinal tract; daily doses are the same for oral or intravenous administration.
What is the antimicrobial spectrum of itraconazole?	Blastomycosis and histoplasmosis. Itraconazole may have a role for *Aspergillus* infections when amphotericin B fails or cannot be administered.
What is the antimicrobial spectrum of ketoconazole?	Histoplasmosis and blastomycosis. Ketoconazole is not used commonly because of its side effects. Itraconazole is equally or more effective and less toxic.

ANTIVIRAL AGENTS

Which viruses are treated with acyclovir?	Systemic acyclovir is effective in treating HSV infections. If treatment is begun within 24 hours after a varicella zoster rash first appears, it decreases the severity of varicella in children and adults.
What are indications for amantadine and rimantidine?	When treatment is begun before exposure to influenza A virus, these agents are 70%–90% effective in preventing influenza. If begun within 2 days of the onset of illness, they may decrease the duration of symptoms by 1–2 days.

What are indications for ganciclovir?	Treatment and chronic suppression of CMV retinitis, pneumonia, and gastroenteritis in immunocompromised patients.
What toxicities are frequently associated with ganciclovir?	Reversible granulocytopenia and thrombocytopenia
What are indications for foscarnet?	Progressive CMV disease due to ganciclovir-resistant strains. It is used most often in AIDS patients with refractory CMV retinitis.
What are common side effects of foscarnet?	Renal toxicity, which is usually reversible

PATHOGENS

BACTERIA

What are bacteria?	A heterogeneous group of unicellular organisms (prokaryotes)
What is the difference between gram-positive and gram-negative bacteria?	There are structural differences in the cell wall of bacteria, so the staining properties on Gram stain are different.
What general histologic types of bacteria are there?	Gram-positive cocci, gram-positive bacilli, gram-negative cocci, and gram-negative bacilli
How can bacteria be further classified?	As aerobes or anaerobes
What are the following organisms and the common syndromes that go with each of the following:	
Gram-positive cocci	Staphylococci (*S. aureus*, coagulase negative), streptococci, enterococci *S. aureus*—bacteremia, infective endocarditis, skin and soft-tissue infection, pneumonia Group A streptococci—skin infection, pharyngitis *S. pneumoniae*—pneumonia, meningitis, otitis media

Enterococci—UTI, bacteremia, endocarditis

Viridans streptococci—infective endocarditis, abscess, dental infection

Gram-positive bacilli   *Bacillus, Corynebacteria, Listeria, Clostridium, Rhodococcus, Erysipelothrix*

Gram-negative cocci   *N. meningitidis, N. gonorrhoeae, M. catarrhalis*—genitourinary tract, respiratory, CNS, gastrointestinal, and abdominal infections and BSI. The cell wall contains lipopolysaccharide.

Gram-negative bacilli   *Shigella, Haemophilus, Enterobacteriaceae, Pseudomonas, Vibrio, Campylobacter, Brucella, Gardnerella, Pasteurella, Francisella, Helicobacter, Acinetobacter, Salmonella, Yersinia, Bordetella, Streptobacillus, Legionella, Capnocytophaga*

Which organisms are the anaerobes?   Peptostreptococci, *Clostridia, Bacterioides, Prevotella,* and *Fusobacterium.* Anaerobes cannot grow in typical concentrations of oxygen; some are strict anaerobes whereas others are facultative.

How do anaerobic infections occur?   Anaerobes gain access to usually sterile spaces or decreased vascular supply provides a lower oxygen tension, allowing colonizing anaerobes to proliferate. Usually, more than one type of organism is present in infection.

When should you suspect an anaerobic infection?   When there are both gram-positive and gram-negative organisms identified on Gram stain, there is foul-smelling pus, and gas is present. Some gram-negative bacilli can also produce gas.

Which are the higher bacteria and their common sites of infection?   *Actinomyces*—mouth, lung, abdomen
Nocardia—pneumonia, brain abscess

What are the sites of mycobacterial infection?	*Mycobacterium tuberculosis*—pulmonary disease is most common, but extrapulmonary disease can occur at any site. Atypical mycobacteria—a number of different organisms produce different diseases.
What are the spirochetes and their associated diseases?	*Treponema pallidum* (syphilis), *Leptospira*, *Borrelia* (Lyme disease, relapsing fever), *Spirillum minus* (rat-bite fever).
How are most of the rickettsial diseases transmitted, and what are the general diseases that they cause?	Most are transmitted by the bite of ticks—Rickettsiae, *Coxiella burnetii*, *Ehrlichia*. They produce multisystem disease, with most organisms producing a vasculitis.
What does *Bartonella* cause?	Bacillary angiomatosis and cat scratch disease

VIRUSES

How are viruses classified?	1. Type and structure of nucleic acid and method of replication 2. Type of symmetry of virus capsid 3. Presence or absence of an envelope

Herpesviruses

Name the herpesviruses.	HSV 1 and 2, VZV, CMV, EBV, human herpesviruses 6 and 7, and herpesvirus simiae
What is the pathogenesis of herpesvirus infection?	After acute infection, herpesviruses remain latent and can cause reactivation disease when a person becomes immunosuppressed.
What are routes of transmission for herpesviruses?	In humans only by direct contact, HSV 1 is spread via oral secretions, and HSV 2 is spread by sexual contact.
What are clinical manifestations of the following: **Primary HSV-1 infection?**	Gingivostomatitis and pharyngitis; patients are usually less than 5 years old.

Incubation is 2–12 days, followed by fever, sore throat, and development of vesicles, which persist for 10–14 days and then resolve.

Primary HSV-2 infection?

Genital infection. Incubation is 2–7 days, followed by fever, malaise, and lymphadenopathy with vesicular or ulcerative lesions on the genitalia. Lesions may last several days.

Recurrent HSV-1 infection?

Usually a prodrome of hours, after which lesions develop on the vermilion border of the outer lip, accompanied by significant pain. Lesions persist for 8–10 days.

Recurrent HSV-2 infection?

Less severe symptoms and less extensive disease than with primary infection. Prodrome is common, and virus can shed even when no lesions are present.

What are other manifestations of herpesviruses?

HSV encephalitis (typically HSV-1), neonatal infection, or infection in an immunocompromised host, resulting in severe infections of gastrointestinal tract, respiratory tract, or CNS

How is the diagnosis of herpesvirus infection made?

By growth of tissue culture (cytopathic effect is seen in 24–48 hours), demonstration of monoclonal antibody to viral antigen, immunohistochemistry, Tzanck smear of skin lesions, and serologic testing

What is the cytopathic effect of herpesvirus infection?

Changes in the normal appearance of cells in tissue culture due to infection with a virus

What is the treatment for herpesvirus infection?

Acyclovir. The dose, route, and duration vary with the type of infection.

Varicella Zoster Virus

What diseases are associated with VZV?

Primary infection—varicella (chickenpox)
Recurrent infection—herpes zoster (shingles)

What is the incidence of VZV infection?	Chickenpox, 3–4 million per year; zoster, 500,000 per year
What is the route of transmission for VZV?	Humans are the only reservoir. Varicella is assumed to be spread via the respiratory route; epidemics occur in late winter and early spring. Because zoster results from reactivation of latent virus in dorsal root ganglia, it does not require new contact. Zoster is contagious and can be spread by direct contact with lesions.

What are clinical manifestations of the following:

Varicella?	Prodrome of 1–2 days, followed by malaise, fever, and rash. Rash is maculopapular with vesicles (dewdrop on a rose petal) that form scabs. It is characteristic for lesions to be at various stages at one time. Rash starts on the face and trunk, and then spreads. New lesions develop over 2–4 days.
Zoster?	Unilateral vesicular lesions in dermatomal distribution. Thoracic and lumbar distributions are most common. Zoster can involve the eye (herpes zoster ophthalmicus). Disease is marked by acute neuritis and postherpetic neuralgia.

What are complications of the following:

Varicella?	Bacterial superinfection of lesions, encephalitis, cerebellar ataxia, and pneumonitis. Varicella is associated with Reye's syndrome.
Zoster?	Meningoencephalitis and disseminated disease in immunocompromised patients
What is the treatment for VZV?	Acyclovir for adolescents and adults (and for children if disease is severe), but there is no real effect on postherpetic neuralgia.

What is the Ramsay Hunt syndrome?

Pain and vesicles on the external auditory meatus, loss of taste on the anterior two thirds of the tongue, ipsilateral facial palsy, and involvement of the geniculate ganglion

How is the diagnosis of Ramsay Hunt syndrome made?

History and physical examination

How can Ramsay Hunt syndrome be prevented?

Immunocompromised patients exposed to varicella should receive varicella zoster immune globulin vaccine, which is particularly useful for seronegative, immunocompromised children and adults.

Cytomegalovirus

What are routes of transmission for CMV?

Blood, sexual contact, and perinatal exposure

What are clinical manifestations of CMV infection?

Congenital infection—three fourths of patients are asymptomatic. Symptoms include jaundice, hepatosplenomegaly, petechiae, and CNS involvement.
CMV mononucleosis—like EBV-related mononucleosis, with fever, mild lymphadenopathy, lymphocytosis, increased liver enzymes, and splenomegaly

What are complications of CMV infection?

The following complications are more common and more severe in the immunocompromised host: interstitial pneumonitis, hepatitis, Guillain-Barré syndrome, meningoencephalitis, myocarditis, thrombocytopenia and hemolysis, retinitis, and gastrointestinal disease.

How is the diagnosis of CMV infection made?

By viral culture or elevation in antibody titer. Rapid methods involve demonstration of monoclonal antibody to immediate early antigen in infected tissue, PCR, and nucleic acid probes.

What is the treatment for CMV infection?	In immunocompromised patients, ganciclovir or foscarnet

Epstein-Barr Virus

By what routes is EBV transmitted?	EBV is found in oropharyngeal secretions, but contagiousness is minimal. Intimate personal contact or contact with blood is necessary to spread EBV.
What are clinical manifestations of EBV infection?	Acute mononucleosis—sore throat, fever, lymphadenopathy, malaise, anorexia, and headache—which resolves over 2–3 weeks.
What are clinical manifestations in patients with EBV infection who are given ampicillin?	A maculopapular pruritic rash develops in 90%–100% of such patients.
What are complications of EBV infection?	Autoimmune hemolytic anemia, thrombocytopenia, splenic rupture (rare), encephalopathy, and other, less common, CNS manifestations
What other diseases are associated with EBV?	Burkitt's lymphoma, other lymphomas, nasopharyngeal carcinoma, and EBV-related lymphoproliferative syndrome
How is the diagnosis of EBV made?	Clinical manifestations and lymphocytosis with atypical lymphocytes are usually all that is required for diagnosis.
What are the laboratory findings in EBV infection?	Heterophile antibodies in > 90% of cases. Culture is not routinely available.
What is the time course or use for the following virus-specific antibodies: **Viral capsid antigens**	Occur early in disease and are seen at presentation in 80% of cases
IgM antibodies	Persist for only 4–8 weeks. Their presence is virtually diagnostic of acute EBV infection.

IgG antibodies	Persist for a lifetime
Early antigens and Epstein-Barr nuclear antigen?	These antibodies remain positive for life and are not helpful in diagnosing acute infection.
What is the treatment for EBV infection?	Treatment is supportive.
How are corticosteroids used in treatment of EBV infection?	Most authorities reserve use of steroids for specific indications, including impending airway obstruction, hemolytic anemia or severe thrombocytopenia, CNS involvement, myocarditis, or pericarditis.

Papillomaviruses

What are routes of transmission for papillomaviruses?	Close personal contact; anogenital warts are most commonly STDs.
What are clinical manifestations of papillomaviruses?	Plantar warts, flat and common warts, anogenital warts (certain types of papillomaviruses are associated with benign warts and some with cervical cancer), and recurrent respiratory papillomatosis.
How is the diagnosis of papillomavirus infection made?	Physical examination
What is the treatment for papillomavirus infection?	In general, most therapies involve physical or chemical destruction of visible lesions. For cutaneous lesions, salicylic acid, lactic acid, or cryotherapy is used. For anogenital lesions, podophyllin, podophyllotoxin, cryotherapy, trichloroacetic acid, electrosurgery, or 5-fluorouracil is used.

Mumps Virus

What is mumps virus infection?	Usually a benign, self-limited, acute viral infection that occurs typically in children and adolescents and involves nonsuppurative swelling and tenderness of the salivary glands, usually involving one or both parotids

How is mumps virus spread?	Direct contact, droplets, or fomites
What are clinical manifestations of mumps virus infection?	Incubation is 2–4 weeks. A nonspecific prodrome is followed by earache and pain over the parotid on the affected side. The gland enlarges and is tender. Fever to 40 degrees Celsius may occur. Meningitis occurs in up to 10% of patients with parotitis, but only 50% of patients with meningitis due to mumps have parotitis. Other neurologic syndromes occur but are more uncommon. Epididymo-orchitis is the most common finding in adult men, occurring in 20% of men with mumps.
How is the diagnosis of mumps infection made?	History of exposure and typical clinical findings
What is the treatment for mumps virus infection?	Treatment is supportive.

Measles

What are measles?	Acute viral infection caused by rubeola virus
How are measles spread?	Direct contact with infected respiratory secretions
What are clinical manifestations of measles?	Incubation is 10–14 days. Prodrome includes fever, anorexia, conjunctivitis, and respiratory symptoms. Koplik's spots appear just before the rash does. The erythematous, maculopapular rash starts on the face and spreads down the body to the extremities and finally to the palms and soles. Illness lasts approximately 7–10 days.
What are Koplik's spots?	Pathognomonic of measles, Koplik's spots are blue-gray lesions on a red base that appear on the buccal mucosa, often next to the second molars.
What are complications of measles?	Pneumonia and encephalitis

How is the diagnosis of measles made?	History and physical examination. The most common laboratory diagnosis is by serologic testing.
What is the treatment for measles?	Treatment is supportive. Oral vitamin A has been shown to decrease the severity of measles.

Influenza

What is influenza?	An acute febrile illness caused by influenza A or B that occurs in outbreaks during the winter
How is influenza virus spread?	Contact with respiratory secretions
What are clinical manifestations of influenza virus infection?	In uncomplicated influenza, incubation is 1–2 days followed by abrupt onset of fever, chills, headache, myalgias, malaise, and anorexia. Severity of symptoms correlates with the severity of fever and lasts 3 days. Respiratory symptoms of cough, nasal congestion, and sore throat last 3–4 days.
Describe the clinical situations for the following complications:	
Primary influenza pneumonia	More common in persons with cardiovascular disease. After initial symptoms of influenza, rapidly progressive pulmonary findings consistent with adult respiratory distress syndrome develop. Mortality rate is high.
Secondary bacterial pneumonia	Very similar to usual bacterial pneumonia. Elderly persons or those with underlying chronic diseases are at highest risk. Several days after a typical bout of influenza, fever and symptoms of bacterial pneumonia develop. Pathogens include S. pneumoniae, H. influenzae, and S. aureus.
What other complications of influenza can occur?	Other pulmonary processes, myositis, TSS, Guillain-Barré syndrome, and Reye's syndrome

How is the diagnosis of influenza made?	Isolation of virus or detection of viral antigen from respiratory secretions. Serologic testing is not clinically useful because there is a delay in making a diagnosis.
What is the treatment for influenza?	For uncomplicated influenza, amantadine or rimantidine; for pulmonary complications, supportive care, amantadine or rimantidine (consider ribavirin), and treatment of bacterial pathogens if present
How is infection with influenza virus prevented?	Immunization with trivalent inactivated vaccine against influenza A and B
Who should receive the influenza vaccine?	Persons at increased risk of complications from influenza, including persons older than age 65 years, residents of chronic care facilities, and persons with underlying chronic pulmonary or cardiovascular disease, significant metabolic disorders, hemoglobinopathies, renal dysfunction, or immunosuppression. Health care workers and other persons who provide care to individuals at risk should also be immunized.
How should chemoprophylaxis against influenza be administered?	Consider giving amantadine or rimantidine for high-risk individuals who have not received vaccine for the 5- to 7-week period of an outbreak. If vaccine is given simultaneously, give chemoprophylaxis for 2 weeks. It can also be used for individuals who are thought to have a weak response to vaccine or for those in whom vaccine is contraindicated.
What is Reye's syndrome?	CNS and hepatic complication of influenza infection (more common after influenza B infection). Almost all cases occur in children, and the mortality rate is 10% to 40%.
When does Reye's syndrome occur?	Usually 4–6 days after a viral infection

What are symptoms and signs of Reye's syndrome?	Nausea, vomiting, and altered mental status consistent with encephalopathy. Hepatomegaly and respiratory arrest occur. Ammonia level is commonly elevated. Hypoglycemia and elevated transaminases, bilirubin, CPK, and prothrombin time also occur.
What is the main cause of death from Reye's syndrome?	Cerebral edema. The pathophysiology is uncertain, but there appears to be a relation to aspirin. The use of aspirin should be avoided in children with fevers from influenza or varicella.

Enteroviruses

What are enteroviruses?	Coxsackieviruses, echoviruses, and enteroviruses
What are clinical manifestations of enterovirus infection?	Acute aseptic meningitis (group B coxsackie virus and echoviruses cause > 90% of cases), encephalitis, exanthems, acute respiratory disease (summer upper respiratory infections in children), herpangina (fever, sore throat and difficulty swallowing, macular lesions on soft palate evolve to vesicles), epidemic pleurodynia, myopericarditis, acute hemorrhagic conjunctivitis
How is the diagnosis of enterovirus infection made?	Virus can be isolated from the throat or feces.
What is the treatment for enterovirus infection?	Treatment is symptomatic.

Hepatitis viruses (see Chapter 5)

What are symptoms and signs of viral hepatitis?	The symptoms of acute hepatitis A, B, and C are indistinguishable. Anorexia, fatigue, myalgia, and nausea occur 1–2 weeks before the onset of jaundice. Patients may experience weight loss, headaches, arthralgia, vomiting, and right upper quadrant pain. Less commonly, cough, pharyngitis, rash, arthritis, and glomerulonephritis are seen. On physical examination, jaundice, hepatomegaly, or splenomegaly may be noted.

What level of bilirubin must be achieved for jaundice to be seen?	Greater than 2.5 mg/dl

Hepatitis A

What type of virus is associated with hepatitis A infection?	RNA picornavirus
How is hepatitis A transmitted?	Fecal–oral route, person to person contact, and contaminated food or water

Hepatitis B

What type of virus is associated with hepatitis B infection?	DNA virus
How is hepatitis B transmitted?	Parenterally (IVDA, blood transfusions), sexual contact, and perinatally. It is not transmitted by the fecal–oral route.

Hepatitis C

What type of virus is associated with hepatitis C?	Single-stranded RNA virus similar to flaviviruses; the cause of most cases of non-A, non-B hepatitis
What is the leading cause of transfusion-related hepatitis?	Hepatitis C, although the incidence is decreasing rapidly as a result of effective blood screening
What other ways is hepatitis C transmitted?	IVDA, sexual contact, and perinatal transmission

Hepatitis D

What type of virus is associated with hepatitis D?	A defective RNA virus that requires co-infection with hepatitis B virus (specifically HBsAg) for replication
What is the mode of transmission of hepatitis D?	Primarily the parenteral route, less often by sexual contact, and rarely perinatally

FUNGI

Candidiasis

What is the normal distribution of candidiasis?

Pathogens of candidiasis are common colonizers of mucocutaneous body surfaces that often become invasive with alterations in host status (e.g., in patients with indwelling catheters or in cases of diabetes mellitus, steroid and antibiotic use, mucosal damage, and immunosuppression).

What are major sites of candidal infection?

Oropharyngeal thrush and esophagitis (particularly in immunocompromised hosts), vaginitis, cutaneous infections, BSI, and disseminated disease

What are risk factors for disseminated candidiasis?

1. Being an impaired host (e.g., patients with neutropenia or HIV infection, transplant recipients, burn victims, and users of corticosteroids)
2. Having a central venous catheter
3. Receiving broad-spectrum antibiotics
4. Undergoing hyperalimentation
5. Having abdominal surgery

What are symptoms of disseminated disease?

Often, fever of unclear origin or septic shock with high fevers, hypotension, and end-organ damage. Multiple organs may be involved, including kidney, brain, myocardium, and eye.

What is found on physical examination in cases of candidiasis?

Macronodular skin lesions and endophthalmitis are clues that may lead to the diagnosis of disseminated disease. Endophthalmitis has been found in 15% of nonneutropenic patients with candidemia; therefore, in clinical situations in which candidemia is suspected, careful fundoscopic examination with ophthalmology consultation is advised.

How is the diagnosis of candidiasis made?

There must be a high index of suspicion. Premortem blood cultures are negative in up to 50% of autopsy-proven cases.

What are treatment principles for candidiasis?	1. Any patient with candidemia should receive treatment. 2. If disease is associated with intravascular catheters, then the catheters should be changed. 3. Nonneutropenic patients with clinically stable, uncomplicated line-related candidemia may be treated with intravenous fluconazole (or amphotericin B). 4. Patients who are clinically unstable or have evidence of hematogenous dissemination should be treated with amphotericin B.

Histoplasmosis

What is the organism associated with histoplasmosis?	A highly infectious dimorphic fungus found in soil called *H. capsulatum*. It grows particularly well in soil contaminated with bird or bat excreta.
What areas are endemic for histoplasmosis?	The central United States, especially the Ohio River and Mississippi River valleys, and certain other river valleys in temperate zones around the world
What is the incidence of histoplasmosis?	250,000 persons infected per year in the United States. Most cases are asymptomatic.
Name the three clinically important histoplasmosis syndromes.	APH, CPH, and PDH
What are risks for development of symptomatic acute pulmonary histoplasmosis (APH)?	Inhalation of a large inoculum and defective cell-mediated immunity
What are clinical features of acute pulmonary disease?	Patients are asymptomatic in 90% of cases. Symptoms include fever, headache, malaise, and nonproductive cough after a 3- to 21-day incubation period.

What do chest radiographs show in APH?	Typically, one or more patchy pneumonic infiltrates (more commonly in lower lung fields where the ventilation distribution is greater) with frequent hilar and mediastinal adenopathy. With heavier exposure, more confluent areas of pneumonitis may be seen.
What is the setting for chronic pulmonary histoplasmosis (CPH)?	Typically, CPH occurs in men older than 50 years of age with chronic obstructive pulmonary disease.
What are symptoms of CPH?	Persistent cough, weight loss, malaise, low-grade fevers, and night sweats over several weeks. Symptoms may mimic those of tuberculosis.
What are the chest radiographic findings in CPH?	Initially, interstitial infiltrate in apicoposterior area of lung; 20% eventually cavitate, whereas others contract, leading to scar formation and volume loss.
What is the setting of progressive disseminated histoplasmosis (PDH)?	PDH usually occurs in association with an underlying immunocompromised state, such as AIDS, lymphoma, leukemia, advanced cancer, or corticosteroid therapy. It also occurs in infants and young children.
What are clinical manifestations of PDH?	Severity of PDH ranges from acute illness to more chronic disease lasting for months to years. Manifestations may include hepatosplenomegaly with abnormal LFTs, gastrointestinal mucosal ulcerations, oropharyngeal ulcers, adrenal insufficiency, anemia, interstitial pneumonitis, and renal involvement. More rarely, CNS disease, lytic bone lesions, and lymphadenopathy occur.
How is the diagnosis of PDH made?	Culture—particularly of sputum, blood, bone marrow, or other suspected site of infection Diagnostic staining of yeast, which forms in tissue

Acute and convalescent serologic testing—may not be useful in immunocompromised patients

Antigen detection in urine and serum—useful in immunocompromised patients with suspected disseminated disease

What is the treatment for the following:

APH?

Often, no treatment is necessary. With more severe illness, itraconazole or amphotericin B may be used.

CPH?

Depending on the clinical course, amphotericin B or itraconazole

PDH?

In immunocompromised patients, amphotericin B; in other patients with milder subacute or chronic PDH, itraconazole

Blastomycosis

What is blastomycosis?

A relatively rare infection with the dimorphic fungus *B. dermatitidis*. Disease is usually confined to skin or lungs; rarely, it is disseminated.

What areas are endemic for blastomycosis?

In the United States, mostly the Mississippi River and Ohio River valleys and the mid-Atlantic and south central states

What are pulmonary manifestations of the following:

Acute pulmonary blastomycosis?

Manifestations are typically influenza-like with fevers, arthralgias, myalgias, and cough. Chest radiograph is nonspecific, often with localized consolidation; hilar adenopathy is rare.

Chronic pulmonary blastomycosis?

Manifestations include cough, sputum production, weight loss, hemoptysis, dyspnea, pleuritic chest pain, and nonspecific radiographic findings.

What are extrapulmonary manifestations of blastomycosis?

Cutaneous—40%–80% of cases (most common extrapulmonary site). Papulopustular eruptions may evolve into verrucous lesions; others become ulcerative.

Bone—one third of cases. Most commonly involved are ribs, vertebrae, and long bones, often with contiguous soft-tissue abscesses or chronic draining sinuses

Genitourinary tract—10%–30% of cases in men, primarily involving prostate, epididymis, or testis

Other sites—subcutaneous nodules, CNS, liver, spleen (adrenal insufficiency is rare)

How is the diagnosis of blastomycosis made?

Culture of fungus. A presumptive diagnosis can be made from some histopathologic specimens based on morphology and staining characteristics of fungal elements.

What is the treatment for blastomycosis?

Ketoconazole or itraconazole for immunocompetent patients with mild to moderate disease; amphotericin B for patients with life-threatening disease, CNS involvement, or those who are immunocompromised

Sporotrichosis

What organism is associated with sporotrichosis?

A saprophytic fungus called *Sporothrix schenckii*

What are clinical manifestations of sporotrichosis?

Primarily cutaneous. A papule, chancre, or subcutaneous nodule develops at the site of a traumatic inoculation. Secondary nodules, which often ulcerate and drain, develop along regional lymphatics. Osteoarticular involvement is the most common extracutaneous manifestation.

What hobbies and occupations put individuals at risk for sporotrichosis?

Gardening and farming

How is the diagnosis of sporotrichosis made?

Histopathologic examination of biopsy specimens may be suggestive but not diagnostic. Definitive diagnosis requires culture.

What is the treatment for sporotrichosis?

Saturated potassium iodide solution or itraconazole is usually effective. Because the organism is sensitive to higher temperatures, heat may be a useful adjunct therapy.

HOST DEFENSES

What are host defenses?

Specific and nonspecific responses to foreign substances (including microorganisms)

What are the nonspecific defenses?

Normal host flora, hereditary factors, natural antibodies, skin and mucosa, complement (via the alternative pathway), fibronectin, and phagocytosis

What are the specific defenses?

Antibodies and cell-mediated immunity

HUMORAL IMMUNITY

What are antibodies?

Glycoprotein immunoglobulins that bind specifically to proteins or polysaccharide antigens and are found circulating and on mucosal surfaces. There are five classes.

What are the five classes of antibodies?

1. IgM—first to appear (5–10 days) after an immune response to a new antigen
2. IgG—75% of all immunoglobulins in serum; also found in tissues
3. IgA—includes secretory IgA, which is the primary antibody in the secretions of the gastrointestinal and respiratory tracts
4. IgE—immediate-type hypersensitivity responses
5. IgD

What are the functions of antibodies?	1. Activation of complement 2. Performance of phagocytosis 3. Performance of antibody-dependent cellular cytotoxicity actions 4. Neutralization of toxins and viruses 5. Antiadhesion 6. Agglutination
What are the consequences of antibody deficiencies?	Increased risk of respiratory infections with *S. pneumoniae, H. influenzae, N. meningitidis* (encapsulated pathogens), and mycoplasma and increased incidence of sinusitis, otitis, and gastrointestinal infections

COMPLEMENT

What is complement?	30 proteins whose activation triggers various proteins to produce an inflammatory response and eliminate pathogens and immune complexes
How is complement activated?	Antigens and antibodies activate the classic pathway; polysaccharides, lipopolysaccharides, and teichoic acid activate the alternative pathway.
What is the result of complement deficiency?	The result depends on which component is deficient and whether that component is absent or reduced. The most common pathogen seen is meningococcus, which is responsible for 80% of infections.

PHAGOCYTOSIS

What cells are involved in phagocytosis?	Granulocytes—neutrophils, eosinophils, basophils
What is the function of neutrophils?	Phagocytosis of organisms followed by oxidative burst and degranulation
What types of neutrophil defects are there?	Decreased number—neutropenia (most common). With < 500 cells, there is a significantly increased risk of infection. Abnormal function—altered chemotaxis, ingestion, or microbicidal function

Defects can be inherited or acquired (e.g., through chemotherapy, drug reaction, splenic sequestration, aplastic anemia, or hematologic malignancy).

What pathogens occur in neutropenic patients?

Staphylococci, gram-negative bacilli, and fungi (*Candida, Aspergillus, Mucor*)

CELL-MEDIATED IMMUNITY

What is cell-mediated immunity?

Part of the immune response that is carried out by T lymphocytes, NK cells, and mononuclear phagocytes. T lymphocytes can be divided into cells that help other parts of the immune system (T helper cells), which are characterized by the CD4 receptor, and cells that mediate cytotoxicity (cytotoxic T cells, CD8 cells).

What are cytokines?

Proteins or glycoproteins secreted by cells that act as signals between cells of the immune system and mediators of response to infection. Cytokines include the interleukins, the interferons, and tumor necrosis factor. Different cytokines are produced by different cells and have different functions.

What are NK cells?

Closely related to T lymphocytes, NK cells can lyse target cells without major histocompatibility complex restriction or presensitization. They may play a role against intracellular pathogens, especially herpesviruses.

What are mononuclear phagocytes?

Bone marrow progenitors, circulating monocytes, and tissue macrophages

What are the kinds of defects in cell-mediated immunity?

Primary— genetic
Secondary— drug therapy (immunosuppressive medications including corticosteroids), radiation therapy, organ transplantation, lymphoreticular malignancies, malnutrition, and infections (viral, most notably HIV infection)

What are the pathogens that result from defects in cell-mediated immunity?	Think intracellular organisms including mycobacteria, *Legionella, Salmonella, Chlamydia, Brucella, Yersinia, Nocardia, Rickettsia, Listeria,* fungi (histoplasma, *Candida, Cryptococcus*) protozoa, and viruses.

MAJOR CLINICAL SYNDROMES

FEVER AND FEVER OF UNKNOWN ORIGIN

What constitutes a fever?	Any oral temperature of more than 37.8°C
Physiologically, how do fever and hyperthermia differ?	With fever, a new temperature set point is established; hyperthermia, on the other hand, does not involve changes in the set point; rather it involves heat production that exceeds heat loss, as occurs with malignant hyperthermia or heat stroke.
What are criteria for defining FUO?	As defined by Pertersdorf and Beeson: 1. Febrile illness of more than 3 weeks' duration 2. Temperatures in excess of 38.3°C on several determinations 3. Lack of a specific diagnosis after 1 week of inpatient investigation Note: "Updated" criteria allow 3 days of inpatient investigation or three outpatient visits to replace the original requirement of 1 week of inpatient investigation.
What are the major causes of FUO?	Infection (30%–40% of cases), neoplasms (20%–30% of cases), collagen vascular diseases (10%–15% of cases), and miscellaneous (10%–20%)
What are common infectious causes of FUO?	Tuberculosis, intra-abdominal infections, bacterial endocarditis, and pyelonephritis
What are common neoplastic causes of FUO?	Lymphomas, leukemias, solid tumors, and disseminated carcinomatosis

What are common collagen-vascular causes of FUO?

Rheumatoid arthritis, rheumatic fever, systemic lupus erythematosus, temporal arteritis, polyarteritis nodosa, and Wegener's granulomatosis

What are common miscellaneous causes of FUO?

Granulomatous hepatitis, drug fever, inflammatory bowel disease, factitious fever, and pulmonary embolus

How is FUO evaluated?

History, thorough physical examination, CBC with differential, urinalysis, blood cultures, tuberculosis skin testing with anergy panel, cultures of involved sites, and specific serologic tests as directed by history and physical examination

What additional diagnostic tests should be ordered for FUO?

Radiographs, ultrasound, CT, MRI, radionuclide scans, and angiography, depending on symptoms and physical findings

What invasive tests should be ordered for FUO?

Always attempt symptom-directed workups. Biopsy of bone marrow, liver, and involved organs should be considered in all FUO patients. In addition, consider bronchoscopy, endoscopy, or laparoscopy if other studies suggest pulmonary, gastrointestinal, or abdominal disease, respectively.

SYSTEMIC FEBRILE SYNDROMES

Sepsis

What is sepsis?

A systemic response to infection manifested by two or more of the following conditions: temperature $> 38°C$ or $< 36°C$, pulse > 90 bpm, respiratory rate > 20 or $Paco_2 < 32$ mm Hg, WBC $> 12,000$ or $< 4000/mm^3$ (or $> 10\%$ bands)

What is the incidence of septic shock?

$> 200,000$ cases per year in the United States

What is sepsis syndrome?	Sepsis with evidence of altered organ perfusion including at least one of the following: hypoxemia, elevated lactic acid, oliguria, or altered mentation
What is septic shock?	Sepsis syndrome and hypotension despite adequate fluid resuscitation attempts
What is SIRS?	Systemic inflammatory response syndrome is a broad descriptive term reflective of clinical sepsis syndrome, but is not limited to infectious origins.
What are the noninfectious causes of SIRS?	Burns and pancreatitis
What are the leading bacterial causes of BSI?	Infection with staphylococci and streptococci, followed by infection with *E. coli*, *Enterobacter* species, and *Pseudomonas aeruginosa*
List the common symptoms and signs of sepsis by bacterial infection.	Fevers, chills, hyperventilation, hyperthermia, changes in mental status, hypotension, bleeding, leukopenia, thrombocytopenia, and organ failure
What are predisposing factors for sepsis?	Surgery, chemotherapy, trauma, transplantation, and splenectomy
What is the workup for sepsis?	1. Meticulous history and physical examination for clues to the source and extent of an infectious process 2. Microbiologic studies including blood cultures and culture of any potential source of a systemic infection (draw blood cultures before initiating antibiotics) 3. If CNS signs are present, lumbar puncture
What is the treatment for sepsis?	1. Empiric antimicrobial regimens (modified based on culture results) should include broad gram-negative and gram-positive coverage with antianaerobic coverage in patients without a urinary tract source. For nosocomial and neutropenic sepsis,

coverage should also include *Pseudomonas.* If an indwelling vascular catheter infection is suspected, vancomycin should be considered.

2. Supportive therapy includes fluid and electrolyte management and sympathomimetic agents (dopamine, dobutamine, and norepinephrine) as needed to maintain adequate blood pressure.

Is there a role for empiric steroids in sepsis?

No, controlled clinical trials have failed to confirm any beneficial effects of corticosteroids in septic shock. However, if a patient is suspected of adrenal insufficiency, replacement doses of corticosteroids are appropriate.

List the organisms associated with post-splenectomy sepsis.

Encapsulated organisms including *S. pneumoniae, H. influenzae,* and *N. meningitidis*

Staphylococcal and Streptococcal Toxic Shock Syndromes

What is TSS?

A multisystem disease mediated by toxins of either *S. aureus* or group A streptococci and commonly characterized by rapid onset of high fever, hypotension, mental confusion, diarrhea, renal failure, erythroderma, and delayed desquamation

What are major risk factors for staphylococcal TSS?

Menstruation and tampon use are linked to two thirds of cases. Nonmenstrual-associated TSS is seen in a broad range of clinical settings including surgical and postpartum wound infections, deep abscesses, burns, and abrasions, among others.

To make the diagnosis of staphylococcal TSS, what four criteria must be met?

1. Fever—temperature > 38.9°C
2. Rash—diffuse macular erythroderma
3. Hypotension—systolic blood pressure < 90 mm Hg; orthostatic decrease in diastolic blood pressure > 15 mm Hg; orthostatic symptoms or dizziness

4. Desquamation—1–2 weeks after onset of illness, particularly of palms and soles

What body systems must be involved (three or more) in TSS?

1. Gastrointestinal—vomiting or diarrhea at onset
2. Muscular—severe myalgia or CPK twice normal
3. Mucous membranes—vaginal, oropharyngeal, or conjunctival hyperemia
4. Renal—blood urea nitrogen or creatinine twice normal or pyuria (> 5 WBC/HPF)
5. Hepatic—bilirubin or transaminases twice normal
6. Hematologic—platelets < 100,000/ mm^3
7. CNS—disorientation or alterations in consciousness without focal neurologic signs when fever and hypotension are absent

What test results must be negative (if performed) in TSS?

Blood, throat, or CSF cultures (blood culture may be positive for *S. aureus*); serologic tests for Rocky Mountain spotted fever, leptospirosis, or rubeola

What is the treatment of staphylococcus TSS?

1. Aggressive monitoring and management of circulatory shock and its complications
2. Removal of potentially infected foreign bodies
3. Drainage and irrigation of infected sites
4. Administration of antistaphylococcal β-lactamase–resistant antibiotic, such as nafcillin

What are symptoms of streptococcal TSS?

Pain is the most common initial symptom, often involving a site of minor local trauma; 20% of patients have an influenza-like syndrome. Fever is a common early sign, and 80% of patients have clinical signs of soft-tissue infection. In 50% of patients, blood pressure is normal on admission, but hypotension develops within 4 hours.

How is the diagnosis of streptococcal TSS made in the following cases:

Definite case?

1. Isolation of group A streptococci from a sterile body site
2. Hypotension
3. More than two of the following: renal impairment, coagulopathy, liver abnormalities, acute respiratory distress syndrome, extensive tissue necrosis (i.e., necrotizing fasciitis), and erythematous rash (may desquamate)

Probable case?

Same as for a definite case without isolation of group A streptococci from a nonsterile body site

What is the treatment of streptococcal TSS?

1. High-dose intravenous penicillin G with or without clindamycin
2. Prompt and aggressive exploration and débridement of deep-seated infection
3. Aggressive monitoring and management of circulatory shock and its complications

Rocky Mountain Spotted Fever

What is Rocky Mountain spotted fever?

A seasonal tickborne systemic illness caused by *Rickettsia rickettsii*, which, unless treated early, is usually clinically severe and frequently fatal

What is the incidence of Rocky Mountain spotted fever?

Depends on geographic location. In the United States, prevalence is highest in the southern Atlantic states and in the southwestern central region.

How is Rocky Mountain spotted fever transmitted?

During the season of activity of *Dermacentor variabilis* (American dog tick) and *Dermacentor andersoni* (Rocky Mountain wood tick), usually between April and October, *Rickettsiae* are inoculated into the dermis from which the tick has fed for 6–10 hours.

What is the incubation period for Rocky Mountain spotted fever?	2–14 days (median, 7 days)
What are initial symptoms of Rocky Mountain spotted fever?	Fever, headache, malaise, myalgia, nausea, vomiting, and rash
Describe the rash of Rocky Mountain spotted fever in terms of the following: Timing	Seen in fewer than 15% of patients on the first day of illness and in 50% by day 3. It usually appears 3–5 days after the onset of fever. Rash is absent in 10%–15% of cases.
Morphologic appearance	Initially, erythematous macules 1–5 mm in diameter appear and become maculopapular with time. Petechiae may develop (secondary to progressive vascular injury with hemorrhage) in up to 75% of cases on or after day 6.
Distribution	Ankles and wrists are affected first, then the trunk, palms, and soles.
What are additional clinical manifestations of Rocky Mountain spotted fever?	Neurologic abnormalities—focal deficits, altered consciousness, seizures, meningismus Renal failure Pulmonary involvement—alveolar infiltrates, interstitial pneumonia, pleural effusion Skin necrosis or gangrene
What laboratory findings are characteristic for Rocky Mountain spotted fever?	Normal WBC count, anemia, thrombocytopenia, coagulopathy, and hyponatremia. Increased lactate dehydrogenase, CPK, and other tissue enzymes are not uncommon.
What are characteristic CSF findings in Rocky Mountain spotted fever?	Pleocytosis (10–1000 cells) in one third of patients, increased protein in one third of patients, and normal glucose

How is the diagnosis of Rocky Mountain spotted fever made?	Most laboratory tests are not diagnostic during the acute stage of illness; hence, a prompt diagnosis is primarily clinical. Certain epidemiologic clues such as appropriate season and region as well as a history of a tick bite (60% of patients report a tick bite during the 2 weeks before the onset of illness) may help to raise clinical index of suspicion. Direct fluourescent antibody test can be performed on a biopsy sample of the skin rash, providing the diagnosis in a few days. Serologic test results showing a significant increase in antibody titers 7–10 days after the onset of illness confirm the diagnosis.
What is the treatment for Rocky Mountain spotted fever?	Doxycycline. Chloramphenicol is an alternative for patients who are pregnant or allergic to doxycycline. In pediatric patients, some investigators recommend chloramphenicol over doxycycline, which may cause staining of teeth; others argue that a short course of doxycycline is more appropriate.

Lyme Disease

What is Lyme disease?	A multisystem, often multistaged, tickborne disease. The first sign of illness, usually seen in the summer, begins with erythema migrans at the site of the tick bite. Within days to weeks, the disease may be manifest at other skin sites, joints, nervous system, or the heart. Persistent disease may be manifest months to years after infection.
What is the causative organism in Lyme disease?	The spirochete *B. burgdorferi*
What is the mode of transmission of Lyme disease?	*Ixodes* ticks
What are the epidemiologic characteristics of Lyme disease?	The most common vector-borne infection in the United States. Incidence depends on geography. Major foci in the United States include the northeast

(Massachusetts to Maryland), midwest (Wisconsin and Minnesota), and West (California and Oregon).

What are symptoms and signs of erythema migrans?

A characteristic erythematous plaque expanding centrifugally and fading centrally (bull's eye), occurring 3–32 days after the tick bite. Erythema migrans is present in nearly 85% of cases and is virtually pathognomonic for Lyme disease. Often, erythema migrans is accompanied by malaise, fatigue, headache, fever, chills, arthralgias, and regional adenopathy.

What are musculoskeletal symptoms and signs of Lyme disease?

In 80% of patients, joint symptoms develop weeks to years after the illness begins if the infection goes untreated. True arthritis usually does not occur until months after the onset of illness.

What are neurologic symptoms and signs of Lyme disease?

Symptoms range from headache and stiff neck to meningitis and encephalitis, occurring at varied times after infection. In patients with meningitis, lymphocytic pleocytosis of > 100 cell/mm^3 with normal glucose and elevated protein is characteristic. Facial nerve palsy may be the presenting symptom.

What are cardiac symptoms and signs of Lyme disease?

Cardiac involvement develops in 5% of cases, usually as some degree of atrioventricular block within several weeks of onset of illness. Because the duration of cardiac involvement is usually brief, permanent pacing is not necessary.

What are the usual laboratory abnormalities?

Laboratory abnormalities are nonspecific.

How is the diagnosis of Lyme disease made?

Characteristic clinical features, exposure in endemic area, and elevated antibody response to *B. burgdorferi*. Diagnosis is confirmed by Western blot assay. Spinal fluid may be tested with PCR.

What is the treatment for Lyme disease?

Specific regimen and duration depend on symptoms. Effective agents include doxycycline, amoxicillin, and ceftriaxone.

Should Lyme disease be treated in seropositive patients without classic clinical features?

For most seropositive patients who lack a history of classic clinical features, the risks of empiric intravenous antibiotic therapy outweigh the benefits. False-positive antibody tests do occur.

CENTRAL NERVOUS SYSTEM INFECTIONS (SEE CHAPTER 12)

RESPIRATORY INFECTIONS

COMMON COLD

What is the common cold?

A mild, self-limited catarrhal syndrome

What pathogens are associated with the common cold?

Primarily rhinovirus. Other pathogens include coronavirus, parainfluenza virus, respiratory syncytial virus, influenza, and adenovirus.

What is the incidence of the common cold?

Adults, 2–4 colds per year; children, 6–8 colds per year

What are symptoms and signs of the common cold?

Incubation is 24–72 hours, followed by nasal discharge and obstruction, sneezing, sore throat, and cough, which lasts approximately 1 week. Physical findings may be minimal.

How is the diagnosis of a common cold made?

Symptoms are fairly diagnostic; however, colds should be distinguished from bacterial sinusitis, otitis media, and allergic rhinitis.

What is the treatment for a common cold?

Treatment is symptomatic.

PHARYNGITIS

What is pharyngitis?

Inflammation of the pharynx

What pathogens are associated with pharyngitis?

Group A streptococci and a number of viruses

What are symptoms and signs of streptococcal pharyngitis?	Pain, odynophagia, fever, headache, chills, exudative pharyngitis, abdominal pain, cervical adenopathy, and leukocytosis. It may be difficult to distinguish viral from streptococcal (or uncommon causes of) pharyngitis, but exudate is rare in viral pharyngitis.
What diagnostic tests are done for pharyngitis?	Rapid antigen detection has a specificity of > 90% but sensitivity of only 60%–95%. If the antigen test is negative, a throat culture should be done.
What is the treatment for pharyngitis?	Streptococcal—penicillin for 10 days Viral—symptomatic therapy Influenza—amantadine

OTITIS MEDIA

What is otitis media?	Inflammation of the middle ear characterized by fluid in the middle ear with signs and symptoms
What is the incidence of otitis media?	Approximately 24 million episodes per year in the United States
What pathogens are associated with otitis media?	*S. pneumoniae, H. influenzae,* group A streptococci, *S. aureus, M. catarrhalis,* and viruses. In some cases, no pathogen is identified.
What are symptoms and signs of otitis media?	Ear pain and drainage, decreased hearing, fever, irritability, lethargy, vertigo, nystagmus, tinnitus, and fluid in the middle ear
How is the diagnosis of otitis media made?	Pathogens identified are so consistent that no specific culture is required unless the patient is gravely ill or has a focus of infection outside the middle ear.
What is the treatment for otitis media?	Coverage of the common pathogens with amoxicillin, amoxicillin/clavulanate, cefuroxime axetil, cefpodoxime proxetil, trimethoprim-sulfamethoxazole, and others

OTITIS EXTERNA

What is otitis externa?

Infection of the external auditory canal with pain and itching

What are symptoms and signs of otitis externa?

Acute localized pustule associated with a hair follicle

What pathogens are associated with otitis externa?

S. aureus is most common.

What are the symptoms and signs of acute diffuse otitis externa (swimmer's ear) and what are the associated pathogens?

Itching and pain with edema and erythema. Gram-negative bacilli, especially *P. aeruginosa*, are found most commonly.

What are the symptoms and signs of chronic otitis externa and what are the associated pathogens?

Chronic otitis externa is caused by irritation from middle ear drainage in patients with chronic suppurative otitis media. Therefore, the associated pathogens are related to those that cause otitis media. Chronic otitis externa is rarely seen in association with tuberculosis, symphilis, yaws, leprosy, or sarcoid.

What are the symptoms and signs of malignant otitis externa and what are the associated pathogens?

Spreads from the skin to soft tissue and bone. Severe pain with purulent drainage develops. Malignant otitis externa occurs in patients with diabetes mellitus, in immunocompromised patients, and in elderly patients. The pathogen is almost always *P. aeruginosa*.

MASTOIDITIS

What is mastoiditis?

Infection in the mastoid that typically follows otitis media

What are symptoms and signs of mastoiditis?

Appears initially to be otitis media; then swelling, erythema, and tenderness develop over the mastoid. Pinna of the ear may be displaced down and away from the head.

How is the diagnosis of mastoiditis made?

Radiographs may reveal cloudiness and loss of the sharp margins of the mastoid secondary to inflammation. CT can clearly define the anatomic abnormalities.

What is the treatment for mastoiditis?

Similar to that for otitis media. If mastoiditis is chronic, consider *S. aureus* or gram-negative pathogens, including *P. aeruginosa*.

SINUSITIS

What is sinusitis?

Infection of more than one of the paranasal sinuses, typically after a viral infection of the respiratory tract (including the common cold)

What are the pathogens in the following cases:
Acute sinusitis?

S. pneumoniae, H. influenzae, anaerobes, *S. aureus, S. pyogenes, M. catarrhalis,* gram-negative bacilli, rhinovirus, influenza virus, parainfluenza virus, and adenovirus

Chronic sinusitis?

Anaerobes, *S. aureus,* and *Viridans* group streptococci are most common, but a variety of pathogens have been isolated; however, infection is not the primary problem in chronic sinusitis.

What are risk factors for sinusitis?

Common cold, dental infections in maxillary teeth, anatomic abnormalities, indwelling nasal tubes, and packing material

What are symptoms and signs of sinusitis?

May be difficult to differentiate from the primary viral illness. The most helpful finding is the presence of respiratory symptoms that persist for longer than 1 week. Other symptoms including purulent nasal discharge, nasal obstruction, and facial tenderness are variably present.

What are complications of sinusitis?

Orbital extension from ethmoidal disease, intracranial extension leading to meningitis or brain abscess, and osteomyelitis of the frontal bone

What laboratory and diagnostic tests are performed for sinusitis?

Sinus radiographs are more sensitive than physical examination, but limited sinus CT scans are usually no more expensive and provide a more detailed view of the paranasal sinuses than plain films. However, neither imaging technique can differentiate bacterial infection from inflammation due to another cause. The gold standard for the diagnosis of sinusitis is culture of an aspirate or puncture of the involved sinus, but this procedure is not required in typical cases of acute sinusitis (sinus radiographs do correlate with culture findings in patients with acute sinusitis).

How is the diagnosis of sinusitis made?

History and physical examination, including transillumination of the sinuses and imaging studies

What is the treatment of sinusitis?

Treat as a bacterial infection empirically with antibiotics that will effectively treat *S. pneumoniae* and *H. influenzae*. Possible agents include trimethoprim–sulfamethoxazole, amoxicillin/clavulanate, and cefuroxime axetil. Treatment should be for 14 days. Additional therapy should include decongestants and phenylephrine nose drops.

What is the role of surgery in sinusitis?

Complications including intraorbital or intracranial extension may require surgery in addition to antibiotics.

EPIGLOTTITIS

What is epiglottitis?

Cellulitis of the epiglottis characterized by rapid progression and the potential for causing sudden, complete airway obstruction. It is most common in boys between the ages of 2 and 4 years.

What are symptoms and signs of epiglottitis?

Fever, irritability, dysphonia, dysphagia, and marked sore throat. Patients often sit leaning forward and may have difficulty swallowing their oral secretions. Airway obstruction may develop rapidly over the course of minutes.

What laboratory and diagnostic tests are used for epiglottitis?

Leukocytosis is common. Blood cultures should be obtained. Although lateral neck radiographs may reveal findings characteristic of epiglottitis, their use is not recommended because there is the possibility that airway obstruction will develop during the delay required to obtain the films.

How is the diagnosis of epiglottitis made?

History and physical examination. In children in whom the diagnosis of epiglottitis is suspected, the patient should be taken to the operating room and examined in a controlled setting where rapid management of the airway is possible. A cherry red epiglottis is diagnostic. Blood cultures are positive in virtually all children with epiglottitis caused by *H. influenzae*.

What pathogens are associated with epiglottitis?

H. influenzae is the number one cause in children, producing almost all episodes; it is also common in adults. Other pathogens include *S. pneumoniae*, staphylococci, and streptococci.

What is the treatment for epiglottitis?

Maintaining an adequate airway is the number one concern and children should be intubated as soon as the diagnosis is made. Antibiotics directed against *H. influenzae* should be given intravenously for 7–10 days. Possible agents include third-generation cephalosporins (e.g., cefotaxime, ceftriaxone).

BRONCHITIS (SEE ALSO CHAPTER 3)

What is bronchitis?

Inflammation of the tracheobronchial tree

PNEUMONIA (SEE ALSO CHAPTER 3)

What is pneumonia? Infection of the lung parenchyma

What is the incidence of pneumonia? Approximately 4 million episodes per year with 1 million hospitalizations and approximately 50,000 deaths

MYCOBACTERIUM TUBERCULOSIS (SEE ALSO CHAPTER 3)

What is the incidence of *Mycobacterium tuberculosis* infection? More than 1.7 billion people in the world are infected with *Mycobacterium tuberculosis*. There are 8 million new cases of tuberculosis per year and 3 million deaths per year.

INFECTIVE ENDOCARDITIS (SEE ALSO CHAPTER 2)

What is infective endocarditis? Infection of the endocardial surface of the heart, most commonly the valves, with the implication that microorganisms are present

PROSTHETIC VALVE ENDOCARDITIS (SEE ALSO CHAPTER 2)

What is the incidence of prosthetic valve endocarditis? Occurs in < 3% of valve replacements—2% in the first year, 1% per year thereafter

GASTROENTERITIS

What is diarrhea? Stool that conforms to the shape of its container; liquid or watery stool that occurs at least three times in 24 hours

What is the incidence and impact of diarrhea? In the United States, rates range from 1.5 illnesses per person per year in communities and day care facilities to 5 illnesses per person per year in a day. Worldwide, diarrheal disease ranks second only to cardiovascular disease as a cause of death. Diarrhea is the cause of death for an estimated 3.3 to 6 million children annually, mostly in Asia, Africa, and Latin America.

What are risk factors for diarrhea?	Involvement with day care centers, travel, immunocompromised status, antibiotic use, and homosexual practices
What features distinguish inflammatory from noninflammatory diarrhea?	In inflammatory diarrhea, the patient is often febrile, the character of the stool is mucopurulent, and fecal leukocytes and lactoferrin are present in the stool. In noninflammatory diarrhea, the patient is usually afebrile, the character of the stool is watery or bloody, and fecal leukocytes and lactoferrin are not present.
What do fever and tenesmus suggest?	Inflammatory proctocolitis
What is the initial diagnostic test of choice for diarrhea?	Assessment for inflammation by examining stool for fecal leukocytes or fecal lactoferrin. If there is inflammation, check stool culture (and *C. difficile* toxin assay if clinical history dictates).
What are causes of inflammatory diarrhea?	*Shigella, Salmonella, Campylobacter jejuni, C. difficile, Entamoeba histolytica,* and enteroinvasive *E. coli*
What is empiric treatment for inflammatory diarrhea?	Oral rehydration therapy. Therapy with a fluoroquinolone (e.g., ciprofloxacin) may shorten the duration of symptoms if *C. difficile* and *E. histolytica* are not suspected.
What is the disadvantage of treating uncomplicated *Salmonella* infections?	The carrier state is prolonged.
What antibiotics are associated with *C. difficile* diarrhea?	Almost all; however, clindamycin, ampicillin, and cephalosporins are most commonly implicated.
What is the treatment for *C. difficile* diarrhea?	1. Discontinuation of the offending antibiotic, if possible 2. Therapy with oral metronidazole (If the patient is refractory to or intolerant of metronidazole, use oral vancomycin.)

What are causes of noninflammatory diarrhea?	Rotavirus, Norwalk virus, *Giardia*, *Cryptosporidium*, *S. aureus*, *Bacillus cereus*, *Clostridium perfringens*, *Vibrio cholerae*, and enterotoxigenic *E. coli*.
What is the treatment for noninflammatory diarrhea?	Oral rehydration therapy

INTRA-ABDOMINAL INFECTIONS (SEE ALSO CHAPTER 5)

PERITONITIS

What is peritonitis?	Inflammation of the peritoneal cavity
What are the types of peritonitis?	1. Primary—spontaneous, no clear cause 2. Secondary—underlying abdominal disease
What are risk factors for peritonitis?	Ruptured viscus, postoperative intestinal anastomotic leaks, pelvic inflammatory disease, ruptured abscess, peritoneal dialysis catheters, and ascites
What are symptoms and signs of peritonitis?	Pain, vomiting, rigid abdomen, rebound tenderness, and hypoactive bowel sounds
How is the diagnosis of peritonitis made?	Clinically. The underlying cause (such as perforated appendix) must be identified immediately. Often, laparotomy is necessary to identify an unclear source of peritonitis.
What are the usual pathogens in peritonitis?	Usually polymicrobic activity. The most commonly isolated aerobes include *E. coli*, *Klebsiella*, *Streptococcus*, *Proteus*, and *Enterobacter* species. The most commonly isolated anaerobes are *Bacteroides*, *Peptostreptococcus*, and *Clostridium* species.
What is SBP?	Spontaneous (i.e., without any evidence of bowel rupture or contamination of the peritoneal cavity) bacterial peritonitis
What are the risk factors for SBP?	Primarily, cirrhotic and nephrotic ascites

How is the diagnosis of SBP made?	Ascitic fluid demonstrating > 500/mm³ leukocytes (with > 50% PMNs), Gram stain, and culture
How does the microbiology of SBP differ from other cases of peritonitis?	In addition to seeing coliforms and anaerobes, pneumococci may be seen, especially in patients with nephrotic ascites.
In general, what should be covered in the empiric antibiotic treatment for peritonitis?	Enteric gram-negative organisms, anaerobes, and, in the seriously ill patient, *Enterococcus*
What are the possible regimens for secondary peritonitis?	Metronidazole plus ampicillin and an aminoglycoside Ampicillin-sulbactam plus an aminoglycoside Ticarcillin-clavulanic acid plus an aminoglycoside Imipenem-cilastatin Metronidazole plus a third-generation cephalosporin
What regimen should be considered for spontaneous peritonitis?	Third-generation cephalosporin (cefotaxime or ceftriaxone)

INTRA-ABDOMINAL ABSCESSES

Intra-abdominal abscesses are divided into which three classifications?	Intraperitoneal, retroperitoneal, and visceral

INTRAPERITONEAL ABSCESSES

What are the most common sites of intraperitoneal abscess?	Subphrenic, midabdominal, and pelvic areas, secondary to the effects of gravity
What are the most common causes of intraperitoneal abscess?	1. Subphrenic—secondary to complications of abdominal surgery (> 90% of cases) 2. Midabdominal—secondary to complications of acute appendicitis, colonic diverticulitis, colonic perforation, or Crohn's disease 3. Pelvic—secondary to acute salpingitis, acute appendicitis, or diverticulitis

What are symptoms and signs of intraperitoneal abscess?	Fever, localized pain, anorexia, weight loss, nausea, vomiting, change in bowel habits, and palpable mass. In subphrenic abscess, diaphragm irritation may cause shoulder discomfort.
What are the laboratory findings in intraperitoneal abscess?	Leukocytosis and elevated ESR
How is the diagnosis of intraperitoneal abscess made?	Ultrasound or abdominal CT scan
What are the most common microbes associated with intraperitoneal abscess?	Anaerobes play a major role, especially *B. fragilis*. Enteric aerobes may also be involved.
What is the treatment of intraperitoneal abscess?	The mainstay of therapy is drainage of pus either surgically or percutaneously. Initial antimicrobial therapy should include one of the regimens discussed for secondary peritonitis and should be tailored after culture and sensitivity data are available.
What are complications of subphrenic abscesses?	Atelectasis, pleural effusion, and basilar pneumonia

VISCERAL ABSCESS

Hepatic Abscess

What are the two major types of liver abscesses?	1. Bacterial or pyogenic (most common in the United States) 2. Amebic (most common in the world)
Are most liver abscesses single or multiple?	Single

Pyogenic Liver Abscess

What are the risk factors for liver abscesses?	1. Biliary tract disease (ascending cholangitis most commonly) 2. Systemic bacteremia with hematogenous spread via the hepatic artery

3. Appendicitis, diverticulitis, or irritable bowel disease causing spread via the portal vein
4. Trauma (penetrating and nonpenetrating wounds)
5. Infection outside the biliary tract with contiguous spread

What are the symptoms and signs of pyogenic liver abscess?	Fever, chills, nausea, vomiting, fatigue, anorexia, and weight loss. In approximately 50% of patients, right upper abdominal pain and hepatomegaly are present. Occasionally, pleuritic chest pain occurs.
What are the laboratory findings in pyogenic liver abscess?	Leukocytosis, anemia, and elevated ESR
How is the diagnosis of pyogenic liver abscess made?	Clinical presentation and confirmation via CT or ultrasound-guided aspiration
What are the usual microbes involved in pyogenic liver abscess?	Greater than 50% of cases are mixed flora with the most common organisms being anaerobes, *E. coli*, *Klebsiella* species, *S. aureus*, and streptococci.
What is the usual treatment for pyogenic liver abscess?	Pathogen-specific antimicrobial therapy with drainage of pus percutaneously or surgically. Antibiotics should be continued several weeks after drainage.
What is the mortality rate associated with pyogenic liver abscess?	In treated cases, the mortality rate is approximately 30%.

Amebic Liver Abscesses

What is the typical history for amebic abscess?	Travel, acute presentation, age younger than 50 years, and history of intestinal amebiasis
Which lobe of the liver is more frequently involved in amebic abscess?	The right lobe

What are the symptoms and signs of amebic liver abscess?	Right upper quadrant pain, fever, chills, and night sweats
What are the laboratory findings in amebic liver abscess?	Leukocytosis, elevated LFTs, and elevated serum bilirubin levels
How is the diagnosis of amebic liver abscess made?	Clinical presentation. Aspiration may reveal "anchovy paste" fluid.
What is the most common pathogen in amebic liver abscess?	*E. histolytica*, usually secondary to intestinal amebiasis
What is the treatment for amebic liver abscess?	Amebicides (such as metronidazole plus diloxanide furoate or paromomycin) with or without CT-directed aspiration

Splenic Abscess

Are most cases of splenic abscess single or multiple?	Most cases are small, multiple, and clinically silent. Clinically important abscesses tend to be large and solitary.
What are the causes of splenic abscesses?	1. Infection via hematogenous route secondary to trauma, or secondary infection or infarction seen in hemoglobinopathies (sickle cell) 2. Systemic bacteremia 3. Extension from a contiguous site
What are symptoms and signs of splenic abscess?	Subacute onset with fever, left-sided pain (sometimes pleuritic in nature), left shoulder pain, and splenomegaly
What are the laboratory findings in splenic abscess?	Leukocytosis
How is the diagnosis of splenic abscess made?	CT scan
What are the microbiologic findings in splenic abscess?	Staphylococci, streptococci, anaerobes, and gram-negative rods, including *Salmonella*

What is the treatment for splenic abscess?	Appropriate antimicrobial therapy, drainage of pus, splenotomy, or splenectomy

Pancreatic Abscess

What is the cause of pancreatic abscess?	Usually occurs in a necrotic pancreas following pancreatitis
What are symptoms and signs of pancreatic abscess?	Approximately 2 weeks after improvement from acute pancreatitis, the patient experiences fever, abdominal pain and tenderness, nausea, and vomiting. A mass is occasionally palpable. Chest radiographs may reveal pleural effusion (most often left-sided), atelectasis, or pneumonia.
What are the laboratory findings in pancreatic abscess?	Elevated serum amylase, elevated alkaline phosphatase, and leukocytosis
How is the diagnosis of pancreatic abscess made?	CT scan is the most accurate. For definitive diagnosis, pancreatic gas must be visualized.
What are the microbiologic study findings in pancreatic abscess?	Enteric gram-negative bacilli, staphylococci, streptococci, and anaerobes
What is the treatment for pancreatic abscess?	Secondary peritonitis regimens

ACUTE CHOLECYSTITIS (SEE ALSO CHAPTER 5)

What is cholecystitis?	Inflammation of the gallbladder
What causes cholecystitis?	Acute inflammation of the gallbladder, usually secondary to biliary tract obstruction by a stone

APPENDICITIS (SEE ALSO CHAPTER 5)

What age-group has the highest incidence of appendicitis?	20–30 year olds

What is the cause of appendicitis?	Obstruction of the appendiceal lumen is identified in 30% of cases. Appendicitis is thought to result in bacterial multiplication, necrosis, and ultimately perforation.

DIVERTICULITIS (SEE ALSO CHAPTER 5)

What is diverticulitis?	Inflammation of a diverticulum (outpocketing of colonic mucosa through the muscularis). Diverticulitis occurs more often with increasing age.
What is the most common anatomic location of diverticulitis?	Sigmoid colon secondary to increased intraluminal pressures

GENITOURINARY INFECTIONS

What are the major causes of vaginitis?	Candidiasis, trichomoniasis, and bacterial vaginosis

VULVOVAGINAL CANDIDIASIS

What is the incidence of vulvovaginal candidiasis?	Three fourths of women suffer from at least one episode in their lifetime, and nearly half of these women have recurrent episodes.
What are risk factors for vulvovaginal candidiasis?	Oral contraceptive use, recent antibiotic therapy, corticosteroid therapy, pregnancy, poorly controlled diabetes mellitus, and tight-fitting undergarments. Infection with HIV has been associated with an increased incidence of persistent or recurring infections.
What organisms are most commonly associated with vulvovaginal candidiasis?	*Candida albicans* (80%–90%). *Candida tropicalis* and *Torulopsis glabrata* also cause vaginitis.
What is the cardinal symptom of vulvovaginal candidiasis?	Pruritus

What are other symptoms and signs of vulvovaginal candidiasis?	External dysuria, vaginal discharge, dyspareunia, premenstrual onset, vulvar erythema, and cheesy, white, thick vaginal discharge
How is the diagnosis of vulvovaginal candidiasis made?	Identification of pseudohyphae in vaginal secretions mixed with 10% KOH confirms the diagnosis. Vaginal pH is normal (< 4.5).
What is the sensitivity of the KOH prep in vulvovaginal candidiasis?	Approximately 50%–75%
What is the utility of culture in vulvovaginal candidiasis?	Culture is more sensitive than KOH microscopic examination, but it does not prove an etiologic role; at least 20% of healthy women harbor vaginal *Candida*.
What is the treatment for vulvovaginal candidiasis?	Topical antifungal agents such as miconazole, clotrimazole, terconazole, or a single dose of oral fluconazole

TRICHOMONIASIS

What risk factor is associated with trichomoniasis?	Having an increased number of sexual partners
What are symptoms of trichomoniasis?	Yellow vaginal discharge (75% of patients), dysuria (25%–50%), vulvar itching, dyspareunia, and occasionally lower abdominal pain
What are clinical findings of trichomoniasis?	Purulent frothy discharge with foul odor; vaginal pH > 5.0.
What is the etiologic organism associated with trichomoniasis?	The protozoan parasite *Trichomonas vaginalis*
How is the diagnosis of trichomoniasis made?	Motile trophozoites, often accompanied by polymorphonuclear cells, are seen on wet mount examination.
What is the sensitivity of the wet mount in trichomoniasis?	60%–80% in symptomatic women

What is the treatment for trichomoniasis?	Metronidazole, 2 g by mouth as single-dose therapy. All sexual partners of the index case should also be treated.

BACTERIAL VAGINOSIS

What are symptoms of bacterial vaginosis?	Vaginal discharge with or without vaginal odor and pruritus
What are signs of bacterial vaginosis?	Homogenous, frothy discharge, elevated vaginal pH, and a positive whiff test
What is the whiff test?	Detection of a fishy odor (caused by amines) when vaginal secretions are placed in 10% KOH.
What is seen on wet mount in bacterial vaginosis?	Clue cells and the absence of leukocytes, trichomonads, and the normal flora of rods
What are clue cells?	Squamous epithelial cells with ragged borders and stippling caused by colonization with bacteria
How is the diagnosis of bacterial vaginosis made?	At least three of the following are required: 1. Thin homogenous vaginal discharge 2. Elevated vaginal pH (> 5.0) 3. Clue cells 4. Positive whiff test
What is the treatment for bacterial vaginosis?	Metronidazole, 500 mg by mouth twice daily for 7 days

MUCOPURULENT CERVICITIS

What are etiologic agents of mucopurulent cervicitis?	*Chlamydia trachomatis* and *N. gonorrhoeae*
What are symptoms of mucopurulent cervicitis?	Most women are asymptomatic; approximately 30% of women with gonorrhea and 30% with chlamydia cervicitis note a vaginal discharge.
What are signs of mucopurulent cervicitis?	Friability and erythema of the cervix, with or without yellow mucopurulent discharge from the endocervix, or > 10 WBC per high-power field of a Gram stain endocervical smear

What is the treatment for mucopurulent cervicitis?

Mucopurulent cervicitis should always be treated, with coverage of both *N. gonorrhoeae* and *C. trachomatis*. Effective regimens include ceftriaxone, ciprofloxacin, or ofloxacin single-dose therapy for *N. gonorrhoeae* and doxycycline 100 mg by mouth twice daily for 7 days for chlamydia.

What are complications of mucopurulent cervicitis?

Pelvic inflammatory disease; in pregnant women, preterm delivery and premature rupture of membranes

PELVIC INFLAMMATORY DISEASE

What is PID?

A clinical syndrome resulting from cervical microorganisms ascending to the endometrium, fallopian tubes, and contiguous structures

What are risk factors for PID?

Being a teenage woman, having multiple sex partners, using intrauterine devices, and having prior PID

What are the usual pathogens in PID?

Usually polymicrobic agents: *N. gonorrhea, C. trachomatis*, and mixed aerobic and anaerobic bacteria

What is the classical triad of symptoms and signs in PID?

Pelvic pain, increased vaginal discharge, and fever (found in only 20% of women). Asymptomatic PID may also occur.

What are the sequelae of PID?

Infertility, ectopic pregnancy, chronic pelvic pain, and recurrent episodes of PID

How is the diagnosis of PID made?

Clinical findings suggested by direct abdominal tenderness, cervical motion tenderness, and adnexal tenderness plus one or more of the following: temperature > 38°C, WBC count > 10,000/mm^3, and pelvic abscess found by manual examination or ultrasonography

What is the differential diagnosis for PID?

Ectopic pregnancy, acute appendicitis, ruptured ovarian cyst, endometriosis, and torsed ovary

What is the treatment for PID?	Outpatient therapy: 1. Ceftriaxone, cefotaxime, or cefoxitin plus probenecid intramuscularly once 2. Ofloxacin twice daily plus clindamycin 3. Metronidazole plus doxycycline, 100 mg twice daily for 10–14 days Inpatient therapy: 1. Cefoxitin (2 g intravenously every 6 hours) or cefotetan (2 g intravenously every 12 hours) plus doxycycline (100 mg twice daily for 14 days). Both cefoxitin and cefotetan should be continued for at least 48 hours after significant clinical improvement is noted. 2. Clindamycin plus gentamicin followed by doxycycline for 14 days

URETHRITIS

What are the two types of urethritis?	GC, caused by *N. gonorrhoeae*, and NGU, usually caused by *C. trachomatis* or *Ureaplasma urealyticum*, or occasionally by *T. vaginalis*, *Mycoplasma* species, and HSV
What are symptoms of urethritis?	Dysuria and urethral discharge (in GC more so than in NGU)
What is the incubation period for urethritis?	In 75% of men with GC, symptoms develop within 4 days. In nearly 50% of men with NGU, symptoms develop within 4 days, although they more likely develop between 7 and 14 days.
What are signs of urethritis?	Spontaneous purulent urethral discharge is more suggestive of GC; a clear urethral discharge suggests NGU.
How is the diagnosis of GC made?	PMNs with gram-negative intracellular diplococci are shown on urethral smear. Culture is also useful.
How is the diagnosis of NGU made?	PMNs are seen in the absence of gram-negative intracellular diplococci.

What is the treatment for GC?	Uncomplicated GC—Cextriaxone (125 mg intramuscularly) or cefixime (400 mg orally) or ciprofloxacin (500 mg orally), or ofloxacin (400 mg orally), plus azithromycin (one dose of 1 g orally) or doxycycline (100 mg orally twice daily for 7 days). There are other regimens as well, but azithromycin or doxycycline is administered in all cases to cover chlamydia. Disseminated GC—There are various regimens for patients with disseminated GC. Pharyngitis—Ceftriaxone or ciprofloxacin is recommended.
What other pathogens should be treated empirically in patients with gonorrhea?	Chlamydiae
What is the incidence of chlamydia co-infection with GC?	10%–30% in heterosexual men; 40%–60% in women
What is the treatment for NGU?	Doxycycline, azithromycin (1 g by mouth once) or erythromycin

HERPES GENITALIS

Which HSV type is associated with genital herpes?	HSV type 2 (70%–95% of cases)
Clinically, how does primary herpes infection differ from recurrent infection?	Initial infection is usually more severe.
What is the incubation period for herpes infection?	2–20 days; mean, 6 days
What is the natural history of herpes infection?	Grouped vesicles on an erythematous base progress to painful shallow ulcers and crust over.

What are additional symptoms of herpes infection?	A prodrome of itching or burning may precede the appearance of lesions; regional lymphadenopathy may develop toward the end of the first week of illness.
How is the diagnosis of herpes infection made?	Diagnosis is usually made on clinical grounds. Tzanck smear may demonstrate multinucleated giant cells; culture remains the gold standard.
What is the treatment for herpes infection?	Oral acyclovir is most useful in the initial infection. It may lessen the duration of recurrent disease if taken very early in the course of relapse.
What is the role of suppressive therapy in herpes infection?	Frequent recurrences may be controlled with daily suppressive therapy, but this does not prevent viral shedding.

SYPHILIS

What is the etiologic agent associated with syphilis?	The spirochete *T. pallidum*
What is the incubation period for syphilis?	10–90 days; mean, 3 weeks
What are the stages of syphilis?	Primary—chancre Secondary—disseminated (mean of 6 weeks after contact) Latent—diagnosed only by serologic testing; early and late stages Tertiary—may or may not be clinically apparent; develops in 30% of untreated patients and involves the aorta and CNS
What are manifestations of primary syphilis?	One or more chancres (ulcerated lesions with heaped-up margins) which are minimally painful and nontender regional adenopathy
What are features of secondary syphilis?	Maculopapular, symmetric, generalized rash primarily involving the oral mucous membranes and genitalia but often with involvement of palms and soles; generalized lymphadenopathy; sometimes alopecia

What are condylomata lata?	Hypertrophic broad, flat lesions of secondary syphilis, occurring primarily in moist areas especially around the anus and external genitalia
What are major manifestations of tertiary syphilis?	Lymphocytic meningitis, dementia, tabes dorsalis (posterior spinal column and ganglion disease), aortic disease, or destructive lesions of skin and bone
What are the names of both treponemal and nontreponemal tests for syphilis?	Nontreponemal tests include VDRL and RPR; treponemal tests include the FTA-ABS and MHA-TP.
What are the advantages of the nontreponemal tests for syphilis?	The nontreponemal tests are inexpensive and useful for following titers during treatment.
What are the advantages of the treponemal tests for syphilis?	The treponemal tests are more specific and more sensitive in primary and tertiary syphilis.
What are the disadvantages of the nontreponemal tests for syphilis?	The nontreponemal tests lack specificity and a positive test needs a confirmatory treponemal test.
What are the disadvantages of the treponemal tests for syphilis?	The treponemal tests are expensive and not useful for serial follow-up.
What are the causes of false-positive nontreponemal tests?	Acute viral illnesses, collagen-vascular diseases, pregnancy, intravenous drug use, and leprosy, among others
When are nontreponemal tests least sensitive?	In primary and late syphilis. In these settings, a treponemal test should be ordered to confirm the nonreactive nontreponemal test.
How do serologic tests change with treatment?	Following adequate therapy, a fourfold drop in titer of nontreponemal tests should be observed within 3 months of early syphilis and within 6 months for latent syphilis. Treponemal tests are not quantitative and often remain positive after adequate treatment.

How is the diagnosis of syphilis made?

Primary—demonstration of spirochetes on dark-field microscopy or a positive serologic test

Secondary—serologic tests (almost always reactive in high titers)

Tertiary—serologic tests

What is the treatment for:

Early syphilis (primary or secondary)?

Benzathine penicillin G (2–4 million U intramuscularly weekly for 2 or 3 doses), alone or with oral regimens OR

Procaine penicillin (2.4 million U intramuscularly daily) plus probenecid (1 g orally daily for 10 days) OR

Doxycycline (200 mg orally twice daily for 21 days) OR

Amoxicillin (3 g orally twice daily) plus probenecid (1 g orally daily for 14 days) OR

Ceftriaxone (250 mg intramuscularly or intravenously daily for 5 days, or 1 g intramuscularly daily for 14 days)

Late syphilis (tertiary), neurosyphilis, or concomitant HIV infection?

Aqueous crystalline penicillin G (2–4 million U intravenously every 4 hours for 10 days) OR

Amoxicillin (3 g) plus probenicid (0.5 g) orally twice daily for 15 days OR

Doxycycline (200 mg orally twice daily for 21 days) OR

Ceftriaxone (1 g intramuscularly or intravenously for 14 days) OR

Procaine penicillin G (2.4 million U intramuscularly) plus probenicid (1 g orally daily) for 10 days

Syphilis in a pregnant woman?

The regimens are the same, but only penicillin is reliable for the treatment of the infant.

What should be done about contacts to syphilis?

For the first 90 days after exposure, the RPR may be negative, so contacts should be treated epidemiologically.

What is a Jarisch-Herxheimer reaction?

Fever, rash, adenopathy and sometimes hypotension, occurring 1–6 hours after initial therapy for syphilis. The reaction is seen in approximately 50% of patients with primary syphilis and virtually all patients with secondary syphilis.

What is the natural history of the Jarisch-Herxheimer reaction?	Self-limited and usually easily treated with antipyretics

URINARY TRACT INFECTIONS (SEE ALSO CHAPTER 4)

What is considered significant bacteriuria?	Greater than or equal to 10^5 bacteria/ml in a voided urine specimen. Fewer numbers of bacteria are generally thought to represent contamination from the anterior urethra.
What anatomic structures are affected in lower UTIs?	Lower UTIs may involve the bladder or urethra.
What anatomic structures are affected in upper UTIs?	Kidneys

SOFT TISSUE, BONES, AND JOINTS

CELLULITIS

What is cellulitis?	Superficial, spreading, warm, erythematous inflammation of the skin
What is erysipelas?	An indurated, warm, erythematous, and edematous spreading lesion with an advancing elevated margin that is sharply demarcated
What are the etiologic agents of erysipelas?	Usually, group A β-hemolytic streptococci, although, rarely, S. aureus produces the same clinical picture
What is impetigo?	Initially a vesicular, then a crusted, superficial infection of the skin, usually caused by group A streptococci or S. aureus

What are predisposing factors for cellulitis?

Previous trauma, underlying skin lesion, and lymphedema

How is the diagnosis of cellulitis made?

Aspirates and skin biopsy from the advancing edge of cellulitis and blood cultures reveal potential pathogens in approximately 25% of patients. Often, no specific agent is isolated and therapy is presumptive.

What are the etiologic agents for cellulitis?

Group A streptococci and S. aureus

What is the presumptive therapy for cellulitis?

Because it is difficult to distinguish clinically between staphylococcal and streptococcal skin infections, initial therapy should adequately cover both organisms. Penicillinase-resistant penicillins or first-generation cephalosporins are antibiotics of choice. Erythromycin and vancomycin are alternatives for mild and severe infections, respectively, in penicillin-allergic patients.

What is necrotizing fasciitis?

Fulminant necrotic infection of the superficial and deep fascia causing thrombosis of subcutaneous blood vessels and ultimately gangrene of underlying tissues

What are the two types of necrotizing fasciitis?

Type 1—involves at least one anaerobic species in combination with more than one facultative anaerobic species
Type 2—typically caused by group A streptococci (with or without S. aureus). It may be associated with the streptococcal TSS.

What is the therapy for necrotizing fasciitis?

Surgical débridement and antibiotics, which are ultimately guided by bacteriologic data. Depending on clinical circumstances, presumptive therapy may include combinations of the following:
  Ampicillin, gentamicin, and clindamycin

Ampicillin, gentamicin, and
metronidazole
Ampicillin-sulbactam and gentamicin

What is gas gangrene?

A necrotizing, gas-forming infection of
muscle

**What are the principal
agents that cause gas
gangrene?**

C. perfringens type A and other
Clostridium species

**What are predisposing
factors to gas gangrene?**

Traumatic injuries, diabetes, vascular
disease, neutropenia, intra-abdominal
infection, and colon cancer

**What are symptoms of gas
gangrene?**

Systemic toxicity and severe pain that is
often disproportionate to physical
findings

**What are signs of gas
gangrene?**

Edematous skin, often with hemorrhagic
bullae, and sometimes associated with
brownish, foul-smelling, watery
discharge and crepitation

**How is the diagnosis of gas
gangrene made?**

Physical examination with multiple
gram-positive rods on Gram stain. CT
demonstrates muscle compartment
involvement with gas in the muscle and
fascial planes. Cultures reveal *C.
perfringens* in most cases.

**What is the treatment for
gas gangrene?**

1. Emergent surgical débridement
2. Antibiotic therapy, usually including
   penicillin and additional agents to
   cover possible anaerobic and gram-
   negative copathogens

OSTEOMYELITIS

What is osteomyelitis?

Infection in bone characterized by
inflammatory destruction and necrosis
with new bone formation

**What is the difference
between acute and chronic
osteomyelitis?**

Acute osteomyelitis evolves over several
weeks; chronic osteomyelitis represents
long-standing infection, evolving over
months or years, and is associated with
persistent microorganisms and
inflammatory response.

What are modes for development of osteomyelitis?	Contiguous spread, hematogenous spread, and direct inoculation
What are features of hematogenous osteomyelitis?	Bone seeding from bacteremia is seen most commonly in prepubertal children and in the elderly. It most often involves the metaphyseal area of long bones or the vertebrae.
How is the diagnosis of osteomyelitis made?	Early bone biopsy for culture and histopathology not only establishes the diagnosis but also often provides the etiologic agent for which susceptibility data can ultimately direct therapy.
Are cultures of sinus tracts useful in osteomyelitis?	These cultures reflect colonization of the tract and do not correlate with the underlying bone infection. However, if *S. aureus* is isolated from an open sinus tract, the likelihood is high (> 80%) that *S. aureus* is also present in bone.
What radiographic changes are associated with osteomyelitis?	Plain films show soft-tissue swelling, periosteal thickening, and focal osteopenia occurring as early as 2 weeks after onset of infection, but, more often, these changes take months.
What are the laboratory findings in osteomyelitis?	Often, elevated WBC and ESR
What other imaging studies are useful in osteomyelitis?	MRI, CT, and radionuclide studies
What is the treatment for osteomyelitis?	1. Débridement of necrotic, avascular infected bone 2. Removal of all foreign objects 3. Pathogen-specific antimicrobial therapy
What is the duration of therapy for osteomyelitis?	Acute—4–6 weeks intravenous therapy Chronic—6 weeks intravenous therapy, then several months of oral therapy

What are reasons for lack of response to therapy in osteomyelitis?	1. Associated undrained abscess (subperiosteal, intramedullary, or subcutaneous) 2. Formation of sequestra 3. Presence of foreign body 4. Development of resistance 5. Altered pharmacokinetics or inadequate dosing of antibiotics 6. Undiagnosed or untreated pathogens
What are complications of chronic osteomyelitis?	Squamous cell carcinoma of draining sinus tract and amyloidosis

INFECTIOUS ARTHRITIS (SEE ALSO CHAPTER 11)

What are predisposing conditions to infectious arthritis?	Preexisting arthritis, trauma, systemic illnesses (e.g., diabetes mellitus and malignancy), and infections elsewhere

ACQUIRED IMMUNE DEFICIENCY SYNDROME

What is HIV?	Human immunodeficiency virus is a chronic infection with a retrovirus that causes progressive dysfunction of the immune system. Patients are predisposed to opportunistic infections and malignancies.
What is AIDS?	Acquired immune deficiency syndrome (AIDS) is caused by infection with HIV and is defined as advanced immunodeficiency with a CD4 count of less than 200 cells/mm^3, a percentage of CD4 cells below 14%, or 1 or more of 26 different opportunistic diseases (occurring when at least moderate suppression of cell-mediated immunity is present)
What is the prevalence of HIV infection and of AIDS?	HIV infection—more than 18 million people worldwide; more than 1 million people in the United States AIDS—more than 4 million people worldwide, accounting for 2.5 million deaths; more than 400,000 in the United States, accounting for over 250,000 deaths

Projected for the year 2000—at least 40 million people infected worldwide

What are risk factors for HIV infection and AIDS?

Homosexual and bisexual activity (40% of AIDS cases in the United States), injection drug use (30%), homosexual activity plus injection drug use (5%), heterosexual activity (10%), blood transfusion or hemophilia (2%), perinatal exposure (1%), and no identified risk (12%, includes those under investigation)

How is HIV transmitted?

Contact with blood and body fluids, not by casual contact

How is the diagnosis of HIV infection made?

Serologically, antibodies against viral antigens are detected. Two enzyme-linked immunosorbent assays and one Western blot assay must be positive for a person to be reported as HIV positive.

What is the natural history of HIV infection?

Normal CD4 count is > 1000 cells/ mm^3. In HIV-positive patients, the CD4 count decreases by 60–100 cells/ mm^3/yr, on average. The median time to development of AIDS is longer than 10 years, but this number varies dramatically among individuals. In addition, approximately 5% are long-term nonprogressors. Although often considered in stages, HIV infection is a continuum—HIV infects and replicates in CD4+ T lymphocytes. HIV antigen appears in the blood within weeks of infection and an immune response develops. The "window period" is the time between infection and development of anti-HIV antibodies when usual serologic diagnostic tests are negative.

What is acute HIV serocoversion?

The time right after infection before there is an immune response. An acute mononucleosis-like illness (fever, headache, pharyngitis, rash, gastrointestinal symptoms, and, occasionally, aseptic meningitis) develops. Almost all patients have anti-HIV antibodies by 6 months.

What characteristics are seen in early to mid infection?

A normal CD4 count decreases to approximately 200–300 cells/mm³. At baseline, most patients have minimal or no symptoms. Some do have fever, fatigue, and lymphadenopathy. Anergy becomes more common when the CD4 count is < 400 cells/mm³. Episodes of VZV, thrush, seborrheic dermatitis, skin and nail infections, and bacterial infections develop. Neurologic symptoms, including peripheral neuropathy and early dementia, may occur. Kaposi's sarcoma and tuberculosis are also seen.

What is seen in advanced HIV infection?

A CD4 count below 200 cells/mm³. Opportunistic infections such as PCP occur and systemic symptoms may be prominent without a defined cause.

What is seen in late-stage HIV infection?

A CD4 count below 50 cells/mm³; increase in the types of opportunistic infections, including toxoplasmosis, CMV, *C. neoformans*, MAC, and CNS lymphoma. Other infections more easily disseminate.

What is the role of antiretroviral treatment in HIV infection?

Recommendations are always changing. Currently available agents include reverse transcriptase inhibitors (AZT, DDI, DDC, D4T, and 3TC) and protease inhibitors (saquinavir, ritonavir, and indinavir). Consider starting therapy when the CD4 count decreases to below 500 cells/mm³, especially if the patient is symptomatic. If the patient is intolerant or progresses, switch to another agent. Combination therapy (usually AZT plus 3TC and a protease inhibitor) is currently the standard of care and is clearly superior to monotherapy.

What are side effects of the following:

AZT (zidovudine, Retrovir)

Primarily, bone marrow suppression. Initially, patients may complain of fatigue, headache, nausea, restlessness, and insomnia. These symptoms often resolve if therapy is continued. Bone marrow suppression may involve either leukopenia, neutropenia, or anemia. In patients who undergo treatment for more than 1 year, myopathy may develop.

DDI (didanosine)

Peripheral neuropathy, pancreatitis, and diarrhea

DDC (dicalcitibine)

Peripheral neuropathy, pancreatitis (less common), and esophageal ulcers

3TC (lamivudine, Epivir)

Fever, malaise, gastrointestinal upset, neuropathy, musculoskeletal pain, sleep or depressive disorders, and pancreatitis

D4T (stavudine)

Peripheral neuropathy

Indinavir (Crixivan)

Asymptomatic hyperbilirubinemia (10% of cases), nephrolithiasis (4%), abdominal pain, nausea, vomiting, diarrhea, and headache

Ritonavir (Norvir)

Abdominal pain, nausea, vomiting, diarrhea, and asthenia

What medications are contraindicated because of interference with hepatic metabolism when using the following protease inhibitors:

Both ritonavir and indinavir

Astemizole (Hismanil), cisapride (Propulsid), midazolam (Versed), terfenadine (Seldane), and triazolam (Halcion)

Ritonavir

All benzodiazepines [including zolpidem (Ambien)], amiodarone (Cordarone), bepridil (Vascor), bupropion (Wellbutrin), encainide, flecainide, propafenone, quinidine, meperidine, piroxicam, propoxyphene, and rifabutin

Indinavir	Rifampin

When should PCP prophylaxis be initiated in a patient with HIV infection?

It should be initiated in patients with a CD4 count of less than 200 cells/mm^3 or a CD4 percentage of 14%, and in patients who have developed thrush or persistent fevers.

Which agent should be used as PCP prophylaxis in HIV infection?

Trimethoprim–sulfamethoxazole DS 3 days weekly or daily allows the fewest breakthroughs. If the patient is intolerant, the first alternative is dapsone, 50–100 mg/day. (Check for G6PD deficiency in blacks and in persons of Mediterranean heritage). Inhaled pentamidine can be used in patients who cannot tolerate either oral regimen. Patients on pentamidine have more episodes of PCP and atypical disease.

What are the most common opportunistic infections in HIV infected persons?

Candidal esophagitis, PCP, MAC, CMV, toxoplasmosis, cryptococcal meningitis, and *M. tuberculosis*

What is MAC?

Mycobacterium avium complex is an atypical mycobacterium that produces disseminated disease in patients with advanced AIDS— the CD4 count is usually less than 50 cells/mm^3. Patients have fever (to 40°C), night sweats, and weight loss, and they may have abdominal pain or diarrhea. Diagnosis is made by blood culture. Treatment is clarithromycin plus ethambutol.

What is the most common cause of retinitis in AIDS patients?

CMV is the most common cause of retinitis in AIDS. It develops late, when CD4 counts are less than 100 cells/mm$^3.$

How does CMV retinitis present?

Initially, patients may be asymptomatic (disease begins peripherally) but progressive visual loss develops. CMV retinitis has the appearance on

	fundoscopy of "cottage cheese and ketchup."
How is CMV retinitis treated?	Patients with CMV retinitis require lifelong therapy with ganciclovir or foscarnet.
What is the most common malignancy in AIDS?	Kaposi's sarcoma
What is the most common focal CNS lesion in AIDS?	Toxoplasmosis
What are the most common causes of pneumonia in AIDS?	PCP, bacterial pneumonia, tuberculosis, fungi (*Cryptococcus*, histoplasmosis)
What are the most common causes of diarrhea in AIDS?	Causes vary geographically and include cryptosporidia, CMV, *C. difficile*, microsporidia, *Salmonella*, *Shigella*, MAC, and HIV enteropathy.
What is the most common cause of dysphagia and odynophagia in AIDS?	*Candida*
How does the course of HIV infection differ in women?	Women suffer recurrent vaginal candidiasis and increased risk of cervical cancer. PID is more likely to require hospitalization and have complications. There is also risk of vertical transmission to infants during pregnancy and delivery.
What is the rate of vertical transmission of HIV?	25%–30%
What is the rate of vertical transmission of HIV when AZT is used during pregnancy?	10%. Other antiretroviral agents have not yet been evaluated in pregnancy.

NOSOCOMIAL INFECTIONS

What is a nosocomial infection?	An infection that was not present or incubating at the time of hospital admission

What are types of nosocomial infections?	Virtually any infection can be nosocomial.
What is the incidence of nosocomial infection?	Occurs in more than 5% of patients admitted to acute care hospitals

NOSOCOMIAL BLOODSTREAM INFECTION

What is nosocomial BSI?	A clinically important blood culture obtained longer than 48 hours after hospital admission that is positive for bacteria or fungus. It may be primary (without a defined source, related to an indwelling line) or secondary (due to infection elsewhere).
What is the incidence of nosocomial BSI?	> 250,000 episodes per year
What are risk factors for nosocomial BSI?	Indwelling venous catheters, extremes of age, underlying disease, malnutrition, increased length of hospital stay, invasive procedures, intensive care unit care
What pathogens are associated with nosocomial BSI?	Coagulase-negative staphylococci, *S. aureus*, enterococci, *Candida, E. coli, Enterobacter, Proteus, Klebsiella,* and other bacteria (less commonly)
What laboratory and diagnostic tests are performed to diagnose nosocomial BSI?	CBC and blood cultures drawn peripherally and through an indwelling line
What is the treatment for nosocomial BSI?	Antibiotics directed against the pathogen. The choice of empiric antibiotics depends on the patient. If BSI is primary, gram-positive cocci should be covered (include coverage for gram-negative bacilli if there is increased risk). If BSI is secondary, treat the underlying cause of bacteremia. Some cases may require removal of the indwelling line.

NOSOCOMIAL PNEUMONIA

What is the incidence of nosocomial pneumonia?

> 250,000 episodes per year. It is the second leading cause of nosocomial infection and the number one cause of death from nosocomial infection in the United States.

NOSOCOMIAL URINARY TRACT INFECTION

What is the incidence of nosocomial UTI?

400,000 to 1 million infections per year; 40% of all nosocomial infections

SURGICAL WOUND INFECTION

What are the two types of surgical wound infections and how do they present?

1. Incisional—pain, erythema, purulent exudate, tenderness, swelling, and wound dehiscence at a surgical incision. It involves the skin, subcutaneous tissue, or muscle above the fascia.
2. Deep wound—infection at an operative site within 30 days after surgery if no implant is in place or longer if a foreign body is present (e.g., meningitis after neurosurgery, abdominal abscess after abdominal surgery)

What is the incidence of surgical wound infection?

> 325,000 cases per year in the United States

What pathogens are associated with surgical wound infection?

S. aureus, other gram-positive cocci, *E. coli, P. aeruginosa, Enterobacter, Proteus,* and *Klebsiella*

What are risk factors for surgical wound infection?

"Dirty" or contaminated procedures, experience of the surgeon, length of operation, poor nutrition, older age, presence of underlying diseases (e.g., diabetes mellitus and rheumatoid arthritis), and use of steroids influence the risk.

How is the diagnosis of surgical wound infection made?

History and physical examination

What is the treatment for surgical wound infection?	Because skin pathogens are most common, consider nafcillin or vancomycin. Cover gram-negative anaerobes if there is deep wound infection or if the patient is at risk. Surgery is often needed for deep infection.

NOSOCOMIAL GASTROINTESTINAL INFECTIONS

What is nosocomial gastrointestinal infection?	Acute gastrointestinal illness in a hospitalized patient; more specifically, a positive stool culture for a pathogen or unexplained diarrhea for more than 2 days or infectious diarrhea beginning in the hospital
What is the incidence of nosocomial diarrhea?	10 per 10,000 hospital discharges
What pathogens are associated with nosocomial diarrhea?	Bacteria cause > 90% of episodes, and *C. difficile* causes 90% of episodes in which a pathogen is identified. Rotavirus is the second most common pathogen and is seen in 1 of 20 infections.
What are risk factors for nosocomial diarrhea?	Patients at the extremes of life or with achlorhydria are at highest risk. Impaired immunity; altered intestinal motility; altered enteric flora (such as after antibiotic therapy); admission to the intensive care unit, and other factors that alter host defenses or increase the risk of colonization also play a role.
What laboratory and diagnostic tests are done in the workup of nosocomial diarrhea?	Stool culture and examination for fecal leukocytes and *C. difficile* toxin
How is the diagnosis of nosocomial diarrhea made?	History, physical examination, and stool studies
What is the treatment for nosocomial diarrhea?	Stop antibiotics if possible, hydration, and supportive care. Treat with metronidazole (by mouth is preferred to intravenous therapy) if the pathogen is *C. difficile*.

TRAVELERS SYNDROMES

What is the most common vaccine-preventable infection of travelers?

Hepatitis A

In what percentage of persons traveling to underdeveloped countries does traveler's diarrhea develop?

30%–50%

What is the predominant microbial pathogen in traveler's diarrhea?

Enterotoxigenic *E. coli*

What is the treatment for traveler's diarrhea?

1. Rehydration
2. Antibiotics, usually ciprofloxacin or ofloxacin
3. Antimotility agent (such as Imodium), if needed

What are contraindications for antimotility agents in traveler's diarrhea?

High fever, bloody stools, or other evidence of an inflammatory colitis or dysentery. (Toxic megacolon has been reported with the use of antimotility agents with inflammatory diarrhea.)

What are the most common causes of febrile illness in returning travelers?

Malaria, enteric fever, hepatitis, and amebic liver abscess

What are major causes of eosinophilia in travelers?

Helminths including filariasis, schistosomiasis, and strongyloidiasis

How can malaria be prevented?

1. Avoid mosquito bites by use of mosquito nets, DEET-containing insect repellents (20%–35% DEET), and wearing permethrin-sprayed clothing
2. Use chemoprophylaxis with chloroquine, mefloquine, or doxycycline. Current Centers for Disease Control (CDC) information should be obtained to establish the proper region-specific regimen.

9

Endocrinology

ABBREVIATIONS

ACTH	Adrenocorticotropic hormone
ADH	Antidiuretic hormone
CRH	Corticotropin-releasing hormone
CT	Computed tomography
DCCT	Diabetes Control and Complications Trial
DHEA-S	Dihydroepiandrostenerone-sulfate
DI	Diabetes insipidus
DTR	Deep tendon reflex
FSH	Follicular stimulating hormone
GH	Growth hormone
GnRH	Gonadotropin-releasing hormone
GRH	Growth hormone–releasing hormone
hCG	Human chorionic gonadotropin
IDDM	Insulin-dependent diabetes mellitus
LH	Luteinizing hormone
MEN	Multiple endocrine neoplasia
MRI	Magnetic resonance imaging
MSH	Melanocyte-stimulating hormone

NIDDM	Non-insulin–dependent diabetes mellitus
PCOS	Polycystic ovary syndrome
PO	By mouth
PRL	Prolactin
PTH	Parathyroid hormone
PTU	Propylthiouracil
RAI	Radioactive iodine
SIADH	Syndrome of inappropriate ADH
T3RU	T3 resin uptake
TB	Tuberculosis
TBG	Thyroxine-binding globulin
TRH	Thyrotropin-releasing hormone
TSH	Thyroid-stimulating hormone
TSS	Transsphenoidal surgery

ANTERIOR PITUITARY

PHYSIOLOGY

What hormones are produced (synthesized)?	GH, PRL, LH, FSH, TSH, ACTH
What are the actions of GH?	In children and adolescents, GH regulates growth and influences metabolism.
What is the role of PRL?	Production of lactation
What are the actions of LH and FSH?	To control gonadal function
What is the function of TSH?	To control the production of thyroid hormone by the thyroid gland

What is the response to ACTH?	Control of glucocorticoid secretion by the adrenal cortex
What is the normal feedback system between the anterior pituitary and the following:	
Gonads?	When the gonads fail or are removed, there is an increase in FSH and LH levels.
Thyroid	When the thyroid fails and there is low thyroxine, TSH secretion is increased. Increased thyroxine inhibits TSH secretion.
Adrenal	When the adrenal fails, the low cortisol level results in ACTH secretion. Increased cortisol feeds back to inhibit ACTH.
How is the anterior pituitary controlled?	The hypothalamus synthesizes many peptides that stimulate pituitary hormone secretion. GRH stimulates GH release, somatostatin inhibits GH release, GnRH stimulates LH and FSH, TRH stimulates TSH, CRH stimulates ACTH, and dopamine acts as a PRL-inhibiting factor.

DISEASES OF THE ANTERIOR PITUITARY

Do adenomas always cause symptoms?	No. Apparently asymptomatic microadenomas are found in 15%–25% of patients in autopsy series.
What are the more common adenomas?	Nonsecretory adenomas and prolactinomas
What are the symptoms and signs of pituitary adenomas?	Mass effects include headache and altered vision (bitemporal hemianopsia). Hormonal effects include hypopituitarism including hypogonadism, adrenal insufficiency, hypothyroidism and DI. Alternatively, hypersecretion of pituitary hormones is observed.

What are symptoms and signs of GH excess if it occurs before puberty?

Gigantism—very tall, arthralgias, cardiomegaly, hypertension

What are symptoms and signs of GH excess if it occurs after puberty?

Acromegaly—frontal bossing, arthralgias, spacing between teeth, soft tissue swelling, increased hand and shoe size, diabetes mellitus, hypertension, skin tags, coarse features

What are symptoms and signs of PRL excess?

Lactation (galactorrhea) and amenorrhea in women, hypogonadism in men

What are symptoms and signs of ACTH excess?

Cushingoid appearance, diabetes, hypertension, hyperpigmentation

What are symptoms and signs of TSH excess?

Hyperthyroidism

Is enlargement of the pituitary ever normal?

The pituitary doubles in size during pregnancy.

How is the diagnosis of pituitary tumors made when the following are involved:
    GH excess

GH stimulates production of insulin-like growth factor 1, which is increased along with GH in acromegaly. As a result of its pulsatile secretion, increased GH may be difficult to document with single samples. In response to an oral glucose load, GH secretion increases in patients with acromegaly, but not in normal subjects.

    PRL excess

A single serum PRL value is usually sufficient. Occasionally, this value must be remeasured.

    ACTH excess (Cushing's disease)

Useful screening tests for excess ACTH and cortisol production include a 24-hour urine collection for free-cortisol and the overnight dexamethasone suppression test (1 mg by mouth at 11 p.m. with measurement of an 8 a.m. cortisol level). If results are abnormal (either an increased urine free cortisol and/or a serum cortisol greater than 5 mg/dl after dexamethasone), then low-dose and high-dose dexamethasone suppression tests are used to distinguish obesity or depression (low dose) and pituitary tumors (high dose) from adrenal tumors or ectopic ACTH, which do not generally suppress.

What are the more common causes of ectopic ACTH production?

Small-cell lung cancer and bronchial carcinoids

What is Cushing's disease?

Pituitary ACTH hypersecretion with increased cortisol production

What are the treatment options for a GH adenoma?

TSS

Conventional pituitary radiation (4500 cGy), which decreases GH levels to < 5 ng/ml in 50% of cases by 5 years

Gamma knife radiation focused to the pituitary gland

Bromocriptine, a dopamine agonist that causes clinical improvement in 90% of patients at doses of 20–60 mg/day. A GH level of less than 10 ng/ml occurs in only 35% of patients, and a GH level of less than 5 ng/ml occurs in 15%.

Octreotide, a synthetic somatostatin analog that reduces GH secretion in most patients but has variable effects on tumor size

What is the cure rate for TSS?

The cure rate for TSS is 75% if the preoperative GH level is less than 40 ng/ml and 35% if the preoperative GH level is more than 40 mg/ml. These results vary with the experience of the neurosurgeon.

What are the side effects of bromocriptine?

Nausea, fatigue, nasal stuffiness, postural hypotension

What is the treatment for a prolactinoma?

Treatment depends on the size of the tumor and the skill of the neurosurgeon. Small tumors may be resectable. Large tumors (> 1 cm) are treated medically with bromocriptine at a dosage of 1.25

mg qHS, increasing slowly to 2.5 mg
three times a day.

What is the treatment of ACTH, LH, FSH, and TSH adenomas?

TSS. If TSS is unsuccessful, then
treatment includes adjuvant conventional
pituitary radiation or gamma knife
radiation.

What is Nelson's syndrome?

Decreased negative feedback of cortisol
caused by surgical removal of the
adrenal glands, resulting in ACTH-
producing pituitary tumors

POSTERIOR PITUITARY GLAND

PHYSIOLOGY

What hormones are released from the posterior pituitary?

ADH, which controls water
conservation, and oxytocin, which is
necessary for milk let-down during
lactation

Where are ADH and oxytocin produced?

The paraventricular and supraoptic
nuclei of the hypothalamus. They are
transported by way of neuronal axons to
the posterior pituitary.

What stimulates release of ADH?

Decreased plasma volume, increased
plasma osmolarity, nausea, and exposure
to hot temperatures

What are the causes of central DI?

Trauma and postoperative state
(neurosurgical)
Anatomic—tumors and infiltrative
diseases (e.g., histiocytosis X)
Infectious—meningitis and encephalitis
Hereditary
Vascular—pituitary apoplexy

What are symptoms and signs of DI?

Polyuria, polydipsia

What are the differential diagnoses for central DI?

Psychogenic polydipsia and nephrogenic
DI

What are the laboratory findings in DI?

Increased plasma osmolarity and
decreased urine osmolarity

What is the water deprivation test?

Water is withheld from the patient to induce dehydration and to assess urinary water retention. In DI, the plasma osmolarity increases without a urinary response to retain water. In central DI (hypothalamic), treatment with ADH concentrates the urine. In nephrogenic DI, ADH has no effect.

What is the treatment for DI?

For central DI, intranasal ddAVP (ADH analog); for nephrogenic DI, thiazides (diuresis causes ablation of medullary gradient and thus decreases urine volume output)

What are causes of SIADH?

Central nervous system disorders—skull fracture, subdural hematoma, subarachnoid hemorrhage (SAH), acute encephalitis, TB meningitis, Guillain-Barré syndrome

Malignant neoplasms—oat cell cancer (lung), cancer of the pancreas, lymphosarcoma, reticulum cell sarcoma, Hodgkin's disease, cancer of the duodenum, thymoma

Nonmalignant pulmonary disease—TB, lung abscess, pneumonia, viral pneumonitis, empyema, chronic obstructive pulmonary disease

Drugs—chlorpropamide, vincristine, vinblastine, cyclophosphamide, carbamazepine, oxytocin, narcotics

Other—hypothyroidism, positive pressure ventilation, possibly postoperative pain

What are symptoms and signs of SIADH?

Confusion, seizures, and coma largely attributable to brain edema secondary to osmotic water shifts

What are the laboratory findings for SIADH?

Decreased Na^+ (< 130 mEq/L), decreased plasma osmolarity (< 270 mOsm/kg), and hypertonic urine

What is the treatment for SIADH?

Correction of the underlying cause of SIADH

Water restriction to 800–1000 ml/day

Demeclocycline (interferes with renal action of ADH)

3% saline given slowly over several hours (if severe hyponatremia is present)

What is a complication of correcting serum Na⁺ too quickly?

Central pontine myelinolysis

How is the release of oxytocin controlled?

By estrogen or manipulation or distention of breasts or female genital tract

What is the function of oxytocin?

It acts on membranes of myometrial cells to cause increased force of contraction, exerts contractile action in myometrium postpartum, and contracts myoepithelial cells of mammary alveoli to cause expulsion of milk.

What are the clinical uses of oxytocin?

For induction of labor and control of hemorrhage after delivery

HYPOPITUITARISM

What are symptoms and signs of the following:

GH deficiency

In children, decreased linear growth; in adults, fine wrinkling around eyes and mouth

Gonadotropin deficiency

Amenorrhea, infertility, altered libido, decreased facial hair growth in men

TSH deficiency

Hypothyroidism with fatigue, cold intolerance, and puffy skin in the absence of a goiter

ACTH deficiency

Cortisol deficiency manifested by fatigue, decreased appetite, weight loss, abnormal response to stress characterized by fever, hypotension, hyponatremia, and a high mortality rate

How is the diagnosis of GH deficiency made?

Insulin tolerance test. Insulin is injected and GH measured at specific time intervals thereafter. GH should normally increase to greater than 9 ng/ml after insulin injection. Other stimulation studies include oral L-dopa and arginine infusion for adults and oral clonidine and intramuscular glucagon for children.

How is the diagnosis of ACTH deficiency made?

Insulin tolerance test. The cortisol level should be greater than 20 ml/dl after adequate hypoglycemia.
Metyrapone test. Administration normally causes an increase in ACTH and cortisol.

How is the diagnosis of thyrotropin deficiency made?

Serum T4, free-T4, and TSH are decreased or inappropriately "normal."

How is the diagnosis of gonadotropin deficiency made?

Measurement of estrogen and FSH and LH levels in women; measurement of testosterone and FSH and LH levels in men. In postmenopausal women, FSH and LH levels should be elevated because there is no longer any negative feedback from the ovaries to secrete estrogen; therefore, "normal" FSH and LH levels suggest gonadotropin deficiency in these women.

What is the treatment for GH deficiency in adults?

Currently, GH replacement is not indicated.

What is the treatment for gonadotropin deficiency?

Estrogen and progesterone for women, testosterone for men

What is the treatment for TSH deficiency?

Thyroxine

What is the treatment for ACTH deficiency?

Hydrocortisone

What is Sheehan's syndrome?

Ischemic pituitary necrosis follows episodes of severe hypotension during pregnancy. It results from hemorrhagic infarction of pituitary adenoma, causing hypopituitarism.

What are other causes of Sheehan's syndrome?	Inflammatory lesions—TB, sarcoid, adenoma pushing and destroying normal tissue, metastasis, histiocytosis X, craniopharyngioma, hemorrhage, hemochromatosis
What is the empty sella syndrome?	The sella has little, if any, obvious normal tissue, and it is filled with cerebrospinal fluid. This is likely either the result of a prior pituitary tumor (that spontaneously regressed) or it is congenital.
What is the pituitary function in empty sella syndrome?	In most cases, normal pituitary function is observed, but some patients do have sporadic pituitary hormone deficiencies.

ADRENAL GLAND

PHYSIOLOGY

What is the negative feedback loop of the hypothalamus–pituitary–adrenal axis for cortisol production?	CRH is released by the hypothalamus in a circadian rhythm and in response to stress. The anterior pituitary, in turn, releases ACTH, which stimulates the adrenal production of cortisol. Cortisol feeds back to the hypothalamus and pituitary to suppress CRH and ACTH.
At what time of day in normal individuals are ACTH and cortisol secretion highest?	Early morning at time of wakening (before 8 a.m.)
At what time of day in normal individuals are ACTH and cortisol secretion lowest?	One hour after beginning sleep (before 1 a.m.)
What factors stimulate ACTH secretion?	Hypocortisolism, hypoglycemia, CRH, and ADH
Pro-opiomelanocortin is the precursor molecule for what four peptides?	ACTH, lipotropin, MSH, beta-endorphin

What are the three layers of the adrenal cortex and their corresponding hormone products?	1. Glomerulosa—aldosterone (mineralocorticoid), "salt" 2. Fasciculata—cortisol (glucocorticoid), "sugar" 3. Reticularis—DHEA, DHEA-S, androstenedione (androgenic steroids), "sex"
What are the main stimuli for aldosterone secretion?	Angiotensin II (hypotension, hyponatremia) and hyperkalemia

CUSHING'S SYNDROME

What is Cushing's syndrome?	Glucocorticoid excess
What are clinical manifestations of Cushing's syndrome?	Centripetal obesity, moon facies, dewlap (under chin), buffalo hump, and supraclavicular fat pads Protein catabolism, thin extremities from muscle wasting, weakness, and proximal myopathy Atrophic skin, facial plethora, violaceous striae, easy bruising, and slow wound healing Hyperglycemia and glucose intolerance Psychological problems (depression, psychosis, suicidal tendency, mania, anxiety, and insomnia) Osteoporosis (vertebral compression fractures, aseptic necrosis, hypercalciuria, and renal calculi) Immune suppression, cutaneous fungal infections, lymphopenia, decreased eosinophils Hyperpigmentation, lymphopenia, decreased eosinophils (if ACTH-dependent Cushing's syndrome)
What is the most common cause of Cushing's syndrome?	Exogenous steroids used to treat nonendocrine disorders. The patient should be asked about receiving intraarticular injections and dermatologic preparations.
What are the four endogenous causes of Cushing's syndrome?	1. Cushing's disease (pituitary tumor), 70%–80%

2. Adrenal tumors (adenoma or carcinoma), 10%–15%
3. Ectopic ACTH and CRH secreted by nonpituitary tumor, < 5%
4. Primary adrenal dysplastic disorders (pigmented micronodular hyperplasia and macronodular dysplasia), rare

What are causes of ectopic ACTH secretion?

Small-cell lung cancer (50%), pancreatic islet cell carcinoma, thymoma, carcinoid tumors, medullary thyroid carcinoma, and pheochromocytoma

What is the usual presentation of ectopic ACTH syndrome?

Rather than the typical cushingoid habitus, ectopic ACTH syndrome tends to present with rapidly progressive hypokalemia, metabolic alkalosis, hyperpigmentation, hypertension, edema, and weakness.

What two screening tests are used to confirm hypercortisolism?

Overnight dexamethasone suppression test and 24-hour urine free-cortisol test

How is the dexamethasone suppression test performed?

Dexamethasone, 1 mg, is taken at 11 p.m. and serum cortisol is measured at 8 a.m. the next morning. Normal response is suppression of cortisol to less than 5 µg/dl.

How is the urine free-cortisol test performed?

A 24-hour urine collection for free-cortisol and creatinine is used to integrate the episodic cortisol secretory patterns.

What are the causes of abnormal screening tests for hypercortisolism?

Pathologic hypercortisolism, noncompliance, stress, obesity, depression, alcoholism, and increased metabolism of dexamethasone from anticonvulsants or rifampin

How is pathologic hypercortisolism confirmed?

Low-dose dexamethasone suppression test

How is a low-dose dexamethasone suppression test performed?

After measuring basal 24-hour urine free-cortisol, 8 a.m. plasma cortisol, and ACTH, dexamethasone, (0.5 mg) is given by mouth every 6 hours for 48 hours. A 24-hour urine for free-cortisol is collected during the second day and serum cortisol is measured at 48 hours. In patients with pathologic hypercortisolism, urine free-cortisol and cortisol levels are not suppressed.

A suppressed ACTH (< 5 pg/ml) suggests what causes of endogenous Cushing's syndrome?

Primary adrenal tumor or nodular dysplasia

Which causes of hypercortisolism are associated with an inappropriately normal or elevated ACTH level (at 1 a.m.)?

Cushing's disease, ectopic ACTH, or CRH syndrome

What test is used to differentiate Cushing's disease from ectopic ACTH syndrome and adrenal tumor?

High-dose dexamethasone suppression test

How is a high-dose dexamethasone suppression test performed?

Dexamethasone (2 mg) is given by mouth every 6 hours for 48 hours. Urine is collected for free-cortisol on the second day and serum cortisol is measured 6 hours after the final dose of dexamethasone is given. In Cushing's disease, the abnormal corticotropes maintain some degree of responsiveness to steroids, so the urine-free cortisol and serum cortisol are suppressed by at least 50% from baseline values. Ectopic ACTH and adrenal tumors are not suppressed with high-dose dexamethasone.

Why is a chest CT scan obtained in some cases in which there is suppression of cortisol by high-dose dexamethasone?

Some ACTH-secreting bronchial or carcinoid tumors can be suppressed with dexamethasone, thereby mimicking Cushing's disease.

What is the radiographic test of choice for identifying suspected pituitary adenomas?	MRI of the sella with and without gadolinium
What causes Cushing's disease?	Pituitary adenomas in 90% of cases. Of these, 90% are microadenomas (< 10 mm), with an average size of approximately 6 mm. Some patients have diffuse corticotropic hyperplasia.
What is the treatment for Cushing's disease?	TSS. If a microadenoma is identified, microadenomectomy is performed and pituitary function is preserved. If a microadenoma cannot be identified, near total anterior hypophysectomy is performed.
What is the cure rate when TSS is used in Cushing's disease?	90% with microadenomas; 50% with macroadenomas
How is cure of Cushing's disease assessed after TSS?	An 8 a.m. cortisol level is drawn 24 hours after the last postoperative dose of hydrocortisone is discontinued. If "cure" has been achieved, the patient's cortisol level is less than 5 μg/dl. Normal levels may indicate surgical failure.
What are three options for treatment in patients who are not cured after TSS?	Repeat TSS, pituitary irradiation, and medical or surgical adrenalectomy
Name four adrenal inhibitors and their site of inhibition.	1. Aminoglutethimide—blocks side chain cleavage enzyme needed for conversion of cholesterol to pregnenolone 2. Metyrapone—inhibits IIβ-hydroxylase, which catalyzes the final step in cortisol and aldosterone synthesis 3. Ketoconazole—blocks both side chain cleavage enzyme and IIβ-hydroxylase 4. Mitotane—a cytotoxic drug that preferentially destroys zona fasciculata and reticularis cells

| **What is the treatment for adrenal adenomas and carcinomas?** | Surgical resection of the tumor. Adrenal carcinomas may also require mitotane therapy, although this is controversial. Adrenal enzyme inhibitors can be used to control refractory Cushing's syndrome. |

ADRENAL INSUFFICIENCY

What is the cause of primary adrenal insufficiency?	Destruction of the adrenal cortex
What is the cause of secondary adrenal insufficiency?	Deficient pituitary ACTH secretion
What is the cause of tertiary adrenal insufficiency?	Deficient hypothalamic CRH secretion
What are the most common causes of adrenal insufficiency?	Prior exogenous glucocorticoids Metastatic disease (lung and breast carcinoma, melanoma, and colon cancer) Granulomatous diseases (TB, histoplasmosis, coccidioidomycosis, and sarcoid)
What are clinical manifestations of polyglandular autoimmune syndrome type I?	Hypoparathyroidism, mucocutaneous candidiasis, and adrenal insufficiency
What is the inheritance pattern of polyglandular autoimmune syndrome type I?	Autosomal recessive
What are clinical manifestations of polyglandular autoimmune syndrome type II?	Adrenal insufficiency, autoimmune thyroid disease (Hashimoto's or Graves' disease), insulin-dependent diabetes mellitus, gonadal failure, and alopecia
In which forms of adrenal insufficiency is mineralocorticoid secretion intact?	Secondary and tertiary. The adrenal cortex maintains responsiveness to the renin–angiotensin system.

Which form of adrenal insufficiency is associated with hyperpigmentation?

Primary

What is the mechanism of hyperpigmentation?

Hypocortisolemia causes increased secretion of ACTH and other proopiomelanocortin-derived peptides such as MSH. These peptides stimulate melanin production, resulting in hyperpigmentation of the skin and mucous membranes.

What are clinical and laboratory features of adrenal insufficiency?

Nausea, vomiting, weakness, fatigue, lethargy, weight loss, anorexia, hyperpigmentation (primary), hyponatremia, hyperkalemia (primary), azotemia, hypoglycemia, hypercalcemia, eosinophilia (TB), and normocytic and normochromic anemia

What are additional clinical features of acute adrenal crisis?

Fever, abdominal pain, hypovolemia, hypotension and shock, confusion, and coma

What initial tests are used in the workup of primary adrenal insufficiency?

Short ACTH stimulation, morning cortisol, and ACTH level

What form of adrenal insufficiency is associated with an elevated ACTH?

Primary

What forms of adrenal insufficiency are associated with a low ACTH?

Secondary and tertiary

What test differentiates secondary from tertiary adrenal insufficiency?

CRH stimulation test. Patients with secondary adrenal insufficiency have little or no ACTH response to CRH, whereas patients with tertiary adrenal insufficiency have an exaggerated ACTH response to CRH.

What is the treatment for primary adrenal insufficiency?

Glucocorticoid replacement—
hydrocortisone (10 mg by mouth every morning, 10 mg at noon, and 5 mg every evening)

Mineralocorticoid replacement—
Florinef, 0.1 mg by mouth every day
Liberal salt intake

How should patients with adrenal insufficiency adjust their medications during a minor febrile illness?

Increase glucocorticoid dose 2- to 3-fold for the few days of the illness

What is the "stress dose" of steroids and when is it indicated?

Hydrocortisone, 100 mg intravenously every 8 hours for 1–2 days until the stress has resolved. This dose is indicated for any adrenally insufficient patient with severe illness or who undergoes major surgery.

How is adrenal crisis managed?

The initial goal of therapy is reversal of hypotension and electrolyte abnormalities, with normal saline (2–3 L) given as quickly as possible. Glucocorticoid replacement with dexamethasone, 4 mg intravenously, or hydrocortisone, 100 mg intravenously, is also given immediately. Mineralocorticoid therapy can be started when the patient is taking PO and the saline infusion is discontinued.

ALDOSTERONE

The following questions define the renin–angiotensin–aldosterone system.

Where is renin produced?

Juxtaglomerular cells of the renal cortex

What are renin stimuli?

Hypovolemia and β-adrenergic stimulation

What does renin do?

Converts angiotensinogen (hepatic origin) to angiotensin I

What does angiotensin-converting enzyme do?

Converts angiotensin I (cleaved) to angiotensin II

What are the effects of angiotensin II?

Directs vasoconstriction and stimulates secretion of aldosterone from the zona glomerulosa of the adrenals

What is the feedback to suppress renin?

Aldosterone and angiotensin II feed back to the juxtaglomerular cells.

What is the principal action of aldosterone in the kidney?

Stimulation of the distal tubule Na^+/K^+ ATPase

What is the effect of aldosterone?

Na^+ retention and K^+ excretion

What is hyperaldosteronism?

Inappropriate secretion of aldosterone

What are the causes of primary aldosteronism?

Adrenal adenoma (60%), bilateral adrenal hyperplasia (40%), macronodular adrenal hyperplasia, glucocorticoid-suppressible hyperaldosteronism, and adrenal carcinoma

What are the causes of secondary hyperaldosteronism?

Volume depletion, renal artery stenosis, malignant hypertension, estrogen, and salt-wasting nephropathy

What is the clinical presentation of hyperaldosteronism?

Diastolic hypertension, hypokalemia, polyuria, and metabolic alkalosis

What laboratory results help distinguish primary aldosteronism from other cases of hypertension?

Elevated aldosterone levels in the setting of suppressed plasma renin activity

What aldosterone and renin levels are suggestive of an adrenal cause of hyperaldosteronism?

A plasma aldosterone to plasma renin activity ratio greater than 50 is suggestive of either an aldosteronoma or bilateral adrenal hyperplasia and warrants further investigation. Also, secondary hyperaldosteronism is dependent on volume status–renin secretion, and levels of aldosterone should decline with saline infusion or blockade of converting enzyme.

How do aldosterone-secreting adenomas and bilateral hyperplasia differ in their response to upright posture?

After 4 hours of upright posture, plasma aldosterone increases significantly in bilateral hyperplasia. Aldosterone does not increase in patients with adenomas and may even paradoxically decrease.

What diagnostic procedures can aid in localization of an aldosterone-secreting adenoma?

CT or MRI and adrenal venous sampling

What is the incidence of nonsecretory incidental adrenal masses detected on abdominal CT scan?

1%

How is adrenal venous sampling performed?

Both adrenal veins and a peripheral site are catheterized. A continuous infusion of ACTH is administered while samples for aldosterone and cortisol are obtained from all three sites. The concentration of aldosterone from the adenoma-containing adrenal is typically 10 times greater than in the opposite adrenal.

What is the treatment for an aldosterone-secreting adrenal adenoma?

Unilateral adrenalectomy

What is the cure rate for surgical removal of the aldosteronoma?

90%

What medical therapies can be used in primary aldosteronism that has failed surgical management or in the nonsurgical candidate?

Spironolactone (200–400 mg/day), amiloride, and calcium channel blockers

PHEOCHROMOCYTOMA

How common are pheochromocytomas?

Not common, occurring in 0.1% of all patients with diastolic hypertension

Where is the most common site for pheochromocytomas?	90%, adrenal medulla; 8%, other chromaffin tissue; 2%, extrathoracic (neck or thorax)
What are common sites of extramedullary pheochromocytomas?	Most are associated with sympathetic ganglia in the mediastinum or abdomen.
What syndrome does multiple, extramedullary, or bilateral pheochromocytoma suggest?	Sipple's syndrome (MEN type 2, with pheochromocytoma plus medullary carcinoma of the thyroid, with or without parathyroid tumors)
What is the presentation of pheochromocytomas?	Depends on the catechol secreted If the catechol secreted is norepinephrine (as it is in the majority of patients), the patient presents with hypertension (sustained with paroxysms), palpitations, headache, pallor, flushing, diaphoresis, and anxiety. If the catechol secreted is epinephrine or dopamine, then the patient may present with hypotension.
Which patients with hypertension should be screened for pheochromocytomas?	1. Patients with severe, sustained, or paroxysmal hypertension or grade 3 or 4 retinopathy 2. Patients with MEN II or III syndromes and their first-degree relatives 3. Patients with hypertension during labor, anesthesia, or receipt of radiographic contrast 4. Patients with worsening hypertension on β-blockers, guanethidine, or ganglionic blockers (e.g., trimethaphan) 5. Patients with unexplained pyrexia and hypotension 6. Supraadrenal masses
Can there be multiple pheochromocytomas?	Yes. 10% are bilateral or multiple

How commonly are pheochromocytomas malignant?	10%
In patients with pheochromocytomas, what may provoke paroxysms of hypertension?	Ingestion of tyramine-containing foods, especially in patients taking monoamine oxidase inhibitors, iodine-containing contrast agents, abdominal examination, and glucagon
Can patients with pheochromocytomas present with only sustained hypertension?	Yes; 50% present in such a manner.
How is the diagnosis of pheochromocytomas made?	Clinical suspicion, demonstration of urinary metabolites (catechols, metanephrines, and vanillylmandelic acid), plasma catechols, CT scanning, or MRI
What special diet or medication adjustments are needed before urinary catechols are measured?	Products containing vanilla and caffiene, and β-blockers must be withheld for 72 hours.
How are plasma catechols measured?	Patients should be supine and resting in comfortable settings. Plasma catecholamine levels are then drawn.
What factors affect plasma catechol levels?	Anxiety, pain, dehydration, congestive heart failure, smoking, and beta-blockers
What is the clonidine suppression test?	Plasma catechol levels may be elevated in both essential hypertension and with pheochromocytomas. Clonidine (0.3 mg by mouth) suppresses the blood pressure in both groups and brings the plasma catechol levels back to the normal range in patients with essential hypertension but not in patients with pheochromocytomas.
What is the treatment for pheochromocytomas?	Surgical removal of the tumors. All patients should be given alpha-blocking agents. Calcium channel blockers may also be helpful, and beta-blockers should be considered before surgery.

THYROID GLAND

PHYSIOLOGY

What is the normal histologic makeup of the thyroid gland?	The thyroid gland is made up of follicles that contain colloid in their lumen. Thyroglobulin is the major protein contained in colloid, and it is the precursor for all thyroid hormones. Iodide is needed to synthesize thyroid hormones and is attached (X4) to tyrosine residues. The wall of the follicle is made up of follicular cells. The parafollicular cells secrete calcitonin.
What are the main forms of thyroid hormone?	Thyroxine (T4) is made only in the thyroid. Triiodothyronine (T3) is made mostly from peripheral conversion of T4 to T3.
How are thyroid hormones transported?	The majority of T4 (> 99%) is bound to TBG with less than 1% circulating "free." T3 does not bind as tightly to TBG. Hence, there is 10 times as much free-T3 as free-T4.
What is T3RU?	An indirect way to measure free-T4. The patient's serum, which contains TBG, is mixed with radiolabeled T3. A resin is added to "take up" any unbound T3. The T3 (radioactive) bound to the resin is proportional to the free-T4 and inversely proportional to the TBG.
What causes a low T3RU?	Hypothyroidism—there is reduced T4 and T3, hence more unoccupied sites on TBG; radiolabeled T3 binds to TBG more than resin, hence a reduced T3RU. Increased TBG—seen most commonly in pregnancy, estrogen treatment, and acute liver disease. Total T4 is increased because of binding to TBG while the "free concentration" is normal.

What are the causes of a high T3RU?	Hyperthyroidism—there is increased T4 and T3, hence fewer unoccupied sites on TBG; radiolabeled T3 binds to resin more than TBG, hence an increased T3RU. Reduced TBG—seen most commonly in androgen treatment, acromegaly, glucocorticoid excess, and chronic liver disease
What are antithyroid antibodies and when are they present?	Antimicrosomal and antithyroglobulin antibodies. The former are present in nearly all cases of Hashimoto's thyroiditis and 80% of Graves' disease.
What is the incidence of a solitary thyroid nodule?	Occurs in up to 5% of the population, with a female to male ratio of 4:1. Incidence increases with age.
What is the differential diagnosis of a solitary thyroid nodule?	Benign colloid nodule (50%–70%), benign adenoma (15%–30%), malignant nodule (5%–10%), and cysts (5%)
What is the most common clinical history of a thyroid nodule?	Asymptomatic
What are risk factors for malignancy in a thyroid nodule?	History of external irradiation, male gender, extremes of age, family history of thyroid cancer (e.g., medullary carcinoma of the thyroid in MEN), rapid growth of the nodule, firm texture of the nodule, and solitary lesion
What are approaches to evaluating the solitary thyroid nodule?	Fine needle aspiration—can identify malignant cells, but a negative cytologic study does not rule out a malignancy. This test is probably most favored for nonsurgical first tests. Ultrasound—can be used to find multiple nodules or document cystic structure that confers a more benign course. It cannot rule out malignancy. Thyroid scan—a "hot" (functioning) nodule is nearly always benign. Conversely, most benign and nearly all malignant lesions are "cold" (hypofunctioning), making

differentiation difficult. This test is
rarely used.

**What are therapies for
thyroid cancer?**

For follicular and papillary cancers,
debate continues as to the most effective
therapies. The larger malignant lesions,
follicular cancers, and medullary
carcinoma likely need near total
thyroidectomies, because they are more
likely to be advanced or multifocal. For
metastatic disease, RAI can be used.

HYPERTHYROIDISM

**What are the causes of
hyperthyroidism associated
with a high radioiodine
uptake?**

Graves' disease, toxic multinodular
goiter, toxic adenoma, trophoblastic
tumor-secreting hCG, and TSH-
secreting pituitary tumor

**What are the causes of
hyperthyroidism associated
with a low radioiodine
uptake?**

Subacute thyroiditis (de Quervain's
thyroiditis), thyrotoxicosis factitia
(exogenous thyroid hormone ingestion),
ectopic thyroid tissue (struma ovarii),
and iodine-induced (jodbasedow
reaction)

**What are signs and
symptoms of
hyperthyroidism for the
following systems:**
   Skin

Warm, moist, diaphoretic, clubbing of
fingers and toes (thyroid acropachy), and
pretibial myxedema (only in Graves'
disease)

   **Head, ears, eyes, nose,
   and throat**

Lid tremor, infiltrative ophthalmopathy
(Graves' disease) with proptosis,
chemosis, lid lag, and periorbital edema

   Cardiovascular

Wide pulse pressure, sinus tachycardia,
cardiomegaly, and high-output
congestive heart failure

   Pulmonary

Dyspnea and tachypnea

   Gastrointestinal

Frequent bowel movements

Neurologic	Hyperkinesia, resting tremor, emotional lability, and proximal muscle weakness
Skeletal	Osteoporosis, hypercalcemia, and hypercalciuria
Reproductive	Irregular menses and gynecomastia
What are the thyroid function test findings in a patient with hyperthyroidism?	A high T4 radioimmunoassay, a high T3RU, and a low (suppressed) TSH
What is a thyroid scan?	Imaging study to localize areas that accumulate radioactive iodine or technetium (a functional iodine substitute)
What is the thyroid scan picture for the following:	
Hyperthyroidism	The uptake of tracer by the gland is usually high.
Hypothyroidism	The uptake of tracer by the gland is generally low.
What are indications for a thyroid scan?	To assist in determining the cause of hyperthyroidism and to screen for metastatic lesions in thyroid cancer
What is Graves' disease?	Graves' disease is the most common cause of hyperthyroidism, in which there is development of an antibody that activates the TSH receptor.
What are the features of Graves' disease?	Diffuse goiter, ophthalmopathy, and dermopathy (although not all features need be present)
What is the age of onset of Graves' disease?	30–40 years
What is the gender distribution of Graves' disease?	More women than men are affected, and there is a positive familial component.

What is thyroid storm?

A life-threatening condition manifested by marked increase in the signs and symptoms of hyperthyroidism

In what diseases does thyroid storm occur?

Thyroid storm is seen most often with Graves' disease, but it may occur in other causes of hyperthyroidism, such as toxic multinodular goiter.

What factors precipitate thyroid storm?

Infection, trauma, emergency surgery, diabetic ketoacidosis, and radiation thyroiditis

What are symptoms and signs of thyroid storm?

Fever, diaphoresis, tachycardia, congestive heart failure, nausea, vomiting, abdominal pain, altered mental status, and hypotension (late)

What are the thyroid hormone levels in thyroid storm?

The diagnosis is based on the history and physical findings and can occur with only modest increases in thyroid hormone levels.

Among treatment options for patients with hyperthyroidism, what are the common antithyroid medications, their actions, and their dosing frequency?

PTU—inhibits synthesis of T4, blocks peripheral conversion of T4 to T3, given three times per day
Methimazole—inhibits synthesis of T4, 10 times more potent than PTU, given once daily

Why are PTU and methimazole used?

They have a rapid onset of action (hours) and data suggest that they may reduce the risk of development of Graves' ophthalmopathy when used as initial treatment.

What are side effects of PTU and methimazole?

Rash and leukopenia (which is reversible by stopping the drug). PTU is the drug of choice in pregnant women with Graves' disease.

How do β-blockers work in patients with hyperthyroidism?

They block peripheral actions of T4 and T3.

How does RAI (^{131}I) work?	It ablates active tissue. Actions are observed over weeks.
What are side effects of RAI?	Many patients have resultant hypothyroidism; it cannot be used in pregnant women.
How does potassium iodide work?	It blocks release of preformed T4 and thereby acts more rapidly than PTU or methimazole. Most patients "escape" from its action within 1 week, making it a short-term therapy.
When is surgery favored for hyperthyroidism?	Surgery is usually reserved for patients who fail RAI, but it is the most rapid way to reduce T4 levels.
What are risks of surgery for hyperthyroidism?	Risk of hypothyroidism and hypoparathyroidism developing postoperatively and damage to the recurrent laryngeal nerve

HYPOTHYROIDISM

What is hypothyroidism?	Inadequate thyroid hormone effect on body tissues
What is cretinism?	Hypothyroidism at birth, resulting in developmental abnormalities
What is myxedema?	Severe hypothyroidism with deposition of mucopolysaccharides in the dermis, leading to doughy appearance of the skin
What are causes of hypothyroidism?	Autoimmune disease (Hashimoto's thyroiditis, postpartum thyroiditis), postradioiodine ablation, secondary hypothyroidism (pituitary disease with reduced TSH), subacute thyroiditis (usually transient), and following thyroid hormone withdrawal
What are symptoms and signs of hypothyroidism?	Development is insidious, and early symptoms are nonspecific—nonpitting edema, dry hair, temporal thinning of brows, fatigue, hoarse voice, expressionless face, large tongue, constipation, ileus, cold intolerance,

decreased appetite, weight gain, muscle cramps, stiffness, carpal tunnel, prolonged relaxation phase of DTRs, sleep apnea, menorrhagia, slowing of intellect, depression, and cardiac enlargement (dilation and pericardial effusion).

What diagnostic tests are useful in hypothyroidism?

TSH—increased in primary hypothyroidism and normal or low in secondary hypothyroidism

T4, free-T4 index—low in both primary and secondary hypothyroidism

What is the treatment for hypothyroidism?

Levothyroxine (T4) is most commonly used, because it does not cause a rapid increase in T3, which has associated risks in elderly patients and patients with cardiac disease.

What is the starting dose of levothyroxine?

In elderly patients or patients with cardiac disease, a low dose is given to start, then the dose is increased gradually (e.g., a 25-µg dose is increased by 25–50 µg every 4 weeks until thyroid function tests normalize, which usually occurs at a dosage of 125 µg/day).

How is therapy initiated in patients with secondary hypothyroidism?

Hydrocortisone is administered before starting thyroid hormone to avoid precipitating potentially fatal adrenal insufficiency.

MYXEDEMA COMA

What is myxedema coma?

A stuporous, potentially fatal state caused by severe hypothyroidism

What are risk factors for myxedema coma?

Advanced age, exposure to cold, infection, trauma, and central nervous system depressants

What are symptoms and signs of myxedema coma?

Hypothermia, areflexia (or delay in DTRs), clouded sensorium, seizures, respiratory depression, and myxedema (doughy skin and symptoms of severe hypothyroidism)

How is the diagnosis of myxedema coma made?	Often, the diagnosis is not obvious, and suspicion is based on clinical presentation.
What is the treatment for myxedema coma?	Because underlying hypothyroidism causes variable absorption from the gut, intravenous administration of thyroid hormone is preferred. The starting dose of L-thyroxine is 500 μg/day; the dose is then reduced to 100 μg/day. Improvement is usually seen within hours. Hydrocortisone, 100 mg/day, may be added if there is a possibility of associated adrenal insufficiency.

MULTIPLE ENDOCRINE NEOPLASIA SYNDROMES

What are the MEN syndromes?	Familial syndromes associated with multiple endocrine tumors
What is the inheritance pattern for MEN syndromes?	Autosomal dominant
What are the associated tumors and findings of MEN type I (Wermer's syndrome)?	Hyperplasia or tumors of the parathyroid, pituitary, adrenal cortex, and pancreatic islet cells Peptic ulceration Gastric acid hypersecretion
What are the associated tumors of MEN type II (Sipple's syndrome)?	Medullary thyroid carcinoma, pheochromocytoma (often bilateral) and hyperplasia of the parathyroid (hypercalcemia rarely seen). No involvement of the pancreas or peptic ulceration.
What are the associated tumors of MEN type III?	Medullary thyroid carcinoma and pheochromocytoma (often bilateral). A marfanoid body habitus develops as do benign neuromas of the eyelids, lips, tongue, buccal mucosa, intestines, bronchus, and bladder.

BONE AND MINERAL DISORDERS

CALCIUM HOMEOSTASIS

What is a normal calcium level?	8.5–10.5 mg/dl
What is the normal ionized calcium level?	4.5–5.0 mg/dl
What percentage of calcium is bound to plasma proteins?	Approximately 50%, mostly albumin. The other half circulates as free ionized calcium.
Which form of calcium is active?	Ionized calcium is physiologically active; therefore, alterations in serum albumin can result in changes in total calcium, although the ionized concentration remains constant.
How can calcium levels be corrected for albumin levels?	By adding or subtracting 0.8 mg/dl to the total calcium for every 1.0 mg/dl change in albumin
What hormones regulate calcium homeostasis?	PTH, 1,25-dihydroxyvitamin D, and possibly calcitonin. These hormones regulate the activity of osteoclasts, distal renal tubules, and intestinal epithelium.
What is the calcium cycle of homeostasis?	When ionized calcium levels decrease, the chief cells of the parathyroid gland release PTH, which, in turn, stimulates osteoclastic bone resorption and distal tubular calcium resorption. PTH also stimulates increased 1,25-dihydroxyvitamin D production, which, in turn, promotes intestinal calcium absorption.

HYPERCALCEMIA

What are the signs and symptoms of hypercalcemia?	"Stones, bones (bone pain), groans, and psychiatric overtones"
What are neurologic signs and symptoms of hypercalcemia?	Altered concentration, somnolence, depression, confusion, weakness, and coma (psychiatric overtones)

What are gastrointestinal signs and symptoms of hypercalcemia?	Constipation, anorexia, nausea, vomiting, pancreatitis, and peptic ulcer disease (seen in primary hyperparathyroidism) [groans]
What are genitourinary signs and symptoms of hypercalcemia?	Polyuria (nephrogenic diabetes insipidus) and nephrolithiasis (stones)
What are cardiac signs and symptoms of hypercalcemia?	Shortening of the QT interval, bradycardia, and first degree AV block
What is the treatment of hypercalcemia?	Hydration with isotonic saline and loop diuretics. In extreme settings, mithramycin, bisphosphonates (pamidronate), or calcitonin are used.

HYPOCALCEMIA

What are neurologic signs and symptoms of hypocalcemia?	Numbness and tingling in extremities and perioral region Spasm of the circumoral muscles with tapping of the facial nerve (Chvostek's sign) Carpal spasm within 3 minutes of inflation of the sphygmomanometer to 20 mm Hg above systolic pressure (Trousseau's sign) Muscle cramps, laryngospasm, bronchospasm, neuromuscular irritability, and seizures
What are cardiac signs and symptoms of hypocalcemia?	Prolonged QT interval and congestive heart failure
What is the differential diagnosis of hypocalcemia?	Hypoparathyroidism— idiopathic, postsurgical, severe hypomagnesemia, radiation, infiltrative disease like hemochromatosis, and DiGeorge syndrome PTH-independent vitamin D deficiency from diet, sun, malabsorption, renal disease, or liver disease Pseudohypoparathyroidism—tissue resistance to PTH

Vitamin D resistance
Pancreatitis
Rhabdomyolysis
Drugs—mithramycin, bisphosphonates,
   phenobarbital

What is the treatment of significant hypocalcemia?

Calcium gluconate, 1–2 amps over 5–10 minutes every 12 hours intravenously, and oral calcium carbonate, 1.5–3.0 g in 3–4 divided doses daily

OSTEOPOROSIS

What is the difference between osteopenia and osteoporosis?

Osteopenia is characterized by a low bone mass, whereas osteoporosis is characterized by a low bone mass with the subsequent development of nontraumatic fractures.

What are symptoms of osteopenia and osteoporosis?

Osteopenia is asymptomatic, whereas symptoms in osteoporosis are due to the fractures that develop.

Where are the most common fractures seen in osteoporosis?

The distal forearm (Colles' fracture), thoracic and lumbar spine, and proximal femur

What is the incidence of osteoporosis?

There are at least 275,000 new osteoporotic hip fractures each year in the United States. As many as one third of postmenopausal women sustain at least one osteoporotic fracture in their lifetime. Men also suffer from osteoporosis but at a much lower rate than women. One fourth to one fifth of all osteoporotic hip fractures and one seventh of all vertebral compression fractures occur in men.

What are risk factors for osteoporosis?

Increasing age, female gender, Caucasian or Asian extraction, early menopause, poor calcium intake, thin body habitus, alcohol abuse, hyperthyroidism, glucocorticoid excess syndromes, and perhaps type I diabetes mellitus

What is the pathogenesis of osteoporosis?

Osteoporosis results from a progressive decrease in the bone mass over time. Once peak bone mass is achieved (in the third or fourth decade of life), the formation of new bone lags the resorption of old bone, and, with each successive remodeling cycle, more bone is lost, placing the patient at risk for fractures.

How is the diagnosis of osteoporosis made?

Determination of bone mineral density. The best test is a dual energy x-ray absorptiometry scan, which measures bone density at the hip and lumbar vertebrae.

What are common therapeutic strategies for osteoporosis?

Therapy includes calcium supplementation (1 g/day), weight-bearing exercise, and hormone replacement therapy. If the latter is contraindicated (usually by a history of breast cancer or thromboembolic disease), there are several alternatives, including bisphosphonates [e.g., etidronate (cyclic therapy) and alendronate (continuous therapy)]. Bisphosphonates inhibit bone resorption.
Calcitonin can stabilize bone mass and may have additional beneficial actions on reducing bone pain from fractures.

OSTEOMALACIA

What is osteomalacia?

A defect in the mineralization of osteoid (bone matrix) in adults (the juvenile equivalent is rickets). The demineralization results in a loss of bone mineral density and bone strength.

What are symptoms and signs of osteomalacia?

Diffuse bone pain that may be localized to the hip area. A waddling gait is often present, attributable to pelvic deformation and bowing of the long bones of the legs. Thin radiolucent pseudofractures (Looser's zones), which are focal accumulations of nonmineralized osteoid, are a distinguishing feature.

How is the diagnosis of osteomalacia made?	Bone biopsy reveals increased osteoid and delayed mineralization.
What is the differential diagnosis of osteomalacia?	Vitamin D deficiency with resulting calcium and phosphate deficiency caused by malabsorption syndromes, hepatic disease with fat malabsorption, pancreatic disease with exocrine insufficiency, and renal disease
What is the treatment for osteomalacia?	Correction of the underlying disorder and vitamin D replacement. If hypocalcemia is severe, calcium replacement may also be indicated.

PAGET'S DISEASE

What is Paget's disease?	A disorder of bone remodeling that results in the formation of an unorganized mosaic of woven and lamellar bone that is less compact and weaker than normal bone
What are symptoms of Paget's disease?	Most patients are asymptomatic. Some experience pain in the affected bones, especially after fractures, which can occur with little trauma. Affected limbs may feel excessively warm because of the increased vascularity. Neurologic complications, including deafness, are due to compression of nerves by abnormal bone. The bony deformities also lead to secondary arthritic problems.
What is the incidence of Paget's disease?	Paget's disease is most common in persons older than 50 years, with a slight male predominance. Paget's disease may have a genetic component, in that 15%–30% of patients have a family history of Paget's disease.
How is the diagnosis of Paget's disease made?	Biochemically, Paget's disease is characterized by an increase in markers of bone turnover, including increased urinary excretion of hydroxyproline, an elevated serum alkaline phosphatase and osteocalcin.

What are the radiographic findings in Paget's disease?	Affected bones show cortical thickening, expansion, and areas of mixed lucency and sclerosis. The skull of affected patients is often described as having a cotton wool appearance.
How are bone scans helpful in Paget's disease?	They are the most sensitive method to identify affected areas of bone; however, they are not specific because they show all areas of increased bone turnover.
What is the therapy for Paget's disease?	Suppression of the activity of osteoclasts by calcitonin, etidronate, and plicamycin: Calcitonin is given as a subcutaneous injection or by nasal inhalation. Etidronate is effective but may alter normal mineralization and should be given on an intermittent basis. Plicamycin is a potent inhibitor of resorption but has a number of toxicities and should be reserved for refractory cases.

REPRODUCTIVE ENDOCRINOLOGY

FEMALE

What are the two types of amenorrhea?	1. Primary amenorrhea—no history of menses and age older than 16 years 2. Secondary amenorrhea—cessation of menses after menarche
What are causes of primary amenorrhea?	Genotype disorder (e.g., testicular feminization and 5-alpha reductase deficiency) Anatomic defect (e.g., müllerian agenesis, Asherman's syndrome [intrauterine adhesions], and imperforate hymen) Ovarian failure (e.g., gonadal dysgenesis and autoimmune disease) Metabolic (e.g., weight loss and chronic illness) Hormonal (e.g., polycystic ovarian disease, congenital adrenal hyperplasia, hyperprolactinemia, and hypopituitarism)

What studies are helpful in the evaluation of primary amenorrhea?

LH, FSH, and estradiol for identification of hypergonadotropic hypogonadism seen in gonadal failure

Testosterone, whose levels are elevated in androgen resistance syndromes and polycystic ovarian disease

PRL for identification of hypogonadotropic hypogonadism seen in hyperprolactinemia

Antiovarian antibodies, which are positive in autoimmune disease

Trial of estrogen and progesterone, which is useful to test for a functional uterus

What is PCOS?

A group of findings including obesity, hirsutism, irregular or absent menses, infertility, and insulin resistance

What are the laboratory findings in PCOS?

Elevated androgen levels (usually testosterone); increased LH:FSH ratio (seen in 75% of cases)

Women with amenorrhea are often at risk for osteoporosis. Is this true for women with PCOS?

Generally, no. Women with PCOS are overweight and have high androgen levels, both of which appear to protect bone mass.

What is the most common cause of secondary amenorrhea in women age 40–65 years?

Menopause

What is the most common cause of secondary amenorrhea in women age 15–40 years?

Pregnancy

What is hirsutism?

Excessive growth of androgen-dependent hair.

What is virilization?

Changes in body habitus as a result of hyperandrogenism, including acne, hirsutism, menstrual irregularities, temporal balding, deepening of the voice, increased muscle mass, and clitoral enlargement

What are causes of androgen excess syndromes?	Ovarian—PCOS, tumors (e.g., arrhenoblastoma), insulin resistance Adrenal—congenital adrenal hyperplasia, tumors (benign or malignant) Exogenous use or abuse of androgens
What are the three common types of enzyme deficiencies causing congenital adrenal hyperplasia and what hormonal intermediate is most elevated with each?	1. 21-hydroxylase and 17-hydroxy progesterone 2. 11-hydroxylase and 11-deoxy cortisol 3. 3-β-hydroxysteroid dehydrogenase and 17-hydroxy pregnenolone
Adrenal androgen excess usually results in increased levels of what compound?	DHEA-S
Ovarian androgen excess usually results in increased levels of what compound?	Testosterone

MALE

What are causes of hypogonadism in adult men?	Genetic (e.g., Klinefelter's syndrome) Orchitis (e.g., after mumps infection as an adult) Trauma, irradiation Autoimmune—hypergonadotropic hypogonadism Hypogonadotropic hypogonadism—hyperprolactinemia, chronic disease, hypopituitarism
What is Kallmann's syndrome?	An inherited abnormality in the GnRH-secreting neurons, resulting in hypogonadotropic hypogonadism. It is associated with anosmia.
What is impotence?	The inability to attain an erection of sufficient rigidity for vaginal penetration
What are common causes of erectile dysfunction?	Vascular insufficiency (either arterial or venous), neuropathic disease (e.g., diabetic autonomic neuropathy), psychogenic causes, hypogonadism, and medications

What is gynecomastia?	Enlargement of the male breast tissue
What are causes of gynecomastia?	Associated with adolescence Pathologic hyperestrogenism—liver disease (reduced estrogen metabolism), testicular tumors, hCG-producing tumors, adrenal tumors Medications (e.g., cimetidine, digoxin, tricyclic antidepressants, marijuana, spironolactone, and alpha methyldopa) Breast carcinoma Hypogonadism with reduced androgens (relative increase in estrogens) Idiopathic cause

DIABETES MELLITUS

PHYSIOLOGY

What is diabetes mellitus?	A disorder characterized by either absolute insulin deficiency or relative insulin deficiency in the setting of insulin resistance, either of which result in hyperglycemia. The elevated blood glucose level is the result of both increased gluconeogenesis in the liver and reduced glucose uptake by peripheral tissues.
What are the physiologic actions of insulin?	Insulin promotes glucose uptake, prevents lipolysis, prevents proteolysis, and suppresses glucagon secretion.
What are the counterregulatory hormones (those with actions opposing insulin)?	Glucagon, cortisol, catecholamines (epinephrine), and GH
What are the physiologic actions of glucagon?	Glucagon promotes gluconeogenesis, promotes ketogenesis, and glycogenolysis.
What criteria are used to diagnose diabetes mellitus?	Fasting plasma glucose > 140 mg/dl on at least two occasions or a single value > 200 mg/dl Oral glucose tolerance test (75 g), where fasting plasma glucose < 140 mg/dl and 2-hour plasma glucose > 200 mg/dl with one intervening value > 200 mg/dl

What is a glycosylated hemoglobin?	During their 90-day life span, red blood cells are permanently glycosylated (a nonenzymatic reaction) at a rate dependent on the prevailing plasma glucose level. Therefore, the higher the percentage of cells with glycosylation products, the higher the plasma glucose levels over the past weeks to months.
What is type I diabetes mellitus (also known as juvenile onset or IDDM)?	Autoimmune destruction of the pancreatic islet beta cells with resultant insulin deficiency
What are the insulin requirements in type I diabetes mellitus?	Patients are dependent on exogenous insulin to prevent ketoacidosis and for utilization of glucose.
What are general characteristics of patients presenting with type I diabetes mellitus?	Younger ages (< 20 years of age), Caucasian race, thin body habitus, often no family history of diabetes mellitus, usually an abrupt presentation (days) with polyuria, polydipsia, nocturia, weight loss, and hypotension (as seen in ketoacidosis)
Are there genetic linkages in type I diabetes mellitus?	There are HLA haplotypes (e.g., DR3 and DR4) associated with a higher incidence of type I diabetes mellitus. There is a 50% concordance in identical twins. At the time of presentation (and likely for some time before presentation), there are islet cell autoantibodies detectable in the circulation.
What is type II diabetes mellitus (also known as adult onset or NIDDM)?	A combination of insulin resistance and delayed insulin secretion after a glucose challenge, producing a relative insulin deficiency
What are the insulin requirements in type II diabetes mellitus?	Patients are not dependent on exogenous insulin for survival, but may require insulin for adequate control of hyperglycemia.

What are general characteristics of patients presenting with type II diabetes mellitus?

Older ages (> 40 years of age), African-American descent, heavier body habitus, strong family history of diabetes mellitus, subtle presentation (months) with polyuria, polydipsia, and nocturia. Many patients gain weight before presentation. Individuals with type II diabetes mellitus do not develop ketoacidosis.

Are there genetic linkages in type II diabetes mellitus?

There is nearly a 100% concordance in identical twins. There are no HLA markers.

What is syndrome X?

A constellation of clinical problems including glucose intolerance, hyperinsulinemia (insulin resistance), hyperlipidemia, and hypertension

What is MODY?

Maturity onset diabetes of the young. This has a greater familial penetrance than type II diabetes and presents with hyperglycemia (no ketosis) in children.

TREATMENT

What are the pharmacodynamics of each type of insulin used to treat diabetes mellitus?

Regular insulin—onset in 30–60 minutes, peak in 2–3 hours, duration of action of 6–8 hours

NPH or Lente insulin—onset in 1–2 hours, peak in 8–10 hours, duration of action of 12–18 hours

Ultralente insulin—onset in 4–8 hours, peak (minor) in 16–24 hours, duration 36–48 hours

What is the split–mixed conventional regimen of administering insulin?

A regimen containing an intermediate-acting insulin (e.g., NPH) and regular insulin given as two daily subcutaneous injections before breakfast and dinner. The total amount of insulin required for most patients with type I diabetes mellitus is 0.6 U/kg/day and, for patients with type II, 1 U/kg/day (or more). Two thirds of the total is given in the morning and one third in the evening. Of the morning dose, two thirds is given as NPH (or Lente) and one third as regular insulin. In the evening, the amounts of regular and NPH are usually even.

What is meant by intensive therapy for diabetic patients?

Any regimen that attempts to mimic the normal diurnal profile of endogenous insulin release. This is usually accomplished with 2–4 injections of insulin per day or with a subcutaneous continuous insulin infusion device. Frequent monitoring of circulating glucose levels and a consistent dietary intake are needed for this regimen.

What is the dawn phenomenon?

A state of relative insulin resistance in the early morning hours caused by normal diurnal variation of counterregulatory hormones. This can result in morning hyperglycemia and is the reason for increased insulin requirements in the morning hours.

What was the DCCT and what were the significant findings?

The Diabetes Control and Complications Trial (*N Engl J Med* 329:977–986, 1993) was pivotal to understanding the importance of strict glycemic control. It examined the effect of intensive therapy (average blood glucose of 155 mg/dl) versus conventional therapy on long-term microvascular complications in type I diabetes mellitus. The following findings were reported:
1. The risk of development of retinopathy declined by 76%.
2. The risk of progression of retinopathy declined by 54%.
3. The occurrence of microalbuminuria (an early sign of renal damage) declined by 39%.
4. The occurrence of overt proteinuria declined by 54%.
5. The risk of development of neuropathy declined by 60%.

The major adverse event associated with the strict glycemic control was a twofold to threefold increase in severe hypoglycemia.

What therapeutic options are available in type II diabetes mellitus?

Dietary restriction (all patients) and weight reduction (if obese), sulfonylureas, biguanides, insulin, and combinations of these agents

What is the mechanism of action of the sulfonylureas?

They stimulate insulin release, increase beta cell sensitivity, and improve insulin sensitivity in target tissues.

What are the side effects of the sulfonylureas?

Hypoglycemia, bone marrow suppression, hemolytic anemia, rash, nausea and vomiting, disulfuram reaction with alcohol, and hyponatremia (SIADH)

What are the mechanisms of action of the biguanides?

They decrease hepatic glucose production, decrease intestinal absorption of glucose, and improve insulin sensitivity.

What are the side effects and contraindications for use of biguanides?

Lactic acidosis can develop in patients with renal insufficiency, making it a contraindication. Similarly, a history of liver disease may be associated with development of a metabolic acidosis. Other side effects include nausea, flatulence, anorexia, rash, and vitamin B_{12} deficiency.

DIABETIC EMERGENCIES

What are the incidence and mortality rates of diabetic ketoacidosis?

There is a 1%–2% incidence rate with a mortality rate of less than 5%.

What are symptoms of diabetic ketoacidosis?

Frequent urination, excessive thirst, weight loss, nausea, vomiting, weakness, muscle aches, headache, abdominal pain, shortness of breath, drowsiness, and eventually stupor and unresponsiveness

What are signs of diabetic ketoacidosis?

Dry mucous membranes, orthostatic hypotension, poor skin turgor, tachycardia, fruity odor on the breath, and Kussmaul's respirations

What are precipitating causes of diabetic ketoacidosis?

Think **five I's:**
Infection (acute or occult, viral or bacterial)
Ignorance (missed insulin dosage)
Infarction
Ischemia (cardiac or mesenteric)
Intoxication (alcohol)

What are common laboratory abnormalities in diabetic ketoacidosis?

Blood glucose greater than or equal to 300 mg/dl, serum bicarbonate less than or equal to 15 mEq/L, arterial blood pH less than or equal to 7.30, anion gap greater than or equal to 15, positive serum acetone, hyperkalemia or hypokalemia, hyperphosphatemia or hypophosphatemia, prerenal azotemia, and hypertriglyceridemia

What is the treatment for diabetic ketoacidosis?

1. Volume repletion (3–5 L total— the first 1–2 L of isotonic saline are given rapidly over 1–2 hours; 5% dextrose is added when the blood glucose decreases below 250 mg/dl)
2. Insulin administration (usually given as a 10 IU bolus intravenously, then 5–10 IU/hour continuous intravenous infusion)
3. Correction of electrolyte abnormalities. Treatment of hyperkalemia at initial onset is accomplished by fluid hydration, insulin administration, and correction of the acidosis, all of which reduce the potassium level. Later, hypokalemia resulting from reduced total body potassium stores is treated with potassium chloride added to the intravenous infusion.
4. Administration of bicarbonate when the pH is less than or equal to 7.0 and the serum bicarbonate level is less than or equal to 5 mmol/L
5. Investigation of precipitating causes

When is the insulin infusion discontinued in diabetic ketoacidosis?

Intravenous insulin is continued for 6–12 hours after the anion gap acidosis and ketonuria has cleared.

Why is glucose administered along with insulin as the blood glucose declines to 250 mg/dl?

Insulin reverses the ketosis, and the simultaneous administration of insulin and dextrose prevents hypoglycemia and allows resolution of the ketosis.

What is nonketotic hyperosmolar coma?

Uncontrolled type II diabetes mellitus and progressive osmotic diuresis lead to severe dehydration. Mental obtundation and seizures result at the later stages.

What are the laboratory findings in hyperosmolar coma?

Blood glucose often greater than or equal to 600 mg/dl, hyperosmolarity greater than or equal to 320 mOsm/L, and azotemia

How is plasma osmolarity calculated?

$2(Na^+)$ + (glucose/18) + (BUN/2.8), with the normal range being 285–295 mOsm/L

Hyperglycemia interferes with measurement of sodium. How is sodium concentration corrected for the glucose concentration?

[(measured glucose – 100) × 1.6/100] + measured sodium = corrected sodium

What is the usual fluid deficit in hyperosmolar coma?

As much as 10 L. Because large volumes of fluid are required for resuscitation, central venous pressure monitoring is almost always needed if there is coexisting cardiac or renal disease.

How is fluid deficit calculated?

$(0.6 \times$ weight in kg$) \times ([Na^+/140] - 1) =$ water deficit (in L)

How is fluid deficit repleted?

One half of the estimated fluid deficit is replaced with normal saline over the first 6–8 hours. Normal saline, 0.45%, is then used to correct the remaining deficit over the next 24 hours.

How is insulin administered for hyperosmolar coma?

Treatment is similar to that for diabetic ketoacidosis.

DIABETIC COMPLICATIONS

What are microvascular complications of diabetes mellitus?	Retinopathy, nephropathy, and neuropathy
What are macrovascular complications of diabetes?	Atherosclerosis—coronary artery disease and peripheral vascular disease
What lesions are characteristic of nonproliferative retinopathy?	Microaneurysms, dot and blot hemorrhages, hard exudates, and "cotton-wool" spots
What lesions are associated with preproliferative retinopathy?	Intraretinal microvascular abnormalities, intraretinal hemorrhages, and venous beading, all signs of severe retinal ischemia
What is the most common cause of visual loss in nonproliferative and preproliferative retinopathy?	Maculopathy including macular edema, hard exudates, hemorrhages, ischemia, or traction on the macula
What are lesions of proliferative retinopathy?	Neovascularization of the disc and neovascularization elsewhere
What are complications of proliferative retinopathy?	Preretinal and vitreous hemorrhages, retinal tears, retinal detachments, neovascular glaucoma, and blindness
What are current recommendations for referral of a diabetic patient to an ophthalmologist?	Patients with type I diabetes mellitus at 5 years' disease duration, patients with type II diabetes mellitus within the first year of diagnosis, any woman with type I diabetes who is planning pregnancy within the next 1 year, and any diabetic patient who complains of persistent decreased visual acuity or with preproliferative changes on a nondilated examination
What are other ophthalmologic complications of diabetes mellitus?	Cataracts, glaucoma, refractory changes, and cranial nerve palsies

What medical intervention can prevent progression of retinopathy?

The DCCT showed that intensive insulin therapy decreased the incidence and progression of retinopathy in type I diabetes mellitus.

What interventions are currently available in the treatment of high-risk proliferative retinopathy and clinically significant macular edema?

Panretinal photocoagulation for proliferative retinopathy and focal laser photocoagulation for clinically significant macular edema

DIABETIC NEPHROPATHY

What is the prevalence of nephropathy in type I diabetes?

One third of all patients with type I diabetes

What is the characteristic pathologic lesion of diabetic nephropathy (Kimmelstiel-Wilson disease)?

Mesangial expansion with the formation of hyaline nodules, glomerular basement thickening, and afferent and efferent arteriosclerosis

What are the five stages in the progression of diabetic nephropathy?

Stage 1—glomerular hyperfiltration, increased glomerular filtration rate (up to 140% normal), and renal enlargement

Stage 2—early glomerular lesions. Expansion of the glomerular mesangium and thickening of the glomerular basement membrane occurs from 4 or 5 years to 15 years after onset of diabetes mellitus.

Stage 3—incipient diabetic nephropathy. Microalbuminuria (defined as urinary protein excretion between 30 mg/day and 200 mg/day) develops and precedes later nephropathy and the development of end-stage renal disease. Glomerular filtration begins to decline once the microalbuminuria exceeds 70 μg/min. Hypertension often is noted.

Stage 4—clinical nephropathy with proteinuria and declining glomerular filtration rate. Glomerular filtration rate declines below normal and proteinuria > 300 mg/day develops. Signs of reduced oncotic pressure (e.g., anasarca) become evident. Hypertension is universal. Overt nephrotic syndrome with proteinuria, hypoproteinemia, and hyperlipidemia can develop. Nearly all patients with azotemia from diabetic nephropathy have coincident retinopathy. End-stage renal disease usually develops within 5 years of clinical proteinuria.

Stage 5—end-stage renal disease. Uremic signs and symptoms are apparent and "renal replacement therapy" is necessary.

What clinical interventions can help slow the progression of diabetic nephropathy?

Aggressive treatment of hypertension with combinations of angiotensin-converting enzyme (ACE) inhibitors, calcium channel blockers, vasodilators, and β-blockers to a target diastolic blood pressure of 85 mm Hg

Dietary protein restriction to 0.6–0.8 g/kg/day once proteinuria reaches > 1 g/day

Strict glycemic control

Early treatment of urinary tract infections to avoid pyelonephritis

Avoidance of radiocontrast dyes

What options for controlling uremia are available for diabetic patients with end-stage renal disease?

Hemodialysis, peritoneal dialysis, and renal transplantation

DIABETIC NEUROPATHY

What are the clinical manifestations of the following diabetic neuropathies:
  Radiculopathy

Dermatomal pain and sensory loss

  Mononeuropathy

Pain, weakness, hyperreflexia, muscle wasting, and sensory loss along the distribution of a mixed spinal nerve.

Nerves most often involved include ulnar, median, radial, femoral, lateral cutaneous, and peroneal

Abdominal polyradiculopathy

Abdominal, thoracic, and lower back pain; weight loss; weakness and atrophy of abdominal muscles; diminished reflexes

Polyneuropathy

Loss of ankle reflexes; stocking and glove loss of vibration, temperature, light touch, and pinprick sensation; distal lower extremity pain and paresthesias; mild peripheral weakness and wasting of intrinsic muscles; foot ulcers; and Charcot's joints

Diabetic amyotrophy

Marked proximal leg weakness, severe weight loss, anterior thigh pain, and diminished patellar reflexes

Cranial neuropathy

Intense periorbital pain preceding either third nerve palsy with sparing of the pupil or sixth nerve palsy. Recovery of function usually takes 6–12 weeks.

Autonomic neuropathy

Gastrointestinal disturbances including esophageal dysmotility, gastroparesis, atonic gallbladder, diabetic diarrhea or constipation, steatorrhea, neurogenic bladder, impotence, retrograde ejaculation, tachycardia, reduced beat-to-beat variability of heart rate with respirations, painless myocardial ischemia, absence of sweating, abnormal vasoconstriction or vasodilation (orthostatic hypotension), and hypoglycemic unawareness

What are high-risk characteristics for the diabetic foot?

The presence of peripheral anesthetic neuropathy, arterial insufficiency, and intrinsic muscle atrophy with "hammer-toe" deformities

What organisms are found in diabetic foot ulcers?

Shallow ulcers contain skin organisms with *Staphylococcus* species and *Streptococcus* species. However, classic diabetic foot ulcers are polymicrobial with gram-positive organisms, gram-negative organisms, and anaerobic organisms that require broad-spectrum antibiotics.

What are the hallmarks of the Charcot foot?

Gradual swelling, shortening and widening of the foot with diminished arches, eversion and external rotation. Radiographs reveal marked osteopenia with bony fragments, spurs, and pathologic fractures.

What are treatment options for painful diabetic peripheral neuropathy?

Optimization of glycemic control, tricyclic antidepressants, carbamazepine, capsaicin cream, and mexiletine

What are treatment options for gastroparesis?

Optimization of glycemic control, small and frequent feedings, low-fat diet, metoclopramide, cisapride, domperidone, erythromycin, and jejunostomy tube feedings in refractory cases

What are treatment options for diabetic diarrhea?

Codeine, loperamide, diphenoxylate, cholestyramine and clonidine, and treatment of bacterial overgrowth

What are treatment options for autonomic neuropathy?

Fluorocortisone and compression stockings

What are treatment options for neurogenic bladder?

Bethanecol and intermittent self-catheterization

What are treatment options for neurogenic impotence?

Papaverine injections, vacuum-constriction, and prostheses. Prostaglandin gels placed in the urethral meatus are under study.

10 Allergy and Immunology

ABBREVIATIONS

ADA	Adenosine deaminase deficiency
APC	Antigen-presenting cell
C1INH	C1 esterase inhibitor
CHF	Congestive heart failure
CVID	Common variable immunodeficiency
FESS	Functional endoscopic sinus surgery
HIM	Hyperimmunoglobulin M
HIV	Human immunodeficiency virus
HLA	Human leukocyte antigen
IFN	Interferon
IL	Interleukin
MHC	Major histocompatibility complex
NARES	Non-allergic rhinitis with eosinophilia
NK	Natural killer
NSAID	Nonsteroidal anti-inflammatory drug
PCP	*Pneumocystis carinii* pneumonia
PSS	Progressive systemic sclerosis
RAST	Radioallergosorbent test

SCID   Severe combined immunodeficiency

XLA   X-linked agammaglobulinemia

HISTORY AND PHYSICAL EXAMINATION

What is the most common disorder of the immune system?

Allergy, affecting 1 in 5 of the population in the United States

What six questions should be asked of patients with allergy complaints?

1. How do symptoms begin?
2. What is the pattern (e.g., regular, paroxysmal, or seasonal) of episodes?
3. What is the response to treatment, if any?
4. What are inducing factors (e.g., inhalants, ingestants, injectants, and irritants)?
5. What is the changeover time of progression to remission?
6. How severe are symptoms?

What should be included in the allergic history for any person?

Think **I DARE U:**
Insect stings
Drug or food allergies
Asthma and anaphylaxis
Rhinitis
Eczema
Urticaria

What are the important features of a family history?

Any atopic disease including asthma, rhinitis, and atopic dermatitis
History of deaths early in childhood
Autoimmune diseases

What are common causes of dyspnea?

Think of **9 P's:**
Pulmonary bronchoconstriction (asthma)
Pneumonia
Pulmonary embolus
Pneumothorax
Pump failure (CHF)
Pericardial tamponade
Psychogenic
Poison (carbon monoxide)
Peak seekers (high altitude)

What are important indoor allergens?

Dust mites, cockroaches, cats, dogs, and mold

What are important outdoor allergens?	Trees, grass, ragweed, and molds

DEFINITIONS

Define the following:	
Specific immunity	The immune system distinguishes between different targets and causes selective destruction.
Clonal selection	Each lymphocyte clone recognizes only one antigen. The specificity of each lymphocyte develops in the absence of antigenic stimulation. The preimmune repertoire can recognize about 1×10^9 different antigens. Clones that can recognize self are deleted or made nonfunctional. Clones that bind an antigen are "selected" and proliferate.
Cytokines	Cytokines are small proteins that are produced by activated cells and that stimulate different functions, depending on what cells bind them. There are many cytokines in several families.
Antigen	An antigen is a protein recognized by the immune system.
Immunoglobulins	Immunoglobulins are protein products of mature plasma cells.
Antibody	Antibodies are immunoglobulins that recognize specific antigens.
Idiotypes	Idiotypes are unique determinants within the antibody combining site.
MHC	Major histocompatibility complex (MHC) is synonymous in humans with HLA. These gene products are prominently displayed on cell surfaces. They were first discovered as impediments for transplantation but they are crucial to the normal immune response because they are necessary for the presentation of foreign protein to T lymphocytes. The absence of MHC results in a severe immunodeficiency.

The presence of different forms (polymorphisms) is associated with the potential for specific disease states (e.g., HLA-B27 and ankylosing spondylitis).

BASIC IMMUNOLOGY

What is the basic function of the immune system?

To destroy foreign proteins and maintain health of organism

What makes the basic function of the immune system possible?

Specific recognition of self from nonself by key effector systems

List some nonspecific immune mechanisms.

Physical barriers (e.g., skin)
Complement
Polymorphonuclear leukocytes
NK cells

Where do lymphocytes arise?

All lymphocytes arise in bone marrow. T cells, however, mature in the thymus, and B cells mature in the bone marrow.

What percentage of circulating lymphocytes are T cells?

80%. The majority of the rest are B cells.

What is the function of T cells (cell-mediated immunity)?

1. To facilitate resistance to facultative intracellular microorganisms (e.g., mycobacteria, viruses, fungi, and parasites)
2. To regulate specific antibody production by B cells

What is the difference between CD4$^+$ and CD8$^+$ cells?

Located on the cell surface, CD4 and CD8 are receptors that are important in determining the recognition of antigen. T cells bearing CD4 can recognize only antigen embedded in MHC class II, which is found only on the surface of a few specialized cells (APCs). T cells bearing CD8 recognize antigen on MHC class I, which is found on all nucleated cells.

Are CD4⁺ and CD8⁺ the same as helper and suppressor cells?

Yes and no. CD4⁺ cells are responsible for most T cell "help"; that is, they help B cells and other cells mount an immunoglobulin or cell-mediated immune response. CD8⁺ cells can be thought of as effector cells that carry out a cell-mediated immune response. The specific cells responsible for suppression are unknown.

What are the two types of helper cells derived from T cells?

Th1 and Th2 cells (mostly CD4⁺ cells) are determined by the cytokines they produce and, therefore, the type of response they help.

What do Th1 cells produce?

IL-2 and IFN-gamma. Th1 cytokines activate macrophages and cytolytic T cells and are associated with cell-mediated immunity.

What do Th2 cells produce?

Predominantly IL-4, IL-5, and IL-10, and they are associated with the production of more immunoglobulin (particularly IgE) and recruitment of eosinophils.

What cell markers might be useful clinically?

CD3—marker used for all T cells
CD4—marker for T helper cells. It generally defines half or more of T cells in the peripheral blood and is the receptor for HIV.
CD8—marker for cytotoxic T cells
CD19 or CD20—B cell markers
CD56—marker for NK cells

What is the difference between T and B cell markers?

T cell markers (e.g., CD4 and CD8) have functional significance, whereas B cell markers (e.g., B1, B2, and B3) are primarily of maturational significance.

What is the function of B cells (humoral immunity)?

To mature plasma cells and produce antibody

What allows specific immunity?

Genetic rearrangement of the DNA in B and T cells, allowing the formation of many different receptors (antibodies and T cell receptors), such that a unique receptor preexists the challenge by any antigen

What are the five major divisions in immunoglobulin?

IgA, IgD, IgE, IgG, and IgM

Where is IgA found?

Most is secreted onto mucosal surfaces. Although IgA is produced in the highest quantities, IgG has higher measurable levels in the blood. Only small amounts of IgA are found in serum.

Where is IgD found?

It is coexpressed with IgM on mature B cells, but its function is not known. It is not a secreted protein.

What is the role of IgE?

It is associated with allergy and with immunity to parasites for which it is thought to assist in antibody-dependent cell cytolysis.

What is the role of IgG?

It undergoes somatic mutation with affinity maturation, is a potent opsonin, and activates complement. It crosses the placental barrier and provides passive immunity for the newborn. It is the most abundant immunoglobulin in the serum and has four subclasses.

What is the role of IgM?

It is the antigen receptor found on mature naive B cells and is the first antibody produced in an immune response. Because it is pentameric, activation of complement is strong. Production does not require T cell help but neither does it generate a memory response.

What is the basic structure of immunoglobulins?

A combination of a heavy chain and a light chain

What are the two types of light chains?

Kappa and lambda

What is the role of immunoglobulin?

Recognition and binding of specific antigens
Activation of cells or of the complement binding system

What are the three phases of the immune response?	Recognition, activation, and execution
Describe each phase of the immune response:	
Recognition	Antigen is bound to specific receptors on B or T lymphocytes. For T cells, this requires passage and presentation through APCs.
Activation	Lymphocytes that have bound a protein proliferate and differentiate into effector cells, all bearing receptors for the protein.
Execution	Stimulating antigen is cleared from the system.
What are APCs?	Antigen-presenting cells that present antigen on their surface in the context of MHC. "Professional" APCs express MHC class II and include dendritic cells, macrophages, and, in a secondary response, B cells.
What is the role of APCs?	To present antigens and to produce soluble immunoregulatory molecules
What is the difference between class I and class II MHC besides location?	MHC class I presents proteins synthesized inside the cell (viral proteins) to CD8$^+$ T cells. MHC class II presents proteins that have been engulfed from outside the cell and processed (most bacterial proteins) to CD4$^+$ T cells.
What are the basic mast cell products?	Vasoactive products (i.e., histamine), chemotactic factors, enzymes, and proteoglycans
What are the histamine receptors?	H1, H2, and H3
What are the circulatory effects of the following:	
H1	Smooth muscle contraction— bronchoconstriction, intestinal motility Pruritus Increased vascular permeability

Arrhythmias
Secretion of mucus

H2

Increased gastric acid secretion
Increased mucus

What are the combined effects of histamine on H1 and H2 receptors?

Hypotension, flushing, and headache

What are leukotrienes and what do they do?

They are products of metabolism of arachidonic acid by mast cells. They cause bronchoconstriction, increase mucus secretion, and cause a potent wheal-and-flare response via increased vascular permeability.

What attracts eosinophils?

C5a, platelet activating factor, histamine, and leukotrienes

In what illnesses are eosinophil counts increased?

Think **NAACP:**
Neoplasms—lymphomas, Hodgkin's disease, hyper-IgE syndrome, Wiskott-Aldrich syndrome
Allergic disorders—drug reactions, atopic dermatitis, allergic rhinitis
Asthma and bronchopulmonary aspergillosis
Collagen-vascular diseases—especially vasculitis and eosinophilic fasciitis
Parasitic infections

What are the roles of the following interleukins?
    IL-6

Induces maturation of B cells to plasma cells

    IL-5

Stimulates growth and differentiation of B cells to select production of IgG and IgA, and stimulates eosinophil colonies and maturation

    IL-4

Enhances B cell production of IgE and IgG1
Activates macrophages and B cells
Induces class II MHC antigens on B cells
Stimulates anti-IgM activated B cells

	Stimulates growth of T and B cells, mast cells, and hematopoietic cells
IL-3	Stimulates B cells and hematopoietic colony formation (includes mast cells and basophils)
IL-2	Promotes growth of NK cells, lymphokine-activated killer cells, B cells, and monocytes Promotes growth of activated T cells Has a potential role in HIV and metastatic cancers
IL-1	Activates T, B, NK, lymphocyte-activated killer cells, and macrophages
What are the effectors of an IgE-mediated response?	Mast cells, basophils, and eosinophils. Mast cells and basophils are the source of histamine and leukotrienes released in an allergic response. Eosinophils are important in the IgE-mediated killing of helminths. IgE and eosinophils are both produced in response to cytokines expressed by Th2 cells.
What proteins are in the cytokine family?	Interleukins (so called because they act between leukocytes) Interferons (because they interfere with viral superinfection in previously infected cells) Hematopoietic growth factors Chemokines (chemotactic cytokines)
What does complement do?	Complement is a form of natural immunity that can lyse pathogens in the absence of specific immunity, opsonize pathogens allowing for more efficient phagocytosis, and enhance the clearance of foreign proteins. Complement is subdivided into activation, amplification, and attack components.
Generally, which immune complexes activate the classic complement pathway?	IgG and IgM

What is the membrane attack complex?	A complex of complement factors C5, C6, C7, C8, and C9 that can cause defects in cell surfaces, thereby causing cell death.
How is the membrane attack complex formed?	The complex is formed after immune complexes activate the classical or alternative complement pathways causing assembly of factors C1, C4, and C2. These factors (or factor B and C3 from the alternative pathway) then act to cleave C3 and C5, which initiates the formation of the membrane attack complex.
What activates the alternative pathway?	Polysaccharides, fungi, and sialic acid–deficient surfaces (this pathway uses factors B, D, and P)
What are the anaphylatoxins?	C4a, C3a, and C5a. These fragments generate an inflammatory response by interacting with mast cells, basophils, and other leukocytes and are formed during complement activation.
Why are C3, C4, and CH50 measured?	These levels can be followed to determine the activity of a variety of autoimmune and inflammatory diseases. CH50 is an indirect measure of the whole complement cascade. C4 measures the crucial component of the classical pathway, and C3 is used in both classical and alternative cascades.

IMMUNODEFICIENCY

How are immunodeficiencies classified?	Primary B cell, T cell, or mixed Complement Phagocytic Secondary Immunosuppression HIV X-linked lymphoproliferative syndrome Malignancy
List the two most common B-cell (humoral) immunodeficiencies.	IgA deficiency and IgG deficiency

How common is IgA deficiency?	Occurs in approximately 1 in 500 persons. It is defined as a serum IgA level of < 15 mg/dl.
What are symptoms and signs of IgA deficiency?	Persons with IgA deficiency may be healthy or may have increased susceptibility to sinopulmonary infections as well as allergic, autoimmune, and malignant diseases.
What is the treatment for IgA deficiency?	Antibiotics for specific infections and, sometimes, prophylactic antibiotics. IgA patients are not given IgG.
Are blood transfusions safe in patients with IgA deficiency?	No. IgA-deficient patients are at increased risk of a severe reaction from immunoglobulin infusions and from blood transfusions (washed packed cells should be given if transfusion is needed).
What constitutes an IgG deficiency?	Total serum IgG < 200–250 mg/dL
What four diseases make up the IgG deficiencies?	1. CVID 2. XLA (1:100,000 live births) 3. HIM 4. Hypogammaglobulinemia associated with thymoma
What infections are seen in IgG deficiencies?	Most common—sinopulmonary infections Common—central nervous system, joint, and gastrointestinal tract infections
What organisms are the most common causes of infection in patients with IgG deficiencies?	Most common—encapsulated bacteria such as *Haemophilus influenzae* or *Streptococcus pneumoniae* Common—*Staphylococcus aureus*, meningococci, *Pseudomonas*, *Campylobacter*, *Ureaplasma*, and *Mycoplasma*
Are persons with IgG deficiencies more susceptible to viral infections?	As a rule, no. However, IgG-deficient patients are susceptible to polio (and should not receive live virus vaccine) and to hepatitis B and C. In patients

with XLA (but not CVID or HIM), a chronic meningoencephalitis, which is ultimately fatal, can develop with ECHO or coxsackievirus infection.

What tests are useful to diagnose infection in patients with IgG deficiency?

These patients have little, if any, of their own antibodies, so diagnosis of infection is made by tests that measure the infectious agent (culture, polymerase chain reaction), not tests of response (enzyme-linked immunosorbent assay, Western blots).

What protozoal infections affect patients with IgG deficiency?

Giardia lamblia infection and, in persons with HIM, PCP

When are patients with CVID first seen?

Patients with CVID, both men and women, generally are first seen in or after the second decade of life.

What are the laboratory and radiographic findings in CVID?

B cells are present in the peripheral blood and sometimes in exuberant lymphoid tissue.

In addition to infection, what are the clinical symptoms of IgG deficiency?

Malabsorption develops in about one half of patients, autoimmune disease in one fourth, and cancer in approximately one sixth.

When are patients with XLA first seen?

Generally, boys with XLA are seen after the first 6 months of life (after maternal antibodies are gone) and within the first 2 years of life.

What are laboratory and radiographic findings in XLA?

XLA patients have essentially no B cells in circulation and no discernible lymphoid tissue (a lateral neck view showing no adenoidal tissue is a diagnostic test in children).

What autoimmune diseases are patients with XLA susceptible to?

A dermatomyositis-like illness or sclerodermatous changes of the skin and joints

Can a patient have a B-cell immunodeficiency with a normal total IgG level?

Yes, there have been reports of patients with B-cell immunodeficiency in spite of a normal total IgG level.

How are patients with B-cell immunodeficiency and normal total IgG level recognized?

Most of these patients have a decreased ability to respond to polysaccharide antigens.

How should patients with recurrent pneumonia or other serious bacterial infections be evaluated?

The patient should receive vaccination with Pneumovax and tetanus; then prevaccination and postvaccination (3–4 week) titers of antibodies to pneumococcal serotypes should be assayed simultaneously. An adequate response is a fourfold increase in antibody titers between the paired serum. Vaccination with the *H. influenzae* (type b) conjugated to a protein may be useful for protecting these patients but is usually not helpful in diagnosis.

Should IgG subclass antibodies be measured?

Prevaccination and postvaccination antibodies are a better functional test of immune status.

What is the treatment for IgG deficiencies?

Monthly infusions of pooled intravenous immunoglobulin. The dose is generally begun at 200–400 mg/kg and is titrated to maintain an IgG trough level of > 400 mg/dl obtained immediately before the next infusion (or sometimes to an adequate clinical response with minimal infections if the dose is prohibitive in terms of time or expense or if the patient continues to have frequent, severe infections). Despite IgG infusions, many patients with CVID require prophylactic antibiotics.

What are other causes of low serum IgG?

Prolonged steroid use, protein-losing enteropathy, nephropathy, and malnutrition

What are the diseases of T-cell (or cellular) deficiency or combined T- and B-cell deficiencies?

Thymic hypoplasia or DiGeorge syndrome
Nezelof syndrome
SCID
ADA

Wiskott-Aldrich syndrome
Ataxia-telangiectasia
Mucocutaneous candidiasis (autoimmune
    polyglandular syndrome type I)
Hyperimmunoglobulin E or Job
    syndrome

For each of the following, list the lymphocyte defect and major abnormality.

DiGeorge syndrome

T cell; cardiac defects (great vessels) and hypocalcemia (failure of development of the parathyroids), absent thymus, abnormal ears, and hypotelorism

Nezelof syndrome

T cell; DiGeorge syndrome without the associated congenital anomalies

SCID

T and B cell; may be X-linked or autosomal recessive. Affected infants rarely survive the severe immunodeficiency state beyond 1 year.

ADA

T and B cells; a form of SCID with deficient purine metabolism (adenosine deaminase)

Wiskott-Aldrich syndrome

Probably B cells with low serum levels of IgM and increased levels of IgE; eczema, thrombocytopenia, repeated infections (encapsulated organisms), lymphoreticular malignancies, and anergy

Ataxia-telangiectasia

T cells, although commonly deficient in IgE and IgA, and sometimes IgG; cerebellar ataxia and oculocutaneous telangiectasia, truncal ataxia, sinopulmonary infections leading to bronchiectasis and lymphomas, and high levels of alpha-fetoprotein and carcinoembryonic antigen

Mucocutaneous candidiasis (autoimmune polyglandular syndrome type I)

Uncertain; superficial candidiasis (not systemic) associated with single or multiple endocrinopathies, iron deficiency, and anergy

Hyperimmunoglobulin E

Uncertain, with increased serum levels of IgE (up to 10 times normal); recurrent infections of the skin and sinopulmonary tract with *S. aureus* and *H. influenzae*, coarse facial features, and chronic eczematous rashes

Do any of the T- and B-cell deficiencies discussed occur in adults?

Mucocutaneous candidiasis and hyperimmunoglobulin E are disorders compatible with living to adulthood. The other T-cell or combined immunodeficiencies listed above are severe and generally present early in life. Without bone marrow transplantation, they are generally fatal.

In general, how are T-cell and combined immunodeficiencies treated?

Bone marrow, fetal liver, and thymus transplantation may have a role. Gamma globulin infusions may be given for patients who are IgG deficient. Fresh-frozen plasma may be given for other immunoglobulin-deficient states. Good postural drainage helps prevent sinopulmonary infections.

What is a simple test for T-cell function?

The "anergy" panel skin test is a measure of delayed type hypersensitivity, and a positive test requires intact T-cell function.

What interferes with an anergy panel?

1. Corticosteroids (topical or systemic)
2. Anticoagulants (induration is the result of fibrin deposition)
3. Technique (failure to place antigen intradermally)

In general, what types of infectious diseases are seen more commonly in HIV patients?

Infections with intracellular pathogens that require intact cell-mediated responses

What infectious diseases in the following categories are seen most commonly in HIV-infected patients?
Virus

Cytomegalovirus and herpes

Parasites	PCP and toxoplasmosis
Fungus	Coccidiomycosis, cryptococcosis, and candidiasis
Mycobacterium	*Mycobacterium tuberculosis* and *Mycobacterium avium* complex
Are bacterial infections uncommon in HIV?	No. Many bacterial infections are more common in HIV-positive persons and are more commonly asssociated with bacteremia.
Is antibody deficiency seen in HIV?	Yes, commonly in young children because T-cell help is required for primary antibody responses. Adult patients may respond poorly to new antigens in late disease.
What is a common complement deficiency?	C2 deficiency is seen in approximately 1:25,000 Caucasians, in whom there is an increased tendency for autoimmune disease. Persons are rarely clinically affected by a decreased ability to opsonize pyogenic bacteria.
In what ethnic groups are terminal complement deficiencies seen and what infections are most common with this problem?	These deficiencies are probably more common in ethnic groups other than Caucasians. People with terminal complement component deficiencies (C5–9) are predisposed to *Neisseria* infections.
What complement deficiency is associated with recurrent episodes of angioedema?	Deficiency of C1 esterase inhibitor
What are other important factors contributing to immunodeficient states?	Protein–calorie malnutrition, burns, malignancy, splenectomy, sickle cell disease, immunosuppression, and uremia

AUTOIMMUNITY

**For the following diseases
caused by antibodies
directed against self,
where are the antibodies
directed?**

    Myasthenia gravis　　　　　Nicotinic acetylcholine receptor at the
　　　　　　　　　　　　　　　neuromuscular synapse

    Goodpasture's syndrome　　Type IV collagen of pulmonary, renal,
　　　　　　　　　　　　　　　and perhaps other basement membranes

    **Autoimmune hemolytic
    anemia (warm)**　　　　　　IgG antimembrane proteins

    **Autoimmune hemolytic
    anemia (cold)**　　　　　　IgM antimembrane oligosaccharides

    **Idiopathic
    thrombocytopenic
    purpura**　　　　　　　　　Platelet glycoprotein IIb/IIIa in some

    Factor VIII inhibitors　　In hemophiliacs, anti-IgG4 predominates

    Pemphigus　　　　　　　IgG antibody to intracellular antigen
　　　　　　　　　　　　　　　localized to the site of acantholysis
　　　　　　　　　　　　　　　(confined to the glycocalyx of the
　　　　　　　　　　　　　　　epidermal cells)

    Pemphigoid　　　　　　　IgG antibody to intracellular antigen
　　　　　　　　　　　　　　　localized to the basement membrane

    Graves' disease　　　　　Anti-TSH receptor

**List the autoantibodies
associated with (but not
necessarily caused by) the
following autoimmune
diseases.**

    Hashimoto's thyroiditis　　Antimicrosomal and antithyroglobulin
　　　　　　　　　　　　　　　antibodies

    **Antiphospholipid
    syndromes**　　　　　　　　Anticardiolipin and lupus anticoagulant

Systemic lupus erythematosus	Antinuclear antibody and anti-dsDNA, among many
Wegener's	Antineutrophil cytoplasmic antibody
Rheumatoid arthritis	Rheumatoid factor
Sjögren's syndrome	Anti-SS-A (Rho) and anti-SS-B (La)
Scleroderma	Anticentromere (CREST) and antitopoisomerase I, also called SCL-70 (PSS)
Dermatomyositis and polymyositis	Anti-Jo-1 (especially with pulmonary fibrosis), anti-PM-Scl (polymyositis and scleroderma), and anti-RNP (polymyositis and mixed connective tissue disease)
Diabetes mellitus	Anti-islet cell antibodies
What are the predominantly T-cell mediated autoimmune diseases?	Polymyositis and multiple sclerosis
Name some predominantly immune complex deposition diseases.	Vasculitides including polyarteritis nodosa Churg-Strauss disease Wegener's granulomatosis Cryoglobulinemia Henoch-Schönlein purpura Serum sickness

ANAPHYLAXIS

What is anaphylaxis?	Anaphylaxis is a life-threatening response, involving more than one organ system, caused by the release of histamine and other mediators from mast cells and basophils by IgE or other mediators.
What are symptoms and signs of anaphylaxis?	Urticaria, angioedema, bronchospasm, diarrhea and abdominal pain, and hypotension

What is the acute treatment for anaphylaxis?	Basic life support and: Epinephrine, subcutaneous injections of 0.2–0.5 ml of 1:1000 every 15–20 min × 3 doses H1 blockers (diphenhydramine, 50 mg) and H2 blockers (cimetidine, 300 mg) intravenously
What other therapy is important in treatment of anaphylaxis?	Corticosteroids may prevent recurrent or protracted anaphylaxis but have no immediate effects. The causative factor should be identified and avoided, if possible. Patients should carry a preloaded epinephrine pen if recurrent exposure is possible.
Why should patients who have had an anaphylactic reaction be monitored after successful therapy?	Episodes can recur for up to several hours after the event.
What are some of the drug and food causes of anaphylaxis?	Drugs—particularly beta-lactams but also NSAIDs, opiates, angiotensin-converting enzyme inhibitors, protamine, insulin, and vaccines Food—shrimp, peanuts (legumes), milk, and eggs (including vaccines made from egg products, such as the influenza vaccine)
What are other common causes and causative agents of anaphylaxis?	Antitoxins, insect venom, Latex, radiocontrast, exercise, systemic mastocytosis, and unknown or idiopathic causes
How is the correct diagnosis of anaphylaxis made?	History is the major diagnostic modality. IgE testing (either by skin testing or by RAST) may be helpful when IgE is suspected. Skin testing should be performed more than 4 weeks after the event, or else false-positive and false-negative tests are more common. If recontact with the causative agent is unavoidable or if no specific diagnosis is made, epinephrine should be prescribed and patients should be instructed in its use.

When can anaphylaxis be prevented?

1. Repeat radiocontrast reactions can largely be prevented by pretreatment with antihistamines and corticosteroids and by using dyes with lower osmotic strength.
2. Insect venom anaphylaxis can be prevented by using venom immunotherapy.
3. The major treatment for other forms of anaphylaxis is avoidance of the causative agent.

MASTOCYTOSIS

What is mastocytosis?

Mastocytosis is a disease of excess mast cells; it can either be localized to the skin or occur in systemic form.

How common is mastocytosis?

Approximately 1 in 5000 patients seen in dermatology clinics has mastocytosis.

What are symptoms and signs of mastocytosis?

Similar to those of anaphylaxis, carcinoid, and pheochromocytoma

What is the most common lesion found on skin examination in mastocytosis?

Urticaria pigmentosa

How is the diagnosis of mastocytosis made?

Bone marrow biopsy and aspirate (for diagnostic and prognostic information)
Urine for 24-hour histamine (5-hydroxyindoleacetic acid, vanilmandelic acid, and metanephrines)
Skin examination (urticaria pigmentosa)
Bone scan, electroencephalogram or neuropsychiatric evaluation, and gastrointestinal studies

What is the treatment for mastocytosis?

H1 antihistamines for pruritus, flushing, and tachycardia
H2 antihistamines for gastric hypersecretion
Epinephrine
Cromolyn (200 mg before meals and at bedtime) may help with gastrointestinal symptoms.

Avoidance of ethanol, NSAIDs, opiates, friction, and physical exertion

What is malignant mastocytosis?

A rarely seen type of mastocytosis in which patients have lymphadenopathy, hepatosplenomegaly, eosinophilia, and malabsorbtion. Without treatment, patients die within 1–2 years.

DRUG ALLERGIES

How common are drug-induced allergies?

Allergies account for 10% of all adverse drug reactions.

Is skin testing helpful for patients with a history of hives to antibiotics?

Penicillin skin testing is reliable for the diagnosis of immediate hypersensitivity; a negative test reduces the risk of an anaphylactic reaction to that of a person with no history of a reaction. A positive skin test indicates a high risk for immediate hypersensitivity reactions.

How common is cross-reactivity in penicillin-sensitive patients?

The history of a reaction to penicillin carries a 5%–15% risk of immediate hypersensitivity to cephalosporins and increases the risk of an adverse response to other, unrelated drugs 10-fold. A positive penicillin skin test increases the risk of a reaction to cephalosporins (and probably imipenem) to 50%.

What drugs interfere with immediate skin tests?

Most antihistamines if used within 3 days of the test (astemizole within 6 weeks) and antidepressants

What is skin testing?

Injection of a small amount of suspected allergen into the skin and looking for a wheal and flare in 15 minutes

Do atopic individuals have an increased risk of anaphylaxis to penicillin?

No. Drug allergies, like venom allergies, occur equally often in atopic and nonatopic subjects.

Are there skin tests for other antibiotics?

Clinically proven skin tests have not been developed for other pharmacologic agents. Testing is sometimes performed for other drugs, but a negative test must be interpreted with caution.

What if there is no alternative agent than the drug allergen?

Desensitization protocols decrease the risk of uncontrolled anaphylaxis. Once therapy is initiated, it cannot be interrupted without resuming the risk of anaphylaxis.

How does desensitization work?

It is not known for certain but there may be a gradual cross-linking of IgE by antigen, causing a controlled anaphylaxis.

Are drug rashes possible with a negative penicillin skin test?

Penicillin skin testing predicts only immediate hypersensitivity. With a negative penicillin skin test, it is still possible for a non-IgE–mediated drug rash, serum sickness, mucocutaneous syndrome, or other adverse side effect to develop.

Is a history of a rash always a contraindication to use of the medication?

It is sometimes possible and necessary to use the medication through a maculopapular rash (e.g., trimethoprim/sulfamethoxazole in HIV), but a history of serum sickness, Stevens-Johnson syndrome, erythroderma, or exfoliative dermatitis are contraindications.

What is serum sickness?

Serum sickness is caused by the deposition of antibody–antigen complexes and the subsequent activation of complement.

What are symptoms and signs of serum sickness?

Fevers, arthralgias, lymphadenopathy, rash (urticarial or maculopapular), nephritis, hepatitis, and other problems in that any vascular bed may be affected. Serum sickness is most commonly seen in response to heterologous serum (e.g., mouse antihuman OKT3 or horse antitetanus). In addition, it is seen in response to drugs, generally after 7–14 days of initial treatment or as early as 3 days with retreatment.

What are mucocutaneous syndromes?

Commonly called Stevens-Johnson syndrome and toxic epidermal necrolysis, these are febrile syndromes that include maculopapular or exfoliating rashes and mucositis. Internal involvement includes the respiratory and gastrointestinal tracts. These syndromes are sometimes fatal.

SKIN

URTICARIA AND ANGIOEDEMA

What is urticaria?

Flat swelling of the epidermis in response to the products of mast cells, such as histamine and leukotrienes

What are symptoms and signs of urticaria?

Pruritic, circumscribed (usually round) areas of dermal edema characterized by a wheal (edema) and flare (surrounding area of hyperemia)

What causes acute urticaria?

Acute urticaria (< 6 weeks) is caused by many things, including allergens, inhalants, ingested or injected drugs (most particularly NSAIDs), viral infections including hepatitis B and Epstein-Barr virus, serum sickness, and pregnancy.

What causes chronic urticaria?

Chronic urticaria (> 6 weeks) is probably caused by many things, but 90% are idiopathic.

What factors should be considered in the evaluation of the patient with urticaria?

Physical urticarias, food sensitivity, drug reaction, chronic infections (sinus, dental, and genitourinary), and collagen vascular disease

How long do episodes of urticaria last?

From minutes to a day

What is angioedema?

Edema of the deep dermal and subcutaneous tissue

What tissue factors cause angioedema?

Like urticaria, histamine and leukotrienes are factors, but bradykinin and other factors also play a role.

What are symptoms and signs of angioedema?

Ill-defined swelling of the skin

What organs other than skin are affected in angioedema?

There is submucosal edema of the gastrointestinal system (lips, esophagus, gastrointestinal tract), nasopharynx, larynx, trachea, or urogenital system.

Is the differential diagnosis different for angioedema than for urticaria?

Angioedema alone as a variant of chronic urticaria accounts for approximately 1 in 10 patients who carry that diagnosis. Other items in the differential diagnosis for angioedema are the use of angiotensin-converting enzyme inhibitors, C1INH deficiencies, either hereditary or acquired, and vasculitis.

How is the cause of angioedema established?

1. If the patient is taking ACE inhibitors, it should be stopped because the side effect of angioedema is life-threatening. This side effect is most commonly seen in the first week of treatment but may occur any time, affecting 3 in 1000 patients.
2. If the C4 level is normal during an episode of angioedema, there is no problem with C1INH because C4 is used up in this process. If the C4 level is low or if a person is seen in an asymptomatic period, C1INH level and functional activity should be measured as should the C1q level. C1q levels are normal in hereditary angioedema and decreased in acquired C1 esterase inhibitor deficiency. Acquired C1INH is associated with malignancy, particularly B-cell lymphomas.
3. If any one lesion lasts for more than 48 hours, a biopsy should be considered to rule out a vasculitis.
4. A workup for chronic urticaria may also be tried.

What is the treatment for urticaria and angioedema?

1. H1 antihistamines. If control is not achieved, H2 antihistamines can be added or doxepin can be used, which has both H1 and H2 antihistaminic activity. Daily steroids are not used.

Epinephrine 1:1000 subcutaneously is used if angioedema is threatening the airway.

2. C1INH deficiency is treated with attenuated androgenic steroids, which increase the production of C1INH. This is effective in patients with deficient production, deficient activity, and increased catabolism of C1INH. Epinephrine may not work in a crisis and a tracheostomy is indicated for laryngeal edema. Antifibrinolytics (epsilon-aminocaproic acid or tranexamic acid) may be helpful.

What is dermatographism?

Appearance of a pruritic linear wheal and flare in response to stroking the skin briskly

What is pressure urticaria?

Painful and pruritic deep swelling in response to pressure over an area

What is cholinergic urticaria?

Small pruritic wheals surrounded by large areas of erythema in response to increases in core body temperature (e.g., from hot baths or showers, exercise, and fever)

ATOPIC DERMATITIS (SEE ALSO CHAPTER 14)

What is atopic dermatitis?

A chronic, relapsing pruritic dermatitis that generally begins in childhood

What are the causes of atopic dermatitis in childhood?

It is frequently associated with food allergies and with inhalant allergies.

What are the causes of atopic dermatitis in adults?

Specific allergies are often more difficult to ascertain because only 20% of substances that produce positive skin tests exacerbate the dermatitis.

What are the usual findings on personal and family history in atopic dermatitis?

A history of eczema, allergic rhinitis, and allergic asthma

What are early skin findings in atopic dermatitis?

Patchy, dome-shaped pruritic papules that are edematous and erythematous

What are late skin findings in atopic dermatitis?

Because the patient rubs and scratches the lesions, they are crusted, excoriated, and scaly (lichenification). Postinflammatory hyperpigmentation and hypopigmentation are commonly seen.

What may vesiculation of the lesions indicate?

Seen in atopic dermatitis but may indicate herpes simplex

What skin diseases need to be excluded on the differential diagnosis of atopic dermatitis?

Seborrheic dermatitis, psoriasis, contact dermatitis, scabies, dermatophyte infections, ichthyosis (multiple causes), mycosis fungoides, Sézary syndrome, and histiocytosis X. Several other rare metabolic conditions may also present similarly.

What underlying conditions should be considered in patients with atopic dermatitis who appear quite ill?

Underlying immunodeficiency states such as Job's syndrome, Wiskott-Aldrich syndrome, XLA, and SCID syndrome

What are the laboratory findings in atopic dermatitis?

Often extremely elevated IgE levels and eosinophilia

What is the treatment for atopic dermatitis?

1. Maintenance of skin moisture
2. Avoidance of pertinent allergens in diet and environment
3. Topical corticosteroids to control inflammation
4. Treatment of skin infections to which such patients are prone, including impetigo caused by S. aureus, viral infections (e.g., herpes simplex, coxsackievirus, and vaccinia), and dermatophyte infections (e.g., Trichophyton, Malassezia, and Candida)

CONTACT HYPERSENSITIVITY (SEE ALSO CHAPTER 14)

What is contact hypersensitivity?	Contact hypersensitivity is a form of delayed-type hypersensitivity to agents that contact the skin. Common agents for contact hypersensitivity include poison ivy, nickel, lanolin, neomycin, P-phenylenediamine, and thimerosal. The differential diagnosis includes photosensitivity dermatitis and irritant dermatitis.
What are skin findings in contact hypersensitivity?	When lesions are due to irritants, they are usually sharp-bordered, erythematous, and may have vesicles that proceed to erosions. When the lesions are due to allergens, they are more indurated with less distinct borders.
What is the treatment for contact hypersensitivity?	Avoidance of the offending agent, topical steroids, or systemic steroids

SINUSITIS AND RHINITIS

What is the differential diagnosis of chronic rhinitis?	Allergic Vasomotor NARES Rhinitis medicamentosa Chronic sinusitis Trauma Cerebrospinal fluid rhinorrhea
What are symptoms and signs of chronic sinusitis?	Documented recurrent episodes of acute purulent sinusitis. Patients frequently complain of frontal headaches, nasal congestion, and pain over the paranasal sinuses.
What is rhinitis medicamentosa?	An inflammatory hypertrophy of cells in the nasal passages as a result of the prolonged use of topical decongestants
What is allergic rhinitis?	A localized immunologic response caused by inhaled allergens

How is the diagnosis of allergic rhinitis made?	Generally by history and physical and by IgE-type response to skin testing
What is seen on cytologic examination of nasal infiltration in allergic rhinitis?	Mast cells, basophils, and eosinophils
What else may cause symptoms suggestive of allergic rhinitis?	Viral or bacterial infections Pregnancy or hypothyroidism Use of birth control pills, reserpine, or methyldopa NSAID sensitivity (often seen with nasal polyps and asthma) Rhinitis medicamentosa Structural or mucociliary defects Atrophic rhinitis
What is chronic sinusitis?	Persistence of symptoms beyond 21 days despite use of antibiotics Recurrence of symptoms less than 1 month after the last episode Three episodes in 6 months or more than four episodes per year
How is the diagnosis of chronic sinusitis made?	Usually, by history Radiographically, by sinus computed tomography scan (plain films are not very sensitive) In rare instances (mostly in research settings), by maxillary puncture
What organisms cause acute sinusitis?	*H. influenzae* (non-typeable) *Moraxella catarrhalis* *S. pneumoniae*
What organisms cause chronic sinusitis?	The same organisms that cause acute sinusitis, plus staphylococci and anaerobes
What is the treatment for sinusitis?	Antibiotics that cover β-lactamase–positive organisms for 14–21 days Promotion of nasal drainage Topical nasal decongestants for 3–5 days Nasal steroids Functional endoscopic sinus surgery (FESS)

What are potential adverse effects of antihistamines?	Somnolence and a possible thickening of mucus, therefore reducing clearance
What are potential adverse effects of the following decongestants?	
Topical	Limited benefit of 3–5 days, possibly leading to rhinitis medicamentosa
Systemic	Hypertension, tachycardia, and agitation

ASTHMA (SEE ALSO CHAPTER 3)

What is asthma?	A disease of airways inflammation characterized by bronchial hyperreactivity
What is the differential diagnosis for wheezing?	Asthma, pulmonary edema, airway obstruction (e.g., laryngospasm, tracheal webbing, tracheomalacia, and foreign body), chronic obstructive pulmonary disease (COPD), congestive heart failure
Is allergy testing useful?	Asthma is an allergic disease in the majority of young adults, and where feasible, allergen avoidance is the treatment with the fewest adverse effects.
What allergens should be tested for?	Indoor allergens, including dust mite, animal dander, and cockroach antigens. Other important allergens include *Alternaria*, which is associated with an increased risk of fatal and near fatal asthma in the Midwest, and *Aspergillus*, because of the syndrome of allergic bronchopulmonary aspergillosis. Pollen allergies are usually more obvious to the patient and therefore less of a problem.
Is allergen immunotherapy useful?	Only in patients with mild to moderate asthma
Is cromolyn therapy useful in the treatment of acute asthma?	Definitely not. Cromolyn works by inhibiting histamine release and it may take as long as 1 week for improvement to occur.

Is aspirin useful in the treatment of acute asthma?

The effectiveness of aspirin is generally tested by escalating challenges. If testing is being performed for asthma, this is quite dangerous and should be done in a monitored unit. Similarly, aspirin desensitization is also performed by graduating doses and is similarly dangerous. Aspirin is, however, effective in controlling asthma in some patients. There is little evidence to suggest that aspirin desensitization is effective for urticaria.

GASTROENTEROLOGY

What are the most common food allergens?

Milk, eggs, nuts (particularly peanuts), shrimp, fish, and wheat

How does food allergy present?

Asthma, urticaria, nausea, vomiting, diarrhea, and oral allergy syndrome (angioedema and sore tongue)

What is celiac disease?

Celiac disease is caused by gluten (specifically gliadin, the alcohol-soluble portion of gluten) hypersensitivity and leads to villous atrophy with malabsorption (lymphocytic and plasma cell infiltration), dermatitis herpetiformis in the skin (with IgA deposition in the skin), and increased risk of GI malignancy.

In what grains is gluten found?

Wheat, oats, rye, and barley

What is eosinophilic gastroenteritis?

An eosinophilic infiltrate of the bowel potentially involving all layers of the gut. Symptoms include nausea, vomiting, diarrhea, malabsorption, obstruction, and ascites.

How is the diagnosis of eosinophilic gastroenteritis made?

Biopsy shows eosinophils in the gut. Involvement is sporadic, so multiple biopsy samples may be required. Usually, patients have a peripheral eosinophilia and very high levels of IgE. IgE testing to foods should be done with a trial of avoidance of positive foods.

What is the treatment for eosinophilic gastroenteritis?	Strict avoidance of any identified offending foods and glucocorticoids

TRANSPLANTATION IMMUNOLOGY

What is a matched graft?	A graft in which the ABO blood group and MHC of the donor and recipient match
Why are grafts matched?	Antibodies against the ABO system and the T-cell responses of the recipient determine whether a graft is accepted or rejected.
Are all grafts matched?	Cardiac, lung, and liver grafts are not MHC matched because other factors such as size, location, and availability limit the transplants much more. Kidney grafting, for which there is the potential for living related and unrelated donors, allows for matching. Bone marrow transplants must be matched, whereas matching in liver transplants may actually decrease survival.
What part of matching is most important?	For most transplants, donor and recipient must be ABO identical or compatible. Matching at HLA-B and DR increases survival in kidney grafts and may increase graft survival in cardiac transplants as well.
What is hyperacute rejection?	Rejection mediated by preformed, complement-fixing antibodies. It takes only hours and is irreversible.
What is accelerated rejection?	Rejection mediated by preformed but not complement-fixing antibodies. Onset is 3–5 days. Treatment is with antithymocyte globulin, which is successful in approximately half of cases.
What is acute rejection?	Rejection mediated by recipient T cells and antibodies as a primary response. It occurs in the first days to months after transplantation and is thought to be directed at passenger APCs. There is

prominent infiltrate of CD8+ cells and polymorphonuclear neutrophils. Immunosuppression is generally successful.

What is chronic rejection?

Mostly antibody deposition leading to hyperplasia and endothelial necrosis. It is slowly progressive and does not respond well to treatment.

What is graft-versus-host disease?

Graft-versus-host disease is an immune response of the donor T cells against the recipient. It is only a problem when transplanting hematopoietic tissue (bone marrow and, very rarely, liver) or when transplanting in neonates.

Why not purge the T cells from marrow before transplantation?

Sometimes, the marrow is purged of T cells, but, without T cells, engraftment is less often successful and the incidence of leukemia increases.

What is the role of immunosuppressives in transplantation?

They decrease T-cell responses to all stimulants, allowing not only organ survival but also opportunistic infections and increased rates of malignancy.

What immunosuppressives specifically target T cells?

Antithymocyte globulin (ATGam) and OKT3, which, in part, bind with the activation sites of T cells via foreign proteins (those of horse and mouse, respectively) and are then selectively cleared by the host's immune system Cyclosporin and FK 506, which decrease IL-2 and interfere with growth and function

Should blood transfusion be avoided?

Yes, for persons likely to need a bone marrow transplant; however, it may enhance renal and cardiac allograft survival by selecting for patients who are hyporesponsive for antibody production.

What infections are common in patients who have undergone organ transplantation?

Same as for HIV (see Chapter 8)

TUMOR IMMUNOLOGY

What are causes of antigenic differences between normal and tumor cells?

1. Chemical carcinogens and ionizing radiation may alter protein synthesis.
2. Viruses may introduce new DNA or RNA into cells.
3. Malignant cells may revert to synthesis of fetal markers such as alpha-fetoprotein or carcinoembryonic antigen, or other fetal proteins.
4. Genetic mutation may lead to expression of inappropriate antigens such as ABO.

Why are antigenic differences potentially important?

If differences between normal cells and malignant cells can be found, then immunotherapy may be effective in curing patients.

What immunotherapeutic agents are currently under investigation?

Interleukins and interferons, monoclonal antibodies, and antitumor vaccines

What are potential uses for monoclonal antibodies?

1. To direct action against tumors through antibody or complement-dependent cytotoxicity
2. To carry cytotoxic substances such as radiolabeled compounds, chemotherapeutic agents (e.g., methotrexate or doxorubicin), or naturally existing toxins, or immunoconjugates, such as ricin

11 Rheumatology

ABBREVIATIONS

ANA	Antinuclear antibody
APS	Antiphospholipid antibody syndrome
AVN	Avascular necrosis
BUN	Blood urea nitrogen
CBC	Complete blood count
CK	Creatine kinase
CNS	Central nervous system
CPP	Calcium pyrophosphate
CTD	Connective tissue disease
CH50	Total complement
CPPD	Calcium pyrophosphate dihydrate deposition disease
dcSSc	Diffuse cutaneous systemic sclerosis
DGI	Disseminated gonococcal infection
DIL	Drug-induced lupus
DIP	Distal interphalangeal joint
DM	Dermatomyositis
ESR	Erythrocyte sedimentation rate
GC	Gonococcal

HIV	Human immunodeficiency virus
HTN	Hypertension
JRA	Juvenile rheumatoid arthritis
lcSSc	Limited cutaneous systemic sclerosis
MCP	Metacarpophalangeal
MCTD	Mixed connective tissue disease
MSU	Monosodium urate
NSAID	Nonsteroidal anti-inflammatory drug
OA	Osteoarthritis
PAN	Polyarteritis nodosa
PM	Polymyositis
PMN	Polymorphonuclear neutrophils
PMR	Polymyalgia rheumatica
PIP	Proximal interphalangeal joint
PsA	Psoriatic arthritis
RA	Rheumatoid arthritis
RF	Rheumatoid factor
RNP	Ribonucleoprotein
ROM	Range of motion
SLE	Systemic lupus erythematosus
SSc	Systemic sclerosis
SjS	Sjögren's syndrome
SCLE	Subacute cutaneous lupus erythematosus
U/A	Urinalysis

WBC	White blood cell

HISTORY AND PHYSICAL EXAMINATION

What five questions should a patient with joint pain be asked?	1. What is the nature of onset (including initiating event)? 2. What is the joint distribution? 3. What is the pattern of activity? 4. How many joints are involved? 5. What are the types of joint symptoms?
What terms describe the following: **Onset**	Insidious, gradual, sudden, explosive
Distribution	Symmetrical or asymmetrical Large joints (hips, knees, and ankles) or small joints (hands and feet) Axial (spine, ribs, and pelvis) or peripheral (arms and legs)
Pattern	Intermittent, migratory, additive Acute versus chronic
Number	Polyarticular, oligoarticular, monoarticular
Symptom type	Arthr*algia* (painful) Arthr*itis* (inflammation—red, hot, swollen, painful)
What are clues to systemic inflammation?	Fatigue, fever, morning stiffness, and weight loss
What are the cardinal clinical features of the following systemic autoimmune diseases? **RA?**	Symmetrical arthritis in hands (MCPs and PIPs) and other joints, morning stiffness
SLE?	Arthralgias, arthritis, rashes (malar, discoid), alopecia, photosensitivity, mouth ulcers, Raynaud's phenomenon

SSc?	Skin changes, sclerodactyly (digital skin tightens and fingers curl), Raynaud's phenomenon
SjS?	Dryness in the eyes and mouth (sicca symptoms), parotid gland fullness
PM?	Proximal muscle weakness, cannot climb stairs or brush hair
DM?	PM with a rash
PMR?	Proximal limb pain, occurring in older people, often associated with giant cell arteritis (i.e., temporal arteritis). Lack of proximal muscle weakness differentiates polymyalgia rheumatica from PM.
How is family history helpful in examining patients with joint pain?	These diseases "cluster"; for example, a woman with RA has an aunt with SLE.
What are causes of AVN?	Think **ASEPTIC:** **A**nemia (sickle cell) **S**teroids **E**tOH (alcohol) **P**ancreatitis **T**rauma **I**diopathic **C**aisson disease (nitrogen emboli) or **C**ongenital

JOINT EXAMINATION

What is ROM?	Range of motion, the extent that a joint can be moved within its particular abilities
What is normal ROM?	Normal can be compared with the examiner's ROM.
What does decreased ROM indicate?	Active inflammation and trauma, or old trauma, chronic arthritis, lack of use, or congenital problems
What tool is used to measure ROM?	A goniometer (a ruler that pivots in the center and is marked in degrees)

What is active ROM?	The patient moves a specific joint.
What is passive ROM?	The examiner moves the joint while the patient relaxes soft tissues (e.g., muscles and tendons).
Why are both passive and active ROM evaluated?	To distinguish muscular and periarticular pain (pain with active, not passive, ROM) from articular (joint) pain (pain with both)

SYNOVIAL FLUID ANALYSIS

What are the classes and qualities of synovial fluid?	Normal—0–200 WBC/mm³, clear to pale yellow, transparent, high viscosity, good mucin clot Noninflammatory—200–2000 WBC/mm³, yellow, clear, good mucin clot Inflammatory—2000–100,000 WBC/mm³, yellow to white, translucent to opaque, poor mucin clot Septic—> 80,000 WBC/mm³ (> 75% PMNs), white, opaque, low glucose, low viscosity, poor mucin clot

BACK PAIN

How common is back pain?	It is almost universal; 80% of persons experience significant back pain in their lifetime.
What are causes of back pain?	Trauma—muscle strain or sprain, subluxed facet joints, compression fractures Degenerative disorders—herniated nucleus pulposus, spondylosis (spinal stenosis), OA Neoplasm—intraspinal tumor Inflammation—sacroiliitis, vertebral body osteomyelitis, disc infection
What structures cause back pain?	Periosteum (compression fractures), posterior longitudinal ligament (disc herniation), nerve roots exiting the intervertebral foramen (dermatomal pain from disc herniation), facet joints (after bending), sacroiliac joints, and paravertebral muscles

What is sciatica?	Irritation of the sciatic nerve as it passes through the foramen
What disc spaces are usually involved in sciatica?	95% are due to disc herniation at L4–5 and L5–S1.
What are presenting symptoms of sciatica?	Pain below the knee that increases with sitting, coughing, and Valsalva maneuver. Pain decreases when the patient is supine.
What are physical examination features for disc disease at the following levels?	
L4–5	Decreased ability to walk on toes
L5–S1	Decreased ability to walk on heels
What are causes of pseudosciatica?	Hip disease, trochanteric bursitis, meralgia paresthetica, diabetic amyotrophy, and vascular claudication

OSTEOARTHRITIS

What is another term for OA?	Degenerative joint disease
What is OA?	"Wear and tear" of cartilage and articular surfaces. It is more mechanical in nature than inflammatory.
What is the incidence of OA?	OA occurs in 30% of adults and is the most common form of arthritis.
What risk factors are associated with OA?	Increasing age, genetics, previous trauma, obesity, and metabolic disorders (e.g., gout, ochronosis)
What are symptoms and signs of OA?	Pain and stiffness. In early disease, involved joints hurt with use and improve with rest; in later disease, involved joints hurt all the time, with worsening of pain at the end of day. Gelling or stiffening occurs with prolonged resting (morning stiffness for less than 30 minutes).

What is found on examination in OA?	Crepitus, bony enlargement, decreased ROM, pain with ROM, and mild inflammation. Distribution is bilateral and asymmetrical, involving hands, feet, knees, and hips and usually sparing shoulders and elbows.
What is found on examination of the hand involved in OA?	Heberden's nodes, enlarged DIPs; Bouchard's nodes, enlarged PIPs; squaring of the first carpometacarpal joints
What are the radiographic findings in OA?	Normal mineralization Non-uniform joint space loss Subchondral new bone formation Subchondral cysts Osteophyte formation
How is the diagnosis of OA made?	History, physical examination, and radiographic study
What is the treatment for OA?	Physical therapy for strengthening of muscles, increased ROM, and stability Education, reassurance Weight loss, cane (to decrease joint stress) NSAIDs, analgesics, capsaicin cream Intraarticular steroids Joint replacement (in advanced disease)

RHEUMATOID ARTHRITIS

What is RA?	An inflammatory, multisystemic disease with flares and remissions, characteristic chronic deformities, systemic features, and RF
What is the incidence of RA?	RA occurs in 1%–2% of all adults. It is the most common autoimmune disease.
What risk factors are associated with RA?	Female gender
What are symptoms and signs of RA?	Morning stiffness for more than 1 hour; symmetrical joint pains; inflammation in hands, feet, knees, hips, shoulders, and elbows; fatigue; weight loss; fever; and subcutaneous nodules

What does examination of the rheumatoid hand find?

Synovitis of MCPs and PIPs (DIPs spared); ulnar drift caused by tendon laxity; subluxation of proximal phalanges under MCP heads; and nodules on bony prominences and extensor surfaces.

What are the laboratory tests findings in RA?

RF present in 80% of cases

What is RF?

An autoantibody (usually IgM) directed against the Fc fragment of IgG

What other conditions are associated with RF?

Subacute bacterial endocarditis, viral infections (e.g., infectious mononucleosis, tuberculosis, Lyme disease), increasing age, and sarcoidosis

What are the radiographic findings in RA?

Periarticular swelling
Juxtaarticular osteopenia, then
    generalized osteoporosis
Uniform joint space loss
Marginal erosions
Subluxations

How is the diagnosis of RA made?

Documentation of inflammatory synovitis by the following:
1. Synovial fluid WBC count > 2000/mm^3
2. Chronic synovitis on histologic study
3. Radiologic evidence of erosions
In the right clinical setting, with symptoms present longer than 6 weeks

What is the treatment for RA?

First line of therapy is with NSAIDs. Second line of therapy is with hydroxychloroquine, methotrexate, gold, azathioprine, and sulfasalazine; physical and occupational therapy; local joint injections with steroids; and surgery for joint stabilization or replacement. Oral steroids should be "temporary" treatment (i.e., while waiting for second-line agents to be effective).

When is treatment of RA urgent?

In cases of severe flares, vasculitis, relative steroid insufficiency, or joint or systemic infections

When is treatment of RA emergent?	When there is severe adrenal insufficiency (addisonian crisis) and atlantoaxial (C1–2) instability
What is adult-onset Still's disease?	Similar to systemic onset JRA, but in adults
What are symptoms and signs of adult-onset Still's disease?	Sudden onset of high, spiking fever, sore throat, and evanescent erythematous salmon-colored rash. Arthritis involves PIPs, MCPs, wrists, knees, hips, and shoulders.

CONNECTIVE TISSUE DISEASE

SYSTEMIC LUPUS ERYTHEMATOSUS

What is SLE?	A disease or collection of syndromes defined by clinical features and autoantibodies directed against various components of cell nuclei
What is the incidence of SLE?	40/100,000, with > 80% occurring in young women
What classification criteria were established by the American College of Rheumatology in 1982 to distinguish SLE from other CTDs?	Think **SOAP BRAIN MD:** **S**erositis—pleuritis, pericarditis **O**ral ulcers—or nasal ulcers as seen by a physician **A**rthritis—nonerosive, symmetrical (hands, knees, wrists) **P**hotosensitivity—skin rash due to unusual sun reaction **B**lood (hematologic)—hemolytic anemia, leukopenia, lymphopenia, or thrombocytopenia **R**enal—proteinuria, RBCs and WBCs or casts **A**NA **I**mmunologic—anti-DNA or anti-Smith antibodies **N**eurologic—seizures, psychosis **M**alar rash—fixed erythema over nose and cheeks **D**iscoid rash—red, raised, scaling plaques that scar

More than four criteria are needed to make a diagnosis, including active serology.

What are other features of SLE?

Protean features, including fatigue, fever, weight loss, myalgias, urticaria, leg ulcers, nonspecific rashes, and peripheral neuropathy

What tests should be ordered for suspected SLE?

CBC, ESR, C-reactive protein, U/A, electrolytes, BUN, creatinine, ANA, anti-DNA, anti-Smith, anti-RNP, CH50, and possibly C3 and C4

Once the diagnosis of SLE is established, what tests are used to follow-up disease activity?

CBC, anti-dsDNA, CH50, U/A, BUN, and creatinine

What are the radiographic features in SLE?

Soft-tissue swelling, juxtaarticular osteopenia, subluxations and dislocations, AVN, and symmetrical distribution, but no erosions

What is the treatment for SLE?

Mild disease—NSAIDs, hydroxychloroquine
Flares and moderate-to-severe disease—oral or intravenous steroids. Steroid-sparing agents include cyclophosphamide, methotrexate, and azathioprine.
Severe lupus nephritis—intravenous pulse cyclophosphamide

What are urgent indications in SLE?

Increasing DNA and decreasing complement, which may herald an acute flare or new complication
Flare
Infection
New signs of renal involvement—decreasing renal function, increasing BUN and creatinine, decreasing creatinine clearance, and increasing proteinuria, urine RBCs, WBCs, and casts

What should be considered in the following SLE emergencies?

Mental status change and headache?

Rule out infection and vasculitis

Acute shortness of breath or chest pain?

Pericardial effusion or tamponade or pulmonary embolus

Leg pain, shortness of breath, pulmonary embolus, and CNS changes?

Rule out hypercoagulable state

Ischemic digits?

Raynaud's phenomenon, APS, vasculitis, and necrosis

Pregnant patient with flare?

Both SLE and toxemia have proteinuria, CNS disease, and HTN; however, SLE has low complement.

Lupus Disease Subcategories

What is APS?

Antiphospholipid antibody syndrome that is either a primary process or part of SLE. APS is a hypercoagulable state that is not always associated with lupus nor is it an anticoagulant. Clinical findings include venous or arterial thrombosis, nonhealing ulcers, livido reticularis, thrombocytopenia, and miscarriage (often in the second trimester). Treatment is with acetylsalicylic acid, heparin, and warfarin.

What laboratory tests are ordered in the workup of APS?

Tests include anticardiolipin antibodies, prothrombin time, partial thromboplastin time, Venereal Disease Research Laboratory tests, and modified Russell's viper venom time, or local test for "lupus anticoagulant."

What is SCLE?

Subacute cutaneous lupus erythematosus, featuring nonfixed, nonscarring rashes, generally in sun-exposed areas, with presence of anti-SS-A (anti-Ro)

What is MCTD?	Mixed connective tissue disease, featuring presence of anti-RNP antibody, myositis, pulmonary disease, Raynaud's phenomenon, arthritis, and vasculitis
What is discoid lupus?	A mostly cutaneous disease with characteristic scarring, scaling plaques that may evolve into SLE
What is neonatal SLE?	Congenital heart block associated with maternal anti-SS-A (anti-Ro) antibody
What is DIL?	Drug-induced lupus. Clinical and serologic signs of lupus appear while the patient is taking a drug, and they disappear when the drug is stopped. DIL is usually less severe disease without renal involvement. Chlorpromazine, methyldopa, hydralazine, procainamide, and isoniazid have been implicated.

SYSTEMIC SCLEROSIS

What is SSc?	A disorder of connective tissue characterized by overproduction of collagen (types I, III) and matrix proteins
What is the hallmark of SSc?	Skin thickening (scleroderma)
What is Raynaud's phenomenon?	Paroxysmal vasospasm of the digits in response to cold or emotional stress. There are three phases: white—pallor, ischemic changes; blue—cyanosis; red—blood flow increases, with warmth, throbbing, and pain.
What are the two main categories of SSc?	1. Limited cutaneous (lcSSc) 2. Diffuse cutaneous (dcSSc)
What are features of lcSSc?	Skin fibrosis that is limited to hands and face; pulmonary HTN, often occurring 20–30 years after diagnosis; esophageal reflux; calcinosis; and telangiectasia

What is CREST syndrome?	**C**alcinosis, **R**aynaud's phenomenon, **E**sophageal dysmotility, **S**clerodactyly, and **T**elangiectasia. This term is often used to describe limited disease.
What are features of dcSSc?	Widespread fibrosis of skin; rapid total progression over several years; 20% incidence of scleroderma renal crisis (malignant arterial HTN with rapidly progressive oliguric renal failure); pulmonary interstitial fibrosis; microstomia; and fibrosis of any part of the gastrointestinal tract
What are the laboratory findings in SSC for:	
lcSSc?	90% of patients have ANA that is mostly anti-centromere antibody.
dcSSc?	95% of patients have ANA that is mostly anti-Scl-70 (an antibody against topoisomerase I)
How is the diagnosis of SSc made?	Often on clinical grounds. Serologic studies are supportive.
What is the treatment for SSc?	There is no treatment for underlying pathophysiology. Renal crisis—Angiotensin-converting enzyme inhibitors, hydralazine Reflux—H2 blockers, omeprazole Lung disease—penicillamine

SJÖGREN'S SYNDROME

What is SjS?	A chronic, progressive autoimmune disease with invasion of exocrine glands by lymphocytes and plasma cells
What is the hallmark of SjS?	Dryness of eyes and mouth caused by decreased lacrimal and salivary gland function
What is the incidence of SjS?	It is the second most commonly recognized autoimmune disease. (It may actually be the most common disease.)

What are symptoms and signs of SjS?	Xerophthalmia (dry eyes), xerostomia (dry mouth), difficulty swallowing and talking, and firm, nontender, enlarged parotids Less common—esophageal mucosal atrophy, atrophic gastritis, dyspareunia
What are extraglandular signs of SjS?	Arthralgia, arthritis, Raynaud's phenomenon, lymphadenopathy, lung involvement, vasculitis, and peripheral neuropathy
What are the laboratory findings in SjS?	ANA, anti-SS-A (anti-Ro), anti-SS-B (anti-La), RF, cryoglobulins, anemia, leukopenia, thrombocytopenia, increased ESR. SjS is known for high levels of multiple antibodies in nonspecific patterns.
What diagnostic tests are obtained for SjS?	Schirmer's test (filter paper in the eye) showing < 5-mm tear wicking in 5 minutes Rose Bengal staining of eye with slit-lamp examination showing keratitis Salivary gland biopsy (lower, inner lip) showing foci of mononuclear cells

AUTOANTIBODY AND DISEASE MATCH

List the diseases associated with the following laboratory tests: **ANA**	SLE, lupus subset, SjS, RA (target—nuclear proteins)
Anti-dsDNA	SLE (target— DNA)
Anti-Sm (Smith)	SLE (target—RNP proteins). This test should not be confused with Sm (smooth muscle antibody) seen in autoimmune hepatitis.
Anti-RNP	SLE, MCTD (target—other RNP proteins)
Anti–SS-A (Ro)	SjS, SCLE, neonatal SLE, SLE (target—proteins associated with RNA)

Anti–SS-B (La)	SjS, SCLE, neonatal LE, SLE (target—other RNA proteins)
Anti-centromere	Raynaud's phenomenon, lcSSc (target—centromere proteins)
Anti–Scl-70	dcSSc (target—antitopoisomerase I)
Anti–Jo-1	Seen in PM>>DM, especially with lung involvement (target—anti-histidyl-tRNA synthetase)
ANCA	c-ANCA (cytoplasmic)—Wegener's granulomatosis (target—proteinase 3) p-ANCA (peripheral)—Polyarteritis nodosa

VASCULITIS

What is vasculitis?	A heterogeneous group of diseases that have in common inflamed blood vessels. This may occur as the primary disease process or in the setting of a CTD.
What is the incidence of vasculitis?	Rare or very rare

POLYARTERITIS NODOSA

In patients with PAN, what is the average age of onset of disease and gender most often affected?	The 5th decade; more common in men than in women
What organ systems are involved in PAN?	Skin, peripheral nerves, joints, intestines, and kidneys; the lungs are usually spared.
What are symptoms and signs of PAN?	Fever, malaise, palpable purpura, joint pains, multiple mononeuropathies, abdominal pain, hematochezia or melena, HTN, and testicular pain
What are the laboratory findings in PAN?	Hepatitis B surface antigen or antibody found in 15% of cases, urine RBCs, RBC casts, and proteinuria

How is the diagnosis of PAN made?	Biopsy of involved organ shows vasculitis and "beads" are seen on mesenteric (or other) angiogram.
What is the treatment for PAN?	High-dose steroids and cyclophosphamide

WEGENER'S GRANULOMATOSIS

In patients with Wegener's granulomatosis, what is the mean age of onset of disease and gender most often affected?	40 years; more common in men than in women
How does Wegener's granulomatosis present?	Presentation usually involves the upper respiratory tract—sinusitis, rhinitis, nasal mucosa with ulcerations, and purulent or bloody nasal discharge.
What are other features of Wegener's granulomatosis?	Arthralgias, fever, cough, hemoptysis, dyspnea, rash, and glomerulonephritis
What are the laboratory findings in Wegener's granulomatosis?	Urinalysis—microhematuria, RBC casts, proteinuria, and increased BUN and creatinine C-ANCA—anti-neutrophil cytoplasmic antibodies in 80% of cases Chest radiograph—bilateral, nodular fixed infiltrates that usually cavitate
How is the diagnosis of Wegener's granulomatosis made?	Clinical features and presence of necrotizing granulomas and vasculitis shown on biopsy (kidney, lung)
What is the treatment for Wegener's granulomatosis?	Oral cyclophosphamide, 2 mg/kg/day, for at least 1 year. This regimen has greatly improved the life expectancy in this disease. Prednisone, 1 mg/kg/day, may be needed at onset.

CHURG-STRAUSS SYNDROME

In patients with Churg-Strauss syndrome, what is the age of onset of disease and gender most often affected?	40 years; more common in men than women

What are the three phases of Churg-Strauss disease?

1. Prodrome lasting more than 10 years. Allergic manifestations include rhinitis, polyposis, and asthma.
2. Peripheral blood and tissue eosinophilia with Löffler's syndrome, which is an eosinophilic endocarditis that should not be confused with Lofgren's syndrome, eosinophilic pneumonia, or eosinophilic gastroenteritis
3. Systemic vasculitis, heralded by fever and weight loss, chest radiograph abnormalities, improvement of asthma, skin lesions, mononeuritis multiplex, congestive heart failure, abdominal symptoms, and renal disease.

What are the laboratory findings in Churg-Strauss syndrome?

Peripheral blood eosinophilia in more than 10% of cases. Biopsy of lung or skin shows eosinophilic necrotizing granulomas and necrotizing small vessel disease.

What is the treatment for Chrug-Strauss syndrome?

Steroids

Name 3–4 distinctive features of each of the following vasculitides: Giant cell arteritis

1. Headache, scalp tenderness, jaw claudication, and ischemic optic neuritis
2. Occurrence in persons approximately 50 years old and more commonly in women than men
3. High ESR (> 80)

Behçet's syndrome

1. Recurrent painful aphthous oral and genital ulcers
2. Uveitis and retinal vasculitis
3. Erythema nodosum, papulopustular skin lesions
4. Possible CNS involvement

Cryoglobulinemia

1. Immunoglobulins that precipitate at cold temperatures, and usually RF

2. Cause of Raynaud's phenomenon, purpura, and ischemic ulcers, which are due to hyperviscosity and plugging of small vessels. Vasculitis is uncommon.

3. Mixed cryoglobulins are associated with CTDs, hepatitis A/B/C, parasites, many infections, and lymphoproliferative diseases.

Takayasu's arteritis

1. Chronic vasculitis of the aorta and its branches
2. Occurrence in young women and in persons of Asian descent
3. Asymmetrically decreased peripheral pulses

Henoch-Schönlein Purpura

1. Occurrence in 5- to 15-year-old children with history of upper respiratory infection
2. Palpable purpura on buttocks and legs (IgA found on biopsy of the skin lesions)
3. Crampy umbilical pain and nephritis

SERONEGATIVE SPONDYLOARTHROPATHIES

Name the five seronegative spondyloarthropathies.

1. Ankylosing spondylitis
2. Reactive arthritis
3. Reiter's syndrome
4. PsA
5. Enteropathic arthritis

What does spondyloarthropathy mean?

Disease of the axial skeleton

What does seronegative mean?

Absence of RF (or other autoantibodies)

What is HLA-B27?

An allele of the HLA-B locus (a "gene"). It has an increased prevalence in most of the seronegative spondyloarthropathies. Its direct role in the pathogenesis of the diseases is unknown.

When is HLA-B27 test ordered?	Generally, it is not. Although HLA-B27 is associated with the seronegative spondyloarthropathies, 10% of Caucasians have it and very few get one of the diseases. The test is not routine, diagnostic, confirming, or used for screening.

ANKYLOSING SPONDYLITIS

What is ankylosing spondylitis?	*Ankylos* means fusion, adhesion; *spondylos* means spinal vertebra
What is the age of onset of ankylosing spondylitis?	Late adolescence, early adulthood
What gender is most often affected?	Male to female, 9:1
What are features of ankylosing spondylitis?	Low back pain or stiffness Chest expansion decreased < 4 cm Enthesitis (inflammation of tendon insertions) Difficulty taking deep breaths Decreased ROM of spine Decreased flexion of lumbar spine (measured distance of 10 cm fails to increase to > 15 cm with flexion) as measured by Schober test Pain in sacroiliac joints as detected by Patrick's test May have peripheral arthritis of the large joints, especially the knees and ankles
What are features of late disease in ankylosing spondylitis?	Fusion of spine (in approximately 10 years) Possible appendicular arthritis Iritis Heart and lung involvement
What are the laboratory findings in ankylosing spondylitis?	Radiographs show symmetrical ankylosis of sacroiliac joints and spine, absence of subluxation and cysts, and generalized osteopenia after ankylosis

How is the diagnosis of ankylosing spondylitis made?	Clinical grounds and radiographic study
What is the treatment for ankylosing spondylitis?	Physical therapy, education, daily posture work, and swimming, with the goal being that the spine fuses straight instead of bent. Medications include NSAIDs (e.g., indomethacin). Sulfasalazine may be effective as a slow-acting second-line drug.
What are emergent considerations in ankylosing spondylitis?	The ankylosed spine is susceptible to fracture, usually transverse, at C5–6 or C6–7, with risk of spinal cord injury.

REACTIVE ARTHRITIS (Reiters syndrome)

What is reactive arthritis?	An acute nonpurulent arthritis complicating an infection at another site
What microbes are associated with reactive arthritis?	*Yersinia, Salmonella, Shigella, Campylobacter* in the gastrointestinal tract; *Chlamydia* in the genitourinary tract
What is the distribution of reactive arthritis?	Asymmetric oligoarthritis of lower extremities (knees, ankles, and MTPs)
What are other features of reactive arthritis?	Urethritis, conjunctivitis, uveitis, circinate balanitis, keratoderma blennorrhagia, oral mucosal ulcers (painless), local enthesopathies, sausage digits, and unilateral (early) or bilateral (late) sacroiliitis
What are the laboratory findings in reactive arthritis?	There are no diagnostic tests, but the clinician should try to isolate pathogens and rule out septic arthritis and gonococcal arthritis.
What is the treatment for reactive arthritis?	NSAIDs (e.g., tolmetin and indomethacin); for chlamydial infection, tetracycline

REITER'S SYNDROME

What is the classic triad of Reiter's syndrome?	Arthritis, urethritis (nongonococcal), and conjunctivitis
What is Reiter's syndrome?	Reactive arthritis
How is the term Reiter's syndrome used?	To describe some cases of full-blown reactive arthritis

PSORIATIC ARTHRITIS

What is the prevalence of psoriasis?	Affects 2% of adults
What percent of persons with psoriasis also have arthritis?	5%
What are the five disease patterns of psoriatic arthritis?	1. Oligoarticular (asymmetric), 50% 2. Spondyloarthropathy, 20% 3. Polyarticular (RA-like), 20% 4. DIP disease ("classic"), 8% 5. Mutilans (deforming), 2%
What is the treatment for psoriatic arthritis?	NSAIDs, methotrexate, and sulfasalazine

ENTEROPATHIC ARTHRITIS

Name several features of the arthritis associated with the following: **Crohn's disease**	1. Occurs in 20% of cases 2. Distribution is pauciarticular, asymmetric, transient, and migratory. 3. Affects large and small joints of lower extremity 4. Causes "sausage digits" (dactylitis) and heel enthesopathies 5. Does not strictly coincide with bowel disease activity 6. Causes sacroiliitis and spondylitis in less than 20% of cases 7. Causes erythema nodosum

Ulcerative colitis	1. Occurs in less than 20% of cases
	2. Arthritis features the same as in Crohn's disease
	3. Has a more distinct temporal relationship between flares of arthritis and colitis than does Crohn's disease

GOUT AND PSEUDOGOUT

GOUT

What is gout?	A disease characterized by the following:
	1. Hyperuricemia
	2. Recurrent attacks of acute arthritis with MSU crystals demonstrated in synovial fluid
	3. Renal stones
	4. Tophi
What is the incidence of gout?	1/4000; prevalence 10/1000
What are risk factors for gout?	Increased age (postadolescent men and postmenopausal women), elevated serum uric acid, use of diuretics, overeating, and alcoholism
What are the four stages of gout?	1. Asymptomatic hyperuricemia
	2. Acute gouty arthritis
	3. Intercritical gout
	4. Chronic tophaceous gout
What is the upper range of normal uric acid levels?	7–8 mg/dl
What are high levels of uric acid?	Men, > 13 mg/dl; women, > 10 mg/dl
What are the two main reasons for uric acid elevation?	Decreased uric acid excretion, 90% Increased uric acid production, 10%
What are common reasons for decreased uric acid excretion?	Decreased renal function, diuretics, HTN, low-dose salicylates, and lead

ACUTE GOUTY ARTHRITIS

Where is the site of first attack of acute gouty arthritis?	First MTP joint, with abrupt onset at night. The joint is warm, red, and very tender.
How are subsequent attacks of acute gouty arthritis characterized?	More frequent occurrence, involving more joints and lasting longer than the first attack
What are attack triggers for acute gouty arthritis?	Alcohol, surgical stress, trauma, acute medical illness, and drugs (diuretics, allopurinol, or probenecid without colchicine)
What is the treatment for acute gout?	NSAIDs, oral or intravenous colchicine, or steroids

CHRONIC TOPHACEOUS GOUT

What is chronic tophaceous gout?	Tophi develop in association with chronic joint pain and sometimes deforming arthritis.
What are tophi?	A core of MSU crystals surrounded by inflammatory cells and a fibrous capsule. Clinically, they are lumpy masses over, on, or in joints and extensor surfaces. They usually appear 10 years after the first attack of gout.
What are complications of chronic tophaceous gout?	Renal stones, proteinuria, HTN, and chronic renal insufficiency
What are the radiographic findings in chronic tophaceous gout?	After years, tophi, punched-out erosions with sclerotic borders, preserved joint spaces, and asymmetric distribution
How is the diagnosis of chronic tophaceous gout made?	Demonstration of MSU crystals in PMNs in synovial fluid
What is the treatment for chronic tophaceous gout?	Allopurinol, colchicine, or both

What is intercritical treatment of chronic tophaceous gout?	Avoidance of alcohol, weight loss, and colchicine; probenecid (uricosuric); and allopurinol (xanthine oxidase inhibitor)
How is the word YUP-pie significant in chronic tophaceous gout?	MSU is birefringent—yellow if parallel to the scope axis, blue if perpendicular, hence, YUP-pie (**y**ellow, **u**rate, **p**arallel)

PSEUDOGOUT

What is pseudogout?	Gout-like arthritis that is not caused by MSU but by CPP, usually, or any other crystal type
What is the incidence of pseudogout?	Approximately half as common as gout
What are risk factors for pseudogout?	Aging, OA, amyloid, hypothyroidism, hyperparathyroidism, and hemochromatosis
What are symptoms and signs of pseudogout?	Characteristics may be gout-like, but subacute and chronic arthralgias and arthritis have been described.
What are the laboratory findings in pseudogout?	In synovial fluid, CPP crystals are short, cuboidal, and blue when parallel to axis.
What are the radiographic findings in pseudogout?	Chondrocalcinosis. CPP is visible on radiograph; MSU is not. Bone is visible on radiograph; cartilage is not. CPP is visible in linear deposits floating in "clear" space above bone; that is, it rests on cartilage.

INFECTIOUS ARTHRITIS*

List the infectious arthritis syndromes.	GC, nongonococcal, Lyme, and viral
What are predisposing conditions for infectious arthritis?	Preexisting arthritis, trauma, systemic illnesses (e.g., diabetes mellitus and malignancy), and other infections

---

* Contribution from C. Sable, N. Theilman, and V. Shami

What are symptoms of infectious arthritis?	Fever, limited joint mobility, joint swelling, and tenderness
What are signs of infectious arthritis?	Elevated temperature, synovial effusion with tenderness, and limited mobility
What pathogens are associated with infectious arthritis?	*Neisseria gonorrhoeae* is most common in sexually active adults. *Staphylococcus aureus* is most common otherwise.
What are the microbiologic findings in nongonococcal bacterial arthritis?	*S. aureus* (60%), streptococci (15%), gram-negative rods (15%), pneumococcus (5%), and polymicrobial (5%)
How is the diagnosis of infectious arthritis made?	Synovial WBC > 50,000/mm^3, > 75% PMNs, low glucose, Gram stain, and culture
What is the differential diagnosis of increased WBCs and PMNs in synovial fluid?	RA and crystalline joint disease
What is the treatment for infectious arthritis?	1. Initial drainage of all purulent material from infected joint 2. Antimicrobial therapy directed by Gram stain and culture results 3. Serial aspirates (or surgical drainage) of infected joint to assess adequacy of therapy and facilitate drainage

GONOCOCCAL ARTHRITIS

What is the incidence of GC?	Of the 1 million cases of GC in the United States per year, 1% have bacteremia and arthritis.
What are general features of DGI?	1. Usually occurs in young, sexually active adults 2. Initial migratory polyarthralgia 3. Tenosynovitis and polyarthritis 4. Dermatitis 5. Purulent arthritis (one or more joints) 6. With or without genitourinary symptoms

What is the distribution of DGI?	Knees, wrists, and ankles
How are skin lesions characterized in DGI?	Multiple vesiculopustular lesions on extremities or trunk
What are the laboratory findings in DGI?	Synovial WBC count may be low. Positive cultures of urethra, cervix, rectum, or oropharynx on Thayer-Martin medium
How is the diagnosis of DGI made?	Usually clinical impression coupled with recovery of organism from genitourinary tract
What is the recovery rate of *N. gonorrhoeae* from synovial fluid?	Less than 25%. Blood cultures are positive in less than 10%.
What is the treatment of DGI?	Intramuscular or intravenous ceftriaxone, intravenous cefotaxime, or intravenous ceftizoxime initially followed by an oral regimen with cefixime or ciprofloxacin. Affected joints are aspirated frequently.
What is the clue to the diagnosis of DGI?	Tenosynovitis and dermatitis are rare in non-neisserial bacterial arthritis.

NONGONOCOCCAL BACTERIAL ARTHRITIS

What are risk factors for nongonococcal bacterial arthritis?	Trauma, surgery, and arthrocentesis Chronic medical illness (e.g., RA, diabetes mellitus, SLE, and chronic liver disease) Age extremes Immunosuppression Prosthetic joints
What are symptoms and signs of nongonococcal bacterial arthritis?	Abrupt onset Acutely swollen, painful joints Loss of motion or function Fever Distribution of 50% in knee, 80% monoarticular (polyarticular cases are usually associated with a risk factor)

What laboratory tests are ordered for nongonococcal arthritis?	Joint aspiration for fluid analysis, Gram stain, and synovial fluid and blood cultures. Missing this diagnosis leads to the risk of disseminated infection and permanent joint deformity.
What are the radiographic findings in nongonococcal arthritis?	Joint space narrowing and erosion of cortex in 7–14 days
What is the treatment for nongonoccocal arthritis?	Intravenous antibiotics, daily aspiration, and daily ROM exercise to prevent joint contractures
Which microbes are usually associated with nongonoccocal arthritis?	*S. aureus,* 60%; β-hemolytic streptococci, 15%; gram-negative rods, 15%; pneumococcus, 15%, and polymicrobial, 5%

LYME ARTHRITIS

What are the three stages of Lyme arthritis and how are they characterized?	1. Early, localized—erythema migrans 2. Early, disseminated—migratory musculoskeletal pain, in joints, bursae, tendons, muscle, and bone 3. Late—in 6 months, onset of brief attacks of oligoarthritis, usually involving large joints (knee). Episodes become longer, with erosion of cartilage and bone.
What laboratory tests are ordered for Lyme arthritis?	Enzyme-linked immunosorbent assay with Western blot to confirm. Both acute and convalescent titers should be evaluated.
What is the treatment of Lyme arthritis?	Doxycycline, 100 mg twice daily for 30 days (stages 1 and 2)

VIRAL ARTHRITIS

Parvovirus B19

What are features of parvovirus B19 illness in adults?	Severe, self-limited flu-like illness with arthralgias and arthritis and a rheumatoid-like distribution

How is the diagnosis of parvovirus B19 made?	Antiparvovirus B19 IgM
What is the treatment for parvovirus B19?	NSAIDs

Hepatitis B Virus

List five arthritis features of hepatitis infection.

1. Infection is immune-complex mediated, occurring early in course.
2. Onset of arthritis is sudden and severe.
3. Distribution is symmetrical, migratory, and additive.
4. Joints involved are hands and knees.
5. Urticaria is a feature.

Human Immunodeficiency Virus

List five articular manifestations of HIV infection.

1. Arthralgia (at any stage)
2. Reiter's syndrome
3. PsA
4. Undifferentiated spondyloarthropathy
5. HIV-associated arthritis that is distinct, oligoarticular, asymmetric, and, in later stages, lasts an average of 4 weeks

List five muscular manifestations of HIV infection.

1. Myalgias
2. PM and DM, HIV induced
3. Myopathy, azidothymidine induced
4. Pyomyositis (a muscle infection)
5. Muscle atrophy

List six rheumatic syndromes seen in HIV.

1. Sjögren-like syndrome
2. Lupus-like syndrome
3. Vasculitis
4. Fibromyalgia
5. Hypertrophic osteoarthropathy
6. AVN

ARTHRITIS SECONDARY TO SYSTEMIC DISEASES

DIABETES MELLITUS

What are nine common musculoskeletal problems seen in diabetes mellitus?

1. Carpal tunnel syndrome
2. Limited hand mobility
3. Frozen shoulder
4. Reflex sympathetic dystrophy

5. Neuropathic (Charcot) joint
6. Septic arthritis
7. Trigger finger
8. Dupuytren's contracture
9. Osteomyelitis

What is shoulder–hand syndrome?

Frozen shoulder, limited hand mobility, and reflex sympathetic dystrophy

What is the differential diagnosis of pain and weakness in the proximal thigh of a diabetic?

Acute mononeuritis (femoral nerve)
Meralgia paresthetica (lateral cutaneous nerve)
Diabetic amyotrophy (polyneuropathy)
Lumbar plexopathy
Herniated disc
Herpes zoster (before eruption)
OA in hip joint
AVN of femoral head
Trochanteric bursitis

THYROID DISEASE

Name five rheumatologic features of hyperthyroidism.

1. Osteoporosis
2. Onycholysis (separation of nail from bed)—differential diagnosis: Reiter's syndrome, psoriasis, PsA
3. Painless proximal muscle weakness with normal creatine phosphokinase—differential diagnosis: PM
4. Frozen shoulder
5. Thyroid acropachy (distal soft-tissue swelling, clubbing, and periostitis of MCPs)

Name four rheumatologic features of hypothyroidism.

1. Carpal tunnel syndrome
2. Polyarthritis
3. AVN of hip
4. Myalgias (may have elevated CK)

What four rheumatic situations are mimicked by hypothyroidism and may be reversible with thyroxine?

1. Carpal tunnel syndrome
2. Seronegative RA
3. Polymyalgia rheumatica with normal ESR
4. PM with normal muscle biopsy

SARCOIDOSIS

What is the incidence of arthritis in sarcoidosis?	10%

What are the two patterns of arthritis in sarcoidosis?	1. Acute:
	    It occurs within 6 months of diagnosis.
	    It occurs more frequently than late arthritis.
	    Ankles and knees are involved.
	    Periarticular swelling is prominent.
	    In 60% of cases, erythema nodosum is present.
	    Radiographs are negative.
	    Lofgren's syndrome may be present.
	2. Late:
	    It occurs 6 months after diagnosis.
	    Knees, ankles, and PIPs are involved.
	    Distribution is less widespread and less dramatic than in acute arthritis.
	    There is association with chronic cutaneous sarcoid.
	    Dactylitis may be a feature.

What is Lofgren's syndrome?	Acute arthritis, erythema nodosum, and bilateral hilar adenopathy; usually a self-limited process of less than 6 months' duration

AMYLOIDOSIS

What is amyloidosis?	A heterogeneous group of diseases characterized by deposition of amyloid, a proteinaceous material
How are types of amyloidosis classified?	By type of amyloid (e.g., AA, AL, Ab2M, and Ab)
Name several features of each of the major clinical syndromes of amyloidosis. **Idiopathic and myeloma associated (AL):**	Mean age at diagnosis 60 years Heart and kidney affected Arthropathy in < 5% Shoulder pad sign—amyloid infiltration of shoulder, a nearly pathognomonic sign

Seen with RA, JRA, and ankylosing
  spondylitis
Extremely rare in SLE, PM
Seen in Crohn's disease; rare in
  ulcerative colitis

Seen in long-term dialysis patients
Carpal tunnel syndrome
Arthropathy
Cystic bone lesions
Pathologic fractures

Localized microdeposits in joints
May be associated with OA and CPPD

ARTHRITIS ASSOCIATED WITH MALIGNANCIES

Name five ways in which musculoskeletal syndromes may be related to malignancies.

1. Metastatic disease to bone
2. Primary malignant disease (rare)
3. Paraneoplastic syndromes (e.g., PM, scleroderma, lupus-like syndrome, and Sweet's syndrome [fever, abrupt onset of painful plaques on arms, neck, and head, and neutrophilia])
4. Increased incidence of malignancy in preexisting CTDs (e.g., SjS)
5. Malignancy as a complication of treatment (e.g., with cyclophosphamide, methotrexate, or radiotherapy) or rheumatic disease

What are features of arthritis resulting from metastatic disease?

1. Rapid reaccumulation of hemorrhagic, noninflammatory effusion
2. Fluid with negative cultures and without crystals
3. Failure of medical therapy
4. Destruction seen on radiograph
5. Long clinical course

ARTHRITIS SECONDARY TO SICKLE CELL DISEASE

What is the incidence of bone or periarticular pain with sickle cell crisis?

20%

What are the most common sites of arthritis in sickle cell disease?	Knees and ankles
What are the most serious complications of arthritis in sickle cell disease?	AVN (hip, 10%); osteomyelitis (salmonella)
What radiographic changes are seen in sickle cell disease?	Cortical bone infarcts with periosteal elevation; widened medullary cavities with thin cortex

ARTHRITIS SECONDARY TO HEMOPHILIA

What is the incidence of hemarthrosis (bleeding into a joint) in hemophilia?	85%. It is the most common major hemorrhagic event in the disease.
What is the natural history of arthritis in hemophilia?	Onset of joint symptoms between ages 1 and 5 years, with repeated events occurring in the first decade, then less frequently
What are features of an acute hemarthrosis?	Swollen, warm, exquisitely painful Held in flexion from muscle spasm Progressive loss of form and function
What are features of a chronic hemarthrosis?	Bony enlargement with atrophic muscle affecting knees, then elbows, ankles, and shoulders Flexion contracture Asymmetric, sporadic distribution

TREATMENT

MEDICATIONS

Name five renal syndromes induced by NSAIDs.	1. Sodium retention and edema 2. Hyperkalemia 3. Acute renal failure 4. Nephrotic syndrome with interstitial nephritis (fenoprofen) 5. Papillary necrosis (aspirin and acetaminophen)

Name eight adverse reactions to intramuscular gold.

1. Mouth ulcers
2. Pruritus and rash
3. Proteinuria
4. Leukopenia
5. Thrombocytopenia
6. Eosinophilia
7. Aplastic anemia
8. Nitritoid reaction (flush)

Name six slow-acting antirheumatic drugs and their time to onset of effectiveness.

1. Intramuscular gold, 4–5 months
2. Methotrexate (MTX), 1–2 months
3. Sulfasalazine (SSZ), weeks to months
4. Hydroxychloroquine (Plaquenil), 3–4 months
5. Cyclophosphamide (Cytoxan, CTX), weeks
6. Azathioprine (Imuran, AZA), weeks

12 Neurology

ABBREVIATIONS

ACA	Anterior cerebral artery
ADC	AIDS dementia complex
AD	Alzheimer's disease
AIDS	Acquired immune deficiency syndrome
ALT	Alanine aminotransferase
AMS	Altered mental status
BPPV	Benign paroxysmal positional vertigo
BUN	Blood urea nitrogen
CBC	Complete blood count
CJD	Creutzfeldt-Jakob disease
CNS	Central nervous system
c/s	Cycles per second
CSF	Cerebrospinal fluid
CT	Computed tomography
EEG	Electroencephalogram
EMG	Electromyogram
ESR	Erythrocyte sedimentation rate
GBS	Guillain-Barré syndrome
GCSE	Generalized convulsive status epilepticus

GTC	Generalized tonic-clonic seizure
HIV	Human immunodeficiency virus
HSV	Herpes simplex virus
ICP	Intracranial pressure
JME	Juvenile myoclonic epilepsy
LEMS	Lambert-Eaton myasthenic syndrome
LP	Lumbar puncture
MCA	Middle cerebral artery
MRI	Magnetic resonance imaging
MS	Multiple sclerosis
NPO	Nothing by mouth
NSAID	Nonsteroidal anti-inflammatory drug
PD	Parkinson's disease
PCA	Posterior cerebral artery
PICA	Posterior inferior cerebellar artery
PML	Progressive multifocal leukoencephalopathy
RAS	Reticular activating system
SAH	Subarachnoid hemorrhage
SE	Status epilepticus
TB	Tuberculosis
TIA	Transient ischemic attack
TLE	Temporal lobe epilepsy
WBC	White blood cell

ALTERED MENTAL STATUS

What is AMS?

Any impairment in a patient's level of consciousness or cognition, varying from mild confusion to coma

What three things should be evaluated immediately in a patient with AMS?

Oxygenation, perfusion (i.e., blood pressure and pulse), and glucose level

What treatment should be given for an impaired level of consciousness of unknown etiology?

Oxygen, naloxone, and glucose. If alcoholism is suspected, thiamine should be given with the glucose.

What are four general causes of AMS?

Toxic/metabolic encephalopathy, anoxic encephalopathy, seizures, and stroke

What are the neurologic examination findings in toxic/metabolic encephalopathy?

Impaired level of consciousness without focal neurologic signs. Patients may also have asterixis.

How do you test for asterixis?

Have the patient extend arms and wrists. Observe for brief downward flaps of the hands.

What is the most common cause of toxic/metabolic encephalopathy in the hospital?

Drugs

List three other general medical conditions that may cause toxic/metabolic encephalopathy.

1. Infection—CNS or systemic infections
2. Organ failure—hepatic or renal
3. Electrolyte imbalance—hypoglycemia, hyperglycemia, hyponatremia, hypercalcemia

What causes lethargy in renal failure?

A uremic substance that loosely correlates with an elevated BUN

What is dialysis disequilibrium syndrome?

Headache, confusion, and somnolence usually associated with large fluid and solute shifts

What is the triad of Wernicke's encephalopathy?

Ataxia, confusion, and ophthalmoparesis

What is treatment for Wernicke's encephalopathy?	Thiamine
What laboratory tests are useful in evaluating a patient with AMS?	Glucose, CBC, liver function tests, electrolytes, BUN, arterial blood gas, drugs of abuse screen and serum drug levels, head CT, and EEG
What is the confusional state that follows a seizure called?	Postictal state, which usually resolves over a few minutes to hours
What is nonconvulsive SE?	A rare type of seizure that presents with prolonged AMS without obvious motor seizures. It is diagnosed with EEG.
How is the confusion from a stroke distinguished from a toxic/metabolic encephalopathy?	A stroke usually has focal neurologic signs such as aphasia or hemiparesis. The AMS associated with a stroke is usually secondary to cerebral edema with mass effect.
What is another vascular cause of AMS, especially in elderly patients?	Subdural hematoma, which is diagnosed by CT scan
What is the most common cause of anoxic encephalopathy?	Cardiac arrest followed by resuscitation. Myoclonus may be associated with the AMS. The prognosis is poor.

COMA AND BRAIN DEATH

What is coma?	An unarousable state of unconsciousness
Place coma on a spectrum with the other "levels of consciousness."	Coma is a more impaired consciousness level than stupor (a state of arousable unconsciousness), obtundation (a markedly impaired but nevertheless alert state of consciousness), lethargy (a moderately impaired state of sustained consciousness), and the "normal" level of consciousness. A level of excited consciousness can be considered as the opposite end of the spectrum.

What are the first steps in management of a comatose patient in the emergency department?	The basic **ABCs** need to be addressed, that is, **A**irway, **B**reathing, and **C**irculation.
What therapy should be given in the emergency department, before the cause of coma is established?	Glucose, thiamine, naloxone, and flumazenil when indicated
What causes should be considered in every comatose patient?	When the examination indicates the brain stem as the locus of the offending lesion, the primary consideration is that of a stroke syndrome (hemorrhage or ischemia) or pressure on the brain stem (herniation). If the brain stem appears intact, stroke syndromes can still be considered, but it is more likely that the cause is toxic/metabolic encephalopathy, seizure, trauma, or infection, all things that can diffusely scramble cortical activity bilaterally.
Coma suggests dysfunction of which brain structures?	Either the midbrain RAS, which "wakes up the cortex," or both cerebral cortices (bihemispheric dysfunction)
What bedside tests help establish whether coma results from dysfunction of the RAS or from bihemispheric dysfunction?	Checking the reflex actions of the cranial nerves, particularly those of the eye movements and the pupillary light response. With bihemispheral dysfunction, these reflexes should be intact and symmetrical. With damage to the midbrain RAS of the brain stem, the normal reflexes or symmetry of the reflexes is lost because the neurologic pathways that mediate these reflexes are located very close to the RAS.
What are four bedside tests of cranial nerve function that are useful in a comatose patient?	(1) Pupillary light reflex, (2) corneal response, (3) vestibulo-ocular reflex (caloric response), and (4) "doll's eyes" (oculocephalic response)
What is the vestibulo-ocular reflex (or cold water calorics test)?	When ice-cold water is instilled against the tympanic membrane of an ear, the normal tendency is for the eyes to

conjugately deviate toward the side of the cold water instillation. The patient's head should be 30 degrees above supine and looking straight ahead. Approximately 100 ml of ice-cold water should be instilled into the ear canal over 1–2 minutes (a butterfly tubing from which the needle has been removed is helpful when placed on the end of a 30-ml syringe). Approximately 5 minutes should elapse before the test is attempted in the other ear. In some circumstances, the patient may display nystagmus with the fast component in the direction opposite to the instilled ear.

The mnemonic **COWS** (**C**old–**O**pposite, **W**arm–**S**ame) is a popular way of remembering the direction of nystagmus, but it does not refer to the direction of eye deviation.

What are doll's eyes?

A less confusing term for this is the "oculocephalic reflex" or the "cervico-ocular reflex." With the patient's eyes open, the patient's head is briskly nodded back and forth (e.g., from left to right and back), activating the same pathways as cold water instillation does in the vestibulo-ocular reflex, partly through causing movement of the endolymphatic fluid in the inner ear (as with cold calorics) and partly through activating proprioceptive receptors in the neck that feed position information to the vestibular system. The "active" part of the reflex is the turning of the eyes away from the direction of head turning, so that eye movement appears to lag behind head movement. The active reflex should not be confused with the passive return of the eyes to midgaze position after the head rotation is complete and there is no more stimulation to the system. Eye movements should be symmetric and conjugate, with equal excursion distances in both eyes.

What are characteristic motor responses of a comatose patient?

The patient cannot respond to command and probably cannot localize noxious stimulation. In response to noxious stimulation, decorticate or decerebrate posturing may be seen.

What is the difference between decorticate and decerebrate posturing?

Decorticate posturing is extension in the legs and flexion at the shoulders, elbows, and wrists. Decorticate flexes the arms up to the chest or "core" of the body. Decerebrate posturing is extension of both the legs and the arms.

What do the different types of posturing indicate?

Posturing usually indicates structural brain damage, in which the cortex is disconnected from the brain stem. In decorticate posturing, the brain stem is probably mostly intact, and the damage is above the midbrain, involving only the cortex. Decerebrate posturing implies a worse injury and prognosis, and indicates not only hemispheral damage but also damage to the top half of the brain stem, involving the whole cerebrum, not just the cortex.

What breathing patterns are characteristic in a comatose patient and may assist in localization of the lesion?

From rostral to caudal (i.e., top to bottom):
Cheyne-Stokes breathing may indicate a metabolic abnormality or disconnection of the cerebral cortex from the diencephalon or brain stem.
Central neurogenic hyperventilation results from irritation to the midbrain.
Apneustic breathing suggests a lesion at the level of the pons.
Ataxic breathing originates from the medulla, suggesting that all higher portions of the CNS above the medulla are dysfunctional.

What are two causes for a seemingly comatose patient whose eyes are open?

Some patients with bihemispheric dysfunction regain their sleep–wake cycle, but do not regain any awareness of their environment. This is the "vegetative" state, and prolonged coma may evolve into this. If it lasts for more than a month, it is a persistent vegetative state. A second possibility is the "locked-in state," in which the patient is not in a coma but has lost all movement of the body and cranial nerve–innervated muscles from a lesion in the pons. Eye movements may be preserved.

What is cerebral "herniation"?

The intracranial compartment is divided into two parts by the tentorium, an invagination of dura mater that is fairly rigid and has a circular opening, or notch, in its center, through which the brain stem passes. When pressure increases in the supratentorial compartment, in which the cerebral hemispheres lie, the brain may be displaced or herniated through the tentorial notch, which causes pressure on the brain stem.

How does the pupil examination indicate when cerebral herniation is occurring?

If pressure increases enough in the supratentorial compartment, the brain stem may be forced further down into the infratentorial space, which can stretch the ipsilateral oculomotor nerve, causing the pupil to dilate. Similarly, as the uncus, the most medial part of the temporal lobe, swells into the tentorial opening, it may compress the third nerve on that side, "blowing" that pupil. Rarely is the side of pupillary dilation contralateral to the side of the lesion causing the herniation.

How is cerebral herniation managed?

Hyperventilation may increase the area for the brain to swell by decreasing the area taken up by intracranial vasculature. The osmotic effects of osmotic diuretics, such as mannitol, may decrease cerebral edema. The only definitive treatment is to address the primary cause of herniation. Some form of craniectomy may be considered, but such a measure implies sacrifice of the portion of brain that is being "unroofed." Other standard conservative measures include elevating the head of the bed, treating hyperthermia, and avoiding high ventilator positive end-expiratory pressures, which can obstruct venous return from the head.

What is brain death?

An irreversible cessation of all cerebral functions, including those of both the hemispheres and the brain stem.

What factors may confound the brain death evaluation?

Barbiturates, drug overdose or sedation, neuromuscular blocking agents, anticholinergics (e.g., atropine), and hypothermia (body temperature less than 32.2-°C).

What findings must be documented on the brain death examination?

No posturing or withdrawal to torso, head, or appendicular noxious stimulation, absent pupillary light response, absent corneal response, absent oculocephalic and vestibulo-ocular reflexes, and absent gag or cough. Absence of spontaneous respiration must also be demonstrated. Deep tendon reflexes may still be present, however.

What is an apnea test?

To rule out the presence of spontaneous respirations, the patient is initially ventilated to a state of hyperoxia (Po_2 > 200) and Pco_2 of < 40. The ventilator rate is lowered to 1 breath per minute (or continuous positive airway pressure of 10). Arterial blood gases are checked every 5 minutes, until the Pco_2 is > 60 and the pH is < 7.3. Spontaneous ventilation during this time is evidence that the brain is not "dead."

What confirmatory tests may be necessary to establish the diagnosis of brain death?

Angiography may demonstrate absent cerebral blood flow, EEG may indicate no electrical brain activity, CT of the head may reveal thrombosed cerebral blood vessels, and radionuclide scanning may reveal no cerebral uptake.

Over what period of time must the status of brain death be demonstrated before brain death can be officially declared?	If no ancillary tests are done (e.g., angiography, CT) to support the diagnosis of brain death, the brain death examination should be confirmed 12 hours after it was initially performed. If an ancillary test is used in the interim, the repeat examination can be done after 6 hours. However, there may be other specific time intervals designated by state law.

DEMENTIA

What is dementia?	A deterioration of intellectual and cognitive functions in multiple areas (one of which is usually memory) that is severe enough to interfere with the ability to accomplish previously performed social or personal occupations or functions. This loss of abilities should not be associated with changes in perception and level of consciousness.
In addition to memory, what are several other areas of cognitive decline that should be evaluated in the workup of suspected dementia?	Judgment, praxis, language, abstract thinking, constructional abilities, and visual recognition
When altered perception or level of consciousness is present along with memory impairment, what diagnosis should be considered?	Delirium, which is primarily a disorder of attention and ability to concentrate. The delirious patient may also be demented (dementia is a risk factor for the development of delirium), but the initial diagnosis of dementia cannot be made while a patient is delirious.
What is the natural history of most dementias?	For the most part, dementias are progressive, but this is not exclusive. Dementia secondary to trauma is not necessarily progressive.
What are the reversible dementias?	Approximately 5%–10% of dementias are reversible. These include dementia secondary to an infection of the CNS (such as neurosyphilis), metabolic and nutritional dementias (B_{12}, folate

deficiencies), inflammatory dementias (vasculitis involving cerebral blood vessels), dementia due to a structural defect impinging on the brain (a subdural hemorrhage or tumor), normal pressure hydrocephalus, and endocrine-related dementia (hypothyroidism).

What is the initial workup of the demented patient?

The workup can be directed by the history and physical examination, but the following initial tests should be considered: B_{12} level, folate level, thyroid function tests, Venereal Disease Research Laboratories (VDRL) or microhemagglutination assay–*Treponema pallidum* (MHA-TP), HIV enzyme-linked immunosorbent assay, ESR, CBC, chemistries, liver enzymes, neuroimaging (CT or MRI), and neuropsychiatric testing.

When should an EEG be obtained in the evaluation of the demented patient?

When onset of dementia is fairly rapid (over months) and when the patient complains of, or is noticed to have, multifocal myoclonic jerks. These symptoms may be due to CJD, which is caused by a prion. In this case, the EEG may reveal periodic epileptiform discharges, which, in this setting, are relatively specific for CJD.

What should the clinician look for when reviewing the neuroimaging of a demented patient?

Large ventricles (that are enlarged out of proportion to whatever cortical atrophy might be present), which could suggest the presence of normal pressure hydrocephalus; evidence of previous strokes that could yield a diagnosis of a vascular dementia; and evidence to rule out existing reversible traumatic sequelae, such as a subdural hemorrhage, or a surgically remedial lesion, such as a neoplasm

When should an LP be considered in the evaluation of dementia?

When chronic meningitis or an inflammatory disease affecting the brain is suspected to be the cause (e.g., in the immunosuppressed patient). Also, in the patient with suspected normal pressure hydrocephalus, a high-volume LP (in which approximately 40–50 ml of CSF are removed) may cause the patient to acutely improve, thus helping to establish the diagnosis.

What common psychiatric syndrome can easily be mistaken for dementia?

Depression may result in or even present with "pseudodementia." In some cases, patients have an organic dementia that appears more severe than it is because of a superimposed pseudodementia. Neuropsychiatric testing can help establish this diagnosis as either the sole cause of symptoms or as a concomitant process confounding an underlying principal dementia.

What is the most common cause of dementia?

The neurodegenerative diseases are the most common cause of dementia. The most important neurodegenerative disease that causes dementia is AD, which accounts for approximately 50%–60% of all dementia. AD has an incidence of approximately 1% per year in persons older than age 65 years and is present in approximately 50% of persons older than age 85 years. Other neurodegenerative diseases that cause dementia or may present with dementia include PD, Huntington's disease, Pick's disease, and progressive supranuclear palsy.

ALZHEIMER'S DISEASE

How is AD diagnosed?

AD is highly suspected from its clinical presentation in the absence of other diagnosable dementias; however, a definitive diagnosis can be made only by brain biopsy or at autopsy.

What laboratory test is useful in diagnosing or predicting AD?

Apo E4 testing. Three different variants of the apolipoprotein E gene exist on chromosome 19 (E2, E3, and E4). E4 is associated with an increased rate of dementia. However, many people with apo E4 never experience dementia, whereas many people without apo E4 do. The use of apo E screening in the relatives of patients with AD should therefore probably be discouraged. As a diagnostic tool, apo E testing is less important than the dementia workup described above.

When the diagnosis of AD is made, approximately how often is the diagnosis correct?

Even when the clinical criteria described above are adhered to, the diagnosis is accurate only approximately 80%–90% of the time.

How is AD managed?

There is no cure for AD, although the drug tacrine (Cognex) has been approved for use in the disease. Tacrine is a long-acting anticholinesterase that crosses the blood–brain barrier. By increasing cholinergic activity in some patients with AD, a temporary improvement (over several months) in memory function may be elicited. Antipsychotic medications may help control some of the behavioral problems (e.g., agitation) that may develop in patients with AD.

How is tacrine used?

It is started at a low dose, 10 mg four times a day. At 6-week intervals, the dose is increased by 40-mg increments, until 160 mg/day is reached (40 mg four times a day). Liver transaminase (ALT) elevations are common (occurring in 25%–50% of patients), so liver function tests should be checked weekly for the first 12 weeks of therapy. The drug should be stopped when the ALT level reaches three times the normal upper limit.

VASCULAR DEMENTIA

What are some of the types of vascular dementia?

Multi-infarct dementia is dementia resulting from multiple strokes that involve both cortical and subcortical brain. Binswanger's disease (subacute arteriolar encephalopathy) is a specific syndrome of pervasive small vessel strokes that are especially prominent periventricularly. There is also a less specific form of small-vessel disease called lacunar infarct vascular dementia.

How common are vascular dementias?

They are the second most common type of dementia and account for approximately 20% of dementia cases.

What is the major risk factor for development of a vascular dementia?

Hypertension

OTHER DEMENTIAS

What is the clinical triad of normal pressure hydrocephalus?

Gait apraxia (a specific form of ataxia), urinary incontinence, and dementia

Does alcoholism cause dementia?

Alcoholism can contribute to dementia. In the alcoholic patient, cognitive impairment may occasionally be limited to problems with memory (particularly short-term memory), which is an "amnestic syndrome" rather than a true dementia. Such patients may demonstrate confabulation.

ENDOCRINE ABNORMALITIES AND VITAMIN DEFICIENCIES

What vitamin deficiency, which is often found in alcoholics, can result in an acute neurologic syndrome when glucose is administered to deficient patients?

Thiamine

What syndrome may be caused by administration of glucose-containing solutions in the presence of thiamine deficiency?

Wernicke's encephalopathy is characterized by confusion, gait ataxia, and eye movement problems. The presence of the complete triad in a particular patient is rare, however, which occasionally confounds the diagnosis.

What chronic amnestic syndrome may follow Wernicke's encephalopathy?	Korsakoff's syndrome is a persistent amnestic syndrome classically associated with confabulation.
How can Wernicke's encephalopathy and Korsakoff's syndrome be avoided?	By routine administration of thiamine, 100 mg intramuscularly or intravenously, to at-risk patients at the time they are seen in the emergency department
What vitamin deficiency causes subacute combined degeneration?	Vitamin B_{12} (cyanocobalamin)
How is subacute combined degeneration characterized clinically?	There is a combination of hyporeflexia, hyperreflexia, diminished proprioception and vibration sensation, and ataxia of gait. Dementia may result, as may optic neuropathy.

In subacute combined degeneration, what causes the:

Hyporeflexia?	Sensorimotor neuropathy
Hyperreflexia?	Degeneration of the corticospinal tract in the CNS
Diminished proprioception and vibration sensation?	Degeneration of the dorsal columns
Who is at risk to develop subacute combined degeneration?	Persons with malabsorption syndromes (secondary to pernicious anemia, gastrectomy, or ileal diseases)
What is the neurologic sequelae of pyridoxine deficiency?	Both excess and deficiency of vitamin B_6 can cause neuropathy. The deficient state tends to cause a mixed sensorimotor neuropathy. In neonates, deficiency may cause seizures.
What is the neurologic sequelae of pyridoxine excess?	The excess state is associated with a specific sensory neuropathy.

What two vitamin supplements should be considered for use in pregnant epileptic patients on anticonvulsants?

Women taking carbamazepine or valproic acid should take 1.0–5.0 mg per day of folate, because of the increased risk of neonatal neural tube defects associated with these medications. Phenytoin, carbamazepine, phenobarbital, and primidone can cause a deficiency of vitamin K–dependent clotting factors in the neonate, so women on these drugs should take 20 mg of vitamin K_1 (phytonadione) per day during the last few weeks of pregnancy. Neonates should be given vitamin K_1 at birth.

What are the neurologic manifestations of vitamin E deficiency?

Decreased cerebellar coordination, peripheral neuropathy, night blindness, and eye movement abnormalities

What neurologic sequelae can result from hypothyroidism?

Myopathy, cramps, neuropathy, mental status changes (including dementia), and coma, if severe

What neurologic sequelae can result from hyperthyroidism?

Mental status changes (including psychosis) and rare cases of myopathy or neuropathy. Hyperthyroidism can also be associated with a form of periodic paralysis. Patients with myasthenia gravis have an increased incidence of hyperthyroidism.

What are two endocrine abnormalities that are associated with an elevated risk of carpal tunnel syndrome?

Excessive growth hormone (acromegaly) and hypothyroidism

Calcifications seen on head CT in the basal ganglia, dentate nuclei of the cerebellum, and the cerebellar cortex suggest what potential endocrine abnormality?

Hypoparathyroidism. Other neurologic effects of hypoparathyroidism result from hypocalcemia and include tetany, cramps, seizures, and paresthesias.

Which is associated with seizures and coma, hypoglycemia or hyperglycemia?

Both

What is the most common neurologic sequela of diabetes mellitus?

Neuropathy. Many different types of neuropathy may manifest, including acute mononeuropathies arising secondary to acute ischemic infarctions of single or multiple nerves (mononeuritis multiplex), a stocking-and-glove distal polyneuropathy, symmetric and proximal motor weakness without pain, a painful thoracolumbar radiculopathy, a lumbar plexopathy causing pain and weakness in one of the thighs (neuralgic amyotrophy), and an autonomic neuropathy.

What drugs can be used to treat the pain and paresthesias that occur from diabetic neuropathy?

Tricyclics (e.g., amitriptyline), selected anticonvulsants (e.g., carbamazepine), and topical capsaicin

What intervention has recently been demonstrated to decrease the incidence and severity of neuropathy in diabetes?

Tight glucose control

Diabetes may cause infarcts of the third cranial nerve, resulting in impaired movement of the affected eye. In such cases, how can third nerve compression by an aneurysm be distinguished on physical examination?

Diabetic third nerve infarcts usually spare pupillary function, whereas compression of the third nerve results in pupillary dilation.

How much is the risk of stroke increased in the diabetic?

By two to four times over baseline

HEADACHE AND FACIAL PAIN

How common is headache?

More than 90% of persons in the United States have had a headache in the past year.

Distinguish between functional and organic headache syndromes.

In functional headache syndromes, there is no discernable structural disease, whereas structural disease is present in organic headache syndromes.

What are two common functional headache syndromes?	1. Tension, or muscle contraction 2. Vascular, including migraine and cluster
What are four important causes of an organic headache syndrome?	CNS infection, elevated intracranial pressure (ICP), SAH, and CNS tumor
Which is more common, functional or organic headache?	Functional headache occurs in 95% of headache patients.
What two features suggest a serious cause for headache (i.e., an organic headache)?	1. Evidence of neurologic deficit by history, neurologic examination, or neuroimaging 2. Recent onset

ORGANIC HEADACHE

What characteristic quality does the pain of SAH have?	Patients complain of the "worst headache in my life."
What symptoms often accompany headache caused by SAH?	Nausea, vomiting, and syncope
What are three important causes of elevated ICP?	1. Mass lesion (such as tumor) 2. Pseudotumor cerebri 3. Hydrocephalus
What distinguishes headache caused by elevated ICP from other headaches?	Presence of papilledema and other focal neurologic signs
What is the likely cause of headache when papilledema is present without a mass lesion?	Pseudotumor cerebri (benign intracranial hypertension)
Who are susceptible to pseudotumor cerebri?	Primarily young obese women
How is the diagnosis of pseudotumor cerebri made?	Elevated opening CSF pressure (greater than 18 cm H_2O), but no mass lesion seen on imaging studies

What additional symptom would be important to detect in pseudotumor cerebri and why?	Deteriorating vision, because increased CSF pressure on the optic nerve may cause blindness.
How should patients with pseudotumor cerebri be followed up?	Regular examination of visual fields and acuity to detect deterioration
How is pseudotumor cerebri treated?	Acetazolamide or surgical fenestration of the optic nerve sheath to release CSF

VASCULAR HEADACHE

What is the characteristic quality of the pain of migraine headache?	Severe, often throbbing, although it may be any character
What are common associated symptoms of migraine headache?	Nausea and photophobia
What distinguishing behaviors do patients exhibit to relieve the pain of migraine?	They lie down in a dark room and go to sleep.
What distinguishes *classic* from common migraine?	A visual aura accompanies or precedes classic migraine.
What distinguishes *complicated* migraines from other migraines?	Complicated migraine is accompanied by a transient neurologic deficit, such as hemiparesis.
What is *common* migraine?	Migraine headache with neither aura nor transient neurologic deficit
What is the usual age of onset of migraine?	School-age or teenage years
What are five frequent precipitants of migraine?	1. Consuming alcohol 2. Consuming soft cheeses 3. Being exposed to bright lights or glare 4. Consuming chocolate 5. Being sleep deprived

What are three prescription drugs used to abort the headache of a migraine attack?

Ergotamine tartrate, sumatriptan, and mixed analgesics (such as Fiorinal)

Where is the presumed action of ergotamine?

Contraction of vascular smooth muscle, which prevents the cycle of vascular relaxation and contraction associated with migraine. Recent evidence suggests it may have other effects, such as antiserotonin effects, which may be more important.

Why is the amount of ergotamine that a patient may take limited to 10 mg per week?

To avoid the risk of "ergotism" with higher doses

What is ergotism?

Excessive vascular contraction, resulting in symptomatic peripheral vascular ischemia or symptomatic coronary artery constriction

What are two contraindications to ergotamine use?

History of coronary artery disease (such as angina pectoris) and peripheral vascular disease

What is the mechanism of sumatriptan?

5-HT1 (serotonin) agonist

How is sumatriptan administered?

At the onset of headache by either a 100-mg injectable syringe or by 25- or 100-mg tablets

What is a contraindication to use of sumatriptan?

Coronary artery disease

What is a common barbiturate used in mixed analgesics?

Butalbital is mixed with caffeine and aspirin or acetaminophen in Fiorinal, Fiorcet, Esgic, and other mixed analgesics.

Why is it important to know about butalbitol?

Because it is a habit-forming barbiturate

What three "prophylactic" drug therapies prevent or reduce the frequency of migraine?	1. Beta-blockers such as propranolol 2. Calcium channel blockers such as verapamil 3. Valproic acid
What is cluster headache?	Clustered attacks of severe orbital headache with nasal congestion and lacrimation
Which gender is most affected by cluster headache?	Males
When do cluster headaches usually begin?	During sleep
Distinguish the behavior of a patient with cluster headache versus migraine headache.	The patient with cluster headache paces; the patient with migraine headache seeks solitude.
What is the first line therapy for cluster headache?	Prophylactic therapy with antimigraine drugs, lithium, and steroids. Analgesics to abort the attack may be helpful, but the attacks may be too brief to treat with abortive therapy.

MUSCLE CONTRACTION–TENSION HEADACHE

Where in the head are the usual locations of tension headache?	Bilateral occipital, nuchal, frontal, or encircling the head
What is the presumed cause of pain in tension headache?	Sustained cranial muscle contraction may be important but the cause is unknown.
Are visual phenomena common in tension headache?	No
Is nausea common in tension headache?	No
What two problems often accompany tension headache?	Psychologic stress and musculoskeletal strain

What two types of drugs are useful for treating tension headache?	1. Tricyclic antidepressants, such as amitriptyline 2. Analgesics, especially NSAIDs
What is another approach for patients with tension headache who fail pharmacologic therapy?	Behavioral medicine (including biofeedback)

FACIAL PAIN

How is the pain of temporal arteritis characterized?	Throbbing, maximal over tender temporal artery
What is an important laboratory finding frequently seen in patients with temporal arteritis?	Elevated ESR
What systemic disorder is frequently associated with temporal arteritis?	Polymyalgia rheumatica
What is the treatment for temporal arteritis?	Corticosteroids
Why is temporal arteritis a relative emergency?	If not treated, it may result in blindness because of involvement of arteries supplying the eye.
What is trigeminal neuralgia?	Paroxysmal, brief pain in the second and third divisions of the trigeminal (fifth) cranial nerve
What is another name for trigeminal neuralgia?	Tic douloureux
What tic is associated with trigeminal neuralgia?	The patient often winces from pain.
What is the course of trigeminal neuralgia?	Usually recurrent for weeks
What initiates a paroxysm?	Sensory stimulus such as touching the lip, smiling, chewing, and shaving

What is the treatment for trigeminal neuralgia?	Anticonvulsants such as carbamazepine or phenytoin, or tricyclic antidepressants
What surgical procedure is used in patients with trigeminal neuralgia who fail medical management?	Chemical ablation of the trigeminal sensory ganglion
Where does temporomandibular joint pain occur?	In front of the ear
What is the usual cause of temporomandibular joint pain?	Trauma or arthritis of the temporomandibular joint, or malocclusion
What are the therapies for temporomandibular joint pain?	Dental treatment, surgical treatment, or treatment of arthritis

OTHER HEAD PAINS

Characterize the post-LP headache.	Pain intensifies when the patient is erect and disappears when the patient is prone.
What is the presumed cause of post-LP headache?	Leak of CSF from the LP site
What is the relationship between post-LP headache and bore of LP needle?	The larger the bore, the greater the risk
How is post-LP headache prevented?	By using a small-bore needle. Keeping the patient supine may help reduce the frequency of post-LP headache.
What is the medical therapy for post-LP headache?	Analgesics, caffeine, and rest
What is definitive therapy for post-LP headache?	A "blood patch." Sterile blood is removed from the patient's arm and injected into the LP site (but not into the dural space) where it presumably patches the leak in the dura.

BACK PAIN

How common is low back pain?	It is the most common pain syndrome causing visits to physicians.
Is most chronic back pain of musculoskeletal or neurologic origin?	Musculoskeletal
What are the most common locations of chronic back pain?	Upper (cervical) and lower (lumbosacral) back
What is the best historical feature distinguishing back pain of neurologic origin from musculoskeletal origin?	Lancinating pain in a dermatomal distribution is a feature of neurologic back pain.
What is the most common cause of acute back pain with neuralgia?	Herniated nucleus pulposus (or "slipped disc")
What findings on neurologic examination support back pain of neurologic origin?	Weakness and sensory loss related to a specific nerve root associated with an absent deep tendon reflex. For example, weakness of plantar flexion with sensory loss in the S_1 dermatome associated with an absent ankle jerk would be consistent with an S_1 radiculopathy.
What two complaints should be urgently evaluated in a patient with back pain?	Leg weakness and urinary or bowel incontinence. These suggest that spinal cord compression may be present.
What laboratory studies are useful in the evaluation of back pain?	MRI, or myelogram and EMG can aid in the diagnosis of back pain of neurologic origin
How is musculoskeletal back pain treated?	Avoidance of the precipitating activity, if known, bed rest, and analgesics, especially NSAIDs. If muscle spasm is present, then muscle relaxants may be useful.

What is the treatment for back pain caused by herniated disc?	If no neurologic signs or symptoms are present, then conservative therapy with rest, analgesics, and muscle relaxants is the initial therapy. If initial therapy fails or if a neurologic deficit is present, then surgery to remove the disc is indicated.

VERTIGO AND DIZZINESS

What is dizziness?	A general term describing a variety of feelings, including light-headedness, vertigo, disequilibrium, and any sensation that the patient interprets as abnormal. It has no specific pathophysiologic or localizing value.
What is vertigo?	A specific term describing a sense of rotational motion indicating dysfunction of the vestibular pathways
What is disequilibrium?	A relatively specific term describing a feeling of "unsteadiness" or of being "about to fall," usually indicating an abnormal gait
Why should dizziness, vertigo, and disequilibrium be distinguished?	They describe different sensations, have different localizing value, and have different pathophysiologic implications.
What is syncope?	Transient loss of consciousness of cardiovascular origin. It is synonymous with fainting.
What is presyncope?	Sensation of being about to faint
What symptoms help distinguish light-headedness attributable to presyncope from disequilibrium?	Presyncope may have transient autonomic symptoms.
What are four CNS locations where dysfunction can cause disequilibrium?	Whole brain (secondary either to primary CNS disorder or systemic illness), causing focal or generalized weakness Cerebellum, causing incoordination Basal ganglia, causing impaired postural reflexes

Sensory tracts or receptors, causing impaired proprioception

Where does peripheral vertigo occur?

Vestibular apparatus and vestibular nerve

Where does central vertigo occur?

Vestibular nucleus and pathways in the brain stem

What are the three most common peripheral causes of vertigo?

1. BPPV
2. Labyrinthitis (also called vestibular neuronitis)
3. Mèniére's disease

What is a distinguishing feature of BPPV?

Vertigo is positional; that is, it is precipitated by specific movements of the head.

What are three classic symptoms of Mèniére's syndrome?

1. Unilateral tinnitus
2. Unilateral deafness
3. Paroxysmal vertigo

List the three most common causes of central vertigo.

1. Vertebrobasilar TIA or stroke
2. Brain stem tumor
3. Cranial nerve VIII tumor

What clinical feature distinguishes central from peripheral vertigo?

Central vertigo is usually accompanied by other brain stem dysfunction.

What are two drugs that are useful in the treatment of all types of vertigo?

Meclizine and benzodiazepines (especially diazepam)

PERIPHERAL NEUROPATHY, NUMBNESS, AND TINGLING

What are some common presenting symptoms of peripheral neuropathy?

Numbness, tingling, burning, or pain that is usually present distally

What findings are present on neurologic examination in patients with peripheral neuropathy?

Loss of pinprick, temperature, joint position, or vibratory sense in the distal extremities, usually in a stocking-and-glove pattern. Muscle weakness and wasting may be present. There may be diminished or absent reflexes late in the course.

What systemic diseases and toxins are associated with peripheral neuropathy?

Diabetes, vasculitis, paraneoplastic disease, uremia, and vitamin B_{12} deficiency
Chemotherapeutic agents
Lead, arsenic, and mercury
Alcohol

What is the most sensitive way to diagnose a peripheral neuropathy?

Neurologic examination, which may show sensory deficits even when the EMG is normal

What laboratory tests are useful in the evaluation of peripheral neuropathy?

ESR, serum glucose, B_{12} level, protein electrophoresis, antineuronal antibodies, rheumatoid factor, HIV, EMG, and possibly urine heavy metal screen, if indicated

What is mononeuritis multiplex?

A condition in which several different peripheral nerves are affected

What is the most common cause of mononeuritis multiplex?

Systemic vasculitis (e.g., polyarteritis nodosa)

What is a compression neuropathy?

Nerve injury caused by trauma or compression

What is the most common compression neuropathy?

Median neuropathy at the wrist (carpal tunnel syndrome)

What are symptoms of carpal tunnel syndrome?

Pain at the wrist and hand; numbness or tingling in the thumb and first finger

What are the neurologic examination findings in carpal tunnel syndrome?

Weakness in the median innervated muscles, including the first and second **L**umbricales, **O**pponens pollicis, **A**bductor pollicis brevis, and **F**lexor pollicis brevis (**LOAF** muscles); sensory loss in the median nerve distribution; positive Tinel's and Phalen's sign

What are Tinel's and Phalen's signs?

Tinel's sign is a tingling sensation in the distal median nerve distribution on percussion of the wrist over the median nerve. Phalen's sign is pain or tingling in the median nerve distribution with prolonged flexion of the wrist.

What is the treatment for carpal tunnel syndrome?

If the case is mild, treatment is usually with NSAIDs and a wrist splint. If initial treatment fails or there is associated denervation seen on the EMG, the patient should have carpal tunnel release surgery.

How can EMG be useful in the diagnosis of peripheral neuropathy?

The EMG can differentiate whether the neuropathy is primarily demyelinating, primarily axonal, or mixed. This aids in establishing a cause. Charcot-Marie-Tooth disease and uremia cause a demyelinating neuropathy. Alcohol and chemotherapeutic agents (e.g., vincristine) cause an axonal neuropathy. Diabetes often causes a mixed neuropathy with both demyelinating and axonal features.

GUILLAIN-BARRÉ SYNDROME

What is another name for GBS?

Acute inflammatory demyelinating polyneuropathy

How does GBS usually present?

Ascending weakness usually begins in the legs, moving upward to involve the arms. The weakness may be associated with or be preceded by mild distal paresthesias.

What are common antecedent illnesses to GBS?

Campylobacter jejuni gastroenteritis is the most common. Patients may have a preceding viral illness such as gastroenteritis or upper respiratory infection.

What are the findings on neurologic examination of patients with GBS?

Symmetrical motor weakness that is usually greater in the distal extremities. Areflexia is invariably present and is therefore necessary for the diagnosis. Sensory function is usually normal, despite sensory complaints.

What laboratory evidence supports the diagnosis of GBS?

CSF shows elevated protein (> 55 mg/dl) without a significant pleocytosis (i.e., "albuminocytologic dissociation"). EMG is normal initially, but eventually shows findings consistent with demyelination.

What is the usual course of GBS?	The paralysis usually is rapidly progressive over 1–4 weeks and is followed by a plateau phase that may last 2–4 weeks or longer. Most patients eventually recover, but 20% have residual weakness at 1 year.
What are serious complications of GBS?	Respiratory compromise, aspiration, arrhythmias, and hypotension. The risks of respiratory compromise and aspiration are associated with diaphragmatic weakness and bulbar weakness, respectively. Arrhythmias and hypotension are secondary to autonomic instability.
What is the proper supportive management of GBS?	Admission to the hospital, possibly the intensive care unit, depending on the symptoms. Patients should have respiratory function monitored closely by measurement of vital capacity. Patients should be intubated when forced vital capacity decreases 12–15 ml/kg or Po_2 decreases below 70. Patients may need intubation for airway protection as well.
What is the treatment for GBS?	Plasma exchange reduces the duration of disability, especially if done in the first 2 weeks of the illness. Patients usually receive 4–6 exchanges on alternate days.
What is the prognosis for GBS?	Approximately 5% of patients with GBS die of complication, despite being given quality care. Most patients recover, but 10% may be permanently disabled.

PARKINSON'S DISEASE

What are the pathologic features of PD?	PD is an idiopathic condition resulting in loss of the pigmented nuclei in the substantia nigra with the presence of Lewy bodies.
What are the three cardinal features of PD?	Rest tremor, cogwheel rigidity, and bradykinesia

What are other clinical features of PD?

Mask facies, loss of postural reflexes, decreased blink rate, small-stepped gait, hypovolemic voice, micrographia, gait arrest, and backward falling

What is the classic tremor associated with PD?

A pill-rolling 4- to 5-Hz tremor seen at rest. This is the most specific clinical sign of PD.

What is the classic triad of symptoms associated with PD?

Bradykinesia (slow movements), resting tremor, and cogwheel rigidity

Describe the classic gait associated with PD.

Short shuffling steps with a festinating or hurried quality. Patients typically require several steps to turn around instead of pivoting.

What is the common age of onset of PD?

Age 40 to 70 years with peak incidence in the 6th decade

Are diagnostic tests necessary to make the diagnosis of PD?

No, unless there are atypical features. In atypical cases, MRI may be useful in evaluating the possibility of cerebrovascular disease, tumor, or multiple system atrophy as potential causes.

What is the difference between PD and parkinsonism?

PD is an idiopathic disorder that is responsive to L-dopa. Parkinsonism has similar features to PD, but is secondary to another cause and is often not responsive to L-dopa.

What are some causes of parkinsonism?

Neuroleptic use (including antipsychotics and antiemetics), cerebrovascular disease, use of the illicit drug methyphenyl-tetrahydropyridine (MPTP), and encephalitis lethargica (von Economo's disease)

What is the main drug used to treat PD?

Sinemet (carbidopa and L-dopa). L-dopa is given in combination with carbidopa, which prevents the peripheral catabolism of L-dopa to dopamine. L-dopa can penetrate the blood–brain barrier, but dopamine cannot. Once in the brain, L-dopa is broken down into dopamine, which alleviates the symptoms of PD.

What is the usual starting dose of Sinemet?	Patients usually start on 100 mg of L-dopa in combination with 25 mg of carbidopa given in two divided doses (one half tablet of Sinemet 25/100 twice daily). This dose is then titrated up to relieve symptoms.
What are common side effects of L-dopa?	Gastrointestinal upset with nausea and vomiting, vivid dreams or nightmares, psychosis, and dyskinesias

STROKE AND SUBARACHNOID HEMORRHAGE

What is a TIA?	A TIA is essentially a stroke that resolves in less than 24 hours. If a stroke-like episode resolves in 24–72 hours, it is a "reversible ischemic neurologic deficit," or RIND. The symptoms and signs of a completed stroke should persist for more than 72 hours.
What are the two most basic types of strokes?	Ischemic strokes (approximately 80%) and cerebral hemorrhages (approximately 20%). Bleeding into an area of primary ischemic stroke is called hemorrhagic stroke.
Based on arterial size, what are the two most basic types of ischemic strokes?	Large vessel strokes (approximately 75%) and small vessel strokes (approximately 25%)
What are the common mechanisms of large vessel stroke?	Embolic (the majority)—artery-to-artery embolization or cardioembolic events Thrombotic—caused by thrombosis of a cerebral vessel Hemodynamic—insufficient cardiac output results in "watershed" or "border zone" infarct Nonatherosclerotic—typically rare, include events such as arterial dissection, drug-induced stroke, and arteritis
What are lacunes?	Small vessel strokes that result from lipohyalinization of a small-caliber artery or arteriole

What is the general name for the cerebrovasculature arising from the carotid arteries?	Anterior circulation
What vessels comprise the anterior circulation?	The internal carotids, their branches (the MCA and ACA), and smaller branches from those vessels
What is the general name for the cerebrovasculature arising from the vertebral arteries?	Posterior circulation
What vessels comprise the posterior circulation?	The vertebral arteries, the posterior inferior cerebellar arteries (PICA), the basilar artery, and the posterior cerebral arteries. The posterior circulation is also called the vertebrobasilar system.
What basic neurologic deficits result from occlusion of the MCA?	MCA stroke results in contralateral head, arm, and some leg weakness associated with aphasia (if on the dominant side of the brain, which is usually the left side) or neglect (if on the nondominant side of the brain)
What neurologic deficits result from occlusion of the ACA?	ACA stroke results in contralateral leg weakness.
What neurologic deficits result from occlusion of the PCA?	PCA stroke results in contralateral hemianopsia.
What neurologic deficits result from occlusion of the PICA?	PICA stroke results in an ipsilateral Horner's syndrome, dyscoordination, and facial sensory loss, but contralateral body sensory deficits. The PICA stroke syndrome is also called the Wallenberg or lateral medullary syndrome.
What are the features of Horner's syndrome?	Unilateral miosis, ptosis, exophthalmos, and anhydrosis

What risk factors are associated with a first stroke?

Hypertension (the most important risk factor), diabetes, smoking, and advancing age. Hypercholesterolemia has not been shown definitively to be a stroke risk factor, but it is usually treated empirically.

What can be done for secondary stroke prevention?

Having had one stroke increases the risk of having another. Aspirin on a daily basis and ticlopidine, another antiplatelet agent, have been shown to decrease the annual risk of restroke by approximately 25%–30%. In patients with carotid stenosis of greater than 70% who are symptomatic (e.g., with TIAs or a history of stroke), and certain asymptomatic patients with tight carotid stenoses, carotid endarterectomy lessens the risk of repeat or completed stroke.

How is stroke prevented in the patient with atrial fibrillation or another cardioembolic source of stroke?

Anticoagulation with warfarin is the most effective treatment and may lessen the risk of cardioembolic stroke in such patients by 60%–80%. However, in patients older than age 75 years, the bleeding morbidity associated with warfarin balances out the decreased risk of stroke. Aspirin, although inferior in preventing cardioembolism in the patient with atrial fibrillation, may be indicated in older persons because of its lower risk of causing bleeding.

What is the role of heparin in stroke?

Heparin may be useful for strokes that appear to be actively progressing (stroke in progress), particularly if progressive thrombosis of the basilar artery is suspected. Heparin may also lower the risk of an imminent repeat cardioembolic event after a primary cardioembolic event has occurred, and it may be helpful in patients with "crescendo TIAs." Even with these limited indications, heparin should not be initiated lightly, because it may convert an uncomplicated ischemic stroke into a more devastating hemorrhagic stroke.

What treatment has recently been demonstrated to improve the ultimate neurologic outcome in ischemic stroke?

If it can be given within 3 hours of the onset of neurologic symptoms, tissue plasminogen activator (tPA) may improve the neurologic outcome.

When a patient is thought to clinically have had a stroke, what initial ancillary test should be performed immediately?

CT of the brain should be performed to distinguish the cause of the perceived stroke as being either ischemic or a hemorrhage. This determination directs subsequent management. Brain damage resulting from an ischemic stroke may take more than 24 hours to manifest on CT, so CT is expected to be normal initially.

What is the initial management of the patient with ischemic stroke?

Administration of aspirin, 325 mg
Judicious control of blood pressure.
    Hypertension should not be aggressively treated, because this may increase the area of infarction. Blood pressures of around 180/100 are acceptable.
Avoidance of hypoglycemia and hyperglycemia and overhydration and dehydration. Non–glucose-containing intravenous solutions should be used.
Electrocardiographic monitoring to check for arrhythmias, left ventricular and atrial hypertrophy/enlargement, and old or new myocardial infarction
NPO status (to decrease the risk of aspiration and hyperglycemia), bed rest, and cardiac telemetry, if possible
Administration of supplemental oxygen as necessary to keep the oxygen saturation of the blood greater than 95%

When is the risk of herniation following a stroke the greatest?

Approximately 2–5 days after the stroke, when the edema around the infarcted area is maximal

When is MRI of the brain indicated in stroke?

MRI has better resolution than CT and may show a small stroke that is not evident on CT. It is superior for imaging the posterior fossa, which is distorted on

CT because of interference from surrounding bone. MRI also allows performance of magnetic resonance arteriography (MRA) to evaluate cerebral blood vessels noninvasively. MRI is not indicated over CT in the patient with an acute stroke, though, because it is inferior to CT in detecting acute bleeding and requires an extended period of time (approximately 30 minutes to 1 hour), during which the patient cannot be observed closely.

What techniques are used to evaluate the status of the blood vessels to the brain?

Carotid ultrasound and Doppler imaging can also noninvasively determine whether there is stenosis in the carotid arteries in the neck and determine the extent of that stenosis if it exists.

MRA can give good quality images of either intracranial blood vessels or extracranial arteries in the neck that supply the brain.

Angiography (via cannulation of a femoral artery) is the gold standard, but it is invasive and carries risks.

In addition to an electrocardiogram, what other cardiac workup should be considered in the patient with a new stroke?

Echocardiography (transthoracic or transesophageal) can help determine whether a cardioembolism was likely to have been the source of stroke. (If so, warfarin would be preferred to aspirin as the treatment for secondary stroke prophylaxis.) Transesophageal echocardiography is more sensitive for detecting left atrial thrombi, but it is costly and invasive.

What is the classic presentation of the patient with SAH?

The acute onset of the "worst headache of my life," with or without focal neurologic deficits

How is the diagnosis of SAH made?

CT of the head reveals a pattern of subarachnoid blood in approximately 90% of cases. If clinical suspicion is high and the CT is negative for blood, then an LP should be performed to look for blood in the CSF.

After the diagnosis of SAH is made, what additional study is essential?

Angiography, to look for a ruptured aneurysm (the most common source of SAH). Rebleeding from the site of a previously ruptured aneurysm can be prevented by surgical clipping of the aneurysm.

What are the most common complications of SAH?

Vasospasm, hydrocephalus, and electrolyte imbalance (particularly hyponatremia)

SEIZURES

DEFINITIONS

What is a seizure?

Temporary alteration of brain function caused by paroxysmal, abnormal cerebral neuronal discharges. Seizures are classified by the International League Against Epilepsy based on their observable clinical manifestations.

What clinical characteristic defines seizures as generalized or partial?

Generalized seizures are associated with a loss of consciousness, while partial seizures are not. This classification reflects whether the whole brain is involved, or only one region.

How are partial seizures classified?

Complex partial seizures are associated with an alteration of consciousness, whereas during simple partial seizures, consciousness is fully preserved. Simple partial seizures are further classified according to whether they have predominantly motor, sensory, autonomic, or psychic symptoms.

Describe a typical complex partial seizure.

Complex partial seizures are characterized by impaired alertness and responsiveness, or "staring unresponsiveness," with amnesia for the event. They are often associated with confused purposeless behavior (automatisms), especially lip smacking, vocalizations, swallowing, and fumbling.

What type of seizure is an aura?

Auras are simple partial seizures that may consist of auditory, visual, gustatory, or olfactory illusions; déjà-vu, jamais-vu; psychic or emotional phenomena; and epigastric sensations. Auras may progress to complex partial seizures which may progress to involve the whole brain or "secondarily generalize." Auras may help localize the site of seizure onset.

What are some common types of generalized seizures?

Generalized tonic-clonic, myoclonic, absence, atonic

Describe a generalized tonic-clonic seizure.

Sudden generalized stiffness of a few seconds duration during the "tonic" phase, followed by rhythmic muscle jerks during the "clonic" phase. Common accompaniments are injury during falling, tongue biting, stertorous respirations, salivation, and peripheral (but not central) cyanosis. Observers may describe only the clonic phase, in which case, strictly speaking, the seizure cannot be termed tonic-clonic, because it may be secondarily generalized. A more general term is convulsion, previously termed major motor seizure.

What is Todd's paralysis?

Todd's paralysis is transient hemiparesis after a seizure, reflecting the location of the most involved area of the brain. It usually indicates a seizure is focal in onset.

What is a provoked seizure?

A seizure occurring in an otherwise normal brain as a result of some transient alteration, such as changes in glucose or sodium levels or drug effects

What is epilepsy?

A continuing tendency toward *spontaneous recurrent seizures* as a result of some persistent pathologic process affecting the brain. The latter criterion excludes patients with provoked seizures, who have an otherwise normal brain. The International League Against Epilepsy has classified epilepsy syndromes according to the type of seizure, EEG changes, age of onset, interictal abnormalities, and natural history.

What is the advantage of using epilepsy syndrome classification rather than identifying a singular seizure type to characterize patients?

Seizures are merely symptoms of brain dysfunction that are not specific to the etiology, just as a cough is a symptom of respiratory system dysfunction. Seizures may be caused by diverse benign or serious causes, just as a cough may be caused by a cold or lung cancer. Patients with a given epilepsy syndrome have a similar natural history, a similar response to treatment, and, presumably, the same pathophysiology.

What is the prevalence of seizures and epilepsy?

Ten percent of the population may experience a seizure sometime during the lifetime, but only approximately three percent of the population has epilepsy.

How are epilepsy syndromes classified?

They are fundamentally based on whether a focal or generalized pathologic process is present, and also whether the process is idiopathic, symptomatic, or cryptogenic.

Of these three epilepsy syndromes:
　　Which is the result of a known histopathologic abnormality in the brain (e.g., a malformation or a brain tumor)?

Symptomatic epilepsies

　　Which presumably have a structural basis because of their association with other neurologic symptoms (e.g., seizures associated with mental retardation)?

Cryptogenic epilepsies

Which are usually inherited and presumably are due to abnormalities of neurotransmission without associated structural abnormalities?

Idiopathic epilepsies

What is the most common generalized epilepsy syndrome arising in childhood?

Childhood absence epilepsy is an idiopathic generalized epilepsy syndrome in which absence seizures begin in early childhood and usually abate by late adolescence. The syndrome is caused by an autosomally dominant inherited abnormality of neurotransmission involving the thalamus and cortex. The EEG characteristically shows generalized 3 c/s spike and wave activity in between and during seizures. The MRI is normal.

What is the most common generalized epilepsy syndrome arising in adolescence or early adulthood?

Juvenile myoclonic epilepsy is an idiopathic generalized epilepsy syndrome in which brief generalized myoclonic jerks and convulsions begin in late adolescence and persist throughout life. It is inherited as an autosomal dominant trait, but the pathologic abnormality is not known. The interictal EEG shows characteristic generalized multiple spike and wave activity in between seizures and occasionally with myoclonic jerks. MRI is normal.

What is the most common epilepsy syndrome of adults?

Temporal lobe epilepsy is a symptomatic partial epilepsy syndrome in which complex partial seizures begin in late adolescence or early adulthood and more or less persist throughout life. It is usually associated with mesial temporal sclerosis, but the etiology is not known. The interictal EEG demonstrates spikes originating from the temporal lobe. MRI may show atrophy and sclerosis of mesial temporal structures.

What epilepsy syndrome does a patient who presents with rare, poorly defined, easily controlled seizures and normal diagnostic test results have?

These findings cannot be classified as belonging to an epilepsy syndrome. Usually the syndrome diagnosis will become clear over time, or the seizures will abate spontaneously and no cause will ever be determined.

What is a pseudoseizure?

A nonepileptic event mimicking a seizure

What EEG findings suggest pseudoseizure?

A normal EEG during an event suspected of being a seizure suggests pseudoseizure. However, the EEG is usually normal during simple partial seizures.

What events could be considered a pseudoseizure?

Hysterical behavior, conversion reaction, malingering, and learned behavior

DIAGNOSTIC TESTS

Why is an EEG indicated in the evaluation of almost all patients with seizures?

To distinguish partial from generalized seizure disorders, to localize the site of seizure onset of partial seizures, and to characterize the epilepsy syndrome

What is the characteristic EEG abnormality present in focal seizure disorders?

Focal spikes and sharp waves. These generally signify a "potentially epileptogenic" area in the brain region originating the epileptiform abnormality. However, focal spikes occur in 1%–2% of the normal population.

What is the characteristic EEG abnormality present in generalized epilepsies?

Generalized epileptiform discharges (spikes, spikes and waves, and sharp waves), which are present over all of the brain regions simultaneously and suggest an epileptogenic process involving all of the cortex simultaneously. Some patients with generalized seizure disorders may have normal EEGs in between seizures.

What is the most sensitive and specific method for determining that a spell is a seizure?

Simultaneous video and EEG monitoring during a spell. However, during simple partial seizures, the EEG may be normal.

| What is the most sensitive neuroimaging study in the evaluation of epilepsy? | MRI defines brain anatomy with greater detail and often identifies subtle abnormalities that are not seen on CT. |

TREATMENT

| What is the treatment of a single seizure? | Treatment depends on the cause. If there is a known provoking factor, the provoking factor is relieved. The treatment of a single seizure of unknown etiology is controversial, but generally antiepileptic drugs are not started until after the second seizure, because many patients do not have a second seizure. If the seizure is attributable to an epilepsy syndrome, then therapy may be initiated, depending on the natural history of the syndrome. |

What is the generic form of each of the following brand-name antiepileptic drugs:

Cerebyx	Fosphenytoin
Dilantin	Diphenylhydantoin or phenytoin
Tegretol	Carbamazepine
Depakene	Valproic acid
Depakote	Divalproex sodium
Zarontin	Ethosuximide
Mysoline	Primidone
Neurontin	Gabapentin
Lamictal	Lamotrigine
Topamax	Topiramate
Valium	Diazepam
Ativan	Lorazepam

Phenobarbital

There is no common brand name.

Which drugs are useful for simple partial and complex partial seizures as part of most epilepsy syndromes?

Simple partial and complex partial seizures are merely different degrees of the same physiologic process so antiepileptic drugs useful for one are useful for the other. All of the drugs listed previously except for ethosuximide are useful for both complex partial and simple partial seizures.

Which drug is useful only for generalized seizures, especially absence seizures in childhood absence epilepsy?

Ethosuximide

Which drug regimen is most useful for both myoclonic jerks and convulsions in patients with juvenile myoclonic epilepsy?

Valproic acid and divalproex sodium

Which drug regimen is the only one useful for partial and generalized seizures?

Valproic acid and divalproex sodium

How long must a patient be seizure-free before drug withdrawal is considered?

The risk of seizure occurrence is determined by the natural history of the epilepsy syndrome. For example, patients with juvenile myoclonic epilepsy generally respond well to medication but almost universally will have seizures when medication is withdrawn. However, when either the natural history of the epilepsy suggests that seizures will not recur or when the diagnosis of epilepsy is not definite, then medication withdrawal may be attempted after approximately 2 years. Risk of seizure recurrence remains 20%–70%, even for patients who are good candidates for drug withdrawal.

PARANEOPLASTIC SYNDROMES

What is a neurologic paraneoplastic syndrome?	A syndrome of neurologic dysfunction that is associated with a specific tumor but is not a direct effect of tumor mass or metastases. Most paraneoplastic syndromes are thought to be secondary to autoimmune-related mechanisms.
What are some paraneoplastic effects on the nervous system that are not autoimmune-related?	Metabolic encephalopathies from organ failure or electrolyte disturbance, stroke from hypercoagulable states
What are four neurologic autoimmune-related paraneoplastic syndromes?	Encephalomyelitis, peripheral neuropathy, cerebellar degeneration, and Lambert-Eaton myasthenic syndrome (LEMS)
What are the most common cancers that result in a paraneoplastic syndrome?	Lung cancer (small cell), ovarian cancer, and breast cancer
What are the specific syndromes in the following cancers:	
Small cell	LEMS, encephalomyelitis, sensory neuropathy, and autonomic neuropathy
Ovarian cancer	Cerebellar degeneration
Breast cancer	Cerebellar degeneration
What is LEMS and how does it present?	Lambert-Eaton myasthenic syndrome is a paraneoplastic syndrome most commonly associated with small-cell carcinoma of the lung. It presents with weakness of the proximal muscles, especially in the legs. The oropharyngeal and ocular muscles may also be affected. Patients also have a degree of autonomic dysfunction and often complain of a dry mouth.

| How is LEMS distinguished from myasthenia gravis? | By EMG. The response to repetitive nerve stimulation in myasthenia gravis patients usually becomes progressively weaker, whereas in LEMS patients, it grows stronger. |

CENTRAL NERVOUS SYSTEM INFECTIONS*

MENINGITIS

| **What is meningitis?** | Inflammation of the meninges (coverings of the brain) that is characterized by an increased number of WBCs in the CSF. Note: Bacterial meningitis is an emergency. |

| **What are the causes of acute meningitis?** | Viruses—enteroviruses, HSV, HIV, arboviruses, lymphocytic choriomeningitis (LCM), mumps, adenovirus
Bacteria—*Streptococcus pneumoniae, Haemophilus influenzae, Neisseria meningitidis, Listeria monocytogenes, Escherichia coli*
Spirochetes—*Treponema pallidum, Borrelia burgdorferi*
Noninfectious—tumors, medications
Protozoa—uncommon
Other—parameningeal, infective endocarditis, postvaccination, postinfectious |

| **What are the causes of chronic meningitis?** | Fungi (*Cryptococcus neoformans, Histoplasma capsulatum, Coccidioides immitis, Sporothrix schenckii*), *Mycobacterium tuberculosis*, carcinoma, vasculitis, sarcoid, Behçet's, and parasites (more commonly with a focal abnormality) |

| **What is the incidence of bacterial meningitis?** | > 3 cases per 100,000 population. *H. influenzae, N. meningitidis,* and *S. pneumoniae* are the offending pathogens in more than 80% of cases. Overall mortality rate is more than 10%. |

---

* In collaboration with V. Shami, N. Thielman, and C. Sable

What is the incidence of viral meningitis?	Exact incidence is unknown because it is underreported and difficult to make an exact diagnosis. One study reported more than 10 cases per 100,000 person-years.
What are the likely pathogens of meningitis in the following:	
Neonates	*E. coli*, group B streptococci, and *L. monocytogenes*
Infants	*E. coli*, group B streptococci, *L. monocytogenes*, *H. influenzae*, and *S. pneumoniae*
Children aged 3 months to 18 years	*H. influenzae*, *N. meningitidis*, and *S. pneumoniae*
Adults aged 18 to 50 years	*S. pneumoniae* and *N. meningitidis*
Ederly persons older than age 50 years	*S. pneumoniae*, *H. influenzae*, *L. monocytogenes*, and gram-negative bacilli
How is the diagnosis of meningitis made?	History, physical examination, and CSF study
What are risk factors for meningitis?	Extremes of age, immunocompromised state, neurosurgical procedures, systemic infections (particularly respiratory), sinusitis, otitis, parameningeal infection, head trauma, cancer, alcohol use, and absent spleen
What are symptoms and signs of viral meningitis?	Headache is commonly the predominant complaint. Fever, malaise, nausea, vomiting, pharyngitis, and meningismus are common. Focal findings are unusual.
What are symptoms and signs of bacterial meningitis?	Headache, fever, meningismus, and CNS dysfunction, usually occurring with or after an upper respiratory infection (> 80%) Nuchal rigidity, Kernig's, or Brudzinski's sign (80%) Obtundation or coma, most suggestive of bacterial meningitis (50%)

	Symptoms lasting less than 24 hours (25%); symptoms lasting 1–7 days (50%)
How is Kernig's sign elicited?	The examiner flexes the patient's leg at the knee and hip and then tries to straighten the leg. The patient resists leg straightening. (Think **K**ernig = **K**nee.)
How is Brudzinski's sign elicited?	The patient's neck is flexed, resulting in the patient flexing at the hips and knees.
Which laboratory tests should be performed for meningitis?	1. LP is crucial. If meningitis is in the differential diagnosis, then an LP should be done. 2. CT scan of the head should be done before an LP if the patient has focal neurologic deficits or if an adequate neurologic examination cannot be performed. (Some clinicians advocate CT in all patients to rule out increased ICP.)
What are the risks of LP?	There is a small risk of infection, bleeding, or brain herniation.
Is herniation likely in meningitis?	No. It is unlikely because the process is diffuse; herniation risk is greatest with focal masses, especially temporal lobe masses.

What factors differentiate bacterial, viral, fungal, and tubercular meningitis?

Table 12–1.   CSF Findings in Acute Meningitis

	Pleocytosis	Glucose	Protein
Bacterial	↑ ↑ ↑ (neutrophils)	↓ ↓	↑ ↑
Viral	↑ (lymphocytes)	. . .	↑
Fungal	↑ ↑ (lymphocytes)	↓	↑
Tuberculous	↑ (lymphocytes)	↓	↑ ↑ ↑

How frequent are positive CSF cultures in bacterial meningitis?	CSF cultures are positive in 75% of cases.
What are normal measurements for CSF?	Opening pressure, 50–195 mm Hg (equivalent to < 18 cm of CSF); WBCs, < 5; polymorphonuclear neutrophil, < 1; glucose ratio to blood, 0.6; protein, 25–40 mg/dl
What can be seen in a traumatic LP?	RBCs:WBCs, > 1000:1; protein increases 1 mg/dl/1000 RBCs
What is the treatment for bacterial meningitis?	Empiric therapy is usually required, because time is needed to make a specific diagnosis. If bacterial meningitis is suspected, the patient should be treated immediately. Therapy can be modified once a specific diagnosis is made.

What is the treatment for bacterial meningitis in the following:

Neonates	Ampicillin with gentamicin or ampicillin plus a third-generation cephalosporin
Infants	Ampicillin plus a third-generation cephalosporin
Children	Third-generation cephalosporin (with or without vancomycin if resistant pneumococci are a problem)
Adults	Third-generation cephalosporin (with or without vancomycin if resistant pneumococci are a problem)
Elderly persons	Third-generation cephalosporin plus ampicillin (with or without vancomycin if resistant pneumococci are a problem)
What is the treatment of viral meningitis?	Supportive, specific treatment exists only for meningitis in which HSV is the precipitating factor. Patients usually have mild disease and recover without specific therapy.

What is the role of steroids in meningitis?

Corticosteroids (dexamethasone) should be administered to infants and children when *H. influenzae* infection is a realistic consideration (0.15 mg/kg intravenously every 6 hours for 4 days). Dexamethasone reduces the incidence of moderate to severe sensorineural hearing loss and may reduce mortality. Data in adults are sparse. There is controversy among experts as to when to give steroids. Steroids should be considered if there are signs of increased ICP or cerebral edema on head CT.

When, in relation to the administration of antibiotics, should corticosteroids be given in the treatment of meningitis?

Before or at the same time as the antibiotics

What is the mortality rate of bacterial meningitis?

Twenty-five percent of patients die with pneumococcal infection, ten percent die with meningococcal infection, and five percent die with *H. influenzae* infection.

What are the complications of meningitis?

Infants and children—sensorineural hearing loss, seizures, mental retardation, focal neurologic deficits, brain abscess
Adults—seizures and focal neurologic deficits

Define the following:
Aseptic meningitis

Meningitis not caused by a common bacterial etiology. Many episodes are caused by viruses, some by noninfectious causes, and some have an unknown cause.

Xanthochromia

Yellow discoloration of the CSF resulting from the breakdown of RBCs or protein. It is seen 2–4 hours after SAH, but it may also be seen with a traumatic LP if the specimen was not centrifuged.

Hypoglycorrhachia	Decreased glucose concentration in the CSF. It is seen in meningitis caused by bacteria, but also with fungal, mycobacterial, and carcinomatous meningitis. It is less common in viral meningitis.

TUBERCULOUS MENINGITIS

What are some common risk factors for tuberculous meningitis?	History of pulmonary TB, alcoholism, corticosteroid use, HIV-positive, impaired immune response, and residence in endemic areas or groups
Which age-groups are at greatest risk for tuberculous meningitis?	The very young and the very old
What organism usually causes tuberculous meningitis?	*M. tuberculosis* and, rarely, *Mycobacterium bovis*
Is tuberculous meningitis usually a primary infection or reactivation of a previous infection?	Usually reactivation
In what percentage of patients with tuberculous meningitis is there active pulmonary TB?	Approximately two thirds
What are the symptoms and signs of tuberculous meningitis?	Fever, confusion, headache, and nuchal rigidity
Over what period of time do the symptoms of tuberculous meningitis develop?	Approximately 2 weeks, compared to hours to days for typical bacterial meningitis
What are the CSF findings in tuberculous meningitis?	Lymphocytic pleocytosis, markedly increased protein, decreased glucose, and increased opening pressure. Acid fast bacilli may rarely be seen.

How long does it take to culture mycobacterium?	Up to 1 month. As much CSF as possible must be submitted to the laboratory because there are usually very few tubercle bacilli.
What are the imaging findings in tuberculous meningitis?	Enhancement of basal cisterns and meninges, and hydrocephalus
What is the prognosis of tuberculous meningitis?	Even with appropriate treatment, 10%–30% of patients die. Coma at the time of presentation is the most significant predictor of a poor outcome.
What are the pathologic findings seen in tuberculous meningitis?	Exudate in the subarachnoid space, especially at the base of the brain involving adjacent brain (causing basal meningoencephalitis), cranial nerves (causing cranial neuropathies), arteries (causing stroke), or obstruction of basal cisterns (causing hydrocephalus)
What is the natural history of untreated tuberculous meningitis?	Confusion progressing to stupor and coma, with cranial nerve palsies, elevated intracerebral pressure, decerebrate posturing, and death in 1–2 months

ENCEPHALITIS

What is encephalitis?	Inflammation of the brain
What is the most common cause of identifiable encephalitis?	HSV (HSV-1 in adults and HSV-2 in neonates)
What are some other causes of encephalitis?	Arboviruses (eastern equine encephalitis, western equine encephalitis, Venezuelan encephalitis) and other viruses. Much less common causes include *L. monocytogenes*, Q fever, Rocky Mountain spotted fever, *Ehrlichia*, toxoplasmosis, *Mycoplasma*, leptospirosis, Whipple's disease, cat-scratch disease, vasculitis, bacterial endocarditis, carcinoma, drug reactions, and other more unusual causes

What age-groups are susceptible to HSV encephalitis?	All age-groups
Are there seasons or geographic areas of increased risk for encephalitis?	No
What are symptoms and signs of encephalitis?	Headache, fever, and stiff neck plus altered consciousness. Seizures and focal neurologic deficits are common. In HSV encephalitis, unusual behaviors, hallucinations, and aphasia may develop related to the temporal lobe involvement of the virus.
What laboratory tests should be performed for encephalitis?	Examination of the CSF is essential. For viral pathogens, a pleocytosis with 10–2000 cells is seen with a mononuclear predominance. A large number of RBCs may be seen with HSV encephalitis. CSF protein is elevated, and glucose is typically normal in viral encephalitis. Serum antibodies may be helpful for some pathogens, but both acute and convalescent (taken 1–3 weeks later) specimens are required. Checking IgM in serum or CSF may be helpful in some cases but is not definitive. Polymerase chain reaction of CSF is available for HSV encephalitis.
What do the following diagnostic tests show in encephalitis?	
CT scan (of the head with contrast)	Often shows enhancement in the region of the brain involved. In HSV encephalitis, the temporal lobes are most commonly involved. *L. monocytogenes* causes a rhombencephalitis (involvement of the brain stem), and focal enhancement in the region of the brain stem may be seen on CT.
EEG	May demonstrate focal abnormalities in the temporal lobe region (periodic lateralizing epileptiform discharges)

MRI of the head	More sensitive than CT and more likely to reveal abnormalities early in the disease process. The combination of CT, EEG, and MRI reveals 99% of cases of HSV encephalitis. MRI is also more sensitive for *Listeria* rhomboencephalitis (because of the improved visualization of the brain stem).
Brain biopsy	May be required for definitive diagnosis. It is typically reserved for patients with severe disease that is not suggestive of HSV encephalitis or that is not responding to acyclovir therapy.
What are the common gross pathologic changes seen in encephalitis?	Hemorrhagic necrosis of frontal and temporal lobes
What microscopic pathologic changes are seen in encephalitis?	Necrosis and inflammation with eosinophilic intranuclear inclusion bodies (Cowdry type A)
What is the treatment for HSV encephalitis?	Treatment is high-dose intravenous acyclovir for 21 days. (Relapses occur with shorter courses of therapy.)
What is the treatment for *Listeria* rhomboencephalitis?	Ampicillin with or without gentamicin intravenously for 21 days
What are the risks of empiric treatment of suspected HSV encephalitis with acyclovir?	Renal failure and erythema at the intravenous infusion site
What are the morbidity and mortality rates of HSV encephalitis?	In untreated cases, 50%–75% of patients die within 18 months. Survival increases to 90% with acyclovir treatment. The most common sequelae are memory and behavior problems.
What are the common complications of HSV encephalitis?	Seizures and focal neurologic deficits

BRAIN ABSCESS

What is a brain abscess?	Focal suppuration within the parenchyma of the brain
What is the incidence of brain abscess?	< 1 in 10,000 hospital admissions. It is more common in males, with a median age of incidence of 30 to 45 years.
What is cerebritis?	Area of low density seen on CT or MRI with an area of ring enhancement that does not decay on delayed scans. This is the early stage of a brain abscess before it develops into a capsule.
What pathogens cause brain abscess in immunocompetent persons?	Streptococci, bacteroides and prevotella, Enterobacteriaceae, *Staphylococcus aureus*, fungi, *S. pneumoniae*, and *H. influenzae*
What pathogens cause brain abscess in immunocompromised persons (i.e., persons with defects in cell-mediated immunity)?	*Toxoplasma gondii*, *Nocardia*, *Listeria*, and *M. tuberculosis* in addition to those listed for persons who are immunocompetent
What pathogens cause focal CNS lesions in AIDS?	*T. gondii*, primary CNS lymphoma, PML, fungi, *M. tuberculosis*, *Mycobacterium avium* complex, and bacteria
What are risk factors for brain abscess?	Brain abscess develops in one of the following four clinical settings: 1. Spread from contiguous focus— sinusitis, mastoiditis, otitis media, tooth abscess, orbital cellulitis 2. Hematogenous spread from a distant focus 3. Trauma 4. Cryptogenic (unknown cause)
What are symptoms and signs of brain abscess?	Headache, fever, AMS, seizures, nuchal rigidity, papilledema, and focal neurologic deficits

What are the laboratory findings in brain abscesses?	Elevated WBC count in approximately 50% of cases; WBC count is greater than 20,000 in only 10% of cases. Blood cultures should also be obtained.
What is the role of the following diagnostic tests in brain abscess?	
Chest radiograph	May help in determining the origin of hematogenous brain abscess
Head CT	Evaluates the sinuses, mastoids, and middle ear in addition to the brain. Brain abscess appears as a focal lesion with a hypodense center surrounded by a ring of enhancement. There may also be another ring of hypodensity corresponding to cerebral edema.
MRI	A more sensitive test early in the disease and can better detect cerebral edema
When is an LP appropriate in the evaluation of a focal CNS lesion?	Never. The information is not helpful (nonspecific inflammation) and may cause the patient's brain to herniate.
How is a diagnosis of brain abscess made?	Clinical history and diagnostic tests. To determine the offending pathogens, a brain biopsy is needed. The need for surgery for diagnosis and treatment should not delay administration of antibiotics once a presumptive diagnosis is made.
What is the most common cause of a focal CNS lesion in patients with AIDS?	*T. gondii.* Empiric therapy for *Toxoplasmosis* is given if the IgG is positive and CT and MRI findings are compatible. A brain biopsy is reserved for patients who fail to respond to empiric therapy or have unusual features.
What is the most common cause of a focal CNS lesion in immunocompromised patients other than AIDS patients?	There is no single predominant cause of a focal CNS lesion and an early brain biopsy is required.

What is treatment for brain abscess?

Aspiration and drainage of the lesion plus antibiotics. Empiric regimens include a third-generation cephalosporin (cefotaxime or ceftriaxone) plus metronidazole or penicillin plus metronidazole intravenously for 4–6 weeks. Therapy may be narrowed after a specific diagnosis is made.

When is medical therapy alone appropriate for brain abscess?

Cerebritis (hemorrhage may result with biopsy)
Underlying condition that greatly increases surgical risk
Abscess that is deep or in a dominant location
Multiple abscesses, especially if remote from each other
Abscess < 3 cm
Early abscess improvement (in many cases cerebritis)
Concomitant meningitis or ependymitis

What is the role of steroids in brain abscess?

The role of steroids is controversial. They are administered in patients with neurologic deterioration associated with an increase in ICP.

What are complications of brain abscess?

Seizures and focal neurologic deficits. Neurologic sequelae occur in 30%–50% of patients.

What is the prognosis for brain abscess?

Mortality rates up to 25% have been reported in different series.

What factors indicate a poor prognosis in brain abscess?

Delayed diagnosis
Poor localization
Multiple, deep, or loculated abscesses
Ventricular rupture
Coma
Fungal abscess
Inappropriate antibiotics

HIV AND THE NERVOUS SYSTEM

What are the four CNS diseases caused specifically by HIV?

HIV meningitis, vacuolar myelopathy, ADC, and HIV-associated cerebral vasculitis (rare)

What are the three peripheral nervous system locations directly affected by HIV?	Muscles (myopathy), nerves (neuropathy), and nerve roots (radiculopathy)
What viral, bacterial, and fungal agents that infect the CNS are commonly secondary to HIV infection?	Cytomegalovirus, HSV, varicella zoster virus, J C virus (PML) TB, neurosyphilis, *Toxoplasma*, and *Cryptococcus*
What is the most common CNS complication of HIV infection?	ADC

HIV MENINGITIS

What are the clinical characteristics of primary HIV meningitis?	Indistinguishable from any other aseptic meningitis
When does HIV meningitis usually occur in the course of HIV disease?	Around the time of seroconversion
What are the CSF characteristics of HIV meningitis?	Mild CSF lymphocytosis and protein elevation as in other aseptic meningitides

ADC

What are the early symptoms and signs in ADC?	Cortical dysfunction—memory loss, behavioral change, impaired motor skills Subcortical white matter dysfunction—upper motor neuron signs Cerebellar dysfunction—ataxia, postural tremor
What are common late symptoms and signs in ADC?	Dementia, psychosis, seizures, incontinence, and spastic paralysis
What are typical CSF findings in ADC?	Mild CSF lymphocytosis, increased protein, and sometimes oligoclonal bands

What do imaging studies in ADC demonstrate?	Cerebral atrophy, ventricular dilation, and subcortical white matter disease (suggesting demyelination)
What is the treatment for ADC?	AZT. However, the current standard of therapy for systemic HIV should also be used (see Chapter 11).
What are the prognosis and clinical course in ADC?	Progressive decline to death within 1 year, usually from secondary infections
What are some of the neurologic adverse effects of AZT?	Headache, generalized weakness and fatigue, myalgia, and mitochondrial myopathy

HIV VACUOLAR MYELOPATHY

What is HIV vacuolar myelopathy?	Vacuolar degeneration of spinal cord white matter
What is the prevalence of HIV vacuolar myelopathy?	It is found at autopsy in approximately 25% of AIDS patients.
What are the most common signs and symptoms of vacuolar myelopathy?	As in other myelopathies, motor and sensory deficits and incontinence
What is the probable causal agent in vacuolar myelopathy?	HIV
What other HIV neurologic disease is comorbid with vacuolar myelopathy?	ADC
What are MRI findings in vacuolar myelopathy?	Typically normal
What is the major differential diagnosis of vacuolar myelopathy?	Cervical stenosis and B_{12} myelopathy, which also affect corticospinal and posterior columns
Is the course of B_{12} myelopathy different from vacuolar myelopathy?	Vacuolar myelopathy usually has earlier incontinence and fewer sensory abnormalities.

PERIPHERAL NERVOUS SYSTEM COMPLICATIONS OF HIV

How common is peripheral nerve disease in patients with AIDS?	Approximately 25% of patients have disease of peripheral nerves at autopsy.
What is the most common myopathy associated with AIDS?	HIV polymyositis
What is the clinical presentation of HIV polymyositis?	Similar to other types of polymyositis (i.e., trunk and proximal limb weakness)
What is the treatment for HIV polymyositis?	Corticosteroids

SOLITARY BRAIN LESIONS AND HIV

What is the differential diagnosis for a solitary brain lesion seen on MRI in AIDS?	Toxoplasmosis, primary CNS lymphoma, and brain abscess
How can CNS toxoplasmosis be differentiated from primary CNS lymphoma?	Radiologically they may be identical.
What is the empiric therapy for a solitary brain lesion in AIDS patients?	Empiric therapy for toxoplasmosis is pyrimethamine plus sulfadiazine or pyrimethamine plus clindamycin. Response (clinical and CT) typically occurs within 2 weeks. If there is no improvement, brain biopsy should be considered.

MULTIPLE SCLEROSIS

To what class of neurologic disease does MS belong?	Demyelinating disease
How common is MS?	In the United States, approximately 1 in 1000 people is affected. Approximately 65% of those with MS are white females, who typically present between the ages of 20 and 40 years.

What does the word "multiple" in multiple sclerosis refer to?	Multiple separate lesions throughout the CNS (brain or spinal cord) arise at multiple points in time.
What duration should a neurologic symptom be to qualify as an "attack?"	More than 24 hours
For attacks to be considered separate in time, how much time should elapse between attacks?	At least 1 month
What is clinical evidence of MS?	Objective neurologic signs that are demonstrable on neurologic examination
What is paraclinical evidence of MS?	Evidence of lesions in the CNS demonstrated by tests or procedures. Potential paraclinical evidence can be obtained by LP, MRI, CT, or electrophysiologic testing (i.e., visual evoked responses, somatosensory evoked responses, and brain stem auditory evoked responses).
How is the CSF of a patient with MS characterized?	In approximately 90% of cases, the CSF contains unique oligoclonal bands (i.e., they are not found in blood). There may occasionally be a slightly elevated leukocyte count (< 25), which tends to be lymphocytic. Mildly elevated protein occurs in approximately 25% of cases. Myelin basic protein can be a good indicator of an acute exacerbation, but it is present only for approximately 2–3 days after an exacerbation occurs.
How often is the MRI abnormal in patients with MS?	In approximately 90% of patients with MS, MRI demonstrates multifocal areas of demyelination. MRI is much more useful than CT in diagnosing and following the course of MS.
Describe the classification scheme upon which the diagnosis of MS is based.	Clinically definite Laboratory-supported definite Clinically probable Laboratory-supported probable

The number of attacks that the patient has had, the clinical evidence that exists on the neurologic examination, and the amount of paraclinical evidence obtained determine the specific category of diagnosis.

What is relapsing–remitting MS?

Approximately 30% of patients with MS have attacks of unpredictable frequency, interspersed with periods of almost complete recovery.

What are other variants of MS?

Relapsing–progressive MS (approximately 40%)—unpredictable attacks or exacerbations associated with some residual deficits between attacks.

Chronic–progressive MS (approximately 20%)—distinctive attacks cannot be discerned, but disability steadily advances.

Benign MS (approximately 10%)—there is only one clinically evident attack, or attacks are separated in time by periods of years and cause no or minimal disability.

What are some of the most common presenting symptoms of MS?

Blurred vision with decreased acuity (possibly due to optic neuritis), double vision, bladder control problems, parasthesias (numbness and tingling) in the extremities, ataxia, fatigue, and focal motor symptoms

What treatment may provide symptomatic relief for patients with an acute exacerbation of MS?

High-dose methylprednisolone at the time of the acute attack. A common dose and schedule is to give 1000 mg daily for 3–5 days, followed by a 2- to 3-week prednisone taper (60 mg for 3 days, 50 mg for 3 days, 40 mg for 3 days, 30 mg for 3 days, 20 mg for 3 days, and 10 mg for 3 days).

What outpatient regimen is often used for MS patients having an acute attack, even though there is only anecdotal evidence of its efficacy?

Oral prednisone tapers, for example, 60 mg for 7 days, then 50 mg for 3 days, 40 mg for 3 days, 30 mg for 3 days, 20 mg for 3 days, 10 mg for 3 days, and 5 mg for 3 days

What treatments, believed to alter the course of MS beneficially, are approved for use in persons with relapsing–remitting MS?

The following drugs decrease the frequency of relapse, but their influence on the long-term prognosis is unknown:
Interferon beta-1b (Betaseron)—Eight million units subcutaneously every other day
Interferon beta-1a (Avonex)—Six million units intravenously weekly
Copolymer 1 (Copaxone)—20 mg subcutaneously daily

What three drugs can be used to treat fatigue in MS patients?

Amantadine, pemoline, and methylphenidate

What drug can be used to help treat urinary urge incontinence?

Oxybutynin

What three drugs are useful in treating spasticity?

Baclofen, dantrolene, and diazepam

To decrease the possibility of a new attack, what should the MS patient avoid?

Elevations of body temperature (e.g., they should swim in nonheated pools and avoid vigorous exercise)

After 10 years, how many MS patients are ambulatory rather than wheelchair bound?

At 10 years, approximately two thirds are ambulatory.

13   Psychiatry

ABBREVIATIONS

CBC	Complete blood count
CBZ	Carbamazepine
CNS	Central nervous system
CPK	Creatine phosphokinase
CSF	Cerebrospinal fluid
CT	Computed tomography
CVA	Cerebrovascular accident
DT	Delirium tremens
ECT	Electroconvulsive therapy
EEG	Electroencephalogram
HIV	Human immunodeficiency virus
LFT	Liver function test
MAOI	Monoamine oxidase inhibitor
MDD	Major depressive disorder
MDE	Major depressive episode
MMPI	Minnesota multiphasic personality inventory
MRI	Magnetic resonance imaging
PTSD	Post-traumatic stress disorder

RPR	Rapid plasmin reagin
SSRI	Selective serotonin reuptake inhibitor
TCA	Tricyclic antidepressant
TFT	Thyroid function test
TLE	Temporal lobe epilepsy
VPA	Valproic acid

PSYCHIATRIC ASSESSMENT

What is a psychiatric history?

Information regarding onset, duration, temporal features, intensity, progression, and alleviating and exacerbating conditions of psychiatric symptoms. Psychiatric symptoms are reflected in a patient's overt behavior or reported internal mental state including features of orientation, mood and affect, cognition, thought content, perceptions, and judgment. Symptoms may include somatic features including any general medical condition, neurologic illness, or neurovegetative function. A thorough history must include a general medical history and review of systems, past psychiatric and medical histories, a developmental and family history, a social history, and a detailed history of substance abuse.

What is a mental status examination?

A detailed description of appearance, behavior and psychomotor activity, speech and language, mood (the patient's subjective expression of internal emotional state, usually a quote), affect (the examiner's objective description of the patient's internal emotional state), thought process, thought content, perceptual disturbances, insight, judgment, estimated intelligence (usually based on vocabulary and use of language), and neuropsychiatric and cognitive function (mini-mental status).

What is a mini-mental status examination?

A standardized screening examination to test cognitive functioning including orientation, attention, memory, language, the ability to identify objects, and the ability to perform different types of sequential movements. A score of 23 or less generally indicates the presence of dementia or delirium. False-positive results may occur in patients with pseudodementia or depression and in elderly patients. False-negative results occur in highly educated professionals with early dementia and in patients with right hemisphere lesions. Table 13-1 is an example of a mini-mental status questionnaire.

Table 13–1. Mini-Mental Status (MMS) Questionnaire

Orientation (Score 1 if correct)
Name this hospital or building.   _____
What city are you in now?   _____
What year is it?   _____
What month is it?   _____
What is the date today?   _____
What state are you in?   _____
What country is this?   _____
What floor of the building are you on?   _____
What day of the week is it?   _____
What season of the year is it?   _____

Registration
Name three objects and have the patient repeat them.   _____
    Score number repeated by the patient. Name the three objects
    several more times if needed for the patient to repeat correctly
    (record trials _____).

Attention and calculation
Subtract 7 from 100 in serial fashion to 65.   _____
    Max. score = 5

Recall
Do you recall the three objects named before?   _____

Language tests
Confrontation naming: watch, pen = 2   _____
Repetition: "No ifs, ands, or buts" = 1   _____
Comprehension: Pick up the paper in your right hand, fold it in half   _____
    and set it on the floor = 3
Read and perform the command "close your eyes" = 1   _____
Write any sentence (subject, object, verb) = 1   _____

Construction
Copy the design below = 1   _____

Total MMS Questionnaire score (Max. = 30)   _____

Adapted from Folstein MF, Folstein S, McHugh PR: Mini-mental state: A practical method for grading the cognitive state of patients for the clinician. *J Psychiatr Res* 12:189, 1975, with permission.

What is the role of the physical examination in evaluating patients with psychiatric disorders?	Without exception, a thorough physical and neurologic examination is required for a complete psychiatric assessment. The brain is the substrate of behavior and can be affected by a myriad of medical illnesses.
What medical illnesses in the following categories can present with psychiatric problems?	
Neurologic	CVA, head trauma, epilepsy (especially complex partial), narcolepsy, normal pressure hydrocephalus, Parkinson's disease, multiple sclerosis, and Huntington's disease
Endocrine	Hypo- or hyperthyroidism; adrenal and parathyroid conditions; hypo- or hyperglycemia; hypopituitarism; pheochromocytoma; and gonadotrophic hormone
Metabolic	Fluid and electrolyte imbalance, hepatic encephalopathy, uremia, porphyria, Wilson's disease, hypoxia, hypotension, and hypertensive encephalopathy
Toxic	Intoxication or withdrawal from alcohol or drugs of abuse, side effects of prescription or over-the-counter drugs, and exposure to environmental toxins
Nutritional	Deficiencies of vitamin B_{12}, nicotinic acid, folate, thiamine, or trace metals; malnutrition; and dehydration
Infectious	AIDS, neurosyphilis, encephalitis, brain abscess, viral hepatitis, infectious mononucleosis, tuberculosis, and systemic bacterial or viral infections
Autoimmune	Systemic lupus erythematosus
Neoplastic	CNS primary or metastatic tumors, endocrine tumors, and pancreatic carcinoma

What common laboratory tests are ordered for psychiatric problems?

CBC, basic chemistries, LFTs, TFTs, RPR, B$_{12}$, folate, toxicology screens, therapeutic drug concentrations, occasionally CSF studies, head CT, head MRI, EEG, and electrocardiogram

Describe the multiaxial categories.

Axis I—clinical psychiatric syndromes

Axis II—personality disorders and specific developmental disorders

Axis III—existing medical, surgical, or neurologic disease

Axis IV—psychosocial stressors

Axis V—global assessment of functioning, reflecting the current or most recent highest level of functioning (social, occupational, psychological) on a scale from 10 (grossly impaired) to 90 (superior function)

PRIMARY THOUGHT DISORDERS

What are primary thought disorders?

Primary psychiatric illnesses characterized by having psychotic symptoms as the defining feature. These include schizophrenia, schizophreniform disorder, schizoaffective disorder, delusional disorder, brief psychotic disorder, and shared psychotic disorder.

What are psychotic symptoms?

Psychotic symptoms include delusions, hallucinations, incoherence, marked loosening of associations, catatonic excitement or stupor, or grossly disorganized behavior. Symptoms may be described as an impairment in reality testing.

SCHIZOPHRENIA

What is schizophrenia?

A chronic, remitting psychotic illness of at least 6 months' duration that includes at least 1 month of two or more active phase symptoms including delusions, hallucinations, disorganized speech, grossly disorganized or catatonic behavior, and "negative" symptoms (e.g., affective flattening, paucity of thought and speech, and paucity of initiation of goal-directed behavior). Impairment in social and occupational functioning is a key feature.

What are the subtypes of schizophrenia?

Paranoid, disorganized, catatonic, undifferentiated, and residual

What is the incidence of schizophrenia?

1/10,000; prevalence, 1/100

What are risk factors for schizophrenia?

Genetic predisposition—twin studies show 50% monozygotic concordance and 18% dizygotic concordance. First-degree relatives have a 5- to 10-fold increased risk. Birth during winter months, obstetric complications, lower socioeconomic status, and immigration have all been associated.

What are symptoms and signs of schizophrenia?

Delusions, hallucinations, disorganized speech, grossly disorganized behavior, and affective flattening

What diagnostic tests are helpful in establishing schizophrenia?

Neuropsychological testing (e.g., MMPI and Rorschach testing)

What is the differential diagnosis of schizophrenia?

Psychotic disorder due to a general medical condition (e.g., Cushing's syndrome and CNS tumor), delirium, or dementia; substance-induced psychotic disorder, delirium, or dementia; substance-related disorder; mood disorder with psychotic features; schizoaffective disorder; schizophreniform disorder; brief psychotic disorder; delusional disorder; and cluster A personality disorder

What is the treatment for schizophrenia?

Hospitalization during acute exacerbation, antipsychotic medications (e.g., haloperidol, chlorpromazine, and clozapine), and behavioral and group therapies. Treatment may be augmented with mood stabilizers (e.g., lithium, CBZ, and valproate).

What other problems are associated with schizophrenia?	Suicide; 50% of schizophrenics attempt suicide, and 15%–20% succeed. Seventy-five percent of schizophrenics smoke cigarettes, 40% are alcoholics, 20% are cannabis users, and less than 10% are cocaine users.

SCHIZOPHRENIFORM DISORDER

What is schizophreniform disorder?	Essential features are the same as those of schizophrenia except (1) total duration of the illness is more than 1 month but less than 6 months and (2) impaired social and occupational functioning is not required for diagnosis. Schizophreniform disorder should be considered a provisional diagnosis.
What is the prevalence of schizophreniform disorder?	Lifetime, 1/500; 1 year, 1/1000
What are risk factors for schizophreniform disorder?	Same as for schizophrenia
What are symptoms and signs of schizophreniform disorder?	Same as for schizophrenia
What diagnostic tests are helpful in establishing schizophreniform disorder?	Same as for schizophrenia
What is the differential diagnosis for schizophreniform disorder?	Same as for schizophrenia plus factitious disorder, HIV infection, TLE, CNS tumors, cerebrovascular disease, and anabolic steroid use
What is the treatment for schizophreniform disorder?	Hospitalization, antipsychotic medications, ECT, mood stabilizers, and psychotherapy

What is the prognosis for schizophreniform disorder?	Prognosis is better with short duration of illness. One third of patients recover completely; two thirds progress to diagnosis of schizophrenia or schizoaffective disorder. There is a high suicide risk.

BRIEF PSYCHOTIC DISORDER

What is a brief psychotic disorder?	Sudden onset of one or more of the following psychotic symptoms: delusions, hallucinations, disorganized speech, and disorganized or catatonic behavior. Duration is at least 1 day but less than 1 month. The patient recovers to premorbid level of functioning.
What is the prevalence of brief psychotic disorder?	Unknown, but considered uncommon
What are risk factors for brief psychotic disorder?	Catastrophic stressors, young adulthood, and associated premorbid personality disorders
What is the differential diagnosis for brief psychotic disorder?	Factitious disorder, malingering, psychotic disorder resulting from a general medical condition, substance-induced psychosis, delirium, epilepsy, dissociative identity disorder, and psychotic episodes associated with borderline and schizotypal personality disorder
What is the treatment for brief psychotic disorder?	Hospitalization, antipsychotic medications, benzodiazepines, and psychotherapy
What is the prognosis for brief psychotic disorder?	No further major psychiatric problems occur in 50%–80% of cases.

SHARED PSYCHOTIC DISORDER (FOLIE À DEUX)

What is a shared psychotic disorder?	A delusion that develops in one person who is involved in a close relationship with another person (the "inducer") who has a preexisting delusion. The patient comes to share the delusional beliefs of

the inducer. Usually, the inducer is dominant in the relationship. The relationship may involve more than two people and has been reported in families (folie à famille).

What is the incidence of shared psychotic disorder?

Rare. It may be more common in women.

What are risk factors for shared psychotic disorder?

Affected individuals often have a family history of schizophrenia.

What is the differential diagnosis of shared psychotic disorder?

Malingering, factitious disorder, psychotic disorder caused by a general medical condition, and substance-induced psychotic disorder

What is the treatment for shared psychotic disorder?

Separation from the inducer and treatment of the disorder of the inducer. Family therapy with nondelusional members of the family and antipsychotic medications may be necessary.

In whom does shared psychiatric disorder develop?

In 95% of cases, two members of the same family are involved; one third involve two sisters and one third involve a husband and wife or a mother and child. The inducer is usually schizophrenic.

SCHIZOAFFECTIVE DISORDER

What is schizoaffective disorder?

A primary psychiatric illness with features of both schizophrenia and mood disorders. It is characterized by an uninterrupted period of illness during which, at some point, there is a major depressive, manic, or mixed mood episode concurrent with psychotic symptoms consistent with schizophrenia. In addition, there is a period of at least 2 weeks during the illness without the presence of mood symptoms.

What are the subtypes of schizoaffective disorder?

Bipolar and depressive

What is the prevalence of schizoaffective disorder?	Lifetime, 0.5%–0.8%
What are risk factors for schizoaffective disorder?	Genetics and female gender. There is increased risk for schizophrenia and mood disorders in first degree relatives.
What are symptoms and signs of schizoaffective disorder?	The presence of symptoms consistent with mania, major depression, or a mixed mood state concurrent with psychotic symptoms consistent with schizophrenia
What is the differential diagnosis of schizoaffective disorder?	Psychotic disorder resulting from a general medical condition, delirium, dementia, substance-induced psychotic disorder, delusional disorder, and mood disorder with psychotic features
What is the treatment for schizoaffective disorder?	Hospitalization, antipsychotic medications, mood stabilizers, antidepressants, and group psychotherapy
What is the prognosis for schizoaffective disorder?	In general, prognosis ranges between that of patients with schizophrenia and those with mood disorders.

DELUSIONAL DISORDER

What is delusional disorder?	An illness characterized by the presence of one or more nonbizarre delusions for at least 1 month. Delusions may be grandiose, erotic, jealous, somatic, or mixed.
What is the prevalence of delusional disorder?	0.03%
What are risk factors for delusional disorder?	Family history of schizophrenia, paranoid personality disorder, or avoidant personality disorder. Onset is usually in middle or late adult life.
What are signs and symptoms of delusional disorder?	Onset of one or more nonbizarre delusions. Hallucinations are not prominent. "Negative" symptoms of schizophrenia are not present. Duration is at least 1 month.

What is the differential diagnosis of delusional disorder?	Delirium, dementia, psychotic disorder caused by a general medical condition, substance-induced psychotic disorder, mood disorders with psychotic features, shared psychotic disorder, hypochondriasis, body dysmorphic disorder, obsessive-compulsive disorder, and paranoid personality disorder
What is the treatment for delusional disorder?	Hospitalization if the patient is agitated, antipsychotic medications, psychotherapy, and family therapy

MOOD DISORDERS

What illnesses comprise the mood disorders?	Major depression, dysthymic disorder, bipolar disorder, and cyclothymic disorder

MAJOR DEPRESSION

What is major depression?	A significant disturbance of mood and neurovegetative function (i.e., appetite, sleep, energy, libido, and concentration), which is persistent and not caused by the direct physiologic effects of a general medical condition or substance abuse
What is the prevalence of major depression?	Lifetime, 15%; as high as 25% in women. Incidence of major depression is 10% in primary care patients and 15% in medical in-patients.
What are risk factors for major depression?	Female sex (up to twofold greater prevalence), divorce, and genetics. First degree relatives have a 1.5–3 times greater chance of development of major depression than the general population.
What are symptoms and signs of major depression?	Persistent presence of depressed mood, diminished interest (anhedonia), significant weight loss or weight gain reflecting appetite disturbance, insomnia or hypersomnia, psychomotor agitation or retardation, decreased energy, excessive guilt, feelings of worthlessness, inability to concentrate, impaired

memory, and suicidal ideation. Anxiety, somatic complaints, or psychotic symptoms may be associated.

What are the laboratory findings in major depression?

TFTs show thyroid dysfunction concurrent with depressive symptoms.

What diagnostic tests are helpful in establishing major depression?

Neuropsychological tests may be helpful.

What is the differential diagnosis of major depression?

Mood disorder resulting from a general medical condition, substance-induced mood disorder, dysthymic disorder, and schizoaffective disorder

What is the treatment for major depression?

Hospitalization for suicidality, psychotic depression, or malnutrition; antidepressant medications (e.g., SSRIs, TCAs, MAOIs), benzodiazepines for short-term treatment of anxiety symptoms; augmentation with lithium or thyroid hormone; and individual psychotherapy

What is the prognosis for major depression?

Up to 15% of patients die by suicide; 50% of patients have a second episode.

DYSTHYMIC DISORDER

What is dysthymic disorder?

A chronic psychiatric illness characterized by the presence of depressed mood more days than not for at least 2 years. Also present are two or more neurovegetative symptoms including poor appetite or overeating, sleep disturbance, decreased energy, low self-esteem, and poor concentration. No major depressive episode is present during the first 2 years.

What is the prevalence of dysthymic disorder?

3%–5%

What are risk factors for dysthymic disorder?

Adolescence and family history of mood disorders

What are symptoms and signs of dysthymic disorder?	Presence of depressed mood that is chronic and associated with neurovegetative dysfunction. It may present with irritability, especially in adolescents, decreased sexual interest, and substance abuse.
What diagnostic tests are useful in establishing dysthymic disorder?	Neuropsychological testing (e.g., MMPI)
What is the differential diagnosis for dysthymic disorder?	Major depression, mood disorder caused by a general medical condition, substance-induced mood disorder, and personality disorder
What is the treatment for dysthymic disorder?	MAOIs, SSRIs, bupropion, and cognitive therapy
How common is double depression and what is it?	Forty percent of patients with MDD also meet criteria for dysthymic disorder ("double depression").
How common is depression before age 25 years?	Fifty percent of patients experience depression onset before age 25 years; 20% of cases progress to MDD.

BIPOLAR DISORDER

What is bipolar disorder?	A chronic, remitting mood disorder characterized by periods of mania, depression, or mixed mood episodes. It may be associated with psychotic symptoms.
What is a manic episode?	A distinct period of persistently and abnormally elevated, irritable, or expansive mood lasting at least 1 week. It is associated with the following: inflated self-esteem, grandiosity, decreased sleep, pressured speech, racing thoughts, distractibility, psychomotor agitation, and enhanced libido.

What drugs are associated with manic episodes?	Amphetamines, baclofen, bromide, bromocriptine, captopril, cimetidine, cocaine, corticosteroids, cyclosporine, disulfiram, hallucinogens, hydralazine, isoniazid, levodopa, methylphenidate, metrizamide, opiates and opioids, procarbazine, and procyclidine
What is a mixed mood episode?	Features of both major depression and mania are present for at least 1 week. Also known as dysphoric mania, a mixed mood episode is thought to be a rapid alteration of mania and depression.
What is the prevalence of bipolar disorder?	0.6%–1.6%
What are risk factors for bipolar disorder?	First degree relatives of bipolar patients have increased rates of mood disorders. Twin and adoption studies support a genetic influence.
What is the differential diagnosis for bipolar disorder?	Mood disorder caused by a general medical condition, substance-induced mood disorder, and cyclothymia
What is the treatment for bipolar disorder?	Hospitalization for acute mania, severe depression, and associated psychosis; mood stabilizers (e.g., lithium, CBZ, and valproate), benzodiazepines, and antipsychotic medications for acute mania and psychosis (antidepressants are avoided because they commonly precipitate mania); ECT for severe, intractable mania; and psychotherapy
Does the frequency of mood disturbances change with age, and how does this affect treatment?	Cycles of mood disturbance increase in frequency with age, and anticonvulsant mood stabilizers tend to be more effective than lithium during later stages of the illness. Completed suicide occurs in 10%–15% of cases, and associated problems include eating disorders, attention deficit hyperactivity disorder, and substance abuse.

CYCLOTHYMIC DISORDER

What is cyclothymic disorder?	A chronic mood disturbance characterized by fluctuating periods of depressive symptoms and hypomanic symptoms. These are present for at least 2 years and none of the episodes meet criteria for a complete manic or depressive episode.
What is the prevalence of cyclothymic disorder?	0.4%–1%
What are risk factors for cyclothymic disorder?	First-degree relatives have an increased incidence of mood disorders. There is an increased family history of substance abuse.
What are symptoms and signs of cyclothymic disorder?	Chronic, persistent presence of mood disturbance with features of hypomania and depression. Substance abuse is common.
What is the differential diagnosis for cyclothymic disorder?	Mood disorder caused by a general medical condition, substance-induced mood disorder, rapid cycling bipolar disorder, and borderline personality disorder
What is the treatment for cyclothymic disorder?	Mood stabilizers (e.g., lithium, CBZ, and valproate), not antidepressants because they may induce manic or hypomanic episodes in 50% of cyclothymic patients, and psychotherapy

ANXIETY DISORDERS

What illnesses comprise the anxiety disorders?	Generalized anxiety disorder, panic disorder, obsessive-compulsive disorder, and post-traumatic stress disorder

GENERALIZED ANXIETY DISORDER

What is generalized anxiety disorder?	Excessive anxiety and apprehensive expectation occurring over a period of at least 6 months. It may be associated with restlessness, easy fatigability, difficulty concentrating, irritability, muscle tension, or disturbed sleep.

What are symptoms and signs of generalized anxiety disorder?	Anxiety, cognitive vigilance, autonomic hyperactivity, motor tension, irritability, disturbed sleep, fatigability, and poor concentration
What is the differential diagnosis for generalized anxiety disorder?	Anxiety disorder resulting from a general medical condition, substance-induced anxiety disorder, mood disorder with anxious features, and adjustment disorder
What is the treatment for generalized anxiety disorder?	Cognitive therapy, benzodiazepines, buspirone, and TCAs

PANIC DISORDER

What is panic disorder?	Recurrent, circumscribed panic attacks, with or without agoraphobia
What is a panic attack?	The sudden development of a discrete period of intense fear or discomfort associated with tachycardia, palpitations, sweating, trembling, shortness of breath, choking sensation, chest pain or tightness, abdominal discomfort, dizziness, derealization or depersonalization, fear of dying, or paresthesias
What is agoraphobia?	Anxiety of being in places where escape is difficult or impossible (e.g., public, crowded places). The fear is usually associated with having a panic attack in an unprotected place.
What is the prevalence of panic disorder?	Lifetime, 1.5%–3.5%
What are symptoms and signs of panic disorder?	Attacks usually begin with a 10-minute period of escalating symptoms and last 20–30 minutes. Syncopal episodes may occur. Respiratory alkalosis may result from hyperventilation.
What is the differential diagnosis for panic disorder?	Anxiety disorder caused by a general medical condition and substance-induced anxiety disorder

What is the treatment for panic disorder?	TCAs, MAOIs, SSRIs, benzodiazepines (e.g., alprazolam, clonazepam, and lorazepam), and cognitive therapies

OBSESSIVE-COMPULSIVE DISORDER

What is obsessive-compulsive disorder?	An illness characterized by recurrent obsessions or compulsions that cause significant distress or impairment in functioning
What are obsessions?	Persistent and recurrent images, impulses, or thoughts that are not merely excessive worries about real-life problems
What are compulsions?	Repetitive behaviors or mental acts (e.g., praying, counting, and repeating phrases) that a person feels driven to perform in order to reduce anxiety or prevent an imagined dreaded event or situation
What is the prevalence of obsessive-compulsive disorder?	Lifetime, 2.5%
What are risk factors for obsessive-compulsive disorder?	Studies show a higher rate of concordance for monozygotic than dizygotic twins; 35% of first degree relatives of patients are also afflicted with the disorder.
What are symptoms and signs of obsessive-compulsive disorder?	Generally, gradual onset of obsessions or compulsions, usually in late teens or early 20s. The patient generally has insight into the unrealistic aspects of the illness. Dermatologic problems may be present due to excessive washing.
What diagnostic tests are used to establish obsessive-compulsive disorder?	Neuropsychological testing may be helpful.

What is the differential diagnosis of obsessive-compulsive disorder?	Anxiety disorder caused by a general medical condition, substance-induced anxiety disorder, body dysmorphic disorder, major depressive episode, hypochondriasis, specific phobia, and tic disorder
What is the treatment for obsessive-compulsive disorder?	Clomipramine, SSRIs, MAOIs, lithium augmentation, and behavior therapy

POST-TRAUMATIC STRESS DISORDER

What is PTSD?	Characteristic symptoms that develop after a person is exposed to a traumatic event involving actual or threatened death or serious injury to self or others and the person's response involved horror, helplessness, or intense fear
What is the prevalence of PTSD?	Lifetime, 1%–14%
What are risk factors for PTSD?	Emigration from an area of considerable civil conflict or social unrest
What are symptoms and signs of PTSD?	Persistent reexperiencing of the traumatic event through recurrent and intrusive images, thoughts, or perceptions; recurrent distressing dreams of the event; flashbacks; avoidance of stimuli associated with the trauma; and hyperarousal and hypervigilance including difficulty sleeping, irritability, difficulty concentrating, and exaggerated startle response
What is the differential diagnosis of PTSD?	Adjustment disorder, acute stress disorder, obsessive-compulsive disorder, schizophrenia, and malingering
What is the treatment for PTSD?	TCAs, SSRIs, MAOIs, CBZ, VPA, clonidine, propranolol, and psychotherapy

ADJUSTMENT DISORDERS

What is an adjustment disorder?	A condition characterized by the development of clinically significant behavioral or emotional symptoms within 3 months of an identifiable stressor. The distress is in excess to what would normally be expected given the stressor. The condition resolves within 6 months.
What are the different types of adjustment disorders?	With depressed mood, with anxiety, with mixed anxiety and depressed mood, with disturbance of conduct, with mixed disturbance of emotions and conduct, and unspecified
What is the prevalence of adjustment disorder?	Common
What is the differential diagnosis of adjustment disorder?	Personality disorder, PTSD, acute stress disorder, bereavement, and nonpathologic response to stress
What is the treatment for adjustment disorder?	Psychotherapy, low-dose antipsychotic medications, and short-term use of benzodiazepines

PERSONALITY DISORDERS

What is a personality disorder?	An enduring pattern of behavior and inner experience that deviates significantly from the expectations of an individual's culture. This pattern may be manifested in the individual's way of perceiving and interpreting self or others; emotional range, intensity, lability, or appropriateness; or impulse control or interpersonal functioning. Onset is generally in adolescence and the patterns are long-standing.
What are the major categories of personality disorders?	Cluster A, cluster B, and cluster C

CLUSTER A PERSONALITY DISORDERS

What are cluster A disorders?	Patterns of inner experience and behavior that are odd or eccentric. They include paranoid, schizoid, and schizotypal personality disorders.

Paranoid Personality Disorder

What is paranoid personality disorder?	Enduring patterns of personality characterized by mistrust and suspiciousness of people in general. It may include anger, hostility, or irritability.
What is the prevalence of paranoid personality disorder?	0.5%–2.5%
What is the treatment for paranoid personality disorder?	Psychotherapy and low-dose antipsychotic medications or benzodiazepines for periods of agitation

Schizoid Personality Disorder

What is schizoid personality disorder?	A lifelong pattern of social withdrawal associated with introversion, bland, restricted affect, and general discomfort with human interaction
What is the prevalence of schizoid personality disorder?	Uncommon
What is the treatment for schizoid personality disorder?	Psychotherapy, antipsychotic medications, antidepressants, and psychostimulant medications (e.g., methylphenidate and dextroamphetamine)

Schizotypal Personality Disorder

What is schizotypal personality disorder?	A disorder characterized by magical thinking, peculiar ideas, illusions, and ideas of reference. Persons with schizotypal personality disorder are described as odd or strange.

What is the prevalence of schizotypal personality disorder?	3%
What is the treatment for schizotypal personality disorder?	Psychotherapy and antipsychotic medications

CLUSTER B PERSONALITY DISORDERS

What are cluster B disorders?	Patterns of inner experience and behavior that appear dramatic, emotional, or erratic. They include antisocial, borderline, histrionic, and narcissistic personality disorders.

Antisocial Personality Disorder

What is antisocial personality disorder?	A pattern of disregard for, and violation of, the rights of others and an inability to conform to social norms. It is associated with impulsivity, aggressiveness, lack of remorse, and deceitfulness.
What is the prevalence of antisocial personality disorder?	3% in men, 1% in women
What is the treatment for antisocial personality disorder?	Psychotherapy. Short courses of psychoactive medications must be given carefully, because there is a high rate of substance abuse.

Borderline Personality Disorder

What is borderline personality disorder?	A pattern of unstable affect, mood, behavior, and self-image. It is associated with "stormy" interpersonal relationships, fear of abandonment, impulsivity, recurrent suicidal gestures, and chronic feelings of emptiness.
What is the prevalence of borderline personality disorder?	2%

What is the treatment for borderline personality disorder?	Psychotherapy, group therapy, and pharmacotherapy including low doses of antipsychotic medications, MAOIs, SSRIs, and anticonvulsants

Histrionic Personality Disorder

What is histrionic personality disorder?	Pervasive and enduring dramatic, attention-seeking, and extroverted behavior associated with an inability to maintain close personal relationships
What is the prevalence of histrionic personality disorder?	2%–3%
What is the treatment for histrionic personality disorder?	Psychotherapy and pharmacotherapy for clear target symptoms

Narcissistic Personality Disorder

What is narcissistic personality disorder?	A disorder characterized by grandiosity, self-importance, need for admiration, and lack of empathy. It is associated with fantasies of success, entitlement, and interpersonal exploitation.
What is the prevalence of narcissistic personality disorder?	< 1%
What is the treatment for narcissistic personality disorder?	Psychotherapy, SSRIs, and lithium

CLUSTER C PERSONALITY DISORDERS

What are cluster C disorders?	Patterns of excessive fearfulness or anxiety. They include avoidant, dependent, and obsessive-compulsive personality disorders.

Avoidant Personality Disorder

What is avoidant personality disorder?	A disorder characterized by social inhibition and withdrawal, feelings of inadequacy ("inferiority complex"), extreme sensitivity to rejection or criticism, and extreme shyness

What is the prevalence of avoidant personality disorder?	0.5%–1.0%
What is the treatment for avoidant personality disorder?	Psychotherapy and beta-blockers (e.g., propranolol and atenolol)

Dependent Personality Disorder

What is dependent personality disorder?	A disorder characterized by a pervasive and excessive need to be taken care of, lack of self-confidence, submissive and clinging behaviors, and fear of separation
What is the prevalence of dependent personality disorder?	2.5% of all personality disorders
What is the treatment for dependent personality disorder?	Psychotherapy, SSRIs, and TCAs

Obsessive-Compulsive Personality Disorder

What is obsessive-compulsive personality disorder?	A disorder characterized by emotional constriction, orderliness, perfectionism, preoccupation with mental and interpersonal control, and inflexibility. Features may include preoccupation with details, rules, lists, or schedules. Perfectionism and inflexibility interfere with task completion.
What is the prevalence of obsessive-compulsive personality disorder?	1%
What is the treatment for obsessive-compulsive personality disorder?	Psychotherapy, clonazepam, and SSRIs

SUBSTANCE-RELATED DISORDERS

What is substance dependence?	A pathologic pattern of substance use manifested by the development of tolerance, withdrawal, and inability to decrease the amount of usage despite repeated attempts. A large amount of

time is spent obtaining the substance, or
an individual gives up social,
occupational, or recreational activities to
obtain or use the substance.

What is substance abuse?   A pathologic pattern of substance use
characterized by recurrent substance-
related legal problems, recurrent
substance use in situations that are
physically hazardous, and failure to fulfill
personal, occupational, and educational
responsibility as a result of substance use

**What is substance
withdrawal?**   The occurrence of a substance-specific
syndrome in the setting of cessation or
decrease in the prolonged and heavy use
of a substance

URGENCIES AND EMERGENCIES

ACUTE PSYCHOSIS

What is acute psychosis?   The acute or subacute onset of psychotic
symptoms

**What are symptoms and
signs of acute psychosis?**   Delusions, hallucinations, incoherence,
loosening of associations, catatonic
excitement or stupor, or grossly
disorganized behavior

**What diagnostic tests are
ordered for acute
psychosis?**   Tests for the variety of organic causes
including head CT, head MRI, EEG,
CBC, blood chemistries, drug screen,
TFTs, HIV screen, LFTs, and CSF
studies. Psychosis is a medical syndrome,
like a fever or a seizure, and may be
caused by a variety of conditions.

**What is the differential
diagnosis for acute
psychosis?**   Primary thought disorders, primary
mood disorders, and organic causes.
Organic causes may include dysfunction
of the CNS for a variety of reasons
including structural CNS lesions (e.g.,
trauma, neoplasm, and CVA), seizures,
delirium, dementia, and causes that are
infectious, inflammatory, toxic,
metabolic, nutritional, iatrogenic (e.g.,
steroids), and endocrine.

What is the treatment for acute psychosis?	Hospitalization, treatment of organic cause, antipsychotic medications, benzodiazepines for acute agitation, and treatment of primary psychiatric illness

NEUROLEPTIC MALIGNANT SYNDROME

What is neuroleptic malignant syndrome?	An extrapyramidal syndrome resulting from antipsychotic medication use
What is the prevalence of neuroleptic malignant syndrome?	Rare
What are risk factors for neuroleptic malignant syndrome?	Use of high-potency antipsychotic medications (e.g., haloperidol and fluphenazine) in high doses when the dosage is increased rapidly
What are symptoms and signs of neuroleptic malignant syndrome?	Hyperthermia, severe muscular rigidity, autonomic instability including tachycardia, hypertension, tachypnea, and diaphoresis, and fluctuating level of consciousness
What laboratory tests are ordered for neuroleptic malignant syndrome?	CPK (elevated in 50% of cases), aldolase, LFTs, white blood cell count, and urine myoglobin
What is the treatment for neuroleptic malignant syndrome?	Discontinue antipsychotic medications; transfer the patient to intensive care unit for supportive measures; dantrolene, initially intravenously 0.8–2.5 mg/kg every 6 hours, then orally 100–200 mg daily when the patient can swallow. Bromocriptine, 20–30 mg daily in four divided doses, may be helpful.
What is the prognosis for neuroleptic malignant syndrome?	20%–30% mortality rate

ACUTE DYSTONIC REACTION

What is an acute dystonic reaction?	An extrapyramidal symptom consisting of intermittent and sustained spasms of muscles of the head, neck, and trunk leading to involuntary movements. It is a

direct result of treatment with
antipsychotic medications.

**What is the prevalence of
acute dystonic reaction?**

10% during the initial phases of
antipsychotic treatment

**What are risk factors for
acute dystonic reaction?**

Male gender, age younger than 40 years,
and high dosages of potent antipsychotic
medications

**What are symptoms and
signs of acute dystonic
reaction?**

Opisthotonos, retrocollis, torticollis,
oculogyric crisis, tongue protrusion,
dysarthria, and dysphagia

**What is the differential
diagnosis of acute dystonic
reaction?**

Tetanus and seizures

**What is the treatment for
acute dystonic reaction?**

Intramuscular benztropine, 2 mg, which
is repeated if not effective in 10–15
minutes; intramuscular
diphenhydramine, 50 mg

ALCOHOL WITHDRAWAL AND DELIRIUM TREMENS

**What is alcohol
withdrawal?**

A physiologic syndrome resulting from
the cessation of prolonged and heavy
alcohol use. The syndrome progresses
soon after the cessation of alcohol use
and may include grand mal seizures or
DTs (alcohol withdrawal delirium).

**What are symptoms and
signs of alcohol
withdrawal?**

Tachycardia, hypertension, diaphoresis,
tremor, insomnia, nausea, vomiting,
anxiety, and seizures. Symptoms of DTs
include severe agitated confusion and
delirium with tactile or visual
hallucinations.

**What are the laboratory
findings in alcohol
dependence?**

Elevated γ-glutamyl transferase (GGT),
mean corpuscular volume (MCV),
magnesium, uric acid, aspartate
aminotransferase (AST), alanine
aminotransferase (ALT), and
triglycerides

What is the differential diagnosis for alcohol withdrawal?	Sedative or hypnotic withdrawal
What is the treatment for alcohol withdrawal?	Thiamine, folate, magnesium intramuscularly; detoxification with oral benzodiazepine (e.g., Librium) taper; intramuscular benzodiazepine (e.g., lorazepam) as needed for autonomic hyperactivity or agitation associated with delirium; and antipsychotic medications for delirium, keeping in mind that they lower the seizure threshold

SUICIDALITY

What is the epidemiologic makeup of suicidality?	0.4%–0.9% of all deaths; 75 suicides per day in the United States
What is the prevalence of suicidality?	12.5/100,000 in the United States
What major factors in the following categories affect suicidal risk?	
Personal and social	Male gender Age older than 40 years Widowed, divorced, or separated marital status Immigrant status Lone dweller or socially isolated Unemployed or retired status
Previous history	Family history of affective disorder, suicide, or alcoholism Previous history of an affective disorder or alcoholism Previous suicide attempt Beginning psychiatric treatment or 6 months after discharge from treatment
Life stresses	Bereavement and separation Loss of job or house Incapacitating or terminal illness
Personality	Cyclothymic or antisocial personality Drug or alcohol dependence

Psychiatric illnesses	Depression Alcohol or drug addiction Dementia, confusion, and organic brain syndromes
What symptoms are worrisome with regard to suicide risk?	Insomnia, weight loss, slowed speech, listlessness, social withdrawal and loss of interest, hopelessness, thoughts of worthlessness, agitation, and suicidal thoughts
What signs are worrisome with regard to suicide attempts?	When the patient takes precautions against discovery, takes preparatory action (e.g., procures means of suicide, makes warning statements, writes suicide notes, and gets personal affairs in order), and uses violent methods or lethal drugs
What is the treatment for suicidality?	Hospitalization and treatment of underlying disorder
What percent of people who attempt suicide have tried before?	40%. Of persons who attempt suicide, 15%–35% make another attempt in the next 2 years.

14 _____ Dermatology

What are the general rules of dermatology?	If it's wet, dry it.
	If it's dry, wet it.
	When in doubt, cut it out.

DEFINITIONS

ANA	Antinuclear antibody
EN	Erythema nodosum
H&P	History and physical examination
HHV	Human herpesvirus
HIV	Human immunodeficiency virus
HPV	Human papilloma virus
HSV	Herpes simplex virus
KOH	Potassium hydroxide
MF	Mycosis fungoides
MM	Multiple myeloma
MMR	Measles, mumps, rubella
NL	Necrobiosis lipoidica
NSAID	Nonsteroidal anti-inflammatory drug
PUVA	Psoralen plus ultraviolet light of A wavelength
RMSF	Rocky Mountain spotted fever
RPR	Rapid plasma reagin

SCC	Squamous cell carcinoma
SLE	Systemic lupus erythematosus
SPF	Sun protection factor
SSSS	Staphylococcal scalded skin syndrome
TEN	Toxic epidermal necrolysis
TPN	Total parenteral nutrition
UV	Ultraviolet
VZV	Varicella zoster virus
VZVIg	Varicella zoster immunoglobulin

TOPICAL THERAPY

What is a lotion?	A powder in water
What is lotion used for?	To cool and dry the skin. It can be used on hairy areas.
What is a cream?	A mix of oil in water
What is cream used for?	To act as an intermediate agent between the strength of lotion and ointment (not particularly drying or lubricating)
What is an ointment?	A mix of water in oil
What is ointment used for?	To lubricate and occlude the skin
What is a gel?	Oil in water and alcohol
What is gel used for?	To act as an agent on hairy areas because it is not as greasy

PRIMARY SKIN LESIONS

What is a macule?	A flat discolored nonpalpable skin lesion < 1 cm in diameter
What is a patch?	A large macule > 1 cm

What is a papule?	An elevated, circumscribed, palpable lesion < 0.5 cm in diameter
What is a nodule?	An elevated, circumscribed, palpable lesion > 0.5 cm in diameter
What is a plaque?	A flat-topped lesion > 0.5 cm in diameter with elevation
What is a pustule?	A circumscribed elevated lesion or papule containing pus
What is a vesicle?	A blister < 0.5 cm
What is a bulla?	A large blister > 0.5 cm
What is a wheal (hive)?	An edematous elevated skin lesion that is usually migratory, lasting 24–48 hours
What is a cyst?	A cavity with an epidermal lining containing fluid
What is telangiectasia?	A dilated superficial blood vessel, usually blanchable

SECONDARY SKIN LESIONS

What is a crust?	A dried skin exudate
What is a scale?	Superficial dead epidermal cells
What is an erosion?	The focal loss of superficial epidermis
What is an ulceration?	Loss of epidermis and some dermis
What is a fissure?	A deep split through the epidermis into the dermis
What is atrophy?	Skin thinning
What is a scar?	Fibrous tissue laid down in response to skin injury
What is an excoriation?	A skin abrasion caused by scratching
What is lichenification?	Thickening of the skin in response to rubbing, with increased skin markings

What are petechiae?	Small nonblanchable lesions caused by extravasated blood
What is purpura?	Larger petechiae

CONFIGURATION AND MORPHOLOGIC TERMS

How are the following lesions shaped?

Nummular	Coin shaped
Serpiginous	Snake-like
Herpetiform	Grouped vesicles resembling herpes simplex (but may also result from noninfectious etiology)
Annular	Ring shaped
Targetoid	Concentric rings
Dermatomal	Follows the distribution of a cutaneous sensory nerve
Verrucous	Warty
Discoid	Oval or round
Morbilliform	Maculopapular, resembling the exanthem of measles

HISTORY AND PHYSICAL EXAMINATION

What key questions should be asked in a dermatologic history?	When did the problem start? Where on the body did the lesion start and where is it now? How did the condition appear at first and how has it changed? What treatments have been tried? Did any treatment help? What are the symptoms? Is anyone else at home affected? Has this or something like it happened before? Does the patient have any chronic medical problems? What medication is the patient taking? Does the patient have allergies?

Are there any diseases that run in the family?

Has there been any occupational or hobby exposures?

Has the patient had any particular life stresses?

What clues on H&P aid in diagnosis of dermatologic conditions?

Age and sex of the patient, and appearance and distribution of the lesion

What six rashes usually involve the palms and soles?

RMSF, secondary syphilis, Stevens-Johnson syndrome, erythema multiforme, toxic shock syndrome, and SSSS

COMMON DERMATOLOGIC DIAGNOSTIC TOOLS

What does a Tzanck prep help diagnose?

Usually HSV and VZV infection

How is a Tzanck test done?

The base of an intact vesicle is scraped with a scalpel blade onto a slide. It is air-dried, fixed in methanol, and stained with Giemsa or Wright's stain, then examined under a microscope.

When are results of Tzanck test positive?

When multinucleated giant cells are seen

What does a KOH prep help diagnose?

Dermatophyte and yeast infections

When should a KOH test be done?

When a lesion has pustules, vesicles, or scales (if it scales, scrape it)

How is a KOH test done?

Skin scales on the roof of a vesicle or pustule are scraped onto a slide with a number 15 scalpel blade or another slide, 1–2 drops of KOH are applied, the sample is covered with a coverslip and gently heated over an alcohol lamp, the sample is allowed to sit for a few minutes, and then it is examined under a microscope.

What does the KOH do in a KOH test?	Dissolves human epithelial cells to clear the background, but does not dissolve the chitin walls of fungi
When are the results of a KOH test positive?	When hyphae, pseudohyphae, or yeast are seen
How is a scabies scraping done?	A papule or burrow is scraped with a number 15 blade and moistened with a drop of oil. The scrapings are transferred to a slide, covered, and examined. A positive result shows mites, eggs, or feces.
What is a Wood's lamp?	A black light with a 360-nm wavelength (UV) filtered through glass
How is a Wood's lamp used?	As the lamp is held over a skin lesion, typical colors are seen. Certain infections fluoresce and hypopigmented lesions are accentuated.
What are Wood's lamp findings for the following diagnoses:	
Erythrasma	Coral red
Tinea capitis (caused by M. canis)	Light, bright green
Pseudomonas	Green
Tinea versicolor	Yellow-gold
Ash leaf macule (tuberous sclerosis)	Accentuated hypopigmentation

TOPICAL CORTICOSTEROIDS

How are topical steroids rated?	From class VII (weakest) to class I (strongest)
What determines the strength of a topical corticosteroid?	Chemical structure, vehicle, and concentration

What are commonly used weak, medium, and potent topical steroids?

Weak   Hydrocortisone

Medium   Triamcinolone acetonide

Potent   Betamethasone dipropionate (Diprolene) and clobetasol propionate (Temovate)

How strong a steroid can be used on the face?

Typically, weak steroids in class VII; rarely, medium or high potency for 2 weeks or less

What are the side effects of topical steroids?

Striae, atrophy, acne, rosacea, perioral dermatitis, pigmentation abnormalities, glaucoma, and systemic absorption

What two factors may promote systemic absorption of topical steroids?

Prolonged treatment and potent topical steroids

INFECTIOUS DISEASES

VIRAL INFECTION

What is an exanthem?

Acute generalized cutaneous eruption, often symmetrical, associated most commonly with viral infection or drug reaction, occasionally with bacterial infection

What are some common exanthems?

Rubella, roseola infantum, adenovirus, echovirus, measles, scarlet fever, coxsackie A and B, and mononucleosis

What is an enanthem?

Lesions on the oral mucosa (e.g., Koplik spots in patients with measles)

Chickenpox and Herpes Zoster

What is chickenpox?

Highly contagious, primary infection of VZV (herpes family)

What is the route of transmission for chickenpox?

Respiratory route with incubation period of 10–21 days. Sensory nerve ganglia harbor latent infection that may later produce herpes zoster (shingles).

What are symptoms of chickenpox?	Fever, malaise, and pruritic rash. The rate of morbidity increases in adults and immunocompromised patients.
What is the appearance of chickenpox?	"Dewdrop on a rose petal." Crops of vesicles with surrounding erythema that are often excoriated and crusted. An important feature is presence of lesions in all stages of evolution.
What is the distribution of chickenpox?	Starts on the head then "rains down" the body
How is the diagnosis of chickenpox made?	Usually clinically. Tzanck smear or culture can verify the diagnosis.
What is the duration of chickenpox?	New lesions erupt for approximately 5 days, then crusting begins.
What is Reye's syndrome?	A sometimes fatal combination of encephalopathy and hepatitis, most often in children with VZV who have received aspirin
How is chickenpox prevented?	Varicella vaccine is available in the United States with promising effectiveness. It is not known what effect vaccination will have on the incidence of shingles. Vaccination is recommended for all adults with a negative titer, whereas the current trend to vaccinate all children is somewhat controversial.
What is herpes zoster (shingles)?	Acute painful reactivation of the VZV from a dorsal root ganglion in a dermatomal pattern. The most common location is thoracic, but special concern should be given to periorbital or nasal lesions because there is common involvement of the eye.
What is the most common complication of herpes zoster?	Post-herpetic neuralgia in which the pain may last for weeks, months, or years after resolution of the rash. This pain tends to be refractory to treatment. One half of 70-year-old persons are affected.

Warts

What are warts?

Also known as verrucae vulgaris, warts are caused by infection of the epithelium by HPV, which causes epithelial hyperplasia. Warts are common in children and immunosuppressed persons.

What is the appearance of warts?

Appearance varies with location. Often, warts appear as firm papules with typical black dots (thrombosed capillaries) and an irregular surface.

What are complications of warts?

Some types of HPV (e.g., 6, 11, 16, 18, 31, 33), especially genital, predispose the patient to malignancy. If warts are perianal, vulvar, or perimeatal, an internal examination is necessary because there may be mucosal involvement.

What is the treatment for warts?

All numerous treatments, including application of liquid nitrogen, topical acids, and carbon dioxide laser, aim to induce inflammation.

Molluscum Contagiosum

What is molluscum contagiosum?

Small papules usually with central umbilication caused by a poxvirus infection. These are very common.

What are risk factors for molluscum contagiosum?

Attendance at day care centers, sexual activity, and HIV infection

What are symptoms of molluscum contagiosum?

Usually none, but the lesions may itch and become eczematized

What is the distribution of molluscum contagiosum?

Anyplace on the body, but the genital area raises suspicion of sexual transmission

What is the duration of molluscum contagiosum?

Months to years. They often spontaneously regress.

How is the diagnosis of molluscum contagiosum made?

Usually clinically. Lesions may also be curetted and placed on a slide for identification of "molluscum bodies."

What is the treatment for molloscum contagiosum?	Curettage and freezing with liquid nitrogen are the most common treatments.
What diagnosis should be considered in a patient with many molluscum in unusual locations?	HIV infection, especially when lesions are on the face. Many molluscum may also be seen in patients with ectopic dermatitis.

Measles (Rubeola)

What is measles?	Paramyxovirus infection that is rarely seen since administration of the MMR vaccine
What is the incubation period for measles?	8–13 days
What are symptoms of measles?	The three C's: cough, coryza, and conjunctivitis plus high fever and rash
What is the appearance of measles?	Petechiae on the soft palate, then white Koplik spots on the mucosa adjacent to the second molars, followed 1–2 days later by erythematous macules and papules
What is the distribution of measles?	The rash starts postauricular, then moves down to the trunk as upper rash fades, in 24–48 hours.
What is rubella and how does it differ from rubeola?	Because of the vaccine, German measles (rubella) has become a rare viral infection. It is milder than rubeola but significant because it can cause serious congenital defects if infection occurs during pregnancy. German measles should be suspected with an exanthem plus posterior cervical lymphadenopathy.

Roseola Infantum

What is roseola infantum?	A common infection in children aged 6 months to 2 years, which is caused by HHV-6 or occasionally HHV-7
What is the rash in roseola called?	Exanthem subitum

How is the diagnosis of roseola made?	Clinical diagnosis is made by "the rash that follows the fever." Fever lasts 3–5 days; then 1–2 days after defervescence, an exanthematous rash appears. Infants generally appear well.

Erythema Infectiosum

What is erythema infectiosum?	An exanthem common in children age 5–15 years old in winter. It is caused by parvovirus B19 infection and is also called fifth disease.
What are symptoms of erythema infectiosum?	Fever, sore throat, and malaise, followed 1–4 days later by a rash
What is the appearance of erythema infectiosum?	Diagnosis is made by the classic "slapped cheek" appearance, which evolves into reticulate erythema on the trunk, proximal arms, and legs.
What is the treatment for erythema infectiosum?	None is necessary; however, infected pregnant women need to be followed for the possibility of fetal complications.

BACTERIAL INFECTION

Folliculitis

What is folliculitis?	A common superficial bacterial infection of the hair follicle
What infectious agents are associated with folliculitis?	Primarily *Staphylococcus aureus*, also *Pseudomonas*, *Candida*, and *Pityrosporum*
What are risk factors for folliculitis?	Trauma, hot tub use (*Pseudomonas*), prior steroid use, and antibiotics (yeast)
What is the appearance of folliculitis?	Pruritic, scattered erythematous papules and pustules around hair follicles
What is the distribution of folliculitis?	Any hair-bearing area (e.g., scalp, extremities, beard area)
How is the diagnosis of folliculitis made?	Clinically or by culture, with antimicrobial choice based on culture result

Cellulitis

What is cellulitis?	A common infection of skin and underlying soft tissue
What infectious agents are associated with cellulitis?	Most common—group A β-hemolytic streptococci, followed by *S. aureus* In the immunocompromised host—gram-negative rods, including *Pseudomonas* Periorbital location in children—*Haemophilus influenzae* After dog or cat bite—*Pasteurella multocida* After salt water trauma—*Vibrio vulnificus*
What are risk factors for cellulitis?	Diabetes mellitus, intravenous drug abuse, immunocompromised state, trauma, venous stasis, and lymphedema
What are symptoms of cellulitis?	Sometimes fever, chills, mild pain, lymphadenopathy, nausea, vomiting, and confusion, especially in the elderly
What is the appearance of cellulitis?	An erythematous, warm, indurated plaque, which may have red streaks extending from it
What is the distribution of cellulitis?	Extremities are most commonly involved.
What is St. Anthony's fire?	Erysipelas—a rapidly spreading superficial cellulitis most often on the face with well-defined margins
What is the most common cause of St. Anthony's fire?	Group A streptococci
What other diagnosis should be considered in the patient with unilateral edema of an extremity?	Deep vein thrombosis, which requires anticoagulation
What clues help determine the need for surgical consultation in cases of cellulitis?	Crepitus (a sign of gas from bacterial metabolism), extreme pain, dusky cyanosis, and superficial gangrene may be signs of necrotizing fasciitis.

What is necrotizing fasciitis in the genitalia called?	Fornier's gangrene
What diagnostic tests are ordered for cellulitis?	Blood cultures, Doppler ultrasound if a severe infection or clot is suspected. The yield from aspiration culture of leading edge is low.
How is the diagnosis of cellulitis made?	Usually clinically
What is the treatment for cellulitis?	In the uncomplicated patient, staphylococcal or streptococcal coverage is needed; broader coverage is needed in patients with medical problems such as diabetes to cover gram-negative rods.

Erythrasma

What is erythrasma?	A common chronic bacterial infection of the intertriginous areas, caused by *Corynebacterium minutissimum*
What is the appearance of erythrasma?	Sharply demarcated pink to brown macules coalesced into confluent patches with a fine scale
How is the diagnosis of erythrasma made?	Wood's lamp shows coral red fluorescence.

Impetigo

What is impetigo?	A contagious superficial bacterial skin infection, common in children in the summer
What infectious agents are associated with impetigo?	Staphylococci, group A β-hemolytic streptococci
What are risk factors for impetigo?	Poor hygiene and trauma
What is the appearance of impetigo?	A honey-colored crusting of erosions. The presence of bullae implies infection with *S. aureus*.

What is the distribution of impetigo?	Face is most common but any site is possible.
How is the diagnosis of impetigo made?	Usually clinically. Occasionally cultures are obtained.
What is the treatment for impetigo?	Usually oral antibiotics for coverage of staphylococci and streptococci. Topical mupirocin (very expensive) may be given if the lesions are localized.
What is the duration of impetigo?	Lesions should clear in approximately 1 week with treatment.
What complication can follow impetigo?	Post-streptococcal glomerulonephritis, which is caused by certain strains of *Streptococcus pyogenes*
What is scarlet fever?	Toxin produced by *S. pyogenes* usually in the setting of streptococcal pharyngitis
What characteristics help in diagnosis of scarlet fever?	Sandpaper texture of the exanthem, "strawberry tongue," linear petechiae in skinfolds (called Pastia's lines), and desquamation that usually follows the rash

FUNGAL INFECTION

Candidiasis—Mucocutaneous and Intertriginous

What are risk factors for candidiasis?	Diabetes, immunosuppression, oral contraceptive use, obesity, pregnancy, and antibiotics
What are symptoms of candidiasis?	Pruritus and occasionally pain. Or, the patient may be asymptomatic.
What is the appearance of candidiasis?	Oral—white patches on mucosal surfaces and tongue that can be scraped off Vaginal— white cheesy discharge with vaginal inflammation Intertriginous—erythematous plaques, papules, and pustules; well-demarcated raw surface with satellite lesions

What is the distribution of candidiasis?	Any mucosal surface, especially oral and vaginal, and intertriginous skin (e.g., groin and under breasts)
What does involvement of the scrotum imply in cases of superficial fungal infection?	Candida affects the scrotum; tinea cruris does not.
How is the diagnosis of candidiasis made?	Clinically, by KOH prep, and sometimes by culture
What is the treatment for candidiasis?	A wide variety of oral and topical antifungal regimens. Griseofulvin is not effective against yeast and nystatin is not effective against dermatophytes.

Tinea (Dermatophytosis)

What is tinea?	A common superficial fungal infection of keratin-containing skin structures
What three genera of fungi commonly cause tinea?	Microsporum, Epidermophyton, and Trichophyton

What is the name for the dermatophyte infection of the following:

Hand	Tinea manum
Foot	Tinea pedis (scaling of soles in a "moccasin" pattern)
Scalp	Tinea capitis
Beard area	Tinea barbae
Body	Tinea corporis
Groin	Tinea cruris (spares scrotum)
Nails	Tinea unguium
What are risk factors for tinea?	Diabetes mellitus and immunosuppression

What is the appearance of tinea?	Scaly erythematous plaque with an active border and central clearing
What are the laboratory findings in tinea?	KOH prep of scraping reveals hyphal elements. In resistant or questionable cases, fungus may be cultured. Some types of microspora fluoresce bright green under a Wood's lamp.
What is the cause of dystrophic nails?	One half of cases are due to dermatophytes, and the other half are caused by inflammatory diseases (e.g., psoriasis) or trauma. Therefore, before initiating systemic treatment for fungus of the nail, positive KOH or culture must be demonstrated.
What is the treatment for tinea?	Topical or oral antifungals depending on location and severity
What is "two foot, one hand" syndrome?	Common pattern of tinea involvement usually caused by *Trichophytron rubrum*
What is a kerion?	A boggy, inflamed mass, usually on the scalp, representing an immunologic reaction to tinea infection. Treatment is with oral antifungals and if the inflammation is severe, prednisone is used.
What is an "Id reaction"?	A hypersensitivity reaction to a dermatophyte infection that is most often manifested as vesicles on the palms and soles

Tinea Versicolor

What is tinea versicolor?	A common superficial yeast infection caused by *Malassezia furfur*. The rash is asymptomatic or, occasionally, pruritic with pigment alterations.
What is the appearance of tinea versicolor?	Scattered sharp round–oval macules with a fine scale made more obvious by scraping. On light or sun-protected skin, lesions are hyperpigmented; on dark or sun-exposed skin, lesions are hypopigmented.

What is the distribution of tinea versicolor?	Usually the upper trunk and back
How is the diagnosis of tinea versicolor made?	KOH scraping demonstrates "spaghetti-and-meatballs" hyphae.
What is the treatment for tinea versicolor?	A 2.5% selenium sulfide shampoo to the affected area is cost effective, although most antifungal agents are adequate. Reinfection is common. Normal pigmentation does not return until there is tanning.

SEXUALLY TRANSMITTED DISEASES

What is the differential diagnosis of genital ulcers?	Think: "**A**lways **S**how **C**aution **G**etting **L**unch **F**rom **T**he **H**ospital:" **A**phthous ulcers **S**yphilis **C**hancroid **G**ranuloma inguinale **L**ymphogranuloma venereum **F**ixed drug eruption **T**rauma (zipper or factitial) **H**erpes

Syphilis

What is syphilis?	A systemic infection caused by *Treponema pallidum*
What is the incidence of syphilis?	Increasing from 40:100,000 in 1992
What are risk factors for syphilis?	HIV-positive state and promiscuity
What are classic skin signs of primary syphilis?	Painless chancre—ulcer with an indurated border
What are classic skin signs of secondary syphilis?	Condylomata lata—soft, fleshy papules in the genital region "Moth-eaten" alopecia Copper penny macules or papules with erythema on the palms, soles, and trunk

What are classic skin signs of tertiary syphilis?	Noduloulcerative syphilides—plaques and nodules with scalloped edges, with or without ulcers and scale Gummatous syphilis—punched out ulcers on an erythematous base on the scalp, face, and lower extremities
What diagnostic tests are ordered for syphilis?	Venereal Disease Research Laboratory, RPR, flourescent treponemal antibody absorption, dark field microscopy for chancres, and HIV tests
How is the diagnosis of syphilis made?	Clinically with laboratory confirmation. Syphilis is called the "great imitator."
What is the treatment for syphilis?	Intramuscular penicillin G for primary syphilis. RPR tests should be repeated periodically to confirm a decreasing titer, which indicates successful treatment.

Gonorrhea

What is gonorrhea?	"The drip," a genitourinary infection caused by *Neisseria gonorrhoeae*, which is common in young, sexually active adults
What are risk factors for gonorrhea?	Sexual activity and other sexually transmitted diseases
What are symptoms of gonorrhea?	In men, urethral discharge; in women, discharge, pain, fever, or no symptoms
What is the appearance of gonorrhea?	In men, periurethral edema and discharge; in women, vaginal discharge, endometritis, and salpingitis
How is the diagnosis of gonorrhea made?	On clinical grounds plus demonstration of gram-negative intracellular diplococci on Gram stain
What is the treatment for gonorrhea?	Ceftriaxone, 125 mg intramuscularly once, plus doxycycline, 100 mg by mouth twice a day for 7 days

What are signs of disseminated gonorrheal disease?	Tenosynovitis, polyarthralgias, and more than 20 papules or pustules with a necrotic center

Herpes Simplex

What is herpes simplex?	Epithelial infection caused by HSV and reactivation of virus stored latent in nerves
What are risk factors for herpes simplex?	Fever blisters are usually obtained in childhood from relatives. Genital infection is transmitted sexually.
What are symptoms of herpes simplex?	Initial symptoms include fever, malaise, pain, headache, or no symptoms. In recurrent cases, symptoms include pruritic or painful lesions (systemic systems are uncommon in recurrent cases).
What is the appearance of herpes simplex?	Clusters of vesicles or erosions on an erythematous base. In immunocompromised patients, atypical presentation and location may occur.
What is the distribution of herpes simplex?	Mucous membranes, lips, and nose, but any location is possible
How is the diagnosis of herpes simplex made?	Clinically or by Tzanck smear or culture
What is the treatment for herpes simplex?	Acyclovir, valacyclovir, and famciclovir may shorten the duration, but they may be ineffective if not started in the first 24 hours. Generalized infection or infection in an immunocompromised host may require higher dosing or intravenous therapy. A vaccine for HSV-2 is in development.
What is the most common cause of recurring erythema multiforme?	A hypersensitivity reaction following herpes infection
What is herpetic infection of the finger called?	Herpetic whitlow, classically seen in dental hygienists who do not wear protective gloves

What is eczema herpeticum?	Widespread florid herpes infection, usually in patients with eczema (atopic dermatitis)
What is the significance of viral shedding?	Herpes can be detected (and probably transmitted) in infected individuals even when they are asymptomatic.

Condylomata Acuminata

What is condylomata acuminata?	HPV infection of the genital epithelium
Which types of HPV are most common?	6 and 11
Which types are more associated with risk of cancer?	16, 18, 31, and 33
What is the incidence of condylomata acuminata?	It may be the most common sexually transmitted disease.
What are risk factors for condylomata acuminata?	Sexual activity. There is a high rate of transmission with contact.
What is the appearance of condylomata acuminata?	Soft, flesh-colored verrucous papule or plaque that may be pedunculated or cauliflower shaped
How is the diagnosis of condylomata acuminata made?	Clinically (confirmation by biopsy in atypical cases)
What is the treatment for condylomata acuminata?	Freezing with liquid nitrogen or application of topical podofilox or podophyllin. Large lesions may require surgical or laser removal. They often recur because the wart virus is in surrounding normal skin. Sexual partners require examination; most do not realize that they are infected. Women require gynecologic examination, and perirectal involvement requires rectal examination. Association with cancer risk should be discussed with the patient.

Human Immunodeficiency Virus

What skin conditions are associated with HIV infection and AIDS and at what CD4 count?

Table 14–1

Skin condition	CD4 count
Seborrheic dermatitis	450
Onychomycosis, candidiasis	400
Pustular cystic acne	350
Herpes simplex and zoster (often generalized)	300
Bullous impetigo	250
Oral hairy leukoplakia	200
Molluscum contagiosum	150
Xerosis	100
Eosinophilic folliculitis	50

What other skin disorders are seen at any CD4 count?

Condylomata acuminata, psoriasis, verrucae, cryptococcosis (mimicking molluscum), and Kaposi's sarcoma

Is there a rash associated with primary HIV infection?

Yes, a morbilliform exanthem in one third of patients

What is Kaposi's sarcoma?

A tumor derived from proliferative endothelial cells. Recent polymerase chain reaction studies have found HHV-8 particles in all types of Kaposi's sarcoma.

What are the three subvariants of Kaposi's sarcoma seen in patients who are HIV-negative?

1. Classic—occurs in elderly Mediterranean men
2. Immunosuppressed—especially occurs with cyclosporine use
3. African

What is the appearance of Kaposi's sarcoma?

Vascular-appearing macules or nodules that may require biopsy for confirmation

What is the distribution of Kaposi's sarcoma?

Any location, especially the face in HIV-positive patients, and lower extremity in classic variants

What is the treatment for Kaposi's sarcoma?	Because all the treatments have side effects and do not provide a cure, treatment varies per patient. Treatments range from observation (if disease is localized) to radiation, surgical excision, intralesional bleomycin, cryotherapy, or alpha-interferon (if disease is extensive or debilitating).
What skin lesions may be confused with Kaposi's sarcoma in AIDS patients?	Skin lesions of bacillary angiomatosis
What is bacillary angiomatosis?	Skin lesions resulting from the proliferation of small blood vessels
What are the two most common causes of bacillary angiomatosis?	*Bartonella henslae* and *Bartonella quintana*
What is the treatment for bacillary angiomatosis?	Doxycycline
What is oral hairy leukoplakia?	White, asymptomatic, verrucous thickening of the inferolateral surface of the tongue caused by Epstein-Barr virus. It is virtually pathognomonic for HIV infection.
How can oral hairy leukoplakia be differentiated from thrush?	Thrush can be scraped off; hairy leukoplakia cannot.

INFESTATIONS

Scabies

What is scabies?	Common infestation of the skin with a burrowing mite, *Sarcoptes scabiei*, transmitted by skin contact
What is seen on physical examination in scabies?	Linear burrows, papules, and excoriations
What are symptoms of scabies?	Extreme pruritus, especially at night

What is the distribution of scabies?	The wrists and ankles and the webs of fingers and toes are the most classic locations, but scabies also occurs in the pubic area (scrotum in men), lower abdomen, trunk, and legs.
What diagnostic tests are performed for scabies?	Scabies scraping
What is the treatment of scabies?	A variety of scabicides are available. Permethrin and lindane are most effective. A single dose of oral ivermectin (which is not yet available in the United States) also appears to be effective.
What is Norwegian scabies?	Whereas typical infestation involves approximately 20 mites, in Norwegian scabies, thousands of mites infest the patient. It is seen in mentally impaired persons, immunosuppressed patients, and patients with decreased sensation.

Pediculosis (Lice)

What is pediculosis?	Three morphologically distinct louse subtypes cause pubic lice (crabs), body lice, and scalp lice.
How are lice transmitted?	Scalp lice can be epidemic in school children, or they may occur in adults, following close contact or sharing of hats, combs, or brushes. Body lice usually are seen in patients with poor hygiene and reside in clothing seams or sheets. Pubic lice are typically sexually transmitted.
What are symptoms of pediculosis?	Pruritus
What is the appearance of pediculosis on the: Scalp?	A few lice and many nits are seen firmly attached to hairs. Nits are glued to hair shafts close to the scalp. If they appear more than 1 cm from the scalp, they are probably hatched eggs.

Body?	Itchy papules may be seen anywhere on the body and tend to occur in a row (breakfast, lunch, and dinner). The lice are rarely seen because they are nocturnal.
What is the distribution of pubic lice?	Pubic lice are seen clinging to individual pubic hairs. They may also be found on axillary hair, chest hair, and eyelashes.
How is the diagnosis of peliculosis made?	On clinical grounds, with visualization of a louse
What is the treatment for lice?	Scalp—Pyrethrin and piperonyl butoxide or lindane is applied for 10 minutes and the nits are combed out after loosening with vinegar. Body—Clothing and bedding are washed in scalding water. Pubic—Pyrethrin and piperonyl butoxide or lindane are applied. (Pregnant women should not use lindane.)

Cutaneous Larva Migrans

What is cutaneous larva migrans?	Lesion caused by migration of a nematode larva (commonly *Ancylostoma braziliense*) under the skin
What is the epidemiology of cutaneous larva migrans?	Common in southeastern United States coastal areas
What are risk factors for cutaneous larva migrans?	Walking barefoot or sitting on infested sand or soil
What are symptoms of cutaneous larva migrans?	Extreme pruritus
What is the appearance of cutaneous larva migrans?	A thin serpiginous, erythematous trail that advances
What is the distribution of cutaneous larva migrans?	Feet and buttocks
What is the duration of infection in cutaneous larva migrans?	Larvae die in 4–6 weeks because humans are not the natural host.

How is the diagnosis of cutaneous larva migrans made?	Clinically
What is treatment for cutaneous larva migrans?	Thiabendazole topically under an occlusive wrap

ECZEMATOUS DERMATITIS

CONTACT DERMATITIS

What is contact dermatitis?	Pruritic acute or chronic inflammation of the skin caused by contact with either a primary irritant or an allergen
What is the difference between an allergen and an irritant?	Allergens cause type IV hypersensitivity reactions and require prior antigen exposure for reaction to develop. Irritants probably represent 80% of contact dermatitis and do not require prior sensitization. Allergic reaction occurs 1–3 days after exposure, whereas irritant responses tend to follow soon after exposure.
What are the most common causes of allergic contact dermatitis?	Poison ivy and Rhus family plants, nickel, leather, and rubber (washed in bleach)
What is the appearance of contact dermatitis?	Irritant—usually sharp-bordered and erythematous, and may have vesicles that proceed to erosions Allergic—may be more indurated with less distinct borders. In dermatitis caused by poison ivy, oxidized black sap is often seen on the lesions.
What is the distribution of contact dermatitis?	Location may give clues to the cause, for example: nickle (earrings)—earlobes; perfume—neck; toothpaste—perioral; leather—feet.
What diagnostic tests are done for contact dermatitis?	Patch testing. A prepackaged kit, the True Test, contains the 24 most common allergens.

What is the treatment for contact dermatitis?	In acute cases, topical corticosteroids three times per day and cool compresses. The precipitant should be identified and avoided. If the case is severe, a prednisone taper may be indicated. The reaction of poison ivy generally lasts 3 weeks from exposure; "new" lesions may develop over time from the same exposure.

ATOPIC DERMATITIS

What is atopic dermatitis?	A chronic, pruritic eczematous skin disease associated with asthma, hay fever, and allergic rhinitis
What is the natural history of atopic dermatitis?	Commonly starts in infancy and usually (but not always) improves with time
What is the major risk factor for atopic dermatitis?	Family history of allergic disease (80% of cases)
What are symptoms of atopic dermatitis?	Pruritus, which may be severe enough to disrupt normal life and which may worsen in winter or with stress. Exposure to allergens (e.g., dust mites, food antigens, and pollens) may exacerbate the condition.
What is the appearance of atopic dermatitis?	Erythematous plaques and papules with excoriations, dry skin, and lichenification of affected skin
What is the typical distribution of atopic dermatitis?	In infants, extensor surfaces and face; in children, flexural areas (popliteal and antecubital fossae), and hands
What tests are helpful in atopic dermatitis?	Scratch test to specific antigens, serum IgE level, and bacterial cultures of infected excoriations
How is the diagnosis of atopic dermatitis made?	Clinically

What is the treatment for atopic dermatitis?	"Soak and grease": avoidance of soap, wool, and fragrance Tepid baths with bath oil and use of lubricants Topical corticosteroids to relieve inflammation Allergen avoidance in the home Antibiotics for secondary infection
What complications may be seen in patients with atopic dermatitis?	Generalized HSV infection and *Staphylococcus aureus* superinfection

STASIS DERMATITIS

What is stasis dermatitis?	Edema with eczematous skin changes of the lower legs resulting from venous insufficiency
What are symptoms of stasis dermatitis?	Pain, pruritus, or no symptoms
What is the appearance of stasis dermatitis?	Edema, mild scale, weeping, hemosiderin deposits, and lichenification. Lesions may progress to ulceration, particularly at the medial malleolus.
What is the treatment for stasis dermatitis?	Leg elevation, oral antibiotics for superinfection, pressure stockings of 30–40 mm Hg (not on active ulcers), Unna's boot (zinc gelatin) to decrease edema and help healing of ulcers, and DuoDerm over ulcers

LICHEN SIMPLEX CHRONICUS

What is lichen simplex chronicus?	Chronic inflammation and thickening of the skin from constant scratching
What is the incidence of lichen simplex chronicus?	It is a common condition, especially in those with atopic dermatitis.
What is the cause of lichen simplex chronicus?	An itch-scratch-itch cycle is set up and the patient cannot stop scratching. Stress exacerbates the condition.

What is the appearance of lichen simplex chronicus?	Solitary or multiple well-demarcated plaques of itchy, thickened, often hyperpigmented, dry skin
What is the distribution of lichen simplex chronicus?	Hairline, wrists, neck, anal area, and extensor forearms and shins
How is the diagnosis of lichen simplex chronicus made?	Clinically
What is the duration of lichen simplex chronicus?	Chronic for years
What is the treatment for lichen simplex chronicus?	Treatment is difficult. The patient should attempt to keep from scratching to break the cycle. Topical corticosteroids are helpful. Topical doxepin and oral antihistamines may also be useful.

NUMMULAR ECZEMA

What are symptoms of nummular eczema?	Localized pruritus
What is the appearance of nummular eczema?	Coin-shaped pink plaques, dull red in color with dry scale; may ooze and form a crust.
What is the distribution of nummular eczema?	Any skin surface, especially lower legs and arms
How is the diagnosis of nummular eczema made?	On clinical grounds after fungus has been ruled out by a KOH preparation
What is the treatment for nummular eczema?	Lubrication of the skin with or without topical hydrocortisone to relieve inflammation and antibiotics for secondary infection. Despite treatment, the condition is likely to recur.

PAPULOSQUAMOUS DISEASES

PSORIASIS

What is psoriasis?	A skin disease of multifactorial causes, in which epithelial proliferation is increased

What is the incidence of psoriasis?	Common, occuring in 2% of whites in the United States
What are risk factors for psoriasis?	Psoriasis is a disease of Western populations and may be hereditary. Severe psoriasis can occur in HIV-infected patients.
What are symptoms of psoriasis?	Possible pruritus, arthritis in 10% of cases, and dystrophic nails
What is the appearance of psoriasis?	Round or oval "salmon pink" plaques with silvery white scale. When scale is removed, typical spots of bleeding occur underneath (Auspitz sign). Pitting of nails and the appearance of "oil spots" underneath may be seen, and there may be generalized exfoliative erythroderma.
What is the distribution of psoriasis?	Elbows, knees, scalp, and buttocks are most common.
What is the Koebner's phenomenon?	Psoriatic lesions may be induced by trauma (a nonspecific sign as may occur in lichen planus).
How is the diagnosis of psoriasis made?	Clinically
What is the treatment for psoriasis?	Topical—tar, anthralin paste, steroids, calcipotriol, salicylic acid, PUVA, UVA and UVB light Oral—methotrexate and etretinate
What is guttate psoriasis?	Explosive eruption of small psoriatic papules and plaques, often following streptococcal pharyngitis

PITYRIASIS ROSEA

What is pityriasis rosea?	A common erythematous scaling eruption of unknown cause, usually occurring in young adults. It is generally asymptomatic.

What is the appearance of pityriasis rosea?	Starts with an erythematous scaly "herald patch" of several centimeters in diameter, then erupts with pink oval macules on the trunk in a "Christmas tree" pattern
How is the diagnosis of pityriasis rosea made?	Clinically
What is the treatment for pityriasis rosea?	None. The condition generally resolves spontaneously in < 6 weeks.
What infection can mimic pityriasis rosea?	Secondary syphilis (which lacks a herald patch) should always be considered in the differential diagnosis. If there is doubt, an RPR should be ordered.

SEBORRHEIC DERMATITIS

What is seborrheic dermatitis?	A chronic inflamed scaling condition of unknown cause. *Pityrosporum ovale* infection has been implicated as a contributing factor.
What is the incidence of seborrheic dermatitis?	Very common, beginning at puberty (common dandruff); also common in the newborn (cradle cap and diaper dermatitis)
What is the appearance of seborrheic dermatitis?	Erythematous, sometimes pruritic greasy scales and plaques
What is the distribution of seborrheic dermatitis?	Scalp, eyebrows, nasolabial fold, ear canal, chest, and groin
How is the diagnosis of seborrheic dermatitis made?	Clinically
What is the treatment for seborrheic dermatitis?	Ketoconazole shampoo three times per week can be applied to scalp, eyebrows, and skin. Topical steroids are used to control inflammation. The goal is control, not cure.
What is the duration of seborrheic dermatitis?	Chronic exacerbations and remissions

What diagnosis should be considered in adults with florid seborrheic dermatitis?	HIV infection. In the elderly, it may be associated with Parkinson's disease.

INFLAMMATORY DISEASE

ACNE

What is acne?	Inflammation of the sebaceous glands with multifactorial cause, including *Propionibacterium acnes* infection and hormones, commonly the first sign of puberty
What are risk factors for acne?	Family history
What is the appearance of acne?	Open (whitehead) and closed (blackhead) comedones, erythematous papules, and pustules Cystic acne—deep nodules and pus-filled cysts. Even though all lesions can cause scarring, it is more common in cystic acne.
What is the distribution of acne?	Face, chest, back, and neck
How is the diagnosis of acne made?	Clinically
What is the treatment for acne?	Mild—topical Retin-A, benzoyl peroxide, erythromycin, clindamycin, azelaic acid, sulfur, and salicylic acid Moderate—topical agents as for mild cases plus oral antibiotics (tetracycline or erythromycin) Severe resistant cystic—isotretinoin

ROSACEA

What is rosacea?	Chronic inflammation of the central face, commonly involving flushing erythema and intermittent acneiform eruptions. There is a wide spectrum of severity from flushing and telangiectasias to disfiguring papules.

Whom does rosacea affect?	Fair-complected persons of Celtic origin
What is the appearance of rosacea?	Erythema with papules, pustules, and telangiectasia, but no comedones
What is rhinophyma?	Rhinophyma is seen almost exclusively in older men. The nose has a bulbous "W.C. Fields" appearance, which is caused by chronic hyperplasia of the sebaceous glands secondary to rosacea.
What are aggravating factors for rosacea?	Conditions that induce flushing—consumption of alcohol (red wine more than beer more than liquor), hot beverages, and spicy foods
What is the treatment for rosacea?	Avoidance of aggravating factors, 250 mg of tetracycline four times per day, topical metronidazole, and many alternative therapies that are similar to acne treatments. Surgical or laser therapy can be used for rhinophyma.

GRANULOMA ANNULARE

What is granuloma annulare?	Chronic granulomatous inflammation of the dermis
Who does granuloma annulare affect?	It most commonly occurs in children.
What are risk factors for granuloma annulare?	An association with diabetes or thyroid disease is controversial.
What are symptoms of granuloma annulare?	None
What is the appearance of granuloma annulare?	Annular dermal papules spreading outward, varying from flesh-colored to pink or violaceous, with no scale present
What is the distribution of granuloma annulare?	Most commonly, lesions occur on the hands, feet, wrists, and ankles, but they may occur in a generalized form.
How is the diagnosis of granuloma annulare made?	On clinical grounds and by biopsy

What is the treatment for granuloma annulare?	Lesions tend to be recalcitrant although many treatments have been tried.

LICHEN PLANUS

What is lichen planus?	A common, usually pruritic inflammation of the skin and mucous membranes, with a characteristic clinical and histopathologic appearance
What is the pathogenesis of lichen planus?	It is usually idiopathic, but it may be associated with hepatitis C. Lichen planus, especially when extensive, has been associated with many drugs (e.g., thiazides).
What is the appearance of lichen planus?	Think the **5 P's:** **P**urple **P**olygonal **P**ruritic **P**apules **P**laque Lesions heal with hyperpigmentation. In the mouth, lacy reticular white lesions are seen. Chronic, painful mucosal ulcerations occur in both the mouth and vagina. There may be nail loss or pterygium formation.
What is the distribution of lichen planus?	Symmetric, most common in flexor areas, wrist, oral cavity, and genitalia
What are Wickham's striae?	White lacy lines on the surface of lichen planus lesions, best visible with a hand lens after applying oil to the surface of the lesion
How is the diagnosis of lichen planus made?	There is a distinctive clinical picture; occasionally, biopsy is done. Lesions demonstrate Koebner's phenomenon at sites of trauma.
What is the treatment for lichen planus?	The condition is poorly responsive to treatment, although most cases resolve spontaneously in less than 1 year; 50% of oral lesions recur.

DERMATOLOGIC MANIFESTATIONS OF SYSTEMIC DISEASE

SKIN METASTASES

Which cancers commonly metastasize to skin?

Breast (number 1 in women), lung (number 1 in men), colon, and lymphoma

To where do the following cancers metastasize?
Breast

Local skin (peau d'orange, en curasse) and scalp

Lung

Trunk along intercostals and scalp

What is Sister Mary Joseph's nodule?

A round, dark periumbilical nodule representing a cutaneous metastasis, usually of gastric cancer

What is erythema gyratum repens?

A "wood grain" pattern of annular, migrating erythematous bands on the trunk associated with internal malignancy

What is necrolytic migratory erythema?

Erythema, pustules, and erosions typically of the groin that mark a glucagon-producing pancreatic tumor. Necrolytic migratory erythema can mimic candidal infection.

CUTANEOUS T-CELL LYMPHOMAS

What is cutaneous T-cell lymphoma?

Cutaneous lymphomas are predominantly T-cell lymphomas. MF is probably the most common and well described; it is a malignancy of the CD4+ helper T cells.

What is the incidence of cutaneous T-cell lymphoma?

Uncommon but not rare. Occurs in middle-aged people, in men more than women, and in blacks more than whites

What are risk factors for cutaneous T-cell lymphoma?

Human T lymphocyte virus has been detected in some patients.

What is the appearance of cutaneous T-cell lymphoma?

Variable, often starting as nonspecific, large, erythematous, superficial patches with fine scale. It can be serpiginous or annular. The lesions may mimic tinea infection. Later MF evolves into plaques and reddish purple nodules with lymphadenopathy. There may also be hyperkeratosis of palms and soles and alopecia.

What is the distribution of cutaneous T-cell lymphoma?

Often starts on buttocks, thighs, and abdomen, and later becomes generalized

What is the course of cutaneous T-cell lymphoma?

Variable progression

What is Sézary's syndrome?

A variation of MF including erythroderma, lymphadenopathy, and more than 10% atypical lymphocytes in the buffy coat

What is large plaque parapsoriasis?

An eczematous condition involving erythematous patches > 5 cm with fine scale. Progression to MF occurs in 10% of cases.

How is the diagnosis of cutaneous T-cell lymphoma made?

On clinical grounds and by biopsy. The diagnosis of MF may require multiple samples over time; biopsy is required for cell typing.

What is the treatment for cutaneous T-cell lymphoma?

No cure
Conservative—topical nitrogen mustard, topical steroids, and UVB therapy
Aggressive—PUVA, electron beam, and extracorporeal photophoresis

ACANTHOSIS NIGRICANS

What is acanthosis nigricans?

A common hyperpigmented, velvety thickening of intertriginous skin, especially at the back of neck and axillae

What conditions are associated with acanthosis nigricans?	Diabetes mellitus, Cushing's disease, oral contraceptives use, Addison's disease, obesity, hypothyroidism, niacin therapy, and malignancies (90% are abdominal)
What is the most common cancer associated with acanthosis nigricans?	Gastric adenocarcinoma
How is the diagnosis of acanthosis nigricans made?	Clinically
What is the treatment for acanthosis nigricans?	Although no treatment is necessary, Lac-Hydrin may be used, and obese patients should be encouraged to lose weight.

NECROBIOSIS LIPOIDICA

What is necrobiosis lipoidica?	Granulomatous disease of unknown cause
Whom does necrobiosis lipoidica affect?	Usually occurs in young adults and in women more than men
What are risk factors for necrobiosis lipoidica?	Diabetes mellitus and trauma. (Whereas less than 1% of diabetics have necrobiosis lipoidica, most patients with necrobiosis lipoidica have diabetes.)
What are symptoms of necrobiosis lipoidica?	Usually none, but lesions are painful if ulcerated
What is the appearance of necrobiosis lipoidica?	Starts as an erythematous macule, then enlarges into a serpiginous yellow-brown plaque with a waxy atrophic center, telangiectasia, and an elevated shiny border
What is the distribution of necrobiosis lipoidica?	Most are pretibial
How is the diagnosis of necrobiosis lipoidica made?	Usually clinically, with biopsy undertaken if there is doubt

What is the treatment for necrobiosis lipoidica?	Minimal success has been achieved with any treatment, including glucose control.

SKIN MANIFESTATIONS OF DIABETES MELLITUS

What skin conditions are associated with diabetes mellitus?	Think **CENTURY:** **C**ellulitis **E**ruptive xanthomas **N**ecrobiosis lipoidica diabeticorum **T**ense bullae on lower legs (diabetic bullae) **U**lcers **R**ubeosis—chronic flushed appearance of face caused by decreased vasoconstrictor tone and pooling of blood **Y**ellow skin—increased beta carotene levels

PRURITUS

What is pruritus?	An unpleasant sensation of itching
What is the differential diagnosis of generalized pruritus?	Think **DOC HELP X THE DAMN ITCHES:** **D**rugs (opiates) **O**nchocerciasis **C**rabs **H**ookworms **E**xpecting (pregnancy) **L**ymphoma (Hodgkin's disease, MF) **P**araproteinemia **X**erosis **T**hrombocytosis **H**epatic disease **E**lusive infections **D**iabetes mellitus **A**llergies (food) **M**ultiple myeloma **N**euroses **I**ron deficiency **T**hyroid (hyper or hypo) **C**hronic renal failure **H**yperparathyroidism **E**rythrocytosis **S**cabies

What is the basic workup for generalized pruritus?	In-depth H&P for symptoms and signs of conditions in the differential diagnosis, biopsy if there are lesions, complete blood count, hepatic enzymes, blood urea nitrogen, creatinine, thyroid panel, stool for blood, and chest films

RHEUMATIC FEVER

What is the classic rash of rheumatic fever?	Erythema marginatum
What is the appearance of erythema marginatum?	Transient, painless, faint, migratory serpiginous rash
What do subcutaneous nodules appear like?	Painless nodules on the extensor surface of large joints

BACTERIAL ENDOCARDITIS

What are Osler's nodes?	Painful purple-red subcutaneous nodules on finger and toe pads
What are Janeway lesions?	Nonpainful petechial and nodular lesions on the palms or soles
Are Janeway lesions more common in acute or subacute bacterial endocarditis?	Acute
What is the most common cause of splinter hemorrhage of the nails?	Trauma. However, bacterial endocarditis is also in the differential diagnosis, especially when multiple nails are involved, and the splinters are near the nailbed.

SARCOIDOSIS

How commonly is the skin involved in patients who have sarcoidosis?	25% of patients have skin involvement. It is possible to have cutaneous sarcoid without systemic involvement.

What are skin signs of sarcoidosis?

Sarcoidosis is considered a "great imitator," with a wide spectrum of appearances. All lesions are "apple jelly" color when blanched with a glass slide:
Erythema nodosum—most common
Lupus pernio
Scarring alopecia, pruritus, ichthyosis, papules, hypopigmented macules, ulceration

What is lupus pernio?

Cutaneous sarcoidosis manifested as small pink, tan, or violaceous papules on the nose and acral areas that are often associated with upper respiratory disease and granulomas in the bones

Are any of the skin signs pathognomonic of sarcoidosis?

No. Even when sarcoid is clinically suspected, biopsy is almost always done for confirmation. Biopsy shows classic noncaseating granulomas.

What is Lofgren's syndrome?

A combination of sarcoid, eosinophilia, erythema nodosum, bilateral hilar adenopathy, and fever. Prognosis is good.

ERYTHEMA NODOSUM

What is erythema nodosum?

The most common panniculitis, it is an acute inflammation of the subcutaneous fat.

In what group is erythema nodosum seen?

More common in young females

What are common causes of erythema nodosum?

Idiopathic, streptococcal infection, oral contraceptives use, ulcerative colitis, and sarcoidosis

What are symptoms of erythema nodosum?

Pain, fever, and malaise

What is the appearance of erythema nodosum?

Diffuse, warm erythematous nodules that are indurated to touch, producing a very characteristic clinical examination

What is the distribution of erythema nodosum?	Pretibial more than arms, and usually symmetrical
What is the duration of erythema nodosum?	Days to weeks
What diagnostic tests are ordered for erythema nodosum?	Culture for *Streptococcus* and chest film for sarcoid
How is the diagnosis of erythema nodosum made?	Clinically, with confirmation by biopsy if necessary
What is the treatment for erythema nodosum?	NSAIDs, rarely systemic steroids, potassium iodide, treatment of the underlying disease, and bed rest. The condition often recurs.

NUTRITIONAL DEFICIENCIES

What is the vitamin C deficiency syndrome?	Scurvy
What are skin signs of scurvy?	Think **RIPE-C:** **R**ed, bleeding gums **I**mpaired wound healing **P**erifollicular petechiae **E**cchymoses on arms and legs **C**orkscrew hairs
What is the zinc deficiency syndrome?	Acrodermatitis enteropathica, which is characterized by acral and perioral eczematous lesions
What are common causes of zinc deficiency/ acrodermatitis enteropathica?	Generally occurs in infants as an inability to absorb zinc (can be fatal) or can be acquired through malnutrition
What is the disease of niacin deficiency?	Pellagra. Certain drugs such as INH (a niacin analogue) can induce a similar state, as can carcinoid (because of tryptophan consumption).
What are symptoms of pellagra?	The **three D's**—**D**iarrhea, **D**ementia, and **D**ermatitis

What are skin signs of pellagra?	Erythematous, hyperpigmented scaling eruption in a photodistribution
What is the rash around the neck called?	Casal's necklace
Can pellagra be a serious problem?	Yes. Patients can die if not treated.
A bright red, atrophic tongue indicates what deficiencies?	Folic acid and B_{12} (among others)
What causes vitamin B_6 deficiency?	Alcoholism and INH use
What are skin signs of vitamin B_6 deficiency?	Seborrheic dermatitis of the face, angular cheilitis, and glossitis
Which essential fatty acid deficiency can result from prolonged total parenteral nutrition use?	Linoleic acid, causing dry, scaly, easily bleeding lesions, which can be treated by rubbing the skin with sunflower oil
What is koilonychia?	Spoon-shaped nails associated with iron deficiency that may be seen in Plummer-Vinson syndrome
What are cutaneous signs of kwashiorkor (protein malnutrition)?	"Flag sign"—alternating bands of light and dark hair "Enamel paint" dermatosis—hard, scaly erythema
What causes a yellow discoloration to the skin in anorexia?	Excessive carrot eating. This may be distinguished from jaundice because there is no involvement of the sclera.

PORPHYRIA CUTANEA TARDA

What is porphyria cutanea tarda?	The most common of the porphyrias, it is a disease of accumulation of porphyrin metabolites in the skin.
What are risk factors for porphyria cutanea tarda?	Alcoholism and other liver disease, iron overload, HIV infection, drugs (e.g., furosemide, tetracycline, estrogens, and chloroquine), and genetic predisposition

What is unique about porphyria cutanea tarda?	It is the only porphyria that can be acquired or genetic.
What is the deficiency in the genetic form of porphyria cutanea tarda?	Heterozygous uroporphyrinogen decarboxylase deficiency
What viral illness is the acquired form of porphyria cutanea tarda associated with?	Strong association with hepatitis C
What is the appearance of porphyria cutanea tarda?	Scarring blisters on the dorsal hands with milia formation, hypertrichosis of the temples, and variable signs (sclerodermal-like plaques, alopecia, and pigmentary changes)
What is the distribution of porphyria cutanea tarda?	Photodistribution—blisters usually first appear on the dorsa of the hands.
What do diagnostic tests demonstrate in porphyria cutanea tarda?	Urine darkens on exposure to air. Samples fluoresce orange-red under Wood's lamp. Quantitative porphyrin analysis shows uroporphyrins to coprophyrins in a 3:1 ratio.
What is the treatment for porphyria cutanea tarda?	Avoidance of hepatotoxins (stop alcohol consumption) Phlebotomy (1 unit per week) until a hemoglobin of 10 is reached; expect improvement in 3–6 months Low-dose hydroxychloroquine

LYME DISEASE

What is the classic rash of Lyme disease?	Erythema chronicum migrans (or erythema migrans)
What is the appearance of Lyme disease?	Expanding annular rash > 5 cm with central clearing at the site of a tick bite. The rash of erythema chronicum migrans takes several days to enlarge; if there is an immediate rash following tick bite, this may be a hypersensitivity reaction to the bite. The diagnosis of Lyme disease is usually made clinically. A minority of patients notice the tick bite.

What type of tick spreads *Borrelia burgdorferi* (the cause of Lyme disease)?	*Ixodes scapularis*—eastern United States *Ixodes pacificus*—western United States
What is the treatment for Lyme disease?	Doxycycline, 100 mg twice a day for 21 days

THYROID DISEASE

What are skin manifestations of hyperthyroidism?	The **10 Ps:** **P**retibial myxedema **P**almar erythema **P**eriorbital swelling **P**ersistent facial flush **P**oor hair growth **P**ink papules, plaques, and nodules **P**igmentation increased **P**roptosis (exophthalmos) **P**alms are sweaty **P**lummer's nails
What are Plummer's nails?	Onycholysis (nails separating from nail bed) and a scoop-like upward curve on nails
What are skin manifestations of hypothyroidism?	Think **COLD MAN:** **C**oarse hair and skin **O**range palms **L**arge tongue **D**ry skin **M**yxedema (may have pretibial myxedema indistinguishable from hyperthyroidism) **A**lopecia of the lateral one third of the eyebrow **N**ails brittle

CUSHING'S DISEASE

What are skin manifestations of Cushing's disease?	Think **STEROID BLAST:** **S**triae **T**elangiectasia **E**cchymoses **R**ound facies **O**besity, central **I**ncreased hair growth **D**ermatophyte infections

Buffalo hump
Large clitoris
Acne
Skin atrophy
Tinea versicolor

NEUROFIBROMATOSIS TYPE I (VON RECKLINGHAUSEN'S DISEASE)

What are skin signs of neurofibromatosis type I?

Café au lait spots—hyperpigmented macules on the trunk and legs
Neurofibromas— soft, fleshy nodules (up to thousands)
Axillary freckling— Crowe's sign
Lisch nodules— hamartomas of the iris (the most common manifestation of neurofibromatosis type I)

What is the buttonhole sign?

Invagination of neurofibromas when pressed

Are café au lait spots pathognomonic for neurofibromatosis?

No. Diagnostic criteria require more than six lesions of more than 1.5 cm; 10% of normal individuals have one to three café au lait spots.

What anatomic location of neurofibroma is almost pathognomonic for neurofibromatosis type I?

Female areola and nipple

What are characteristics of neurofibromatosis type II?

Bilateral acoustic neuromas, schwannomas, and neurofibromas but no café au lait spots or axillary freckling

What diagnosis should be considered with extensive café au lait macules with a "coast of Maine," or irregular, edge?

Albright's syndrome, which is manifested by bone lesions and precocious puberty in girls. The large macules respect the midline and rarely involve the face.

TUBEROUS SCLEROSIS

What is tuberous sclerosis?

A genodermatosis inherited in an autosomal dominant pattern with mental retardation, seizures, and specific skin changes

What are skin manifestations of tuberous sclerosis?	Ash leaf spots—often the first sign, hypopigmented macules shaped like a thumbprint on thighs and leg Adenoma sebaceum Facial angiofibromas Shagreen patches Periungual fibromas on the nails

MISCELLANEOUS SYSTEMIC DISEASE

What is the differential diagnosis of diffuse hyperpigmentation?	Think **HYPERPIGMENTS:** **H**emochromatosis **Y** **P**orphyria **E**xpecting (pregnancy) a**R**senic **P**heochromocytoma **I**atrogenic—drugs, PUVA therapy **G**ut—malabsorption **M**elanoma **E**xcess thyroid hormone **N** **T**umors—adrenocorticotropin hormone and melanocyte stimulating hormone secreting **S**cleroderma
What are Cullen's sign and Grey Turner's signs?	Periumbilical and flank pooling of blood resulting from hemorrhagic pancreatitis (or ruptured tubal pregnancy)

NAIL SIGNS AND SYSTEMIC DISEASE

What are nail signs of cirrhosis?	Terry's nails—opaque white proximal nail plate with normal-colored distal nails Muehrcke's nails—transverse white bands across nails seen in hypoalbuminemia
What are Beau's lines?	Transverse nail ridges secondary to arrested nail growth during severe illness
What are half-and-half nails?	Lindsey's nails—proximal half of nail bed is white and distal half is brown as is seen in chronic renal failure

What are Mees' lines?	White, transverse nail plate lines secondary to arsenic poisoning or renal failure

BULLOUS DISEASE

What is the differential diagnosis of bullae?	Bullous erythema multiforme, SSSS, TEN, dermatitis herpetiformis, porphyria, renal disease, diabetes, carbon monoxide toxicity, barbiturate use, pemphigus vulgaris, bullous pemphigoid, and epidermolysis bullosa

PEMPHIGUS VULGARIS

What is pemphigus vulgaris?	The most dramatic and serious of the family of pemphigus diseases, pemphigus vulgaris is a chronic, life-threatening, autoimmune bullous disease of mucous membranes and skin, with defective cellular adhesion of epidermal cells.
What is the incidence of pemphigus vulgaris?	Uncommon, occurs at any age
What are risk factors for pemphigus vulgaris?	Jewish or Mediterranean ethnicity
What is the appearance of pemphigus vulgaris?	Flaccid blisters that break easily and become weeping erosions
Where does pemphigus vulgaris start?	On mucous membranes in more than 50% of cases, a distinctive feature that helps in the diagnosis
What is the distribution of pemphigus vulgaris?	It may remain localized to mucous membranes or spread to scalp, face, chest, axilla, and groin.
What is Asboe-Hansen's sign?	The ability to extend a pemphigus vulgaris blister by pressing on the lateral edge
What is Nikolsky's sign?	Creation of a new pemphigus vulgaris blister by pressing on uninvolved skin

How is the diagnosis of pemphigus vulgaris made?	Skin biopsy. Histologic examination reveals a suprabasilar blister and immunofluorescence shows intracellular IgG.
What is the treatment for pemphigus vulgaris?	Systemic steroids, azathioprine, and cyclophosphamide
What is the prognosis for pemphigus vulgaris?	Fatal if untreated and 10% mortality rate with treatment. Exacerbations and remissions occur.

BULLOUS PEMPHIGOID

What is bullous pemphigoid?	Seen in older patients, bullous pemphigoid is a chronic autoimmune blistering disease that is usually not life-threatening.
What is the incidence of bullous pemphigoid?	Much more common than pemphigus vulgaris
What is the appearance of bullous pemphigoid?	Large tense bullae on erythematous or normal skin. A minority of patients have mucous membrane involvement.
What is the distribution of bullous pemphigoid?	Common on lower extremities and flexural areas, but can be generalized
How is the diagnosis of bullous pemphigoid made?	Clinical suspicion is confirmed by biopsy. Histologic examination reveals a subepidermal blister. Immunofluorescence shows deposition of IgG and C3 in the epidermis along the basement membrane.
What is the treatment for bullous pemphigoid?	Tetracycline in mild cases; systemic steroids, azathioprine, and methotrexate in more severe cases
What is the prognosis for bullous pemphigoid?	A self-limited disease, it characteristically remits after years.

OTHER BULLOUS DISEASES

What is dermatitis herpetiformis?	An intensely pruritic, vesicular eruption over extensor surfaces

What is associated with dermatitis herpetiformis?	A gluten-sensitive enteropathy. Lesions disappear when a strictly gluten-free diet is followed.
What is the treatment of choice for dermatitis herpetiformis?	Dapsone
What is SSSS?	Staphylococcal scalded skin syndrome infection is caused by *S. aureus*, which releases an epidermolytic toxin that can act at distant sites, causing a generalized desquamative disease in young children whose kidneys cannot clear the toxin.
How can SSSS be differentiated from TEN?	At times, it is difficult to distinguish between the two by clinical examination, but biopsy reveals a higher cleavage plane in SSSS than in TEN.
From where should the culture be obtained in SSSS?	Mucous membranes

BENIGN SKIN TUMORS

KELOID

What is a keloid?	Overgrowth of scar tissue extending beyond the original site of injury, more common in dark-skinned people
What is the appearance of keloid?	Skin-colored, shiny, protuberant firm nodule
What is the distribution of keloid?	Earlobe and areas of high skin tension (chest, shoulders, and knees)
How is the diagnosis of keloid made?	Clinically. Biopsy should be avoided unless necessary because it may cause further overgrowth.
What is the treatment for keloid?	Intralesional triamcinolone or surgery plus intralesional steroids. Pressure dressings using silicone may help.

DERMATOFIBROMA

What is dermatofibroma?	A firm dermal papule or nodule with ill-defined borders. It is skin colored or hyperpigmented, often occurring on the legs. It exhibits "button-holing" when surrounding skin is pinched, and it may form at sites of insect bites or trauma.
What is the treatment for dermatofibroma?	Treatment is not required unless it is desired for cosmetic reasons.

SEBORRHEIC KERATOSIS

What is seborrheic keratosis?	Benign epidermal proliferation with a greasy "stuck on" appearance, which may contain keratin horns. They can be tan, grey, or black and occur most commonly in elderly white patients.
What is the treatment for seborrheic keratosis?	None necessary
What is the sign of Leser-Trélat?	Explosive growth of seborrheic keratoses associated with gastrointestinal malignancy

SKIN TAG (ACHROCORDON)

What is a skin tag?	A benign pedunculated skin growth associated with obesity and aging. Intertriginous sites and eyelids are the most common sites.
What is the treatment for a skin tag?	Removal only for cosmesis

SUN DAMAGE AND CANCERS

How do sunscreens work?	They block UVB (short wavelength) and sometimes UVA (long wavelength) light by either a chemical or physical process
Which range of UV light causes sunburn?	UVB is the most important cause outdoors, but UVA is used in tanning salons; both contribute to aging and skin cancer.

What does SPF 15 indicate?	Protection from sunburn 15 times longer with the sunscreen than without

ACTINIC KERATOSIS

What is actinic keratosis?	Precancer of epidermis caused by chronic sun exposure (actinic = sun)
What is the appearance of actinic keratosis?	1 mm to 1 cm rough scaling pink patches and papules with indistinct margins
How is the diagnosis of actinic keratosis made?	Clinically. The lesion is often more easily felt by palpation than it is seen. If there is induration, biopsy rules out SCC.
What is the treatment for actinic keratosis?	Reduction of sun exposure, freezing with liquid nitrogen, or curetting. If there are many lesions, topical 5-fluorouracil can be used.
What is the prognosis for actinic keratosis?	1:1000 lesions progress to SCC per year, but SCC develops eventually in 20% of patients with actinic keratoses.

BASAL CELL CARCINOMA

What is basal cell carcinoma?	Malignant neoplasm of epidermal basal cells
What is the incidence of basal cell carcinoma?	It is the most common form of cancer in the world.
What are risk factors for basal cell carcinoma?	Sun exposure and fair skin
What are symptoms of basal cell carcinoma?	Bleeding, itching, or no symptoms
What is the appearance of basal cell carcinoma?	A variety of subtypes have a characteristic clinical appearance: Nodular (most common)—pearly translucent papule with surface telangiectasias Pigmented—shiny blue-black nodule Superficial—red scaly eczematoid patch with or without crust or ulcer

What is the distribution of basal cell carcinoma?	Nose, then nasolabial fold, ear, face, back, and chest, but may occur anywhere
How is the diagnosis of basal cell carcinoma made?	Clinical concern necessitates biopsy or excision.
What is the treatment for basal cell carcinoma?	Excision with margin if small Mohs' micrographic surgery if larger or in a difficult area Radiation
What is the prognosis for basal cell carcinoma?	Spread by direct extension, rarely metastasize
What is nevoid basal cell carcinoma syndrome?	An autosomal dominant genodermatosis with a susceptibility to forming many basal cell carcinomas throughout life

SQUAMOUS CELL CARCINOMA

What is SCC?	Malignant neoplasm of epidermis
What is the incidence of SCC?	20% of all cutaneous malignancies
What are risk factors for SCC?	Sun exposure, family history, and immunosuppression following transplantation
What is the appearance of SCC?	Erythematous, scaling, indurated plaque or hard nodule with smooth or ulcerated surface
What is the distribution of SCC?	Sun-exposed skin and in burns and scars
What is the term for SCC arising in a wound or burn scar?	Marjolin's ulcer
What is the term for SCC in situ of the glans penis?	Erythroplasia of Queyrat
What is the term for SCC in situ of the skin?	Bowen's disease, which may also occur in non–sun-exposed skin

How is the diagnosis of SCC made?	Clinical suspicion necessitates biopsy.
What is the treatment for SCC?	Excision
What is the prognosis for SCC?	Metastasis is location dependent, approaching 15% in high-risk areas such as the lip.

MELANOMA*

What is melanoma?	Malignant neoplasm of melanocytes
What is the incidence of melanoma?	There are 32,000 cases per year in the United States, accounting for 6500 deaths per year. The median age of diagnosis is 53 years old. The incidence has tripled in the United States over the past 40 years, increasing faster than any other cancer.
What are risk factors for melanoma?	Caucasian race, red and blonde hair, fair skin, exposure to light (especially UVB), tendency to develop sunburn, frequent sunburn as a child or adolescent, dysplastic nevus syndrome, xeroderma pigmentosum, family history, and immunosuppression
What other factors should raise suspicion of melanoma?	A new pigmented lesion; a change in color, size, shape, or surface (ulcer, scaling, crusting, or bleeding) of an existing mole; and itching, burning, or pain of an existing mole
What characteristics of a mole suggest melanoma?	Think **ABCDE:** **A**symmetry **B**order (irregular, indistinct) **C**olor (variegated or dark black) **D**iameter (> 0.6 cm) **E**levated from skin surface

---

* In collaboration with S. Meisfeldt and D. Woytowitz

What are the four clinical and histologic subtypes of melanoma?

1. Superficial spreading (70%)
2. Nodular (15%–30%)
3. Lentigo maligna (4%–10%)
4. Acral lentiginous (2%–8%)

What is a Hutchinson's freckle?

Lentigo maligna—a large flat brown macule on older patients. In 10 years, MM develops in one third of these patients.

What is Hutchinson's sign?

Periungual pigmentation associated with subungual (under the nail plate) MM

What is the distribution of melanoma?

Anywhere on the body. Legs are the most common site in women; the back is the most common site in men.

What is the approach to biopsy a suspicious cutaneous lesion?

Excisional biopsy. A punch biopsy can be used if the lesion is of a size or in a location that would result in disfigurement if an excisional biopsy was performed. Biopsy should extend to subcutaneous tissue to allow depth measurement because that is the most important prognostic factor.

What is the treatment for melanoma?

Wide excision if the lesion is localized; chemotherapy if the disease has metastasized

What margins are used in excision of melanoma?

For 1-mm thick lesions: 1 cm; for 2-mm thick lesions: 2 cm

What is the staging for melanoma?

The American Joint Committee on Cancer Staging system:
Stage IA—localized to skin, < 0.75 mm in vertical depth
Stage IB—localized to skin, 0.76–1.5 mm in vertical depth
Stage IIA—localized to skin, 1.5–4.0 mm in vertical depth
Stage IIB—localized to skin, > 4.0 mm in vertical depth
Stage III—local lymphadenopathy involving only one nodal basin; < 5 in transit metastases without nodal metastases
Stage IV—advanced regional metastases or distant metastases

What are poor prognostic factors in melanoma?	Depth of vertical invasion (Breslow's thickness and Clark's level); location on scalp, feet, soles, head and neck, and trunk; male gender; nodular and acral lentiginous histologic subtypes; ulceration; increased mitotic rate; larger tumor volume; microscopic satellites of tumor; older age; and DNA aneuploidy
What are common sites of metastases for melanoma?	Subcutaneous tissue, skin, lymph nodes, bone, liver, spleen, and CNS
What is the workup of a patient with early stage melanoma?	H&P, chest film, and liver function tests. If the patient is asymptomatic, then there is no need to look for evidence of metastatic disease with radiographic tests.

What is the 5-year survival rate for melanoma at the following stages:

I and IIA	80%–90%
IIB and III	40%
IV	< 5%

Is there any adjuvant treatment for melanoma?	Yes. Interferon alpha-2b has been approved for the adjuvant treatment of melanoma stages IIB and III. Studies have demonstrated a 30%–40% rate of improvement in survival in patients receiving interferon.
What is the treatment for metastatic melanoma?	The disease is incurable at this time; therefore, palliation of symptoms is the goal. Surgical resection of symptomatic metastases, if possible, is the best option. Melanoma is relatively radioresistant and chemoresistant; however, local radiotherapy can offer some benefit.

IMMUNE AND AUTOIMMUNE DISEASE (See also Chapter 11)

SJÖGREN'S SYNDROME

What is Sjögren's syndrome?	Autoimmune inflammatory disease consisting of keratoconjunctivitis sicca,

xerostomia, and rheumatoid arthritis, possibly associated with evolution of other connective tissue diseases (sicca complex)

What is the appearance of Sjögren's syndrome?

Keratoconjunctivitis sicca (denuded epithelium of the conjunctiva) and purpura of legs

What are symptoms of Sjögren's syndrome?

Dry mouth and eyes, difficulty speaking, and dyspareunia

How is the diagnosis of Sjögren's syndrome made?

On clinical grounds plus biopsy of salivary gland

What is the treatment for Sjögren's syndrome?

Immunosuppressants and artificial lubricants

SYSTEMIC LUPUS ERYTHEMATOSUS

What is SLE?

Systemic autoimmune disease of connective tissue

What are symptoms of SLE?

Pruritus, pain, arthritis, weight loss, fever, and fatigue

What are subtypes of lupus?

SLE (internal involvement)
Chronic cutaneous—includes discoid (95% remain confined to the skin)
Subacute cutaneous—bright annular rash in sun-exposed areas and no scarring. Half of cases meet criteria for SLE.

What is the appearance of lupus?

SLE—Skin involvement in 75% of patients with lesions being photosensitive; brightly erythematous, macular malar butterfly rash; erythematous papules; bullae; Raynaud's phenomenon; palpable purpura (vasculitis); and periungual telangiectases
Discoid—Scarring plaques usually localized above the neck with dilated follicles and horny plugs
Subacute—Polycyclic, annular lesions on sun-exposed surfaces and upper trunk

What is the distribution of SLE?	Face is most common, but symmetric lesions are seen on arms, legs, fingers, chest, and back.
What is the treatment for SLE?	Steroids, immunosuppressants, and antimalarials (for cutaneous involvement)
What drugs may induce SLE?	Whereas dozens of drugs have been implicated to cause SLE, hydralazine, INH, procainamide, and phenytoin are all common. These drugs mimic the cutaneous lesions of SLE and often have a positive antihistone ANA. HCTZ can cause subacute cutaneous lupus erythematosus (SCLE) and penicillamine can induce discoid lupus erythematosus (DLE)-positive dsDNA.
What is neonatal lupus erythematosus?	Infants are born with transient lupus lesions from placental transfer of maternal antibody, usually resolving spontaneously. There is strong association with permanent heart block, especially with presence of Ro antibody.

SCLERODERMA

What is scleroderma?	A serious, chronic systemic fibrosing disease
What are features of the following subtypes of scleroderma?	
Progressive systemic sclerosis	Occurs in elderly women. More than 95% of patients have Raynaud's phenomenon. There is internal involvement, especially of the heart, lung, and kidney. Sclerosis of the skin is a major diagnostic feature.
CREST	*C*alcinosis cutis, *R*aynaud's phenomenon, *e*sophageal dysfunction, *s*clerodactyly, and *t*elangiectasias
Morphea (localized scleroderma)	Violaceous macules advance to hard, smooth ivory-colored "pigskin" lesions, most common on trunk, with possible motion-limiting joint involvement.

Linear	Lines of sclerosis on extremities or scalp (en coup de sabre), with possible bone atrophy beneath
What are symptoms of scleroderma?	Pain and stiffness of joints, especially the fingers, Raynaud's phenomenon, dysphagia, and weight loss
What is the treatment for scleroderma?	No effective treatment
What is the prognosis for scleroderma?	Progressive systemic sclerosis—slow progression of visceral and skin fibrosis over years Morphea—tends to involute over time

PYODERMA GANGRENOSUM

What is pyoderma gangrenosum?	A chronic ulcerative condition of the skin
What are risk factors for pyoderma gangrenosum?	Inflammatory bowel disease, hepatitis, Behçet's disease, rheumatoid arthritis, SLE, and monoclonal gammopathy. One half of cases are idiopathic.
What is the appearance of pyoderma gangrenosum?	Purple progressing to a painful necrotic ulcer with purple overhanging border
What is the distribution of pyoderma gangrenosum?	Legs, buttock, and abdomen
How is the diagnosis of pyoderma gangrenosum made?	Clinically; biopsy may be needed to rule out other diseases.
What is the treatment for pyoderma gangrenosum?	Steroids, dapsone, minocycline, and cyclosporine

VITILIGO

What is vitiligo?	An autoimmune disorder resulting in destruction of melanocytes and depigmentation
What is the appearance of vitiligo?	Depigmented patches that are more disfiguring in dark-skinned patients

What diseases are associated with vitiligo?	Graves' disease and Addison's disease
What is the distribution of vitiligo?	Starts distally on fingers or penis, and may spread anywhere
How is the diagnosis of vitiligo made?	Clinically
What is the treatment for vitiligo?	In light-skinned patients, no treatment may be necessary other than skin protection; in dark-skinned patients, topical steroids may be given for local disease. PUVA therapy may be effective in restoring skin pigment; in severe cases, chemical depigmentation of the remaining skin may be necessary.

ALOPECIA AREATA

What is alopecia areata?	Autoimmune process characterized by localized loss of hair
What is the incidence of alopecia areata?	Most common in young people
What is the appearance of alopecia areata?	Round area of hair loss without skin lesions, with no scarring. There may be diagnostic "exclamation point" hairs, which are thinner at the base than at the end. Alopecia areata can progress to complete body hair loss in alopecia universalis. There may also be nail pitting.
How is the diagnosis of alopecia areata made?	Usually clinically
What is the treatment for alopecia areata?	There is no cure, but intralesional steroid injections may stimulate hair growth at least temporarily. It takes approximately 1 month to see results and new hairs may initially be white. Sometimes oral steroids are used.

What is the prognosis for alopecia areata?	In 75% of patients, hair regrows after treatment. In many patients, regrowth is spontaneous. Younger age, more extensive loss, atopic diathesus, and ophiasis (hatband loss) are poor prognostic indicators.

DERMATOMYOSITIS

What is dermatomyositis?	A systemic autoimmune disease with inflammation of skin and muscles
What is the age of onset for dermatomyositis?	Occurs from infancy to old age
What association is made with dermatomyositis?	In patients older than 60 years, there is a strong association with internal malignancy.
What are symptoms of dermatomyositis?	Fever, weight loss, arthralgias, and proximal muscle weakness
What is the appearance of dermatomyositis?	May have butterfly malar rash, photosensitivity, periorbital heliotrope rash; periorbital edema; periungual telangiectasias; Gottron's papules (flat-topped violaceous papules); calcinosis cutis (more common in juvenile diabetes mellitus); and Raynaud's phenomenon (one third of patients)
How is the diagnosis of dermatomyositis made?	On clinical grounds, plus laboratory findings of elevated CK and ANA
What is the treatment for dermatomyositis?	Steroids plus immunosuppressants

DERMATOLOGIC URGENCIES AND EMERGENCIES

What are some of the dermatologic urgencies and emergencies?	Bullous pemphigoid, pemphigus vulgaris, SSSS, toxic shock syndrome (see Bullous Disease); cutaneous vasculitis; RMSF; and meningococcemia

ERYTHEMA MULTIFORME

What are causes of erythema multiforme?	HSV-1 infection, by far, is the most common cause; other factors include hepatitis A or B infection, pregnancy, drugs, and streptococcal infection.
What are symptoms of erythema multiforme?	Pruritus, fever and malaise, arthralgias and headache, or no symptoms
What is the appearance of erythema multiforme?	Erythematous "target lesions," papules, and plaques
What is the distribution of erythema multiforme?	Often localized to extremities
What is the treatment for erythema multiforme?	Stop any potentially offending drug. Prophylactic acyclovir should be considered in recurrent HSV-induced erythema multiforme
What is the prognosis for erythema multiforme?	Episodes usually resolve in 2–3 weeks. The major concern is progression to Stevens-Johnson syndrome.

STEVENS-JOHNSON SYNDROME

What is Stevens-Johnson syndrome?	Extensive cutaneous and mucosal involvement, often with atypical target lesions, vesicles, and erosions. Stevens-Johnson is predominantly a drug reaction and may be fatal.
Which medications are the most common culprits in Stevens-Johnson syndrome?	Phenobarbital, phenytoin, beta-lactams, sulfonamides, and NSAIDs

TOXIC EPIDERMAL NECROLYSIS

What is TEN?	Severe, extensive full epidermal thickness necrosis associated with a high mortality rate
What is the appearance of TEN?	Bullae, exfoliation, mucosal involvement, and nail loss are common.

What is the cause of TEN?	Generally a drug reaction
What is the treatment of TEN?	Stop all medications, correct electrolyte imbalances, administer pain control, and give antibiotics as needed. Supportive and aggressive skin care in a burn unit is recommended. Use of systemic corticosteroids is controversial.

EXFOLIATIVE ERYTHRODERMA

What is exfoliative erythroderma?	A severe, generalized red inflammation and exfoliation of the skin
What are common causes of exfoliative erythroderma?	Think **D-SCALPP:** **D**rug eruptions **S**eborrhea **C**ontact dermatitis **A**topic dermatitis **L**ymphoma **P**ityriasis rubra pilaris **P**soriasis
What are symptoms of exfoliative erythroderma?	Pruritus, chills, fevers, or no symptoms
What is the treatment for exfoliative erythroderma?	Admit patient to hospital, stop all medications, give topical or oral steroids, "soak and grease," and monitor fluids and electrolytes. Skin biopsy may help confirm the diagnosis.
What severe consequence may follow erythroderma?	High-output cardiac failure from increased blood flow through skin

MENINGOCOCCEMIA

What are skin signs of meningococcemia?	Petechiae and purpura on the lower extremities and trunk. Larger lesions with stellate, sharp, angulated borders with central necrosis are caused by septic emboli.

ROCKY MOUNTAIN SPOTTED FEVER

What is the rash of RMSF?	Petechiae and ecchymoses begin on the wrists and ankles and spread to the palms and soles. They later generalize and become purpuric.

DRUG ERUPTIONS

What are the three most common drug eruptions?	1. Morbilliform exanthem 2. Urticaria 3. Fixed drug eruption
How common are drug eruptions?	Occur in 3% of hospitalized patients

FIXED DRUG ERUPTION

What is a fixed drug eruption?	Inflammation of the skin resulting from ingested drug
What is the incidence of fixed drug eruption?	Common
What are symptoms of fixed drug eruption?	None
What is the appearance of fixed drug eruption?	Well-circumscribed red to purple macule on the skin or mucous membranes
What is the distribution of fixed drug eruption?	Same location each time the drug is taken
How is the diagnosis of fixed drug eruption made?	Clinically
What is the treatment for fixed drug eruption?	Stop the offending drug.

PALPABLE PURPURA

What is palpable purpura?	Vasculitic inflammation (vasculitis)
What is the differential diagnosis for palpable purpura?	Connective tissue disease Henoch-Schönlein purpura Internal malignancy (lymphoma and leukemia) Polyarteritis nodosa Wegener's granulomatosis Infection Cryoglobulinemia Churg-Strauss disease Drugs Idiopathic

15 ___ Pharmacology

ABBREVIATIONS

ABBREVIATIONS

EPS	Extrapyramidal side effects
MBC	Minimum bactericidal concentration
MIC	Minimum inhibitory concentration
PAE	Postantibiotic effect
SSRI	Selective serotonin reuptake inhibitors
TCA	Tricyclic antidepressants

PHARMACOKINETICS AND PHARMACODYNAMICS

What is the difference between kinetics and dynamics?	Pharmacokinetics refers to the effect of the body's function on the absorption, distribution, metabolism, or elimination of a drug; pharmacodynamics is the concentration-related effect of the drug on a body or organism.
What is half-life?	The time required for the serum concentration of a drug to decrease by one half. This may not always correspond to duration of therapeutic effect.
What major factors affect the pharmacokinetics of drugs?	Renal and hepatic function affect elimination and metabolism; protein binding and fluid status affect distribution.
What two plasma proteins are important for protein binding of drugs?	Albumin commonly binds acidic drugs (e.g., phenytoin), and α_1-acid glycoprotein commonly binds basic drugs (e.g., lidocaine).

What parameter is commonly used to estimate renal function?	Serum creatinine
Which laboratory parameters are useful to estimate hepatic function?	There are no reliable indicators of metabolic capacity. In general, bilirubin indicates the ability of the liver to conjugate, and prothrombin time indicates the synthetic capacity of the liver.
What are the two major types of metabolism?	Phase I reactions (e.g., oxidation, reduction, and hydrolysis) usually convert the substances to active metabolites. Phase II reactions (conjugation to form glucuronides, sulfate, or acetates) usually convert substances to inactive metabolites. Phase II reactions generally require less functional metabolic capacity than do phase I reactions.
What are common hepatic enzyme inducers?	Carbamazepine, ethanol (chronic), phenobarbital, phenytoin, rifampin, and tobacco
What are common hepatic enzyme inhibitors?	Cimetidine, ethanol (acute), erythromycin, ketoconazole, omeprazole, ciprofloxacin, and valproic acid
What are common medications that are dependent on hepatic blood flow for clearance?	Lidocaine, theophylline, and cimetidine

What alterations in pharmacokinetics and pharmacodynamics affect drug therapy in elderly patients?	1. Pharmacokinetics
	   Distribution—patients have less lean body mass and total body water, and reduced serum albumin concentrations
	   Metabolism—patients have less capability to metabolize through the phase I pathway
	   Excretion—patients have reduced renal blood flow, glomerular filtration rate, tubular secretion, and creatinine clearance

2. Pharmacodynamics. Changes in receptor sensitivity must be considered for older patients. These alterations occur over a period of years and exhibit great variability between patients.

Does variability in pharmacokinetics affect drug therapy in pediatric patients?

Yes. Changes in absorption (e.g., changes in gastric pH and reduced gastrointestinal motility), distribution (e.g., increased volumes of distribution and reduced serum albumin levels and protein-binding sites), metabolism, and excretion occur throughout the developmental stages in neonates to adolescents.

PHARMACOKINETICS AND PHARMACODYNAMICS IN INFECTIOUS DISEASE

What patient-specific parameters must be considered when selecting and dosing antibiotics?

Identified or suspected organisms
Type and severity of infection
Perfusion at the site of infection
Renal function
Hepatic function
Clinical status

Why are patient-specific parameters important in selecting and dosing antibiotics?

Knowing the specific or suspected organisms determines the appropriate antibiotic selection. Knowing the severity of infection, clinical status, and ability to perfuse the site help the clinician decide the antibiotic dosage, route, and dosing interval. Renal or hepatic dysfunction may alter drug dosing.

What basic pharmacologic concepts must be considered when selecting and dosing antibiotics?

The time that the antibiotic concentration remains above the MIC, hospital susceptibility patterns, and concentration-dependent killing effects of antibiotics

What is MIC?

Minimum inhibitory concentration, that is, the minimum concentration of antibiotic required to inhibit the growth of an organism

What is MBC?

Minimum bactericidal concentration, that is, the minimum concentration of antibiotic required to kill an organism

What is the significance of the MBC:MIC ratio?

The MBC:MIC ratio more accurately reflects the actual bactericidal ratio in vivo. An MBC:MIC ratio greater than 32 indicates that an organism is tolerant to a particular antibiotic. This phenomenon has been known to occur with β lactams (penicillin and cephalosporins) and glycopeptides (vancomycin) against staphylococci, streptococci, and enterococci.

How does the MIC affect drug selection?

The lower the MIC for an organism to an antibiotic, the more susceptible the organism is to the drug. The longer the serum drug concentrations remain above the MIC, the greater the killing effect of the antibiotic.

When susceptibility reports from the laboratory are expressed as MIC, is the antibiotic with the absolute lowest MIC always the best choice?

No. The absolute value of the MIC must be considered in conjunction with factors such as absorption, protein binding, and volume of distribution, all which affect the concentration of the antibiotic at the site of infection.

What is concentration-dependent killing?

Antibiotics that exhibit this phenomenon demonstrate a linear relationship between killing rate and concentrations above the MIC for a particular organism. The higher the peak serum concentration, the faster and more complete the bactericidal effect. Concentration-dependent killing has been demonstrated for aminoglycosides and quinolones. These antibiotics may be more effective when the total daily dose is given in higher doses at less frequent intervals.

What is concentration-independent killing?

For some antibiotics, the relationship between killing and concentration "flattens out" once the concentration exceeds 4 to 5 times the MIC. This is generally true with β lactams and glycopeptides. For these agents, the more rational dosing approach is to maintain the concentration 4 to 5 times the MIC for extended time periods.

What is PAE?

Postantibiotic effect refers to the continued suppression of bacterial growth beyond the time that the antibiotic is present at the site of infection. Examples of antibiotics with PAE are β lactams and aminoglycosides against some gram-negative organisms and the addition of rifampin to aminoglycoside and penicillin regimens in treating some staphylococcal infections.

What are hospital susceptibility patterns?

Susceptibility and resistance patterns of particular antibiotics to selected organisms at specific hospitals or institutions

PHARMACOKINETICS AND PHARMACODYNAMICS IN NEUROLOGY

Why are so many drug interactions associated with antiepileptic agents?

Antiepileptic agents may cause drug interactions through hepatic enzyme induction (e.g., phenytoin, phenobarbital, and carbamazepine), hepatic enzyme inhibition (e.g., valproic acid), or because of increased protein binding (e.g., phenytoin).

Which antiepileptic agents require therapeutic drug level monitoring?

Phenytoin, phenobarbital, carbamazepine, and valproic acid. The newer antiepileptics (e.g., gabapentin, and felbamate) do not have established therapeutic ranges and currently require no drug level monitoring.

Why monitor antiepileptic agents for therapeutic drug levels?

To monitor efficacy and toxicity. The clinician should treat the patient, not the drug level.

What are the therapeutic ranges for:
   Carbamazepine?

4–12 mg/L

Phenobarbital?	10–30 mg/L
Phenytoin?	5–20 mg/L
Valproic acid?	50–100 mg/L

What other therapeutic uses do antiepileptic agents possess?

Treatment for a variety of neuropathies and pain syndromes

Do the same drug level monitoring requirements apply for other uses of antiepileptic agents?

Yes. Again, the clinician should treat the neuropathic or pain syndrome, not the drug level.

PHARMACOLOGIC PEARLS IN PULMONOLOGY

Can all aerosolized oral inhalers be administered on an as-required basis?

No. Only short-acting inhaled β agonists (e.g., albuterol and metaproterenol) may be used as required for dyspnea, because these agents have a rapid onset of action. The long-acting agents (e.g., salmeterol, triamcinolone, beclomethasone, cromolyn, nedocromil, and ipratropium) are most effective when administered on a regularly scheduled basis.

PHARMACOLOGIC PEARLS IN NEPHROLOGY

What types of drugs typically require adjustments for renal failure?

Any drug that is primarily cleared by the kidney requires dosing adjustments in renal dysfunction. Among these drugs are antibiotics and H_2 antagonists. In addition to reduced renal clearance of drugs, renal failure (primarily end-stage renal disease) may also alter the protein binding of drugs and result in higher free (active) serum drug concentrations of such drugs as phenytoin and digoxin. These types of agents may also require dosing adjustments.

Is the response to diuretic therapy altered in patients with decreased renal function?

Patients with a creatinine clearance of approximately 30 ml/min or less may not respond to thiazide diuretics (e.g., HCTZ). As renal function continues to decline, the response to loop diuretics (e.g., furosemide and bumetanide) may also be altered, and the use of the combination of a loop diuretic plus metolazone may be needed. When metolazone is used, it need be administered only once daily (regardless of the frequency of administration for the loop diuretic).

PHARMACOLOGIC PEARLS IN PSYCHIATRY

AGENTS USED FOR SLEEP

What drugs may commonly be used for insomnia?

Benzodiazepines, chloral hydrate, diphenhydramine, and zolpidem

How long should insomnia be treated?

Transient insomnia that is not secondary to an underlying medical or psychiatric illness should be treated on an as-required basis for several nights only.

Of the common agents used for insomnia, is diphenhydramine the safest?

Although the adverse effect profile of diphenhydramine appears relatively benign, diphenhydramine possesses anticholinergic properties that must be considered when given to elderly patients, in whom there may be a paradoxical reaction, and to patients with cardiac conduction abnormalities.

ANTIANXIETY AGENTS

Should outpatients using as-required benzodiazepines be continued on these agents during a hospital stay?

It is important to determine the true frequency of use by the patient at home. If the patient uses the drug frequently at home, failure to continue the drug during hospitalization may result in signs and symptoms of drug withdrawal.

Are antianxiety agents affected by organ dysfunction?

Yes. Most benzodiazepines are metabolized in the liver.

ANTIDEPRESSANTS

What adverse effects are most commonly seen with antidepressants?

Sedation, anticholinergic properties, orthostatic hypotension, cardiac conduction irregularities, and seizures

Which antidepressants are associated with the most anticholinergic effects?	TCAs (e.g., amitriptyline, doxepin, imipramine, nortriptyline, and desipramine)
What antidepressants are associated with the least anticholinergic effects?	Trazodone, bupropion, and SSRIs (e.g., fluoxetine, paroxetine, sertraline, and fluvoxamine)
Which antidepressents are commonly associated with orthostatic hypotension?	Trazodone and some TCAs
Which antidepressants are most commonly associated with irregularities in cardiac conduction?	TCAs
How are seizures associated with antidepressants?	Any of the antidepressants may lower a patient's seizure threshold.
How is sedation associated with antidepressants?	Sedation may occur less frequently with SSRIs and bupropion than with TCAs or trazodone.

ANTIPSYCHOTIC AGENTS

What are the most common adverse effects seen with antipsychotic agents?	EPS effects (e.g., pseudoparkinsonism, dystonia, and akathisia), sedation, anticholinergic effects, and cardiovascular effects (e.g., orthostasis and electrocardiographic changes)
What "rules of thumb" apply in association with psychotropic drug type and adverse reactions?	Low-potency agents (e.g., thioridazine and chlorpromazine) have a greater propensity toward anticholinergic, cardiac, and sedative effects, and possibly less propensity toward EPS. Higher potency agents (e.g., haloperidol) have greater propensity toward EPS. Agents in the midpotency range produce variable adverse drug reactions.

Section III

The Consultant

16   The Consultant

ABBREVIATIONS

BUN	Blood urea nitrogen
CABG	Coronary artery bypass grafting
CBC	Complete blood count
CHF	Congestive heart failure
COPD	Chronic obstructive pulmonary disease
DVT	Deep venous thrombosis
ECG	Electrocardiogram
FEV$_1$	Forced expiratory volume over the first second
FVC	Forced vital capacity
JVD	Jugular venous distention
MI	Myocardial infarction
MRSA	Methicillin-resistant *Staphylococcus aureus*
NPO	Nothing by mouth
PFT	Pulmonary function test
PVC	Premature ventricular contraction
VPB	Ventricular premature beat
VT	Ventricular tachycardia

ROLE OF THE MEDICAL CONSULTANT

What is the role of the medical consultant?

To provide expertise in medical areas of patient care, often when the patient's primary care team specializes in an area other than internal medicine. For example, a patient scheduled for surgery may have a cardiac condition that should be evaluated before the patient undergoes anesthesia.

When is a medical consult called?

When the patient's primary care team requests internal medicine input regarding a specific clinical question or condition

Is the consultant responsible for generating the clinical question?

It is the consultant's job to identify the clinical question under consideration if it is not initially made clear by the primary care team.

When should the consult be carried out?

Consults may be emergent, urgent, or elective. It is important to determine the nature of the consult and to respond appropriately. For example, a patient with dysrhythmias and hemodynamic instability warrants immediate attention. In general, a courteous and rapid response to any consult is appreciated by the primary team.

What data should the consultant use to answer the clinical question?

The consultant gathers established data from the patient's chart and primary care team. The consultant then generates additional information needed to "fill in the gaps" by performing a focused history and physical examination. It is always important to see the patient and gather additional data as a consultant.

How broad are the recommendations generated by the consultant?

The recommendations are usually relatively narrow in scope and limited to those needed to answer the clinical question posed to the consultant. The consult recommendations are considered to be goal directed.

Are any peripheral recommendations appropriate?

Yes. Under some circumstances, it is appropriate to provide contingency plans. In a patient whose condition is changing or who may fail an initial therapeutic recommendation, it may be helpful to include a backup plan.

Should there be any other information included in the consult?

Often, it is appropriate to (tactfully) share one's expertise with the primary team by providing a recent, concise article from a journal that the primary team is unlikely to have been exposed to, such as a frontline specialty journal. This is never a substitute for direct communication with the primary team regarding recommendations but is solely supplemental.

How are the consultant's recommendations reported?

The recommendations are recorded in writing in the patient's chart on the consult note. Specific recommendations including drug dosages and tests to be ordered should be written succinctly and be clearly visible. They should also be communicated directly to the referring attending or resident physician, providing an opportunity for questions and clarification. Medical students involved in calling consults for their team are often eager for the answers to the clinical questions about their patient's care and are grateful to be included when recommendations are reported.

Whose responsibility is it to ultimately decide how and whether or not to carry out a consultant's recommendations?

The patient's primary care team. If patient care is significantly compromised by failure to carry out the recommendations, then it may be appropriate for the consultant to discuss them again with the primary team. It is not appropriate to engage in "chart wars."

How long should the consulting team follow up the patient?

Each case varies, but, generally, the consulting team should not sign off the case in the same day that the consult was called. The patient is generally followed up until the clinical questions at hand are resolved or until the consult team is no longer providing useful input. Until then, appropriate follow up and continuity are appreciated by the primary team. After signing off the case, the consultant should indicate willingness to become involved again if the patient's status changes.

PREOPERATIVE CLEARANCE OF THE SURGICAL PATIENT

Why is it important to clear patients for surgery?

To assess the patient's risk for cardiac and other adverse events. Any existing medical problems can be treated before surgery to maximize the patient's chances of having an uneventful procedure and recovery. This is especially important before elective surgery because clearance is a process of weighing the need for surgery against the risk of surgery. A higher level of risk is tolerated when a patient needs emergency abdominal surgery than when the patient is undergoing elective cholecystectomy.

Other than specific medical illness, are there any general risk factors for patients undergoing surgery?

Yes. Age is a contributor to surgical risk. Patients younger than 65 years of age have a 1% mortality rate, whereas those older than 65 years of age have a 5% mortality rate.

When does death occur during the surgical course?

During surgery, 35%; during induction of anesthesia, 10%; within 48 hours of surgery, 55%

What is the most important tool for assessing risk associated with surgery for cardiovascular patients?

The history and physical examination is the most important element of the evaluation. Many patients need no further workup before surgery.

When is a preoperative ECG indicated?

Patients with a history of cardiac disease, or with history and physical examination findings that suggest cardiac disease (e.g., diabetes mellitus, atherosclerosis, hypertension, dysrhythmias, certain malignancies, collagen vascular diseases, and infectious diseases) should have a preoperative ECG. ECGs should also be obtained in patients undergoing intrathoracic, intraabdominal, aortic, or emergency surgery. Lastly, any patient at risk for electrolyte abnormality, any patient taking a potentially cardiotoxic medication, any man older than age 45 years, or any woman older than age 55 years should have an ECG before surgery.

When should preoperative chest films be obtained?

This study is associated with false-positive results if ordered in the absence of an indication on the history and physical examination. Indications include a medical history of cardiovascular disease (e.g., valvular disease, CHF, and coronary or cerebrovascular disease) or pulmonary disease (e.g., asthma, COPD, occupational lung disease, and tobacco use), or a history of a malignancy. Age greater than 60 years or symptoms and signs of an infection are also indications.

What are the two most important risk factors for significant postoperative cardiac events?

Presence of CHF and MI within the last 6 months

What is a significant cardiac event?

Sudden death, MI, unstable angina, pulmonary edema, or serious dysrhythmia (e.g., such as ventricular tachycardia or ventricular fibrillation)

What is the risk that a patient who undergoes surgery and who has had a prior MI will have another such cardiac event?

The risk depends on how recently the patient experienced the cardiac event. In general, the risk of subsequent MI is approximately 5%. In the first 3 months after an MI, however, the risk is approximately 30%, and, in the following 3 months, the risk is approximately 15%. After the initial 6 months, the risk is assumed to be 5%.

What is the risk of a cardiac event occurring in a surgery patient without a cardiac history?

Approximately 0.5% (10 times less than in a patient with cardiac history)

How does the presence of unstable angina affect operative risk?

Although angina has not been definitively established as an independent predictor of postoperative complication, patients with unstable angina should generally not undergo surgery (except CABG). These patients should have their extent of disease defined and should receive appropriate medical therapy.

Can patients who have undergone CABG then undergo other surgery?

Patients who have undergone CABG have about a 1% incidence of a cardiac event when undergoing surgery.

What important elements of patient history should be discussed with cardiac patients about to undergo surgery?

Previous MI, chest pain, dyspnea, syncope, dysrhythmias, history of rheumatic fever, and history of diabetes

What elements of the physical examination are especially important for cardiac patients about to undergo surgery?

Vital signs are important as are jugular venous distention, bruits, slow carotid upstroke, displaced point of maximal impulse (PMI), murmurs, S3 gallop, and rubs.

What is the Goldman scale?

Developed in 1977, the Goldman scale quantifies operative risk for MI based on several variables assessed by history, physical examination, and simple laboratory data. Each variable is assigned a value based on its contribution to relative risk. The effect of the variables on noncardiac complications is not assessed.

What nine variables are associated with an increased risk of perioperative MI or death in Goldman's work and what were their point values?

Table 16–1

Variable	Point Value
Third heart sound or JVD	11
Myocardial infarction within 6 months	10
Nonsinus rhythm	7
> 5 PVCs per minute	7
Age > 70 years	5
Emergency procedure	4
Hemodynamically significant aortic stenosis	3
Aortic, intraabdominal, or intrathoracic surgery	3
Poor general health	3

How do the point values help determine perioperative risk?

Table 16–2

Points	MI, Pulmonary Edema, VT	Death
0–5	0.7%	0.2%
6–12	5.0%	2.0%
13–25	11.0%	2.0%
>26	22.0%	56%

What is "hemodynamically significant" aortic stenosis?

Indicators of significance (in the absence of echocardiography) are poor exercise tolerance, a history of syncope, CHF or angina, a late-peaking systolic murmur, delayed pulses, and absence of the aortic component of the second heart sound (A2).

Dysrhythmia is more likely to result in complications of what nature?

Dysrhythmias are primarily useful as a marker for patients with ischemic disease and are therefore more associated with ischemic complications rather than dysrhythmic ones.

Is hypertension a marker for an increased risk of cardiac complications?

By itself, no, although diastolic pressure greater than 110 mm Hg is sometimes considered a relative contraindication to elective surgery. When hypertension is a manifestation of other serious illness such as renal artery stenosis, hyperaldosteronism, or pheochromocytoma, the illness should be treated before the patient undergoes elective surgery.

Should patients who are NPO take blood pressure medication on the morning of surgery?

Yes, unless otherwise instructed. By not taking such previously prescribed treatment, the patient is predisposed to perioperative blood pressure variability and postoperative cardiac complications. The major risks of anesthesia are related to hypotension and rebound hypertension.

Does regional anesthesia reduce the rate of postoperative cardiac complications compared to that of general anesthesia?

Except in patients with CHF, the type of anesthesia selected does not alter outcome with regard to cardiac status. However, the notion has intrinsic appeal and regional anesthesia is therefore often used in sicker patients undergoing surgery. The ultimate choice of anesthetic is appropriately left to the anesthesiologist, with input from the primary and consult teams.

PREOPERATIVE EVALUATION OF LUNG FUNCTION

What is the most important element of evaluation of pulmonary function?

Patient history and physical examination

List factors that predispose the patient to pulmonary complications.

Obesity, smoking, COPD, chronic bronchitis, type of surgery or incision, asthma, occupational lung disease, neuromuscular disease, coma, nutritional depletion, acidosis, tracheal intubation, hypotension, hypoxemia and azotemia are all potential contributors to postoperative pulmonary complications.

What are some potential postoperative pulmonary complications?

Postoperative pulmonary complications can be infectious (e.g., pneumonia, empyema, and bronchitis) or noninfectious (e.g., atelectasis, pneumonitis secondary to aspiration, and adult respiratory distress syndrome).

Does a patient benefit from quitting smoking shortly before undergoing surgery?

Yes. Improvement in lung function and mucociliary clearance is detectable in less than 1 month after quitting. Patients who quit smoking 8 weeks before surgery have a statistically significant decrease in the number of pulmonary complications compared with those who do not. This is independent of functional status as assessed by PFTs. In addition, carboxyhemoglobin levels decrease quickly, thus improving oxygen delivery such that quitting smoking even shortly before surgery may be of benefit.

Which patients with predisposing characteristics for pulmonary complications should undergo PFTs?

This is a judgment call. The history and physical examination are important. Functional limitation such as difficulty with walking steps or distances should prompt further evaluation. Any patient with an abnormal lung examination (e.g., wheezing or rhonchi) is likely to benefit from PFTs. Other studies useful for evaluation of pulmonary risk (when indicated by the history and physical examination) are chest radiographs, ECG, and arterial blood gases.

What finding on PFTs is truly predictive of perioperative pulmonary complications?

None. Forced vital capacity, FEV_1, maximum breathing capacity, maximum midexpiratory flow, and arterial blood gas findings have all failed to reliably predict pulmonary complications. No degree of abnormality on PFT is considered prohibitive for non–lung surgery down to an FEV_1 of 450 ml. However, it is clear that patients with clusters of abnormalities on the PFT studies are more likely to suffer complications than those without underlying pulmonary condition. It is in those patients with less numerous or dramatic abnormalities that pulmonary complications are difficult to predict. The studies are valuable for uncovering or quantifying suspected pulmonary problems that may be improved with intervention before surgery.

Are certain PFT findings prohibitive for patients undergoing lung resection?

Advanced age coupled with $FEV_1 < 2$ L, maximum voluntary ventilation < 50% predicted, or an abnormal ECG has been found to portend postoperative difficulties. In general, a patient should have a predicted postoperative FEV_1 of at least 800 ml. As is the case with non–lung surgery, the correlation between the degree of abnormality on PFTs and postoperative complications is poor (at least when predicted postoperative FEV_1 is more than 800 ml).

Does use of anesthesia (other than general anesthesia) decrease respiratory complications?

Yes and no. If the anesthesia is strictly local, as in a nerve block, the answer is yes. But, with spinal anesthesia, the answer is no. The reason is that the anesthesia itself is only a small contributor to pulmonary complications. Other factors such as the type of surgery (e.g., upper abdominal or thoracic), loss of hyperinflation by sighing, pain, and sedation all contribute to the development of pulmonary complications. These factors are present regardless of the type of anesthesia used.

PREOPERATIVE USE OF THE LABORATORY

Should every surgery patient have preoperative laboratory tests?

No. The indications for these are provided by the history and physical examination or by the type of surgery planned. The CBC can be reserved for patients undergoing procedures in which large blood losses are expected or who have indication on history and physical examination of anemia. Others who require a CBC include patients older than 60 years of age.

Is a chemistry profile a routine study before surgery?

This study is appropriate for some individuals, such as those older than 60 years of age with hypertension, diabetes, or renal disease. Also, patients who take diuretics, bowel preparations, or nephrotoxic drugs should undergo a preoperative chemistry study.

In whom should coagulation studies be obtained?

Coagulation studies are appropriate in any patient actively bleeding or with a known or suspected bleeding disorder (including iatrogenic causes such as Coumadin or aspirin therapy). Patients with liver disease or malabsorption may be deficient in clotting factors and should have preoperative prothrombin time and partial thromboplastin time measured.

ANTIBIOTIC PROPHYLAXIS BEFORE SURGERY

What are prophylactic antibiotics?

Antibiotics given perioperatively to decrease the risk of infection and improve outcome.

Are prophylactic antibiotics always indicated before surgery?

No. Antibiotics are indicated when infection would be particularly serious, when prosthetic or artificial material is to be implanted, or when the planned procedure is likely to give rise to infection.

All surgical procedures involve some risk of infection, so why not always use antibiotic prophylaxis?

Use of antibiotics is not without some risk, specifically the risks of toxicity, allergic reaction, superinfection, and the development of resistance.

Should the coverage provided by prophylactic antibiotics be broad or narrow?

The coverage should be focused, that is, directed at the most likely pathogens of potential infectious complication.

Why is cefazolin popularly used as prophylaxis before surgery?

Cefazolin is a first generation cephalosporin that provides good coverage against *Staphylococcus aureus* and *Streptococcus*, both of which are likely pathogens of infection whenever the skin is broken. This drug also has an appropriately long half-life.

When would prophylactic antibiotics other than cefazolin be indicated?

1. When likely pathogens would not be well-covered by cefazolin, as in colorectal surgery or appendectomy. Under these circumstances cefoxitin or cefotetan would provide better protection against anaerobic organisms including *Bacteroides fragilis.*
2. When the patient is allergic to beta-lactam antibiotics
3. In cases of MRSA, which is susceptible to vancomycin. (Use of vancomycin is limited to circumstances that clearly require it.)

In preoperative cases, when should the antibiotic be given?

The antibiotic should be given just before the procedure to ensure that there are adequate drug levels throughout the surgery. In cases of major blood loss or prolonged operation, a second dose might be indicated.

Should antibiotics be continued postoperatively?

Not usually. An exception is when infectious complications are likely, such as when there is accidental spillage of stool during an abdominal procedure. In such a case, antibiotics are no longer considered prophylaxis but rather therapeutic and necessary.

Are prophylactic antibiotics indicated for laparoscopic surgery?

The need for prophylaxis is determined by the type of procedure performed, not by the method of surgery. The use of prophylactic antibiotics in laparoscopic surgery is less well-studied than the use of prophylactic antibiotics in traditional surgical incisions, but currently recommendations are the same for both.

INDICATIONS AND REGIMEN FOR SUBACUTE BACTERIAL ENDOCARDITIS PROPHYLAXIS

What patients require antibiotic prophylaxis for subacute bacterial endocarditis?

Any patient with a murmur caused by structural heart disease (e.g., mitral regurgitation, mitral stenosis, aortic stenosis, aortic insufficiency, and idiopathic hypertrophic subaortic stenosis) or a previous bout of endocarditis is an appropriate candidate. Any patient with prosthetic joints, valves, or vascular grafts or a valve damaged by previous rheumatic disease or valvular surgery is eligible for prophylaxis. Patients with mitral valve prolapse without a murmur probably do not need routine antibiotic prophylaxis.

Do candidates for prophylactic antibiotic therapy for subacute bacterial endocarditis need such therapy for all procedures?

No. Prophylactic therapy should be given for any procedure likely to introduce bacteria into the bloodstream (e.g., dental procedures with expected bleeding from gums and gastrointestinal or genitourinary surgery).

What antibiotics are indicated as prophylaxis against bacterial endocarditis in patients with rheumatic heart disease?

PO—amoxicillin (3 g before and 1.5 g 6 hours after the procedure)

PO and penicillin allergic—erythromycin (dose depends on the preparation) or clindamycin (300 mg before and 150 mg 6 hours after the procedure)

NPO—ampicillin (2 g 30 minutes before and 1 g 6 hours after the procedure)

NPO and penicillin allergic—clindamycin (300 mg intravenously 30 minutes before the procedure and 150 mg intravenously 6 hours after), ampicillin plus gentamicin, or vancomycin

For genitourinary and gastrointestinal procedures—amoxicillin (if low risk) or ampicillin plus gentamicin or vancomycin plus gentamicin (depending on penicillin allergy)

DEEP VENOUS THROMBOSIS PROPHYLAXIS

What are risk factors for DVT?

Age older than 40 years, surgery lasting more than 1 hour, previous DVT or pulmonary embolus, extensive tumor, hip or knee surgery, major trauma or fractures, and stroke are all elements that contribute to highly increased risk of DVT. Other risk factors include MI, CHF, obesity, immobility, and postpartum state.

Do all surgical patients benefit from DVT prophylaxis?

Yes, but not necessarily pharmacologic prophylaxis. Patients at low risk of DVT can wear graduated compression stockings and undertake early ambulation as prophylactic measures. These patients include those younger than 40 years of age who are undergoing procedures less than 1 hour long or patients who are pregnant.

Do all other patients besides those with low risk of DVT need pharmacologic prophylaxis?

Patients with a moderate risk of DVT often are given pharmacologic prophylaxis. These patients include those older than 40 years of age who are undergoing a procedure longer than 1 hour or who have medical conditions such as MI or CHF. Postpartum patients have moderate risk of DVT. Prophylaxis involves the methods used for low-risk patients plus one of the following: subcutaneous heparin (5000 units) twice per day, low–molecular-weight heparin, intravenous dextran, or external pneumatic compression.

Who are patients with high risk of DVT and what prophylaxis is appropriate for them?

These patients are older than 40 years of age, undergoing long procedures, often orthopedic ones, and might have a history of DVT, pulmonary embolism, stroke, or recent trauma. They are eligible for the same prophylaxis that moderate-risk patients receive, except the high-risk patient may receive heparin three times daily. Other therapies used for these patients include warfarin or vena caval interruption.

Why use warfarin only in patients with high risk of DVT?

Warfarin is associated with a higher risk of bleeding complications (approximately 6%) than heparin (approximately 2%).

Is aspirin ever used as prophylaxis against DVT?

Aspirin is not as effective as the other methods discussed; therefore, it is not recommended.

Why are dextrans rarely used as prophylaxis for DVT?	Dextrans have been associated with anaphylactic reactions, they are expensive, and they require intravenous administration.
What other methods of DVT prophylaxis are in development?	The biologically active components of hirudin (which is found in the saliva of the leech) are a promising possibility for DVT prophylaxis based on results of early trials. Also murine monoclonal antibodies that bind the fibrinogen receptor on platelets are in development as is recombinant human factor Xa, which blocks thrombin activity.

PERIOPERATIVE MANAGEMENT OF THE DIABETIC PATIENT

What increased risks does a diabetic patient face in the perioperative period that the nondiabetic patient does not?	Metabolic (hyperglycemia and hypoglycemia), cardiovascular, and infectious risks
Why is the type of diabetes (i.e., type I or type II) important to distinguish during the perioperative period?	Type I diabetic patients are prone to ketoacidosis whereas type II diabetic patients generally are not. Both are subject to variations in glucose control perioperatively, given NPO status (hypoglycemia) and the stress of illness and surgery (hyperglycemia).
How is the type I diabetic managed, in general, perioperatively?	While NPO, the patient is given intravenous glucose and insulin drips at 1–3 units per hour with titration (sliding scale) based on serum glucose levels.
How is the insulin-requiring type II diabetic patient managed perioperatively?	Type II insulin-requiring diabetic patients are generally given one half their usual dose of long-acting insulin on the morning of the surgery. Their blood glucose is then monitored frequently via finger sticks. Infusions or subcutaneous injections of insulin and glucose are adjusted accordingly.

How should the patient whose diabetes is controlled on oral hypoglycemics be managed for surgery?

Patients should have their oral agent discontinued 1 day before surgery. (Chlorpropamide should be stopped 2–3 days before surgery and metformin should be stopped 1–2 days before surgery.) Patients often require no exogenous glucose or insulin, but these may be used if necessary. Serum glucose should be monitored in anticipation of such a possibility.

How is the patient with diet-controlled diabetes managed for surgery?

Diet-controlled diabetic patients can often undergo surgery without any glucose or insulin. Intravenous fluids should lack dextrose, and the patient's blood glucose level should be monitored throughout the procedure. Again, insulin and glucose should be administered if needed.

Why are finger sticks rather than urine glucose tests used to determine blood sugar?

The correlation between urine glucose and blood glucose is not reliable, especially in older patients.

What is a reasonable target range for blood sugars in diabetic patients undergoing surgery?

Generally, 150–250 mg/dl is considered an acceptable range. Patients with infection may require tighter control.

In patients whose blood sugar is difficult to maintain, is it better to be on the high side or the low side of the acceptable range?

It is better to have blood sugars run somewhat high than to risk insulin shock.

How much is risk increased for cardiovascular event for diabetic patients compared with their nondiabetic counterparts?

Two times for male diabetics and four times for female diabetics

Why is the diabetic at increased risk of infection?

The major reason is that small-vessel disease results in tissue ischemia. Also, hyperglycemia impairs phagocytosis and gastroparesis increases the risk of aspiration pneumonia.

Does the presence of palpable peripheral pulses rule out the presence of tissue ischemia in diabetic patients?

No. The pathology in diabetic circulation is microvascular in nature.

How does the medical consultant minimize chances for complications during surgery for diabetic patients?

A good history and physical examination is of primary importance. Important elements of the history include duration of disease, current medications, current diet, typical blood sugar levels, and preexisting complications such as retinopathy, nephropathy, and neuropathy. The consultant should also elicit information regarding angina, previous MI, claudication, activity limitation, and other major cardiac risk factors (e.g., family history, smoking, hypertension, and hyperlipidemia). The type of surgery planned and type of anesthesia are also factors.

What should be observed on physical examination of a diabetic patient?

Especially vital signs, heart and lung examination findings, and condition of extremities. Degree of hygiene, any ulcers, evidence of poor perfusion (e.g., decreased hair growth and decreased pulses), and neurologic findings should be noted. Patients with peripheral neuropathy are much more prone to extremity complications with their attendant morbidity and mortality.

What laboratory evaluations are needed for diabetic patients preoperatively?

Blood glucose level, hemoglobin A1C, electrolytes (especially sodium and potassium), BUN and creatinine, and urinalysis. Thyroid studies may be indicated if history and physical examination suggest any abnormality.

Is chronic renal insufficiency a contraindication to surgery?

No, but it indicates a need for meticulous attention to volume and electrolyte status perioperatively.

Why might a diabetic patient be instructed to fast for a full 12 hours before surgery?

Diabetic gastroparesis predisposes the patient to aspiration during surgery.

POSTOPERATIVE FEVER

What are the common causes of postoperative fever?

The **five Ws** of postoperative fever are as follows:
Wind (atelectasis)
Water (urinary tract infection)
Wound (wound infection)
Walking (DVT)
Wonder drugs (drug reaction)

Which of the five W's is the most common cause of fever?

Atelectasis. Auscultation of the lungs and a chest radiograph are often all that is needed to make a diagnosis. Treatment involves incentive spirometry, chest physical therapy, and ambulation.

Should antibiotics be given to patients with postoperative fever?

Antibiotics should be avoided until a source of infection is diagnosed by repeated careful, comprehensive history and physical examinations. Surgical wounds should be carefully evaluated for evidence of infection. Urinalysis and culture as well as culture of blood and all invasive lines should be carried out.

MISCELLANEOUS MNEMONICS

What is the mnemonic for evaluation of pain?

OLDER QQS:
Onset
Location
Duration
Exacerbation and alleviation
Radiation
Quality
Quantity
Symptoms associated with the pain

What is the mnemonic for altered mental status?

TIPS AEIOU:
Trauma and temperature
Infection
Psychiatric disorder or **P**oison
Sepsis or **S**troke or **S**eizure or **S**pace-occupying lesion

Alcohol intoxication or withdrawal
Electrolyte imbalance
Insulin (hyperglycemia or hypoglycemia)
Overdose or O_2 deficit
Uremia

What is the mnemonic for acidosis without anion gap?	**HEART CCU:** **H**yperaldosteronism **E**xpansion (volume) **A**cid loading **R**enal tubular acidosis **T**urds (diarrhea, pancreatitis) **C**hronic pyelonephritis **C**arbonic anhydrase inhibitors **U**reterojejunostomy
What is the mnemonic for chronic interstitial nephritis?	**POSTCARD:** **P**yelonephritis **O**bstruction **S**ickle cell disease **T**uberculosis **C**arcinoma **A**nalgesics **R**enal vein thrombosis **D**iabetes or **D**iuretics
How do the glucocorticoids compare in potency with respect to hydrocortisone?	**D**on't **S**top **P**rednisone **H**astily: **D**examethasone (25 times more potent) **S**olumedrol (5 times more potent) **P**rednisone (4 times more potent) **H**ydrocortisone

Section IV

Environmental Medicine

17

Diseases Resulting From Environmental and Chemical Causes

ABBREVIATIONS

ACLS	Advanced cardiac life support
ADME	Absorption, distribution, metabolism, or elimination
ALT	Alanine aminotransferase
ARDS	Acute respiratory distress syndrome
AST	Aspartate aminotransferase
AV	Atrioventricular
BUN	Blood urea nitrogen
CNS	Central nervous system
ECG	Electrocardiogram
EtOH	Alcohol
LFT	Liver function test
LSD	Lysergic acid diethylamide
PCP	Phencyclidine
PT	Prothrombin time
SR	Sustained release
TCA	Tricyclic antidepressant

POISONING

GENERAL INFORMATION

What is the incidence of toxic exposures reported in the United States?	According to the 1994 annual report of the American Association of Poison Control Centers, approximately 2 million toxic exposures were reported; approximately 50% of these were reported in children younger than 6 years, roughly 8000 of the exposures were severe, and death occurred in over 760 cases.
What is a toxin?	Toxins can be a variety of substances (e.g., drugs, cleaning supplies, cosmetics, plants, pesticides, and chemicals). Routes of exposure vary, including dermal exposure, ocular exposure, inhalation, and ingestion. In 1994, ingestion accounted for approximately 75% of exposures.
Of the common poisonings that occur, approximately what percentage are due to:	
Medications?	50%
Cosmetics, pesticides, petroleum products, and turpentine?	20%
Cleaning and polishing agents?	15%
Other substances?	15%
What can be done to reduce the incidence of toxic exposure?	Education, proper marking of containers, and removal of poisonous substances from areas with small children
What are some of the sources of information available to investigate diagnosis and treatment of toxic exposures?	Local Poison Control Center; Hospital Drug Information Centers, Pharmacists, and the following computer and text references: Poisindex

Haddad LM, Winchester JF: *Clinical Management of Poisoning and Drug Overdose*, 2nd ed. Philadelphia, WB Saunders, 1990.

Goldfrank LF, et al: *Toxicologic Emergencies*, 4th ed. Norwalk, CT, Appleton & Lange, 1990.

BASIC PRINCIPLES

What physical examination features suggest exposure to the following poisons:	
Cyanide	Cyanide odor
Carbon monoxide	Cherry red flush of the skin and mucous membranes
Lead	Lead line and paralysis of extensor muscles
Cholinesterase-inhibitor insecticides	Pupillary constriction, salivation, and gastrointestinal hyperactivity
What is the first rule to remember in toxic exposure?	First, stabilize the patient using the ABCs: *a*irway, *b*reathing, and *c*irculation. Provide continual monitoring and support of vital signs throughout treatment.
After stabilizing the patient with toxic exposure, what should be done next?	Information about the exposure should be obtained and supportive care should be given. A physical examination should be performed and clinical assessment made. Laboratory screening and analysis should be considered as should gastric decontamination. Improving elimination from the body and checking for antidotes should also be considered.
What are important features of the history of exposure?	Time, type, and amount of exposure, as well as information from the patient's family, friends, pharmacy, physician, and past medical history. Allergies, previous admissions, and access to medication and chemicals are important to know. Ingestions of multiple substances are

common in suicide attempts and gestures, and alcohol is commonly used to wash down pills.

In cases of suicide attempt or gesture, what additional steps are needed once the patient is medically stable?

Psychiatric consultation should be obtained. Patients thought to be at risk to themselves or others should be detained against their will if necessary, but this requires legal intervention.

What are the characteristic physical examination findings in the following common toxic syndromes:

Anticholinergics (e.g., atropine, belladonna alkaloid, TCAs, antipsychotics, antiparkinsonian medications, and antihistamines)

Red as a beet, hot as a hare, dry as a bone, blind as a bat, and mad as a hatter (i.e., dry, flushed skin and mucous membranes, fever, dilated pupils, and delirium)

Cholinergics (e.g., organophosphates)

Think **SLUDGE:**
Salivation
Lacrimation
Urination
Defecation
Gastrointestinal upset
Emesis

Opiates (e.g., morphine, codeine, heroin, and methadone)

Triad of miosis, depressed mental status, and depressed respiration

Barbiturates (e.g., phenobarbital and pentobarbital)

Depressed mental status and respiration, bradycardia, hypothermia, hypotension, pulmonary edema, and areflexia

Stimulants (e.g., amphetamines, cocaine, and aminophylline)

Excitation and agitation, tachycardia and arrhythmias, hypertension, mydriasis, and seizures

Substance withdrawal

Agitation, confusion, mydriasis, tachycardia, hypertension, abdominal pain, nausea and vomiting, and seizures

What should be considered in laboratory screening for drugs?	Cost, false-negative and false-positive results, and time to complete analytical results
When are qualitative tests useful in patients with toxic exposure?	1. When no patient history is attainable 2. When clinical signs and symptoms differ from patient history 3. When multiple toxins are suspected 4. When medicolegal documentation is needed. Such documents can only be used in court if the legal chain of custody is observed.
When are quantitative tests useful in patients with toxic exposure?	1. When the drugs have documented associations between adverse effects and therapeutic concentration 2. When there is rapid analysis time 3. When levels of drug present may direct medical management
Do pharmacokinetic alterations change laboratory parameters or clinical signs?	Yes. Drug pharmacokinetics may be unpredictable in toxic exposures. In general, all parameters—ADME—may be prolonged over those of the normal dose. Volumes of distribution are altered, and metabolism may invoke pathways that are not commonly used for normal doses of substances.
Why consider gastric decontamination in patients with toxic exposure?	To inhibit further adsorption from ingested toxins that may be present in the gastrointestinal tract. This prevents or decreases continued toxicity. The efficacy of gastric decontamination may vary with (1) the substance ingested, (2) length of time for exposure, (3) patient age, and (4) underlying medical problems.
What are the different types of gastric decontamination?	Syrup of ipecac, gastric lavage, activated charcoal, cathartics, and whole bowel irrigation
How does syrup of ipecac work?	It is composed of the alkaloids emetine and cephaeline. These alkaloids act both centrally (through stimulation of the

chemoreceptor trigger zone) and locally (by causing direct irritation of the gastric mucosa).

What are indications for use of syrup of ipecac?

It is useful early in toxic exposure, just after toxic ingestion, and in asymptomatic adults known to have ingested substances with latent toxicities. Syrup of ipecac is available over the counter and can be used at home. It is no longer routinely recommended if lavage and charcoal are available.

What are contraindications to the use of syrup of ipecac?

Unconsciousness; seizure; lack of gag reflex; ingestion of caustic neurotoxins, acids, bases, or hydrocarbons; active gastrointestinal bleeding; known cardiac instability; and age younger than 6–9 months old

What are complications of the use of syrup of ipecac?

Mallory-Weiss tears, pneumomediastinum, gastric rupture, and delay in the administration of activated charcoal

What is the dosing for syrup of ipecac?

Children younger than 1 year: Use is controversial

Children 1–12 years: 15 ml of ipecac followed by 1–2 glasses of water. The dose should be repeated once if no emesis occurs within 30 minutes.

Adults: 15–30 ml of ipecac followed by 3–4 glasses of water. The dose should be repeated if no emesis occurs within 30 minutes.

How is gastric lavage performed?

Typically, with the airway protected, a large-bore tube is used to remove the stomach contents. Serial aliquots of warm lavage solution (saline or tap water) are used. The procedure is repeated until the fluid removed is clear.

In whom should gastric lavage be used?

Patients who are obtunded or intubated, patients with life-threatening ingestions, patients with very recent ingestions, or patients who have ingested a substance that decreases gastric motility (e.g., anticholinergic agents).

What are contraindications to gastric lavage?

Gastric contents are larger than the lavage tube or hose, are alkalotic, or are sharp; airway cannot be protected.

What are complications of gastric lavage?

Accidental tracheal intubation, perforation of the esophagus or gastric area, and adverse cardiorespiratory effects

What is activated charcoal?

A porous substance with a vast surface area to adsorb toxins, created using heated wood pulp, steam, acids, and oxidizing substances. Adsorption of toxins begins within several minutes of contact, unless food is in the gastrointestinal tract.

What are indications for use of activated charcoal?

In most toxic exposures, use as a single agent or after gastric emptying.

What are contraindications, complications, and limitations of activated charcoal?

In cases of caustic ingestion, activated charcoal has questionable efficacy and may complicate endoscopy.

Activated charcoal should be used with caution in patients at risk for aspiration and those with decreased gastrointestinal motility.

Activated charcoal is incapable of adsorbing cyanide, ferrous sulfate, lithium, boric acid, dichlorodiphenyltrichloroethane, and carbamate insecticides.

How is activated charcoal dosed?

Children younger than 12 years: 20–30 g (1–2 g/kg)

Adults: 60–100 g

Administer with 70% sorbitol to reduce gastrointestinal transit time and prevent charcoal from remaining in gut (to decrease time for gut absorption of toxin). An approximate 10:1 ratio of activated charcoal to toxin is needed to adsorb all ingested toxin. This ratio may be unattainable in some ingestions.

Can multiple doses of activated charcoal be used?	Yes. The premise is to disrupt enterohepatic circulation such that available free toxin may be absorbed from the bloodstream back into the gastrointestinal tract for adsorption by charcoal.
What doses are used for multiple dosing of activated charcoal?	1.0–1.5 g/kg, then 0.5–1.0 g/kg every 2–6 hours. Sorbitol is given with the initial dose, but not with every dose. Patient signs, symptoms, and drug levels should be monitored.
What are indications for multiple dosing of activated charcoal?	Large ingestions, ingestion of extended release products, and especially overdose of theophylline and digoxin
What are additional cautions and limitations?	Use may increase the risk of perforation, cause diarrhea (and consequently, electrolyte disturbances), or cause constipation
What is the rationale for whole bowel irrigation?	To shorten gastrointestinal transit time and to reduce the absorption of toxic substrate
In what patients should whole bowel irrigation be used?	Patients in whom toxic substances are not adsorbed by activated charcoal, patients who have ingested a large amount of extended release drug products, and patients who have packed body orifices with drug
What are contraindications of whole bowel irrigation?	Gastrointestinal ileus, obstruction, bleeding, and perforation
What is the dosing for whole bowel irrigation?	Oral or nasogastric polyethylene glycol electrolyte solution (e.g., GoLYTELY or Colyte) is given until rectal fluid is clear. Use up to 0.5 L/hour for children and 2 L/hour for adults.
What is the rationale for cathartic use of whole bowel irrigation?	To shorten gastrointestinal transit time to result in reduced absorption of toxic substances

What types of cathartics are used in whole bowel irrigation?	Most common—saline and osmotic agents (i.e., sorbitol) Other agents—sodium sulfate, magnesium sulfate, magnesium citrate
What are indications for cathartics?	The primary indication is for use of sorbitol with activated charcoal. Otherwise, it is seldom used because of adverse effects and questionable efficacy.
What are complications of cathartics?	Fluid and electrolyte alterations— Sodium products may produce hypernatremia and should be avoided in congestive heart failure; magnesium products may cause magnesium toxicity in patients with renal failure and dehydration.
What methods may be used to promote renal elimination of toxins?	Extracorporeal removal by hemodialysis or hemoperfusion Alterations in urinary pH Forced diuresis
When are extracorporeal methods used for renal elimination of toxins?	When toxins can be removed by hemodialysis or hemoperfusion, when clinical status declines after appropriate initial management, and in cases of life-threatening hyperkalemia with or without renal dysfunction
What types of drugs are removed by hemodialysis?	Drugs with low molecular weight Low plasma protein–binding drugs Drugs with volume of distribution < 1.0 L/kg Un–ionized, uncharged substances
How does hemoperfusion work?	Toxic substances are extracted from blood as it washes over a column of activated charcoal or carbon.
What are complications of hemoperfusion?	Hypotension, thrombocytopenia, hypocalcemia, and embolus (air or charcoal)

What is the premise of forced diuresis?	To increase removal of toxin by reducing the time for renal reabsorption. Forced diuresis can be done with any crystalline fluid with or without altering urinary pH.
Why use alterations in urinary pH with forced diuresis?	To increase urine output. Toxin is trapped as an ion in the urine, therefore inhibiting reabsorption (i.e., weak acids are inhibited by alkalotic urine, and weak bases are inhibited by acidotic urine). Agents used include sodium bicarbonate and ammonium chloride.
What are complications of forced diuresis?	Fluid overload, electrolyte imbalance, altered urinary pH, and serum acid–base disturbances

COMMON PHARMACOLOGIC TOXINS

Acetaminophen

What is the mechanism of acetaminophen toxicity?	When toxic acetaminophen doses are ingested, the normal glucuronidation and sulfation pathways become saturated and approximately half of the dose may form the toxic intermediary (N-acetylimidoquinone) via the cytochrome P-450 system. Glutathione stores are quickly reduced. A decrease in stores to approximately 30% of the normal level results in increased levels of the toxic metabolite and hepatic necrosis occurs.
What are the clinical stages of acetaminophen toxicity?	Stage 1—ingestion to 24 hours after ingestion. Symptoms include nausea, vomiting, gastrointestinal irritation, lethargy, diaphoresis, and malaise. Stage 2—24–48 hours after ingestion (a deceptive asymptomatic phase). There may be slight elevation of hepatic enzymes and right upper quadrant pain. Stage 3—72–96 hours after ingestion. Symptoms include severe nausea, vomiting, jaundice, CNS changes ranging from lethargy to coma,

elevated AST and ALT (may be > 10,000 IU/L), coagulation dysfunction, and renal failure. Stage 4—4–14 days after ingestion. Symptoms and laboratory values resolve.

What dose of acetaminophen causes toxicity?

Typically, toxicity is associated with acute ingestions of > 7.5 g; 13–25 g is typically fatal. Acetaminophen may be found alone or as part of many combination pharmaceutical products.

What is the treatment for acetaminophen toxicity?

Supportive care, gastric decontamination, serum acetaminophen levels to assess the need for acetylcysteine administration

What type of gastric decontamination is used in acetaminophen toxicity?

Ipecac or gastric lavage may be useful if administered within 4 hours of exposure.

Is activated charcoal useful in acetaminophen toxicity?

Activated charcoal effectively adsorbs acetaminophen. It may also reduce the systemic absorption of the antidote acetylcysteine, but it can cause nausea and vomiting, making it difficult to give the acetylcysteine. If administration of acetylcysteine is delayed by at least 1 hour for some reason, then activated charcoal is an appropriate option for decontamination.

What is the role of laboratory assessment of serum acetaminophen concentrations?

Acetaminophen treatment is guided by serum acetaminophen levels. To be reliable, levels must be determined at least 4 hours after ingestion. Levels measured before this time may be falsely low. The most common method of evaluation of acute acetaminophen toxicity is to plot the levels measured against the time since ingestion on the Rumack-Matthew nomogram.

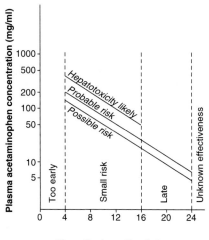

Rumack-Matthew nomogram. Adapted from Lewis RK, Paloucek FP: Assessment and treatment of acetaminophen overdose (review). *Clin Pharmacol* 10 (10): 765 – 74, 1991.

What is the mechanism for acetylcysteine antidotal therapy in acetaminophen overdose?

Acetylcysteine is administered to replace the sulfhydryl substance that detoxifies the N-acetylimidoquinone metabolite. Also, acetylcysteine may prevent liver damage by replenishing the glutathione stores, thereby stopping the accumulation of the toxic intermediary.

What are indications for acetylcysteine antidotal therapy in acetaminophen toxicity?

1. Serum levels of acetaminophen in the possibly toxic range
2. Ingestion exceeding 140 mg/kg

3. Unclear time of ingestion, but a predicted half-life exceeding 4 hours

It is best to substantiate the predicated half-life and the amount of ingestion with serum acetaminophen levels. Delaying initiation of antidote for > 10 hours escalates the risk of toxicity. Acetylcysteine therapy may be ineffective if begun more than 24 hours after ingestion.

What is the antidotal dose of acetylcysteine in acetaminophen toxicity?

140 mg/kg orally, then 70 mg/kg every 4 hours for 17 doses. The solution is manufactured as 10% and 20%. The 20% solution is mixed with soda or orange juice to a 5% solution before administering for oral use. The dose may be increased by 30% if activated charcoal is used. The intravenous form is not available in the United States.

What are additional monitoring concerns in acetaminophen toxicity?

LFTs should be monitored every 24 hours for approximately 3–4 days. Serum bilirubin should be measured in stages 1 and 2. AST and ALT levels typically peak 3–4 days after ingestion; levels > 1000 IU/L may signify liver cell damage. Electrolytes and fluid status should be monitored for supportive care. BUN and creatinine should be measured because kidney damage may also occur.

What are adverse effects of acetylcysteine?

Nausea and vomiting (acetylcysteine has a rotten egg odor)

What is alcohol–acetaminophen syndrome?

People with underlying liver disease, whether clinical or subclinical and usually caused by alcohol use, are at high risk for acetaminophen-induced hepatic necrosis. Less than 1 g of acetaminophen may be toxic. This is an often underrecognized cause of acute hepatic failure.

What is the prognosis for acetaminophen toxicity in alcohol–acetaminophen syndrome?	Serum transaminase levels may reach > 10,000 and do not correlate with prognosis. Because the patient may be acutely encephalopathic and significant hepatic necrosis portends a poor prognosis, transplant consideration should be initiated early in the course of hospitalization.

Cyclic Antidepressant Toxicity

What drugs are cyclic antidepressants?	Traditional tricyclic antidepressants (e.g., amitriptyline, imipramine, doxepin, nortriptyline, desipramine), monocyclics (e.g., bupropion), tetracyclics (e.g., maprotiline), and amoxapine (a dibenzoxazepine).
What are the mechanisms behind cyclic antidepressant–induced toxicity?	Inhibition of norepinephrine and serotonin reuptake, alpha blockade, cardiac membrane stabilization (an anesthetic-like property), and anticholinergic effects. Toxicity is then exhibited through CNS, cardiac, and anticholinergic manifestations.
What are CNS effects of cyclic antidepressant toxicity?	Anticholinergic effects and central adrenergic effects, possibly beginning with agitation and progressing to delirium, hallucinations, lethargy, and coma. Hyperreflexia, myoclonus, and seizures may occur. When seizures develop, they are typically brief, occurring within the initial 6–8 hours.
What are cardiovascular manifestations of cyclic antidepressant toxicity?	Hypotension may result from peripheral alpha blockade and from catechol depletion. Cardiac arrhythmias result from the membrane-stabilizing and anesthetic property. ECG findings may include sinus tachycardia and prolongation of the PR, QRS, and QT intervals.
What are the most frequent signs of cardiac toxicity with cyclic antidepressants?	Sinus tachycardia, QRS prolongation, AV blocks (including complete heart block), and bundle branch blocks

What are anticholinergic effects of cyclic antidepressant toxicity?

Gastrointestinal symptoms (decreased bowel sounds, reduced motility, and prolonged gastric emptying, making absorption of overdose erratic and unpredictable), urinary retention, respiratory depression, mydriasis, blurred vision, tachycardia, dry skin, and flushing

Does the amount of cyclic antidepressant ingested predict severity of toxicity?

No. The dose ingested is a poor indicator of patient outcome.

What is the treatment for cyclic antidepressant toxicity?

Supportive care (a major component), gastric decontamination, and treatment of cardiac, CNS, and respiratory manifestations

What type of monitoring is needed in cyclic antidepressant toxicity?

Depending on clinical presentation: oxygen status, cardiac monitoring including baseline ECG, intravenous access, blood chemistries, CBC, and arterial blood gas

What types of gastric decontamination are used in cyclic antidepressant toxicity?

Gastric lavage, single-dose activated charcoal, multiple-dose activated charcoal, and lavage followed by charcoal. Ipecac may not be an appropriate choice because CNS symptoms may develop rapidly.

Is extracorporeal removal of toxins helpful in treatment of cyclic antidepressant toxicity?

No. Cyclic antidepressants are highly protein bound and have large volumes of distribution, making extracorporeal removal ineffective.

What is the treatment for cardiac toxicity with cyclic antidepressants?

Cardiac toxicity is responsible for most of the deaths. Treatment is with intravenous sodium bicarbonate, 1–2 mEq/kg bolus, then continuous infusion (isotonic-150 mEq sodium bicarbonate/L D5W) titrated to systemic pH 7.45–7.5. Efficacy stems from sodium-loading effect to reverse the inhibition of slow Na^+ channels in cardiac tissue. The benefit of alkalinization may help decrease binding of cyclics to cardiac tissue.

What are indications to treat cardiac toxicity with sodium bicarbonate in cyclic antidepressant toxicity?

Acidosis, resistant hypotension, abnormal cardiac conduction, ventricular arrhythmias, and cardiac arrest. It is unclear at what point of QRS prolongation sodium bicarbonate should be initiated. Some sources recommend use with QRS duration greater than or equal to 0.10 second whereas others recommend use with QRS greater than or equal to 0.16 second.

How should cardiac arrhythmias be treated in cyclic antidepressant toxicity?

Hypoxia, hypotension, and acidosis should be treated, then sodium bicarbonate therapy should begin. Class IA (e.g., quinidine and procainamide) and IC (e.g., flecainide and propafenone) should not be used because they act similarly to the cyclic antidepressants.

Lidocaine may be used for ventricular arrhythmias.

β-Blockers have been used successfully to treat supraventricular and ventricular tachycardias, but adverse effects of hypotension, bradycardia, and cardiac arrest may occur.

Atropine cannot be used to treat cyclic antidepressant bradycardia because these antidepressants inhibit muscarinic receptors. Isoproterenol or pacemakers may be needed for bradyarrhythmias and heart blocks.

How is refractory hypotension treated in cyclic antidepressant toxicity?

Fluids and sodium bicarbonate. If there is no response, then norepinephrine, phenylephrine, and dopamine may be used as pressor agents.

What is the treatment for CNS toxicity in cyclic antidepressant toxicity?

Supportive care. Agitation and seizures respond to benzodiazepines. Second line seizure treatment is phenobarbital.

What is the treatment of respiratory complications in cyclic antidepressant toxicity?

Supportive care, pulse oximetry monitoring, oxygen, and intubation if necessary. Respiratory acidosis adversely affects myocardial function.

Iron—Acute Intoxication

What dose of iron is considered toxic?

Greater than or equal to 20 mg/kg of elemental iron. Doses of 20–60 mg/kg typically produce mild to moderate toxicity; doses exceeding 60 mg/kg produce severe toxicity.

How does iron cause gastrointestinal toxicity?

Locally, iron may cause corrosion in the gastrointestinal mucosa ranging from irritation to ulceration, bleeding, loss of oxygenation, and perforation. Hepatic necrosis may occur as the portal circulation receives the initial toxic iron concentration from the blood.

How does iron cause systemic toxicity?

Multiple systemic effects may occur, including venodilation (decreased systemic and central venous pressures), enhanced capillary membrane permeability (third spacing and hypotension), interference with serum proteases (may increase PT), cellular destruction, and metabolic acidosis.

What are symptoms and signs of iron toxicity for the following stages?

Stage I:

Nausea, vomiting, diarrhea, and abdominal pain. Fluid losses with or without bleeding may result in decreased perfusion, hypotension, and acidosis. Symptoms occur rapidly after ingestion and may be relieved after 6–12 hours.

Stage II:

Lethargy, metabolic acidosis, and possibly hypotension occurring in the period between relief of gastrointestinal symptoms and development of severe systemic effects. Onset is 6–12 hours after ingestion; duration is 12–24 hours.

Stage III:

Multiple organ dysfunction, including cerebral damage, coma, cardiac depression, renal dysfunction, liver failure, and ischemic bowel. Liver failure may result in coagulopathy or decreased blood glucose.

Stage IV:	Gastrointestinal scarring resulting in gastric outlet and small bowel obstruction

What is most important to remember when making the diagnosis of iron toxicity?

Diagnosis is based on clinical presentation regardless of time since ingestion or laboratory test results.

What are important aspects of laboratory data in iron toxicity?

1. Normal serum iron is 50–150 $\mu g/dl$; levels greater than 300–350 $\mu g/dl$ typically result in toxicity; levels greater than 500 $\mu g/dl$ may cause severe toxicity.
2. Peak serum iron levels occur approximately 2–6 hours after ingestion.
3. The blood level of iron is not the cause of toxicity. The intracellular concentration of iron creates the toxicity.
4. Association between level and symptoms varies among patients.
5. Serum level shows only one point in time.
6. Total iron-binding capacity is not a helpful measurement because it may be inappropriately high when serum iron levels are high.
7. Blood glucose levels and white blood cell count may become elevated with serum iron greater than 300 $\mu g/dl$ and may give additional information for severity of toxicity.

What is the treatment for iron toxicity?

1. Stabilization of the patient
2. Gastric decontamination—syrup of ipecac may be useful if ingestion is very recent, gastric lavage may be used, but activated charcoal is ineffective.
3. Chelation therapy with deferoxamine
4. Supportive care—fluid and electrolyte replacement, management of acid–base abnormalities, and coagulopathy

How does deferoxamine work?

It acts as a chelating agent by converting ferric ions in the blood to ferrioxamine, which is renally eliminated.

What are indications for deferoxamine therapy?

1. Serum iron greater than 300–350 μg/dl in symptomatic patients or greater than 400 μg/dl in asymptomatic patients
2. Ingestion of more than 180–300 mg of elemental iron
3. Clinical symptoms and signs worse than passing, minor symptoms (i.e., more than one bout of emesis or more than one soft stool)

What dose of deferoxamine should be used in iron toxicity?

Therapy is most effective if given as 15 mg/kg/hour via continuous intravenous infusion for adults or approximately 4 mg/kg/hour intravenously via continuous infusion for children. Other methods include intramuscular or intravenous therapy of 1 g for one dose, then 500 mg every 4 hours for two doses with additional doses of 500 mg every 4–12 hours, depending on the patient's clinical status. Maximum is 6 g/24 hours for children and adults. Children may receive 20 mg/kg intramuscularly or slow intravenous infusion, with subsequent doses of 10 mg/kg every 4–12 hours as needed, depending on the patient's clinical status. Intravenous administration is preferred for all patients because total dose given may be more accurately controlled.

What are adverse effects of deferoxamine therapy?

These primarily occur with rapid intravenous injection and include flushing, erythema, urticaria, hypotension, shock, and seizures.

What is the appropriate duration for deferoxamine therapy?

Treatment is continued until serum iron levels are within normal limits and the patient has resolution of clinical symptoms and signs. Treatment duration is typically 6–12 hours. Some patients produce vin-rose colored urine during chelation with deferoxamine. When this color resolves, therapy may be discontinued. The vin-rose colored urine is not an absolute marker for presence of toxicity.

Salicylate Toxicity

What is the mechanism for salicylate-induced toxicity?

1. The agent acts centrally to stimulate the respiratory center.
2. Skeletal muscle metabolism is increased, raising the demand for oxygen and elevating production of carbon dioxide, resulting in hyperventilation and further respiratory alkalosis.
3. The agent interferes with central and peripheral glucose metabolism and utilization.

How is salicylate poisoning classified?

Acute or chronic:
Acute intoxication—doses of 150–300 mg/kg typically cause mild to moderate symptoms. Doses greater than 300 mg/kg produce severe toxicity, and doses of greater than 500 mg/kg may be lethal.
Chronic intoxication—typically, greater than 100 mg/kg/day for more than 2–3 days

What is the clinical presentation in acute salicylate toxicity?

Dehydration, hearing loss, tinnitus, tachypnea, nausea, vomiting, elevated PT, alterations in platelet function, electrolyte loss, and proteinuria

What is the usual acid–base abnormality in salicylate toxicity?

Children younger than 4 years old typically present with metabolic acidosis and are acidemic. Older children and adults typically present with mixed acid–base states seen as respiratory alkalosis, elevated anion gap metabolic acidosis, and alkalemia.

What is the clinical presentation in chronic salicylate toxicity?

Same as acute toxicity but may also include pulmonary edema, CNS manifestations (e.g., agitation, confusion, blunted mental status, seizures, and coma), elevated LFTs, and kidney failure

What do salicylate levels indicate for treatment of toxicity?

Plasma levels may not correlate with severity of intoxication. Treatment is guided primarily by the patient's clinical status. Levels should not be obtained sooner than 6 hours after ingestion because they may be falsely low. Salicylate levels may escalate for approximately 24 hours depending on the amount and type of product ingested. If SR products are ingested, peak salicylate levels may be prolonged to 10–60 hours after ingestion. Repeated salicylate levels obtained 4–6 hours after the original level may be useful to monitor or document the status of the blood concentration.

Is there a treatment nomogram for salicylate toxicity?

Yes, the Dome nomogram. First, though, the patient's clinical presentation should be used to determine the severity of toxicity and subsequent treatment.

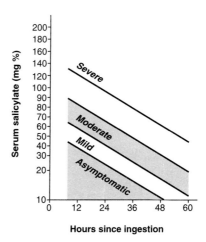

Hours since ingestion

Dome nomogram. Adapted from Watson WA: Clinical Toxicology. In *Applied Therapeutics: The Clinical Use of Drugs.* Edited by Young LY, Koda-Kimble MA, and Kradjan WA. Vancouver, WA, 1995, pp 104.1 – 104.23.

When is the Dome nomogram not an appropriate tool?	1. When the salicylate is taken over several hours or days 2. When the salicylate is enteric-coated or there is SR product ingestion 3. When the product has oil of wintergreen, which causes quick absorption 4. When patients have kidney dysfunction 5. When the time of ingestion is unclear 6. When there is acidemia
What is the treatment for salicylate toxicity?	First, stabilization of the patient. The general steps then include gastric decontamination, fluid therapy, intravenous sodium bicarbonate, possible extracorporeal elimination, treatment of seizure, and treatment of coagulopathy.
What type of gastric decontamination is used in salicylate toxicity?	A variety may be used, including gastric lavage alone or with activated charcoal, activated charcoal alone, or whole bowel irrigation.
Why is sodium bicarbonate used in the treatment of salicylate toxicity?	Acidosis may create an environment for enhanced salicylate movement across the blood–brain barrier and increase salicylate levels in the brain. As the blood becomes more alkalinized, salicylate moves into the ionized form and penetration into all tissues is reduced. Sodium bicarbonate also enhances salicylate elimination through alkalinization of the urine to trap and remove drug in ionized form.
How much sodium bicarbonate is used in the treatment of salicylate toxicity?	1–2 mEq/kg/L intravenous solution. D5W is recommended for solution to keep the intravenous fluid from being hypertonic. Serum pH of 7.55 should not be exceeded. If the clinician is attempting to create alkalotic urine, then urine pH should be greater than 7.5.
What are adverse effects of treatment with sodium bicarbonate?	Hypernatremia, increasing alkalosis in patients with respiratory alkalosis, hypokalemia, and fluid overload

When should bicarbonate therapy be stopped in salicylate toxicity?	When salicylate levels reach 35–40 mg/dl and when the patient's clinical status improves and signs and symptoms resolve
When is extracorporeal elimination appropriate in salicylate toxicity?	When standard management is ineffective, when there is evident damage in vital organs, when the patient is at an extreme of age, or when the liver or kidney cannot clear the drug
What are other supportive care issues in salicylate toxicity?	Patients should be monitored and treated for occurrence of seizures and coagulopathy.

Miscellaneous

What are antidotes (adult dose) for the following?

Opiates:	Naloxone, initial dose of 2 mg, unless the patient has a history of chronic narcotic use, in which case, starting dose is 0.4 mg, which is titrated accordingly. Larger doses may precipitate severe withdrawal.
Methanol or ethylene glycol:	Ethanol—loading dose, 10 ml/kg (10% solution), then continuous infusion of 0.15 ml/kg/hr
Anticholinergic agents:	Physostigmine, 1–2 mg intravenously over 5 minutes
Organophosphates or carbamate:	Atropine, 2 mg intravenously, may be repeated to dehydrate pulmonary secretions
INH and hydralazine:	Pyridoxine g/g
β-blockers:	Glucagon, 5–10 mg intravenously, then 2–10 mg/hr
TCAs:	Bicarbonate, 1–2 mmol/kg
Digitalis:	Digibind (mg of digoxin ingested/0.6 = number of vials)

Benzodiazepines:	Flumazenil, 0.2 mg intravenously; if no effect after 30 seconds, then 0.3 mg is administered intravenously; if no effect after 30 seconds, then 0.5 mg is administered intravenously every minute to a total dose of 3 mg. Seizures may occur during therapy.
Calcium channel blockers:	Calcium chloride, 1 g

ELECTRICAL INJURY

How common are deaths caused by electrical injury?	Approximately 1000 deaths per year are due to electrical current and 200 deaths per year are due to lightning strikes; also, 5% of admissions to burn units are from electrical injuries.
What factors determine the extent of electrical injury?	Duration of contact, alternating current (tetanic contraction does not allow release of the contact), pathway through the body (what is in between), and resistance to the flow of electricity (lowered by moisture)
What renal injuries occur after an electrical injury?	1. Direct injury to the kidney secondary to electrical injury 2. Hypotensive injury 3. Renal tubular damage from myoglobin and hemoglobin secondary to muscle necrosis and hemolysis 4. Rapid volume loss into the destroyed or injured tissue
What other complications may occur in electrical injury?	Swelling may result in compartment syndrome, metabolic acidosis may result from lactate production, and infection may result from inadequately débrided tissue.
What are late neurologic sequelae of electrical injury?	Visual disturbances, peripheral neuropathy, incomplete transection of the spinal cord, reflex sympathetic dystrophies, late convulsive disorders, and intractable headaches

**What are baseline findings
in the following
parameters?**

Hematocrit: Elevated secondary to dehydration

Urinalysis: Myoglobinuria

Lumbar puncture: Elevated pressure, bloody tap

ECG: ST and T wave changes that may persist

Serum potassium   Unexplained hypokalemia after 2–4
                               weeks

**What does acute
management of electrical
injury entail?**

1. Removal of the victim from the
   contact without touching the victim
   directly (unless power is definitely
   terminated)
2. ACLS (there is high risk for cardiac
   arrhythmias)
3. Rapid fluid and electrolyte
   replacement (standard formulas
   estimating replacement based on
   surface burn are inaccurate because
   of the extensive internal injury)
4. Wound management
5. Administration of tetanus toxoid and
   antibiotics

DROWNING

**What is the mechanism of
injury in drowning?**

In "dry" drowning, laryngospasm
develops and the victim dies of hypoxia
caused by mechanical obstruction of
airflow. In "wet" drowning, water
reaches the alveoli and directly
interferes with oxygen exchange or
damages alveoli and causes ARDS.

**Does water temperature
affect prognosis in
drowning?**

Yes. Hypothermia induced by cold water
slows metabolic rate and may induce a
protective mechanism against hypoxia.
Patients should be rewarmed per
hypothermia protocol in addition to
receiving respiratory support. The
presence of hypothermia should lead to
longer resuscitative efforts.

What is the acute management of drowning?

Victims should be removed from the water as soon as possible and given ACLS with particular attention to airway and breathing. If any trauma is suspected, the patient's head and neck should be immediately stabilized. ACLS may be started in the water if immediate removal is impossible. A low threshold for endotracheal intubation is indicated. The patient should be placed on a cardiac monitor as soon as possible.

Should abdominal thrust be administered in the field?

Current ACLS recommendations are that abdominal thrust is not indicated except to remove a foreign body from the airway or to clear the airway if the patient does not ventilate with standard basic cardiac life support procedures. The thrust may lead to aspiration of gastric contents and further alveolar damage.

What else should be done acutely in drowning cases?

Drowning often follows an inciting event such as head trauma, cardiac arrhythmia, myocardial infarction, alcohol intoxication, or drug use. These events should be treated accordingly during resuscitative efforts.

What laboratory abnormalities are common in drowning cases?

Hypoxia dominates over hypercapnia. The victim is often acidotic. Both hypoxia and acidosis may depress cardiac function. Blood chemistries are usually normal.

What is the best treatment for hypoxia?

Mechanical ventilatory support, including continuous positive airway pressure, is indicated for persistent hypoxia. Occasionally, cardiopulmonary support may be needed.

What are poor prognostic indicators in drowning cases?

Prolonged submersion, severe metabolic acidosis (pH < 7.1), asystole, fixed and dilated pupils, and low Glasgow score (< 5)

ALCOHOL

Is alcohol consumption a problem in the United States?	The average American intake is two drinks per day and two-thirds of Americans drink alcohol. Alcohol use, both acute and chronic, is responsible for 10% of all deaths, and 50% of fatal accidents and trauma cases are alcohol-related.
What is alcoholism?	There are four phases of alcoholism: 1. Prealcoholic syndrome 2. Prodrome (marked by guilt, sneaking drinks, and blackouts) 3. Addiction 4. Chronic health decline
What predisposes a person to alcoholism?	There is growing evidence for a genetic cause of susceptibility to alcohol abuse although environmental pressures also play a role. A strong family history of alcohol abuse should lead to a higher index of suspicion.
What are clues to the diagnosis of alcoholism?	The patient becomes suspicious, notes periods of amnesia, disruption of personal life, a downward career drift, gastritis, diarrhea, myopathy, and tremor.
How is the diagnosis of alcoholism made?	1. EtOH level greater than 150 mg/dl without intoxication is a positive indicator. 2. The **CAGE** questions have an 80% sensitivity: Have you ever tried to **C**ut down on drinking? Have you ever felt **A**nnoyed by criticism about your drinking? Have you ever had **G**uilty feelings about drinking? Have you ever taken an **E**ye opener in the morning?
What are common laboratory abnormalities in alcoholism?	LFTs include elevated gamma-glutamyltranspeptidase, AST:ALT ratio > 2:1, or isolated elevated AST

Mean corpuscular volume (MCV) may be elevated with normal or low hematocrit.

PT may be prolonged.

A decreased BUN may signify chronic malnutrition.

What is alcohol withdrawal?

A state of physical and psychologic distress created by a decline in the steady-state alcohol level that a person is accustomed to. A chronic alcoholic may "withdraw" long before the EtOH level reaches zero. The rate of metabolism is influenced by the chronicity of use, amount consumed acutely, and presence of metabolic disorders (e.g., liver disease) or other drugs (e.g., benzodiazepines). Acute abstinence usually leads to symptoms within 7 days (often 48–72 hours).

What are signs of alcohol withdrawal?

Mild withdrawal presents with autonomic excitability (e.g., tachycardia, hypertension, and low-grade fever) and increasing agitation, often with tremor and confusion. In patients with severe withdrawal, autonomic instability and respiratory distress, agitation, and seizures may develop.

What are DTs?

Delirium tremens signify severe withdrawal and have both a physical component (tremors and seizures) and a hallucinatory component. This is a life-threatening condition.

How is risk for alcohol withdrawal assessed?

Any patient with a history of withdrawal or heavy drinking should receive benzodiazepine prophylaxis and careful monitoring.

What is the treatment for alcohol withdrawal?

If liver function is normal, the patient should receive librium, either by mouth or intravenously in a tapering fashion. A good starting dose is 50 mg every 4 hours the first day, then every 6 hours, then the dose is halved and the interval is tapered. If liver disease is present, 1–2 mg of lorazepam is used as a starting dose. The patient must be monitored for excessive sedation and the dose adjusted accordingly.

DRUGS OF ABUSE

What are the current favorite street drugs?

Marijuana remains a popular choice, especially among the teenage and college crowds. Popular drug use is often dictated by geography and cultural influences. Cocaine is still highly prevalent. Methamphetamine and heroin are also making comebacks. PCP and LSD are still used. Glue sniffing is used by teenagers predominantly.

What are signs of chronic drug use?

Development of psychiatric problems such as depression or paranoia may signal abuse problems. As the addiction grows, antisocial behavior in the form of lying, manipulation, and failure to meet personal and business obligations becomes more prominent. Casual users may hide their use indefinitely.

What are the major categories of illicit drugs?

1. Stimulants (e.g., cocaine and methamphetamines)
2. Depressants (e.g., barbiturates, marijuana, opiates, and glue)
3. Hallucinogens (e.g., LSD, PCP, and peyote)

What are the effects of cannabinoids?

Marijuana, the most common cannabinoid, is usually rolled and smoked, although it may be taken orally as well. Acutely, it mimics severe alcohol intoxication with mental depression. It can precipitate a severe depressive state. Physical examination may show conjunctival erythema and tachycardia. Angina may develop even hours after use. Chronic bronchitis may develop as well. It may also cause gynecomastia and infertility and depress the immune system. Withdrawal is marked by tremor, nystagmus, gastrointestinal distress, and sleep disturbance.

Are there any legal uses for illicit drugs?

Cannabinoids are potent antiemetics and can be used for control of intractable nausea in cancer patients in some states. A special dispensation from the Drug Enforcement Administration is required and debate continues over legitimizing its use.

What are the effects of opiates?

Opiates cause CNS depression through several different receptors. They are related to the endogenous endorphins that play a role in analgesia and feeling of well-being. Common findings include lethargy, somnolence, miosis, and respiratory and cardiac depression. Intravenous preparations may cause more rapid and profound effects than oral use. Abuse may develop from illegal street use or medical use of prescribed drugs.

Do opiates cause significant withdrawal?

Yes. Factors influencing severity include the drug half-life, dose, and chronicity of use.

What are signs of opiate withdrawal?

The opposite effects of intoxication, including nausea, diarrhea, lacrimation, rhinorrhea, myoclonus, insomnia, and piloerection

What is the treatment for opiate withdrawal?

Drugs with short half-lives, namely morphine and heroin, may lead to withdrawal within 8–16 hours of last use. Treatment consists of observed, controlled administration of long-acting agents such as methadone. Clonidine (0.1–0.3 mg two to four times daily) may counteract some of the physical symptoms. A mild withdrawal syndrome consisting of autonomic dysfunction and sleep disturbance may persist for up to 6 months and interfere with long-term abstinence.

What are the dangers of intravenous drug use?

The most obvious is transmission of infectious diseases including hepatitis B and C and human immunodeficiency virus due to shared needles.

Endocarditis of the tricuspid valve is seen almost exclusively in this group, and causative agents include normal skin flora (*Staphylococcus*) and unusual organisms such as *Pseudomonas*. Osteomyelitis may also develop, often in vertebral bodies. Intravenous drug abuse should be suspected in patients with sternoclavicular osteomyelitis, often a result of injecting into the jugular or subclavian veins. Injection of contaminated material may also lead to painful local phlebitis.

Are barbiturates similar in action to opiates?

Yes. Both act as CNS depressants. Prescriptions for barbiturates, except to treat seizure disorders, have declined. Because these are usually long-acting agents, withdrawal signs take longer to appear and are generally less severe.

What are the effects of abuse of anxiolytics such as benzodiazepines?

These cross-react with alcohol, which is why they are used to treat alcohol withdrawal. Abuse of anxiolytics is not uncommon; they are often prescribed inappropriately to treat "anxiety" and "nerves." Withdrawal symptoms are similar to those of alcohol withdrawal but do not appear for many days because anxiolytics are longer acting agents.

What are the effects of sniffing glue?

Hydrocarbon-based commercial products such as glue and paint thinner can cause CNS depression and feelings of euphoria. They are often used by younger persons and may create long-term memory and cognitive deficits. Prolonged exposure may lead to life-threatening CNS and respiratory depression.

Why is cocaine abuse dangerous?

Because it creates a high sympathetic discharge, cocaine use increases myocardial oxygen demands and may induce myocardial ischemia. It also induces coronary and peripheral vasospasm, which can cause a myocardial infarction or stroke. This effect may occur up to several days after cocaine use. Hyperpyrexia and malignant hypertension may also occur.

What is the treatment for cocaine-induced myocardial infarction?

Treatment of choice is thrombolysis, not angioplasty.

What is "crack lung"?

ARDS-like damage, often unilateral, that is seen acutely after smoking cocaine

What is "crashing"?

Cocaine products produce a rapid, intense euphoric state, which may occur as quickly as 8–10 seconds after smoking "crack." This is followed by an abrupt drop in mood. Alcohol is often used to modulate this reaction.

What is the treatment for cocaine overdose?

Intravenous diazepam at 0.5 mg/kg over 8 hours. β-Blockade alone should be avoided because it may cause vasospasm secondary to unopposed alpha stimulation.

What are the effects of amphetamines?

Amphetamines are potent metabolic stimulants. Milder forms are legally available and are often used as weight control aids. Overdose causes tachycardia, anxiety, and agitation. A synthetic methamphetamine known as "ice" has recently gained popularity. Overdose may lead to hyperpyrexia, dilated pupils, tachypnea, rhabdomyolysis, hypertensive crisis, seizures, and cardiac arrhythmias. Treatment should be directed at the manifestations and include control of seizures with benzodiazepines and blood pressure control with labetalol or nifedipine.

What are the effects of "acid"?

LSD, or acid, causes hyperpyrexia, tachycardia, tremor, hypertension, pupillary dilatation, labile moods, and visual hallucinations. There are no reports of deaths directly attributable to the physiologic effects of LSD.

What is a "bad trip"?	LSD can provoke a prolonged panic episode lasting up to 24 hours. Supportive care consisting of "talking down" the patient and small doses of anxiolytic drugs may help.
What is "angel dust"?	PCP
What are the effects of PCP?	PCP produces a state of intense agitation and analgesia. It has been described as causing acts of superhuman strength (e.g., ripping off handcuffs), but the effect is more due to the analgesia than enhanced muscle strength. It may cause horizontal or vertical nystagmus, hyperacusis, and diaphoresis. Feelings of estrangement and distorted images of self develop. Overdose may lead to coma, which is treated with gastric lavage and acidification of urine.
Can acute drug use be confused with psychiatric disorders?	Yes. Cocaine may induce a state of paranoid delusions. PCP use may appear to be an acute schizophrenic break. Also, chronic cocaine use can unmask schizoform disorders.

Index

Page numbers in *italics* represent figures; page numbers with *t* indicate tables.

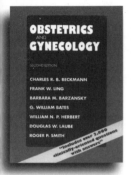